Pathophysiology of Spinal Cord Injury (SCI)

Pathophysiology of Spinal Cord Injury (SCI)

Editors

Cédric Geoffroy
Warren Alilain

MDPI • Basel • Beijing • Wuhan • Barcelona • Belgrade • Manchester • Tokyo • Cluj • Tianjin

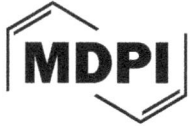

Editors
Cédric Geoffroy
Department of Neuroscience
Experimental Therapeutics
Texas AM University
Collage Station
United States

Warren Alilain
Spinal Cord and Brain Injury
Research Center
University of Kentucky
Lexington
United States

Editorial Office
MDPI
St. Alban-Anlage 66
4052 Basel, Switzerland

This is a reprint of articles from the Special Issue published online in the open access journal *Biology* (ISSN 2079-7737) (available at: www.mdpi.com/journal/biology/special_issues/Pathophysiol_SCI).

For citation purposes, cite each article independently as indicated on the article page online and as indicated below:

LastName, A.A.; LastName, B.B.; LastName, C.C. Article Title. *Journal Name* **Year**, *Volume Number*, Page Range.

ISBN 978-3-0365-5888-2 (Hbk)
ISBN 978-3-0365-5887-5 (PDF)

© 2022 by the authors. Articles in this book are Open Access and distributed under the Creative Commons Attribution (CC BY) license, which allows users to download, copy and build upon published articles, as long as the author and publisher are properly credited, which ensures maximum dissemination and a wider impact of our publications.

The book as a whole is distributed by MDPI under the terms and conditions of the Creative Commons license CC BY-NC-ND.

Contents

Marisa A. Jeffries and Veronica J. Tom
Peripheral Immune Dysfunction: A Problem of Central Importance after Spinal Cord Injury
Reprinted from: *Biology* **2021**, *10*, 928, doi:10.3390/biology10090928 1

Minna Christiansen Lund, Ditte Gry Ellman, Maiken Nissen, Pernille Sveistrup Nielsen, Pernille Vinther Nielsen and Carina Jørgensen et al.
The Inflammatory Response after Moderate Contusion Spinal Cord Injury: A Time Study
Reprinted from: *Biology* **2022**, *11*, 939, doi:10.3390/biology11060939 21

Cristián Rosales-Antequera, Ginés Viscor and Oscar F. Araneda
Inflammation and Oxidative Stress as Common Mechanisms of Pulmonary, Autonomic and Musculoskeletal Dysfunction after Spinal Cord Injury
Reprinted from: *Biology* **2022**, *11*, 550, doi:10.3390/biology11040550 49

Liisa Wainman, Erin L. Erskine, Mehdi Ahmadian, Thomas Matthew Hanna and Christopher R. West
Development of a Spinal Cord Injury Model Permissive to Study the Cardiovascular Effects of Rehabilitation Approaches Designed to Induce Neuroplasticity
Reprinted from: *Biology* **2021**, *10*, 1006, doi:10.3390/biology10101006 65

Michelle A. Hook, Alyssa Falck, Ravali Dundumulla, Mabel Terminel, Rachel Cunningham and Arthur Sefiani et al.
Osteopenia in a Mouse Model of Spinal Cord Injury: Effects of Age, Sex and Motor Function
Reprinted from: *Biology* **2022**, *11*, 189, doi:10.3390/biology11020189 81

Adel B. Ghnenis, Calvin Jones, Arthur Sefiani, Ashley J. Douthitt, Andrea J. Reyna and Joseph M. Rutkowski et al.
Evaluation of the Cardiometabolic Disorders after Spinal Cord Injury in Mice
Reprinted from: *Biology* **2022**, *11*, 495, doi:10.3390/biology11040495 101

Pauline Michel-Flutot, Isley Jesus, Valentin Vanhee, Camille H. Bourcier, Laila Emam and Abderrahim Ouguerroudj et al.
Effects of Chronic High-Frequency rTMS Protocol on Respiratory Neuroplasticity Following C2 Spinal Cord Hemisection in Rats
Reprinted from: *Biology* **2022**, *11*, 473, doi:10.3390/biology11030473 125

Afaf Bajjig, Pauline Michel-Flutot, Tiffany Migevent, Florence Cayetanot, Laurence Bodineau and Stéphane Vinit et al.
Diaphragmatic Activity and Respiratory Function Following C3 or C6 Unilateral Spinal Cord Contusion in Mice
Reprinted from: *Biology* **2022**, *11*, 558, doi:10.3390/biology11040558 143

Gizelle N. K. Fauss, Kelsey E. Hudson and James W. Grau
Role of Descending Serotonergic Fibers in the Development of Pathophysiology after Spinal Cord Injury (SCI): Contribution to Chronic Pain, Spasticity, and Autonomic Dysreflexia
Reprinted from: *Biology* **2022**, *11*, 234, doi:10.3390/biology11020234 157

John R. Walker and Megan Ryan Detloff
Plasticity in Cervical Motor Circuits following Spinal Cord Injury and Rehabilitation
Reprinted from: *Biology* **2021**, *10*, 976, doi:10.3390/biology10100976 195

Jaclyn H. DeFinis, Jeremy Weinberger and Shaoping Hou
Delivery of the 5-HT$_{2A}$ Receptor Agonist, DOI, Enhances Activity of the Sphincter Muscle during the Micturition Reflex in Rats after Spinal Cord Injury
Reprinted from: *Biology* **2021**, *10*, 68, doi:10.3390/biology10010068 213

Emma K. A. Schmidt, Pamela J. F. Raposo, Karen L. Madsen, Keith K. Fenrich, Gillian Kabarchuk and Karim Fouad
What Makes a Successful Donor? Fecal Transplant from Anxious-Like Rats Does Not Prevent Spinal Cord Injury-Induced Dysbiosis
Reprinted from: *Biology* **2021**, *10*, 254, doi:10.3390/biology10040254 229

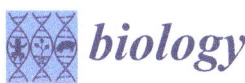

Review

Peripheral Immune Dysfunction: A Problem of Central Importance after Spinal Cord Injury

Marisa A. Jeffries and Veronica J. Tom *

Department of Neurobiology and Anatomy, Drexel University College of Medicine, Philadelphia, PA 19129, USA; maj359@drexel.edu
* Correspondence: vjt25@drexel.edu

Simple Summary: Spinal cord injury can result in an increased vulnerability to infections, but until recently the biological mechanisms behind this observation were not well defined. Immunosuppression and concurrent sustained peripheral inflammation after spinal cord injury have been observed in preclinical and clinical studies, now termed spinal cord injury-induced immune depression syndrome. Recent research indicates a key instigator of this immune dysfunction is altered sympathetic input to lymphoid organs, such as the spleen, resulting in a wide array of secondary effects that can, in turn, exacerbate immune pathology. In this review, we discuss what we know about immune dysfunction after spinal cord injury, why it occurs, and how we might treat it.

Abstract: Individuals with spinal cord injuries (SCI) exhibit increased susceptibility to infection, with pneumonia consistently ranking as a leading cause of death. Despite this statistic, chronic inflammation and concurrent immune suppression have only recently begun to be explored mechanistically. Investigators have now identified numerous changes that occur in the peripheral immune system post-SCI, including splenic atrophy, reduced circulating lymphocytes, and impaired lymphocyte function. These effects stem from maladaptive changes in the spinal cord after injury, including plasticity within the spinal sympathetic reflex circuit that results in exaggerated sympathetic output in response to peripheral stimulation below injury level. Such pathological activity is particularly evident after a severe high-level injury above thoracic spinal cord segment 6, greatly increasing the risk of the development of sympathetic hyperreflexia and subsequent disrupted regulation of lymphoid organs. Encouragingly, studies have presented evidence for promising therapies, such as modulation of neuroimmune activity, to improve regulation of peripheral immune function. In this review, we summarize recent publications examining (1) how various immune functions and populations are affected, (2) mechanisms behind SCI-induced immune dysfunction, and (3) potential interventions to improve SCI individuals' immunological function to strengthen resistance to potentially deadly infections.

Keywords: autonomic dysreflexia; spinal cord injury; immune dysfunction; SCI-IDS

1. Introduction

Spinal cord injury (SCI) is a traumatic injury that results in disrupted bidirectional communication between higher levels of the central nervous system (CNS) and the body below the level of the injury. While SCI is often associated with motor and sensory dysfunction, SCI results in a myriad of other systemic functional changes and deficits, including altered immune function. Immune dysfunction after SCI has long been documented. For instance, SCI individuals exhibit more frequent infections, with pneumonia ranking as a leading cause of death after injury [1]. Even when death is not the eventual outcome, pneumonia and post-operative wound infections are associated with impaired functional recovery in SCI persons [2]. While this increased susceptibility to infection was historically attributed to the medical interventions routinely administered in the acute phase after

SCI [3], it is becoming apparent that the rise in infections is largely due to secondary changes in peripheral immunity that occur after injury [4]. Studies have only recently begun to reveal the underlying biological mechanisms of immune pathology after injury. Individuals with SCI display various immunological changes, including immunosuppression despite concurrent chronic systemic low-grade inflammation, termed SCI-induced immune depression syndrome (SCI-IDS) (Figure 1) [5,6]. Unfortunately, because of our limited understanding of mechanisms that contribute to SCI-IDS, there are no FDA-approved treatments for use in SCI individuals that specifically improve immune function. Therefore, SCI-IDS represents a problem with myriad remaining questions. Importantly, identification of potential therapeutic targets to improve immune function would make a significant and lasting impact on the general health and well-being of the SCI community. In this review, we summarize the current literature describing the chronic peripheral inflammation and increased susceptibility to infection characteristic of SCI-IDS, the mechanisms behind the development of immune dysfunction, and how these pathological changes might be ameliorated therapeutically.

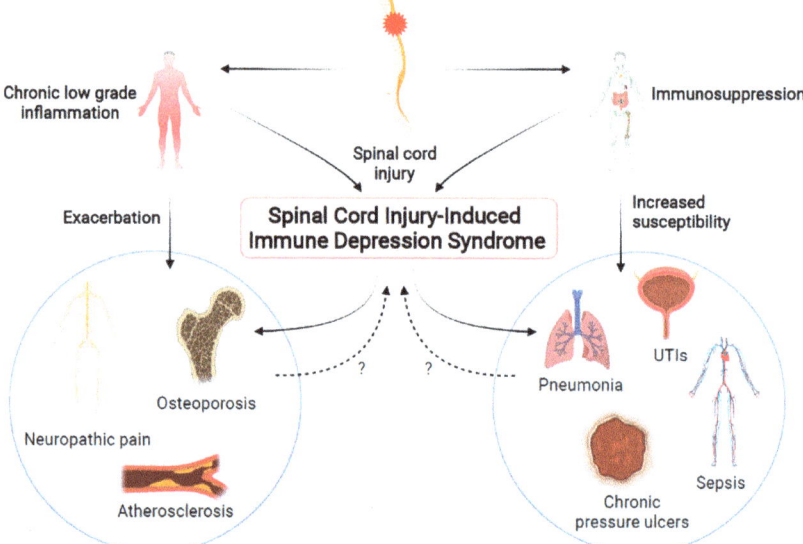

Figure 1. After spinal cord injury (SCI), both chronic systemic inflammation and immunosuppression result in SCI-induced immune depression syndrome (SCI-IDS). Altered immune function results in increased susceptibility to infection and exacerbated secondary complications of SCI. In turn, these secondary complications and infections may create a feedback loop which amplifies immune dysfunction. Created using BioRender.com accessed on 2 September 2021.

2. The Consequences of Peripheral Immune Dysfunction

2.1. Chronic Low-Grade Inflammation

While much research has focused on the resulting neuroinflammation in the spinal cord after SCI, there is also persistent, low-grade, peripheral inflammation that has been identified in SCI individuals (Figure 1) [6,7]. Examination of serum cytokine levels from SCI persons revealed that proinflammatory cytokines IL-2, IL-6, tumor necrosis factor alpha (TNFα), and/or IL-1RA were significantly increased compared to their levels in able-bodied subjects [8,9]. Interestingly, SCI subjects who experienced pain, urinary tract infections (UTIs), or pressure ulcers displayed higher levels of these proinflammatory cytokines than those without [9]. Another study found that C-reactive protein (CRP), IL-2, and granulocyte macrophage colony stimulating factor (GM-CSF) were significantly increased while TNFα,

IL-4, and granulocyte colony stimulating factor (G-CSF) were significantly decreased in SCI persons compared to controls [10]. In men with SCI regardless of injury level, blood serum concentration of CRP, IL-6, endothelin-1, and soluble vascular cell adhesion molecule (sVCAM) were all significantly increased, suggestive of chronic low-grade inflammation [11]. A recent whole-blood gene expression study found significantly upregulated Toll-like receptor signaling pathway genes in participants with chronic SCI compared to those without, supporting the presence of systemic inflammation [12]. Activation of circulating $CD3^+$ and $CD4^+$ T cells was increased after SCI, although $CCR4^+$ $HLA-DR^+$ regulatory T cells were concurrently expanded [12]. The exact roles of regulatory T cells are complex, and the functional implications of increased regulatory T cells are not fully understood. Moreover, it is not yet known if the increase in the CCR4+ HLA-DR+ regulatory T cells causes immune dysfunction or they expand in response to an altered immune environment. Nevertheless, these data reveal immune dysfunction after chronic SCI in humans, and the increased activation of T cells may contribute to long-term inflammation.

2.2. Increased Susceptibility to Infection

Despite a sustained state of inflammation in SCI persons, they experience increased susceptibility to pathogenic infection due to concurrent immunodeficiency (Figure 1). The significance of this is underscored by clinical data examining causes of death in SCI individuals [13–16]. The leading cause of death within the first year after a traumatic SCI in the Czech Republic was found to be pneumonia infection (17.1%), with UTIs making up 7.3% of all deaths [16]. Pneumonia remained the leading cause of death after a year in the SCI population at 14% of all deaths, with UTIs at 10.3%, pressure ulcers at 12.1%, and sepsis of unknown origin at 6.5%, making infections the leading cause of mortality after SCI at over 40% of all deaths [16]. In a 70-year study from Britain, the leading cause of death after SCI was respiratory (29.3%) with infections such as pneumonia making up the vast majority of these (23.5% of all deaths) [15]. Another 7.8% of deaths in this study were attributed to urinary tract infections and sepsis of unknown origin, further demonstrating the gravity of infections in SCI individuals [15].

Why are respiratory infections so prevalent and deadly in the SCI population? Preclinical and clinical studies indicate that injury level and severity contribute to infection susceptibility. Clinically, over 40% of deaths in the tetraplegic population of the long-term study in Britain were attributed to respiratory causes, including infection [15]. In a small study from Germany, pneumonia and influenza ranked in the top three causes of death for tetraplegics, but not paraplegics, and tetraplegic subjects had a significantly reduced life expectancy compared to paraplegics [17]. Part of the problem is that higher-level injuries result in loss of innervation to motor neurons that innervate the diaphragm and intercostal muscles, resulting in compromised respiratory motor control (reviewed in [18]). The lack of mobility in SCI persons also exacerbates this issue since exercise, like walking and running, has been shown to reduce pneumonia-related mortality [19–22]. However, what may make respiratory infections particularly deadly for SCI persons is that higher injuries above the level of thoracic segment 6 (T6) result in disruption of descending supraspinal input to sympathetic preganglionic neurons (SPNs) that innervate immune organs and modulate immune function, which we describe in more detail in a later section. This combination results in a heavily reduced capacity to effectively clear respiratory infections.

Preclinical studies in animal models have further increased our understanding of impaired immune responses and subsequent increased susceptibility to infection following SCI [23–26]. Due to immune impairment, mice with thoracic SCI exhibit reduced ability to clear influenza or mouse hepatitis virus (MHV) infection in the lungs or liver, respectively [23,26]. In fact, mortality rates in infected SCI mice were 40% after influenza infection and 100% after MHV infection. Specifically, these mice exhibited reduced numbers of influenza-specific $CD8^+$ T cells or MHV-specific $CD4^+$ T cells after viral infection [23,26]. In a follow-up influenza study, deficient $CD8^+$ T cell infiltration and numbers were discovered to be mediated via corticosterone signaling, and administration of mifepristone to inhibit corticosterone throughout the experiment rescued numbers of virus-specific CD8$^+$ T cells [27]. In another study, high thoracic (i.e., T3) hemisection in a mouse model of inducible bacterial pneumonia resulted in increased bacterial load in the lungs, indicative of inability to clear infection [25]. Moreover, rats with complete transection at T10 developed UTIs when inoculated transurethrally with a lower dose of *E. coli* than uninjured rats [24]. Histological analysis indicated that while inflammation in the bladder was virtually resolved by 14 days post-infection in uninjured controls, SCI rats displayed chronic inflammation of the bladder with mononuclear cell aggregates located within the lamina propria. Together, these studies demonstrate the independent risk of SCI on infection rates across a wide range of infection types, further underscoring the need for therapeutic advancement in treating SCI-IDS.

2.3. Effects of Immune Dysfunction on Other Physiological Processes

There are common secondary complications after SCI that are likely worsened by the chronic immune dysfunction observed in SCI persons (Figure 1). Osteoporosis is ubiquitous in the SCI population, resulting in acute rapid reduction in bone density after injury that stabilizes after 2–3 years; this bone loss also increases susceptibility to fractures [28,29]. While the role of immune function in the pathogenesis of osteoporosis in the SCI population is not well described, osteoporosis independent of SCI is an inflammatory condition that progresses due to immune dysfunction, cytokine release, and a persistent low-grade inflammatory state typically seen in aging [30–32]. Therefore, it is not unreasonable to suggest that the long-term inflammation observed in SCI individuals would contribute to osteoporosis pathology [33].

Another secondary complication after SCI is neuropathic pain, which presents in anywhere from 18–96% of SCI persons [34–39]. As with osteoporosis, it is well established that both peripheral and central inflammation contribute to the development of neuropathic pain [40–42]. As described above, one study found that SCI persons presenting with neuropathic pain exhibited elevated serum levels of IL-6 and IL-1RA compared to those without neuropathic pain [9]. A recent clinical study indicated that an anti-inflammatory diet in SCI individuals resulted in reduced composite score of proinflammatory mediators IL-2, IL-6, IL-1β, TNF-α, and interferon gamma (IFN-γ) and was associated with decreased neuropathic pain score [43].

SCI individuals are frequently plagued by pressure ulcers due to immobility and resultant tissue ischemia. Data indicate that skin ulcers and cutaneous wounds heal more slowly after thoracic SCI in mice [44]. Cutaneous wounds normally progress through four stages of healing: hemostasis, inflammation and cytokine release, cytokine-induced epithelial and vascular proliferation, and wound resolution [45]. In the general population, wounds such as pressure ulcers often persist chronically in an inflammatory state that inhibits healing progression [45,46]. In line with this, clinical evidence suggests that anti-inflammatory topical treatments, such as TNFα inhibition via infliximab, can improve wound healing of chronic ulcers [47]. However, SCI persons exhibit sustained baseline vasodilation due to sympathetic denervation. This sustained baseline vasodilation and subsequent hypotension has been hypothesized to impair the requisite inflammation phase of wound healing, inhibiting wound healing at an earlier stage of repair [48]. In fact, evidence specifically from SCI models has shown that cutaneous inflammatory stimulation does not elicit appropriate localized inflammation. After complete T3 transection, mice injected subcutaneously with complete Freud's adjuvant emulsion exhibited reduced cutaneous localized inflammation as measured by both fluorescent IVIS imaging and magnetic resonance imaging (MRI) [49]. Therefore, it seems that both persistent low-grade inflammation and immunosuppression after SCI may impair pressure ulcers from recovery.

The general consensus is that SCI increases the risk of atherosclerotic diseases, such as coronary artery disease and cardiovascular disease, via a multitude of secondary complications, from obesity to metabolic syndrome and sustained, low-grade inflammation [11,50–54]. While recent clinical research indicates that presentation of atherosclerotic pathology in

SCI persons is not solely dependent on increased inflammatory markers [55,56], it may be exacerbated by increased inflammation [56]. Preclinical research using a mouse model of atherosclerotic disease ($ApoE^{-/-}$) found that atherosclerotic lesions were significantly increased in mice with a T9 contusion injury compared to uninjured controls [57]. While the development of atherosclerosis was associated with increased plasma levels of IL-1β, TNFα, IL-6, monocyte chemoattractant protein-1 (MCP-1), and C-C motif chemokine ligand-5 (CCL-5), increased MCP-1 and CCL-5 were specifically observed in SCI mice versus uninjured controls. Importantly, the use of an anti-inflammatory salicylate drug was found to prevent SCI-induced exacerbation of atherosclerosis, possibly via the reduction in TNFα, MCP-1, and CCL-5 plasma levels [57].

Research therefore indicates that immune dysfunction in SCI individuals is of pathological consequence and resolution of chronic inflammation and concurrent immunosuppression could prove highly beneficial in improving quality of life.

3. Why Does Peripheral Immune Dysfunction Occur?

3.1. Disruption of Descending Central Pathways

SCI, particularly above the level of T6, can result in loss of modulatory input to immune organs via autonomic innervation and the hypothalamic-pituitary-adrenal (HPA) axis (Figure 2). The spleen, the largest lymphoid organ, has been better studied in relation to SCI-IDS than any other lymphoid tissue and shows dramatic changes after disruption of modulatory innervation [58]. Upon SPN activation, which normally occurs due to stress in the "fight or flight" response, post-ganglionic terminals in the spleen release norepinephrine (NE) directly to splenocytes in the white pulp and the HPA axis is stimulated to release glucocorticoids (GCs) from the adrenal gland (Figure 2) [59,60]. Under homeostatic conditions, splenic lymphocytes express anti-inflammatory β-adrenergic receptors (β-AR) that promote reduced cell proliferation, decreased proinflammatory cytokine release, and reduced antibody production. GCs from the adrenal glands mediate similar anti-inflammatory effects via GC receptors [61]. During inflammation, T cells and B cells highly express α-adrenergic receptors (α-AR) that promote maturation, activation, and migration (reviewed in [58,62]).

After SCI, supraspinal control of the sympathetic system is disrupted and sympathetic activity becomes dysregulated. Acutely, this results in increased GC release from the adrenal glands that impairs immune function (Figure 2) [63]. Over time, maladaptive plasticity of the sympathetic circuitry within the spinal cord below the level of injury develops. In people with severe high-level SCI, the combination of interruption of supraspinal input to sympathetic circuitry caudal to the level of injury and the plasticity of this circuit leads to sympathetic hyperreflexia, which overtly manifests as autonomic dysreflexia (AD) [64–66]. This sympathetic hyperactivity results in abnormally high levels of NE in the spleen and activation of β-ARs on lymphocytes that result in sustained immunosuppression (Figure 2) [67,68]. In turn, this chronic immunosuppression increases susceptibility to infection as described above. Sympathetic innervation and the HPA axis have been identified as both independent and interrelated causes of immune dysfunction after SCI [63,64].

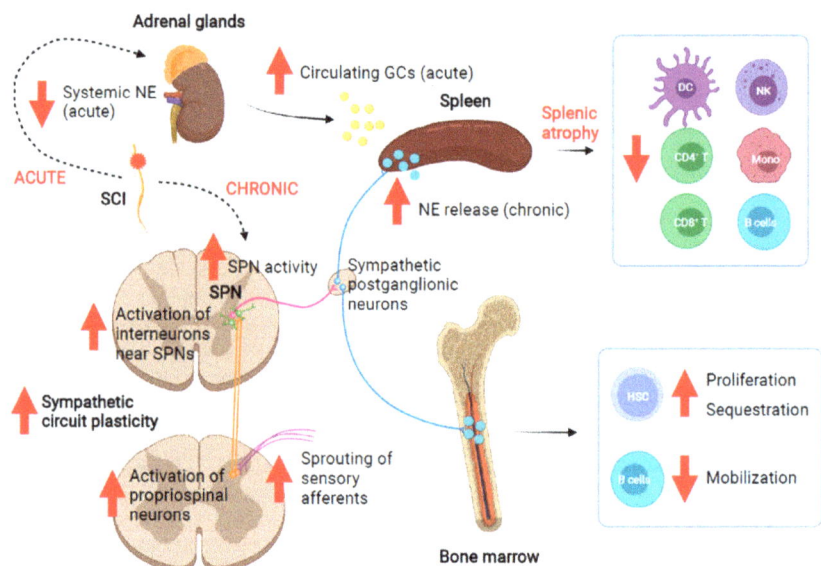

Figure 2. After a SCI, there is an acute drop in systemic norepinephrine (NE) and an increase in plasma glucocorticoids (GCs) released by the adrenal glands. Chronically, increased neural circuit plasticity results in sympathetic hyperreflexia and release of NE by sympathetic post-ganglionic neurons, including those targeting the spleen and other lymphoid organs such as the bone marrow. These changes after SCI result in measurable altered immune profile and function. Created using BioRender.com accessed on 2 September 2021.

3.2. Sympathetic Hyperreflexia

Recent studies have determined that sympathetic hyperreflexia contributes to SCI-IDS. Moreover, because sympathetic hyperreflexia development is correlated with injury level and severity, the extent and nature of immune dysfunction after SCI is injury level and severity dependent [25,58,63–65,67,69]. For instance, in the human SCI population, tetraplegic individuals display exacerbated increases in levels of the proinflammatory marker CRP compared to paraplegic individuals [70]. While chronic SCI persons exhibit fewer circulating $CD3^+$ and $CD4^+$ T cells and increased activation of remaining T cells, increased activation is particularly evident in those with complete or high level (above T6) injuries [71]. One preclinical study using rats showed that both pro-inflammatory and anti-inflammatory markers in plasma were significantly higher following a clip compression injury at T6/7 than at cervical level 6/7 (C6/7) [69]. It was suggested that this difference was due to the development of SCI-IDS in the cervically injured rats, though this was not directly demonstrated. Similarly, mice displayed splenic atrophy and leucopenia after a complete transection injury at T3 but not at T9 [64,65]. By 5 weeks post-injury, 50–70% of leukocytes were depleted, with a 60% reduction in the splenic B cell population. Moreover, T3-transected mice produced significantly lower antibody titers than uninjured controls when immunized with ovalbumin (OVA) antigen. These changes coincided with the development of AD [64]. Splenic white pulp atrophy and loss of B cells was exacerbated in the T3 SCI animals when sympathetic hyperreflexia was experimentally elicited with noxious sensory stimuli, such as colorectal distension (CRD). CRD also worsened the impaired immunological response after OVA antigen inoculation. Underscoring this, there was no significant effect on splenic B cells in the T9 injured group, which did not experience sympathetic hyperreflexia, indicating that sympathetic hyperreflexia is a causative factor in the development of SCI-IDS (Figure 2) [64].

Increased activation of vesicular glutamate transporter 2 (VGLUT2)+ excitatory interneurons in the lateral horn of thoracic spinal cord after injury has been implicated in the development of sympathetic hyperreflexia. These glutamatergic interneurons synapse on SPNs, and the number of presynaptic puncta contacting SPNs increases with time after SCI [65]. Chemogenetics, specifically designer receptors exclusively activated by designer drugs (DREADD), have also been used preclinically with great success to effectively determine the role of these excitatory interneurons in the intermediate and medial grey matter of the thoracic spinal cord after injury [65]. In this study, the researchers performed a T3 SCI in adult mice that expressed Gi/o-coupled human muscarinic M4 (hM4Di DREADD) in VGLUT2+ interneurons within the thoracic spinal cord. Clozapine-N-oxide (CNO) was injected starting two weeks after injury to silence the hM4Di-expressing, excitatory interneurons in thoracic spinal cord. Mice with this treatment exhibited normal splenic size and numbers of $CD4^+$ T cells, $CD8^+$ T cells, and $B220^+$ B cells [65]. While this study did not directly examine whether these immune changes were functionally relevant, it revealed the causative role of maladaptive neural plasticity in immunological changes after SCI and indicated that targeting glutamatergic interneurons specifically may be a promising therapeutic target to ameliorate immune dysfunction.

Concurrent increases in blood endogenous GCs and splenic NE levels also appear to play a role in SCI-IDS (Figure 2). Systemic coadministration of selective antagonists for β-2 adrenergic and GC receptors resulted in reduced splenic atrophy and normal antibody titer after OVA immunization, suggesting the importance of sympathetic control in regulating immune function [64]. Importantly, severing the splenic nerve to obliterate sympathetic innervation prior to T3 SCI in mice abrogated the increased susceptibility to pneumonia infection normally observed in animals after T3 SCI with intact sympathetic signaling [25]. These studies indicate that the severity of immune dysfunction is strongly tied to sympathetic activity.

A notable caveat of preclinical studies using complete SCI models to elicit SCI-IDS is whether this complete loss of supraspinal input to the SPNs is recapitulated in humans with SCI. This is highly relevant because human injuries classified as clinically complete often are anatomically incomplete and have some tissue sparing [72–76]. So then, what happens to immune function after incomplete SCI, particularly below the level of T6? Preclinical studies found that splenic atrophy did not occur in rats with moderate, incomplete injuries at either cervical (C6/7) or thoracic (T6/7) levels [69,77]. However, splenic NE, corticosterone, and leukopenia were significantly increased within a week after the incomplete thoracic injuries but not cervical injuries [77]. Additionally, circulating pro- and anti-inflammatory cytokines and chemokines were increased in thoracic-injured rats compared to those with cervical injuries [69]. In line with this, some preclinical studies already described in this review reported changes in immune profile and function after incomplete SCI, even below T6 [26,27,78]. One factor that may contribute to this is that some of the SPNs that modulate sympathetic input to the spleen are located within T6/T7 spinal cord and are likely directly injured by even a moderate, mid-level SCI.

Our personal observations further support the concept of SCI-induced immune changes in the absence of overt splenic atrophy. While we found measurable splenic atrophy at 8 weeks post-complete T3 transection in rats, we observed that the splenic immune cell profile was already significantly altered by 4 weeks post-complete T3 SCI, though the spleens grossly appeared similar at that point (unpublished personal observations; [79,80]).

As described in earlier sections, one clinical study found that proinflammatory markers, such as CRP, were increased after SCI regardless of injury level [11], while another study found that the severity of increased CRP correlated with injury level [70]. Similarly, while activation of T cells was significantly increased in the general SCI population, individuals with complete or high-level injuries above T6 displayed a more pronounced effect [71]. What is not clear from these aforementioned studies is how injuries at different levels and severities affect sympathetic tone and if this plays a role in the disparate results described. It appears that injury level and severity contribute to the extent of immune dysfunction after SCI, but this is not absolute and the level dependence of SCI-induced immune dysfunction is likely complex.

3.3. Aberrant Activity of the HPA Axis

One recent study found that dysregulated HPA axis function after sympathetic disruption corresponds with more severe acute leucopenia after high thoracic injury. Specifically, mice with a T1 complete transection displayed acute reduction in systemic NE and increase in plasma GCs while those with a T9 complete transection did not [63]. This increase in GCs was due to adrenal gland denervation after the high thoracic complete injury resulted in aberrant hypercortisolism. In line with this, T1-transected mice displayed reduced numbers of CD19$^+$ B cells, CD4$^+$ or CD8$^+$ T cells, CD11b$^+$ monocytes, NK1.1$^+$ natural killer (NK) cells, and CD11c$^+$ dendritic cells (DC) in multiple lymphoid organs, including the spleen (Figure 2).

3.4. Disrupted Bone Marrow Function

Bone marrow is a key hematopoietic organ where bone marrow hematopoietic stem cells reside that give rise to myeloid and lymphoid cells, replenishing immune cell populations daily. Sympathetic innervation to the bone marrow regulates both bone turnover and immune cell production (reviewed in [81,82]). It is worth mentioning that the ubiquitous osteoporosis experienced by the SCI population is exacerbated by sympathetic hyperreflexia, resulting in reduced bone production and increased bone resorption [83–85]. These changes in bone turnover are part of an interconnected loop in which bone denervation promotes osteoporosis and immune dysfunction, which in turn bidirectionally affect each other.

Just how exactly bone marrow-derived immunity changes after SCI has been described in a few publications [86–88]. Clinically, persons with SCI exhibit impaired bone marrow stem cell function [86,87]. In particular, SCI individuals displayed impaired NK cytolytic function, reduced T cell killer function, and lower IgG levels indicative of inhibited B cell function despite normal circulating lymphocyte numbers. When bone marrow aspirates were cultured, the number of long-term culture-initiating cells was significantly reduced in cultures from SCI persons, particularly tetraplegics, indicative of decreased progenitor growth [86]. Preclinically, a recent publication explored the mechanisms behind SCI-induced bone marrow hematopoietic dysfunction [88]. After SCI, mice exhibited increased hematopoietic stem cell proliferation and accumulation in the bone marrow, as well as impaired mobilization regardless of injury level and severity (Figure 2). In T3-transected mice specifically, expression of bone marrow cytokines and chemokines was significantly increased, and C-X-C motif chemokine ligand 12 (CXCL12)/C-X-C motif chemokine receptor 4 (CXCR4) signaling specifically led to sequestration of hematopoietic stem cells and mature B cells. These changes appear to have functional implications, as the bone marrow response to inflammatory stimulation with lipopolysaccharide (LPS) was impaired after SCI [88].

3.5. Obesity

Several aforementioned studies observed increased susceptibility to various infections in rodents with lower thoracic injuries at T9/10, which largely leave descending control of sympathetic circuitry intact [23]. Therefore, while disruption of sympathetic innervation to lymphoid organs strongly contributes to immune dysfunction after SCI, it is not the only cause. Although the primary insult may be in the spinal cord, SCI is an injury of nearly every system in the body, from gastrointestinal to cardiovascular. The multi-system dysfunction observed after SCI results in a clinical population more likely to suffer from complications such as obesity and type 2 diabetes [89–91]. Indeed, while sympathetic hyperreflexia and subsequent AD appear to be a major underlying cause of SCI-IDS, concomitant chronic low-grade inflammation has been strongly linked to neurogenic obesity (reviewed in [92]) as well as other secondary complications of SCI (reviewed in [6,93]). Importantly, these conditions also can contribute to the development of immune dysfunction after SCI.

Obesity, which affects approximately 66% of SCI individuals [94], is thought to be a primary cause of the chronic low-grade inflammation observed after SCI [92]. Adipocytes have been shown to release "adipokines" such as TNFα, IL-6, and MCP-1, resulting in a systemic proinflammatory state in obesity [92,95]. In the SCI population specifically, higher waist circumference is associated with elevated CRP, a proinflammatory cytokine implicated in cardiovascular disease [70,96]. Evidence indicates that exercise to mitigate obesity can reduce systemic inflammation [97,98]. In SCI individuals specifically, plasma levels of proinflammatory cytokines TNFα and IL-6 were reduced after an arm cranking exercise regimen that improved anthropometric index, decreased waist circumference, and decreased plasma concentration of leptin [99]. Similarly, 10 weeks of functional electrical stimulation cycling by SCI persons resulted in increased muscle mass by dual X-ray absorptiometry and significantly reduced levels of proinflammatory cytokines IL-6, TNFα, and CRP [100].

Obesity, in turn, increases the risk of developing type 2 diabetes [101], a condition which is strongly associated with persistent systemic inflammation (reviewed in [102]). Studies have shown that SCI individuals are at higher risk of developing type 2 diabetes [89,91,103]. Interestingly, type 2 diabetes is considered to be immune-driven yet also contributes to immunosuppression via diabetes-mediated hyperglycemia [104,105]. While the role of type 2 diabetes in immune dysfunction specifically in the SCI population has yet to be established, it is highly possible that the known effects of insulin resistance and hyperglycemia on immunity carry over. These secondary complications arising from SCI therefore provide some explanation as to why SCI persons experience chronic low-grade systemic inflammation.

3.6. Repetitive Infections and Wounds

Persistent bacterial infections are thought to manipulate the immune system to prevent clearance [106,107]. In SCI individuals, repetitive infections, namely UTIs and infected chronic pressure ulcers, may contribute to both systemic low-grade inflammation and concurrent immunosuppression. As described in an earlier section, when SCI persons present with UTIs or pressure ulcers, serum levels of proinflammatory cytokines such as IL-6 and TNFα are significantly higher than in SCI persons without these infections [9]. This would suggest that ongoing infection can exacerbate the systemic inflammation observed after SCI. Along with this, SCI persons with an ongoing UTI displayed higher levels of urine IgA concentrations compared to those without infection, and SCI individuals displayed sustained IgG response to bacterial antigens despite no differences in circulating T cells specific to UTI bacterial antigens, compared to controls [10]. Interestingly, AD events have been documented to result in reduced oxygenation and increased perspiration of the skin, which in turn may contribute to increased susceptibility to pressure ulcers [108]. In turn, pressure ulcers and UTIs can both serve as stimuli that elicit AD events, which can further impair immune function after SCI, as described above. While it is still unclear to what degree persistent UTIs and pressure ulcer infections modulate immune activity in SCI individuals, it is apparent that an ongoing infection correlates with additional immunological changes.

4. Potential Interventions to Improve Immunological Function Post-SCI

4.1. A Critical Need for Clinical Therapies

There are no currently approved therapies specifically targeting improving the immune system for SCI individuals. In fact, the routine use of methylprednisolone in acute treatment of SCI persons in the United States is of debatable benefit for various reasons (reviewed in [109,110]), including the known effect of immunosuppression. While some studies have suggested that motor function recovery may be incrementally improved with methylprednisolone treatment, others have not found measurable effects but did note appreciable side effects [111,112]. Therefore, whether using methylprednisolone is of benefit is highly debated, even more so now that attention has turned to its immunosuppressive properties as a corticosteroid [113]. Another standard treatment for SCI individuals is rehabilitative medicine. With respect to systemic inflammation specifically, several studies have found that exercise lowers circulating levels of TNFα, IL-6, and CRP [99,114].

One method to improve quality of life in SCI individuals would be to reduce likelihood of infection. Clinical studies have examined the prophylactic use of antibiotics to prevent UTIs in the SCI population [14,115]. However, while several groups found that prophylactic low-dose clindamycin, sulfamethoxazole, nitrofurantoin, trimethoprim, or cefalexin treatment was effective in significantly reducing the rate of UTIs during extended treatment [116–118], another group found that prophylactic sulfamethoxazole or nitrofurantoin was not effective in reducing UTIs in the SCI population [119]. Additionally, antibiotic-resistant bacterial colonization of the bladder is common with prophylactic use of antibiotics in SCI persons [118,120], suggesting that prevention of infections via this route is unlikely to prove beneficial in the long term. To circumvent this problem, two studies attempted long-term prophylactic use of four antibiotics on a cyclical regimen; this method resulted in fewer yearly UTIs in SCI individuals [121,122]. Prophylactic antibiotic treatment has also been recommended by the North American Spine Society in cases of spinal surgery [123], with clinical studies often, but not always, indicating a reduction in post-operative infections, particularly with multiple days of treatment [124,125]. How these treatments might affect other types of infections in SCI persons remains unknown. Additionally, how recurring use of antibiotics affects the SCI body's gut microbiome (discussed in more detail below) and the downstream consequences of that is not well understood.

Alternatively, therapeutic options could address underlying causes of immune dysfunction. As mentioned above, one cause of SCI-IDS is sympathetic hyperreflexia. There have been multiple preclinical and clinical studies using procedures and pharmacological interventions to both limit the onset of AD and manage it (reviewed in [126,127]). The current medical advice is that persons presenting with AD manage their symptoms using nonpharmacological methods, such as removing the offending stimulus (i.e., blocked catheter, tight clothing, or bowel impaction) and moving to a sitting position [128]. While these methods are typically successful in eventually ending the AD event, sustained high blood pressure can occur that demands further medical attention [66,128]. Commonly used drugs for the treatment of AD solely mitigate hypertensive symptoms [127], and therefore have short-lived effects that do not cure the underlying disorder. These drugs include nifedipine and nitrates, amongst other hypertension medications, such as angiotensin I converting enzyme inhibitors. Epidural stimulation has also been used to stabilize variable blood pressure in SCI persons [129]. Interestingly, preclinical work has revealed mixed data on the use of exercise to mitigate AD. While one study found that passive hindlimb cycling or active forelimb swimming did not change AD severity after T2 contusion injury in rats [130], another study found that passive hindlimb cycling after complete T3 transection did reduce the severity of AD [131]. Other studies have used botulinum toxin, capsaicin, anticholinergics, or surgical procedures to prevent the development or continuation of AD [126]. These treatments have had variable success in reduction in AD events in SCI persons [126,132,133]. However, it is important to keep in mind that sympathetic hyperreflexia affects not only the vasculature but also any organ that receives sympathetic innervation. None of these studies have examined effects on immune function, regardless of observed changes in AD presentation. It is possible that examining immune function after such treatments would reveal immunological changes, which would be of interest given the importance of improving immunity post-SCI. Additionally, there are no approved treatments to prevent the development of sympathetic hyperreflexia from the outset. Therefore, there is a dire need for the identification of treatments that improve immune function after SCI. In the following sections, we summarize recent preclinical research examining potential means to specifically improve immune function after SCI.

4.2. Gabapentin

Some preclinical studies have attempted to reduce the maladaptive neural plasticity that contributes to AD worsening via pharmacological intervention. Gabapentin (GBP), an anti-seizure and neuropathic pain medication known to prevent synaptogenesis at high doses, has been used after SCI in preclinical models to examine its effect on AD. Several studies have indicated that acute treatment with a low-dose of GBP (50 mg/kg) or chronic treatment with a very high-dose of GBP (400 mg/kg/day) starting the day of complete T4 SCI in rats decreased mean arterial pressure in response to CRD [134–137]. However, chronic treatment with this very high-dose of GBP (400 mg/kg/day) also increased the frequency of spontaneous AD events [136]. On the other hand, in another recent study, chronic treatment with a slightly lower dose of GBP (200 mg/kg/day) starting one day after complete T4 SCI in mice prevented excitatory synaptic formation and sprouting of sensory afferents, two examples of spinal plasticity associated with sympathetic hyperreflexia. This resulted in reduced frequency of spontaneous AD events, attenuated induced AD by CRD, and, importantly, mitigated changes in immune profile after SCI (Figure 3) [137]. Additionally, chronic treatment with this dose of GBP resulted in prevention of splenic atrophy and maintenance of $CD3^+$ T cell and $B220^+$ B cell populations in the spleen (Figure 3) [137]. One important difference in these seemingly conflicting studies is that Eldahan et al. did not observe any changes in excitatory or inhibitory presynaptic markers in the lumbosacral dorsal horn at the very high dose of GBP. Species/strain dependent differences may also account for the divergent results. While studies have presented conflicting data on the use of GBP for prevention of AD, the data from Brennan et al. support the notion that suppression of neural plasticity in the sympathetic circuit below the level of injury can improve the immune profile after SCI.

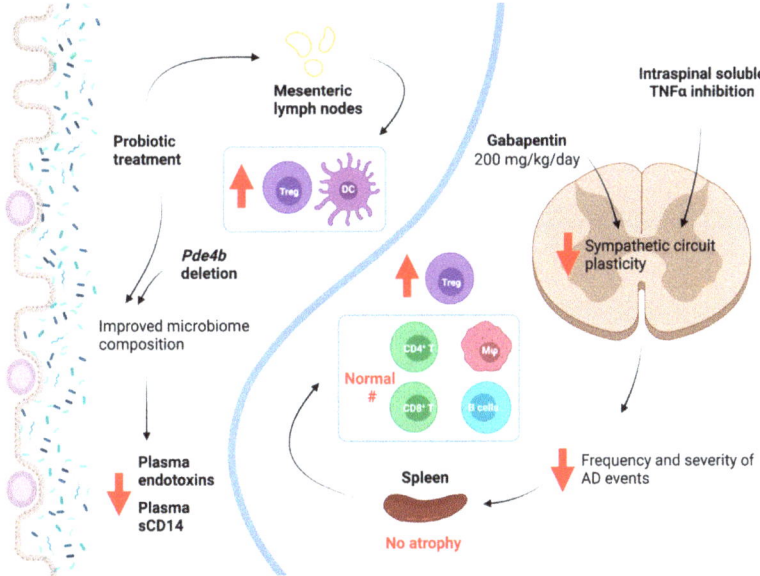

Figure 3. Preclinical studies have revealed that pharmacological inhibition of sympathetic circuit plasticity, either through the use of high-dose gabapentin (GBP) or soluble TNFα inhibition, can reduce autonomic dysreflexia (AD) and improve splenic immune cell profile. Separately, studies have examined the modulation of gut microbiota, either through probiotic treatment or deletion of *Pde4b*, to improve microbiome composition after SCI, which in turn improves anti-inflammatory immune cell profile in gut-associated lymphoid tissues (GALTs), like mesenteric lymph nodes (MLNs), and reduces circulating markers of inflammation. Created using BioRender.com accessed on 2 September 2021.

4.3. Inhibiting TNFα

Other studies have targeted TNFα signaling to improve sympathetic hyperreflexia and splenic function. TNFα expression is persistently upregulated in the spinal cord after injury, contributing to neural plasticity. TNFα exists in two forms; its soluble form is a product of transmembrane TNFα cleavage by TNFα-converting enzyme. While the former is highly proinflammatory and plays a role in neural plasticity below the level of injury [138], the latter has been shown to have neuroprotective effects [139,140]. After SCI, specific central inhibition of soluble TNFα using the experimental compound XPro1595, which inhibits soluble TNFα specifically, resulted in improved functional recovery [141]. Importantly, these effects were not replicated with central administration of etanercept, a pan-TNFα inhibitor that affects both soluble and transmembrane TNFα [141]. This highlights the particular role of soluble TNFα in SCI pathology, and paved the way for examination of how soluble TNFα inhibition after SCI might affect other facets of recovery, including immune function.

We recently reported that continuous intrathecal administration of XPro1595 in rats with complete T3 transections beginning up to 3 days post-injury significantly reduced intraspinal plasticity within the sympathetic circuit and lowered the frequency and severity of AD events (Figure 3) [79,80]. Additionally, in XPro1595-treated rats, splenic atrophy was prevented, and splenic immune cell profile was similar to non-injured control spleens, in contrast to spleens from injured animals without XPro1595 that exhibited an altered immune cell profile. In particular, $CD45R^+$ B cells, $CD8^+$ T cells, and $CD11b/c^+$ macrophages were returned to uninjured numbers, while $CD4^+CD25^+FoxP3^+$ regulatory T cells were significantly increased (Figure 3) [79,80]. Improved splenic immune profile corresponded with reduced sympathetic, noradrenergic sprouting in the spleen [79]. Excitingly, the improved immune profile in turn resulted in reduced susceptibility to pneumonia infection, with no XPro1595-treated injured rats dying while nearly 40% of vehicle-treated injured rats succumbed to infection. While vehicle-treated injured rats that survived exhibited persistent weight loss at 10 days post-infection, those that received XPro1595 returned to baseline [79]. However, when XPro1595 treatment was delayed until 2 weeks post-injury, no beneficial effects on AD were observed, suggesting that administration at some point prior to 2 weeks is vital to the effectiveness of this particular treatment strategy [142]. Nevertheless, the benefit of central soluble TNFα inhibition after subacute injury to attenuate sympathetic hyperreflexia and to improve downstream immune function is particularly promising given the striking increase in resistance to pneumonia infection.

4.4. Modulation of Gut Microbiota

Another possible therapeutic option may exist in gut microbiota. Notably, ~70% of immune cells reside in gut-associated lymphoid tissues (GALTs), where they respond to microbial antigens and metabolites produced in the gut and serve as the first line of defense against pathogens entering via the gastrointestinal route [143]. The links between gut microbiota, neurological function, and immunological pathology are research topics of great interest in diseases ranging from multiple sclerosis to autism [144–147], and the downstream effects of SCI on this complex system are only now beginning to be revealed.

In a landmark study examining microbiota changes after SCI, a T9 contusive injury in mice resulted in immune disruption, e.g., altered numbers of $B220^+$ B cells, $CD4^+$ and $CD8^+$ T cells, $CD11b^+$ macrophages, and $CD11c^+$ DCs in GALT mesenteric lymph nodes and Peyer's Patches [78]. Importantly, the researchers discovered that therapeutic treatment with probiotics in the first month post-injury resulted in a more anti-inflammatory GALT profile, increasing numbers of $CD4^+CD25^+FoxP3^+$ regulatory T cells and $CD11c^+$ DCs in the mesenteric lymph nodes (Figure 3) [78]. Another group examined the gut microbiome composition of humans with SCI and found that bacterial phyla that produce the short-chain fatty acid butyrate—which is associated with having strong anti-inflammatory effects—were significantly reduced [148]. While not directly demonstrated, these gut microbiome changes might contribute to a proinflammatory state in SCI persons [148].

Since these groundbreaking studies, there has been an explosion of interest in how gut microbiota are altered after SCI, and how modulation of the gut microbiome might improve both neurological and immunological outcomes for SCI individuals [149–156]. In regard to peripheral immunity, a recent study demonstrated that after a T9 contusive injury in mice, the gut microbiome displayed a reduced *Firmicutes* to *Bacteroidetes* phyla ratio as well as an increase in the phylum *Proteobacteria* that contains Gram-negative bacteria that produce the endotoxin LPS, which is associated with systemic inflammation [157]. In fact, the researchers found that sCD14, a marker of systemic inflammation, was significantly increased at 42 days post-SCI. Interestingly, deletion of *Pde4b* to disrupt the TLR4/TNFα/PDE4B axis mitigated the microbiome imbalance observed after SCI, and resulted in reduced endotoxin and sCD14 serum levels, suggestive of reduced inflammation (Figure 3) [157]. Taken together, these studies strongly suggest that improving gut microbiota health may in turn improve immunological function in SCI persons, which is particularly exciting given the accessibility of the gut for therapeutic intervention.

5. Conclusions

Immune changes post-SCI have major implications in the quality of life of SCI individuals as well as their treatment. With disruption of descending CNS input to immune organs as well as secondary complications of SCI contributing to SCI-IDS, individuals with SCI are faced with a constant state of inflammation and increased risk of infection. Promisingly, recent preclinical research indicates a wide range of potential interventions that may be able to improve immune function and reduce the risk of infection. However, whether these effects are replicated after chronic immune dysfunction has already occurred, which populations of immune cells should be targeted, and how this affects immunity to various infection types in persons are all unknown facets of immune modulation post-SCI. Importantly, while there are many gaps in knowledge regarding immune function and modulation after SCI that remain to be filled, potential opportunities to identify effective therapeutics to better immune function will undoubtedly result in improved quality of life for those living with SCI.

Author Contributions: Conceptualization; writing—original draft preparation; writing—review and editing; visualization, M.A.J. and V.J.T.; funding acquisition, V.J.T. Both authors have read and agreed to the published version of the manuscript.

Funding: This work was supported by NIH R01 NS106908, NIH R01 NS111761, and NIH R01 NS085426 to V.J.T.

Institutional Review Board Statement: Not applicable.

Informed Consent Statement: Not applicable.

Data Availability Statement: Not applicable.

Conflicts of Interest: The authors declare no conflict of interest.

References

1. Soden, R.J.; Walsh, J.; Middleton, J.W.; Craven, M.L.; Rutkowski, S.B.; Yeo, J.D. Causes of death after spinal cord injury. *Spinal Cord* **2000**, *38*, 604–610. [CrossRef]
2. Failli, V.; Kopp, M.A.; Gericke, C.; Martus, P.; Klingbeil, S.; Brommer, B.; Laginha, I.; Chen, Y.; DeVivo, M.J.; Dirnagl, U.; et al. Functional neurological recovery after spinal cord injury is impaired in patients with infections. *Brain* **2012**, *135*, 3238–3250. [CrossRef]
3. Montgomerie, J.Z. Infections in patients with spinal cord injuries. *Clin. Infect. Dis.* **1997**, *25*, 1285–1290. [CrossRef]
4. Riegger, T.; Conrad, S.; Liu, K.; Schluesener, H.J.; Adibzahdeh, M.; Schwab, J.M. Spinal cord injury-induced immune depression syndrome (SCI-IDS). *Eur. J. Neurosci.* **2007**, *25*, 1743–1747. [CrossRef] [PubMed]
5. Meisel, C.; Schwab, J.M.; Prass, K.; Meisel, A.; Dirnagl, U. Central nervous system injury-induced immune deficiency syndrome. *Nat. Rev. Neurosci.* **2005**, *6*, 775–786. [CrossRef] [PubMed]
6. Allison, D.J.; Ditor, D.S. Immune dysfunction and chronic inflammation following spinal cord injury. *Spinal Cord* **2015**, *53*, 14–18. [CrossRef]

7. Schwab, J.M.; Zhang, Y.; Kopp, M.A.; Brommer, B.; Popovich, P.G. The paradox of chronic neuroinflammation, systemic immune suppression, autoimmunity after traumatic chronic spinal cord injury. *Exp. Neurol.* **2014**, *258*, 121–129. [CrossRef]
8. Hayes, K.C.; Hull, T.C.; Delaney, G.A.; Potter, P.J.; Sequeira, K.A.; Campbell, K.; Popovich, P.G. Elevated serum titers of proinflammatory cytokines and CNS autoantibodies in patients with chronic spinal cord injury. *J. Neurotrauma* **2002**, *19*, 753–761. [CrossRef]
9. Davies, A.L.; Hayes, K.C.; Dekaban, G.A. Clinical correlates of elevated serum concentrations of cytokines and autoantibodies in patients with spinal cord injury. *Arch. Phys. Med. Rehabil.* **2007**, *88*, 1384–1393. [CrossRef]
10. Pavlicek, D.; Krebs, J.; Capossela, S.; Bertolo, A.; Engelhardt, B.; Pannek, J.; Stoyanov, J. Immunosenescence in persons with spinal cord injury in relation to urinary tract infections -a cross-sectional study. *Immun. Ageing* **2017**, *14*, 22. [CrossRef]
11. Wang, T.D.; Wang, Y.H.; Huang, T.S.; Su, T.C.; Pan, S.L.; Chen, S.Y. Circulating levels of markers of inflammation and endothelial activation are increased in men with chronic spinal cord injury. *J. Formos. Med. Assoc.* **2007**, *106*, 919–928. [CrossRef]
12. Herman, P.; Stein, A.; Gibbs, K.; Korsunsky, I.; Gregersen, P.; Bloom, O. Persons with chronic spinal cord injury have decreased natural killer cell and increased toll-like receptor/inflammatory gene expression. *J. Neurotrauma* **2018**, *35*, 1819–1829. [CrossRef]
13. Frankel, H.L.; Coll, J.R.; Charlifue, S.W.; Whiteneck, G.G.; Gardner, B.P.; Jamous, M.A.; Krishnan, K.R.; Nuseibeh, I.; Savic, G.; Sett, P. Long-term survival in spinal cord injury: A fifty year investigation. *Spinal Cord* **1998**, *36*, 266–274. [CrossRef] [PubMed]
14. Garcia-Arguello, L.Y.; O'Horo, J.C.; Farrell, A.; Blakney, R.; Sohail, M.R.; Evans, C.T.; Safdar, N. Infections in the spinal cord-injured population: A systematic review. *Spinal Cord* **2017**, *55*, 526–534. [CrossRef]
15. Savic, G.; DeVivo, M.J.; Frankel, H.L.; Jamous, M.A.; Soni, B.M.; Charlifue, S. Causes of death after traumatic spinal cord injury—A 70-year British study. *Spinal Cord* **2017**, *55*, 891–897. [CrossRef]
16. Kriz, J.; Sediva, K.; Maly, M. Causes of death after spinal cord injury in the Czech Republic. *Spinal Cord* **2021**, *59*, 814–820. [CrossRef]
17. Thietje, R.; Pouw, M.H.; Schulz, A.P.; Kienast, B.; Hirschfeld, S. Mortality in patients with traumatic spinal cord injury: Descriptive analysis of 62 deceased subjects. *J. Spinal Cord Med.* **2011**, *34*, 482–487. [CrossRef]
18. Terson de Paleville, D.G.; McKay, W.B.; Folz, R.J.; Ovechkin, A.V. Respiratory motor control disrupted by spinal cord injury: Mechanisms, evaluation, and restoration. *Transl. Stroke Res.* **2011**, *2*, 463–473. [CrossRef]
19. Ikeda, T.; Inoue, S.; Konta, T.; Murakami, M.; Fujimoto, S.; Iseki, K.; Moriyama, T.; Yamagata, K.; Tsuruya, K.; Narita, I.; et al. Can Daily walking alone reduce pneumonia-related mortality among older people? *Sci. Rep.* **2020**, *10*, 8556. [CrossRef]
20. Williams, P.T. Dose-response relationship between exercise and respiratory disease mortality. *Med. Sci. Sports Exerc.* **2014**, *46*, 711–717. [CrossRef]
21. Ukawa, S.; Zhao, W.; Yatsuya, H.; Yamagishi, K.; Tanabe, N.; Iso, H.; Tamakoshi, A. Associations of daily walking time with pneumonia mortality among elderly individuals with or without a medical history of myocardial infarction or stroke: Findings from the Japan collaborative cohort study. *J. Epidemiol.* **2019**, *29*, 233–237. [CrossRef]
22. Rice, H.; Hill, K.; Fowler, R.; Watson, C.; Waterer, G.; Harrold, M. Reduced Step count and clinical frailty in hospitalized adults with community-acquired pneumonia. *Respir. Care* **2020**, *65*, 455–463. [CrossRef]
23. Held, K.S.; Steward, O.; Blanc, C.; Lane, T.E. Impaired immune responses following spinal cord injury lead to reduced ability to control viral infection. *Exp. Neurol.* **2010**, *226*, 242–253. [CrossRef]
24. Balsara, Z.R.; Ross, S.S.; Dolber, P.C.; Wiener, J.S.; Tang, Y.; Seed, P.C. Enhanced susceptibility to urinary tract infection in the spinal cord-injured host with neurogenic bladder. *Infect. Immun.* **2013**, *81*, 3018–3026. [CrossRef]
25. Brommer, B.; Engel, O.; Kopp, M.A.; Watzlawick, R.; Muller, S.; Pruss, H.; Chen, Y.; DeVivo, M.J.; Finkenstaedt, F.W.; Dirnagl, U.; et al. Spinal cord injury-induced immune deficiency syndrome enhances infection susceptibility dependent on lesion level. *Brain* **2016**, *139*, 692–707. [CrossRef]
26. Bracchi-Ricard, V.; Zha, J.; Smith, A.; Lopez-Rodriguez, D.M.; Bethea, J.R.; Andreansky, S. Chronic spinal cord injury attenuates influenza virus-specific antiviral immunity. *J. Neuroinflamm.* **2016**, *13*, 125. [CrossRef]
27. Norden, D.M.; Bethea, J.R.; Jiang, J. Impaired CD8 T cell antiviral immunity following acute spinal cord injury. *J. Neuroinflamm.* **2018**, *15*, 149. [CrossRef]
28. Battaglino, R.A.; Lazzari, A.A.; Garshick, E.; Morse, L.R. Spinal cord injury-induced osteoporosis: Pathogenesis and emerging therapies. *Curr. Osteoporos. Rep.* **2012**, *10*, 278–285. [CrossRef]
29. Tan, C.O.; Battaglino, R.A.; Morse, L.R. Spinal cord injury and osteoporosis: Causes, mechanisms, and rehabilitation strategies. *Int. J. Phys. Med. Rehabil.* **2013**, *1*, 127. [PubMed]
30. Clowes, J.A.; Riggs, B.L.; Khosla, S. The role of the immune system in the pathophysiology of osteoporosis. *Immunol. Rev.* **2005**, *208*, 207–227. [CrossRef]
31. Pietschmann, P.; Mechtcheriakova, D.; Meshcheryakova, A.; Foger-Samwald, U.; Ellinger, I. Immunology of Osteoporosis: A mini-review. *Gerontology* **2016**, *62*, 128–137. [CrossRef]
32. Srivastava, R.K.; Dar, H.Y.; Mishra, P.K. Immunoporosis: Immunology of Osteoporosis-role of T cells. *Front. Immunol.* **2018**, *9*, 657. [CrossRef]
33. Noller, C.M.; Groah, S.L.; Nash, M.S. Inflammatory stress effects on health and function after spinal cord injury. *Top. Spinal Cord Inj. Rehabil.* **2017**, *23*, 207–217. [CrossRef]
34. Werhagen, L.; Budh, C.N.; Hultling, C.; Molander, C. Neuropathic pain after traumatic spinal cord injury–relations to gender, spinal level, completeness, and age at the time of injury. *Spinal Cord* **2004**, *42*, 665–673. [CrossRef]

35. Lee, S.; Zhao, X.; Hatch, M.; Chun, S.; Chang, E. Central neuropathic pain in spinal cord injury. *Crit. Rev. Phys. Rehabil. Med.* **2013**, *25*, 159–172. [CrossRef]
36. Hagen, E.M.; Rekand, T. Management of neuropathic pain associated with spinal cord injury. *Pain Ther.* **2015**, *4*, 51–65. [CrossRef] [PubMed]
37. Burke, D.; Fullen, B.M.; Stokes, D.; Lennon, O. Neuropathic pain prevalence following spinal cord injury: A systematic review and meta-analysis. *Eur. J. Pain* **2017**, *21*, 29–44. [CrossRef] [PubMed]
38. Li, C.C.; Lin, H.R.; Tsai, M.D.; Tsay, S.L. Neuropathic pain experiences of spinal cord injury patients. *J. Nurs. Res.* **2018**, *26*, 280–287. [CrossRef] [PubMed]
39. Kim, H.Y.; Lee, H.J.; Kim, T.L.; Kim, E.; Ham, D.; Lee, J.; Kim, T.; Shin, J.W.; Son, M.; Sung, J.H.; et al. Prevalence and characteristics of neuropathic pain in patients with spinal cord injury referred to a rehabilitation center. *Ann. Rehabil. Med.* **2020**, *44*, 438–449. [CrossRef] [PubMed]
40. Schomberg, D.; Olson, J.K. Immune responses of microglia in the spinal cord: Contribution to pain states. *Exp. Neurol.* **2012**, *234*, 262–270. [CrossRef]
41. Matsuda, M.; Huh, Y.; Ji, R.R. Roles of inflammation, neurogenic inflammation, and neuroinflammation in pain. *J. Anesth.* **2019**, *33*, 131–139. [CrossRef]
42. Calvo, M.; Dawes, J.M.; Bennett, D.L. The role of the immune system in the generation of neuropathic pain. *Lancet Neurol.* **2012**, *11*, 629–642. [CrossRef]
43. Allison, D.J.; Thomas, A.; Beaudry, K.; Ditor, D.S. Targeting inflammation as a treatment modality for neuropathic pain in spinal cord injury: A randomized clinical trial. *J. Neuroinflamm.* **2016**, *13*, 152. [CrossRef]
44. Kumar, S.; Yarmush, M.L.; Dash, B.C.; Hsia, H.C.; Berthiaume, F. Impact of complete spinal cord injury on healing of skin ulcers in mouse models. *J. Neurotrauma* **2018**, *35*, 815–824. [CrossRef] [PubMed]
45. Zhao, R.; Liang, H.; Clarke, E.; Jackson, C.; Xue, M. Inflammation in chronic wounds. *Int. J. Mol. Sci.* **2016**, *17*, 2085. [CrossRef]
46. Demidova-Rice, T.N.; Hamblin, M.R.; Herman, I.M. Acute and impaired wound healing: Pathophysiology and current methods for drug delivery, part 1: Normal and chronic wounds: Biology, causes, and approaches to care. *Adv. Skin Wound Care* **2012**, *25*, 304–314. [CrossRef]
47. Rosique, R.G.; Rosique, M.J.; Farina, J.A. Curbing inflammation in skin wound healing: A review. *Int. J. Inflamm.* **2015**, *2015*, 316235. [CrossRef]
48. Rappl, L.M. Physiological changes in tissues denervated by spinal cord injury tissues and possible effects on wound healing. *Int. Wound J.* **2008**, *5*, 435–444. [CrossRef]
49. Marbourg, J.M.; Bratasz, A.; Mo, X.; Popovich, P.G. Spinal cord injury suppresses cutaneous inflammation: Implications for peripheral wound healing. *J. Neurotrauma* **2017**, *34*, 1149–1155. [CrossRef]
50. Myers, J.; Lee, M.; Kiratli, J. Cardiovascular disease in spinal cord injury: An overview of prevalence, risk, evaluation, and management. *Am. J. Phys. Med. Rehabil.* **2007**, *86*, 142–152. [CrossRef]
51. Bigford, G.E.; Bracchi-Ricard, V.C.; Keane, R.W.; Nash, M.S.; Bethea, J.R. Neuroendocrine and cardiac metabolic dysfunction and NLRP3 inflammasome activation in adipose tissue and pancreas following chronic spinal cord injury in the mouse. *ASN Neuro* **2013**, *5*, 243–255. [CrossRef]
52. Libin, A.; Tinsley, E.A.; Nash, M.S.; Mendez, A.J.; Burns, P.; Elrod, M.; Hamm, L.F.; Groah, S.L. Cardiometabolic risk clustering in spinal cord injury: Results of exploratory factor analysis. *Top. Spinal Cord Inj. Rehabil.* **2013**, *19*, 183–194. [CrossRef] [PubMed]
53. Solinsky, R.; Betancourt, L.; Schmidt-Read, M.; Kupfer, M.; Owens, M.; Schwab, J.M.; Dusseau, N.B.; Szlachcic, Y.; Sutherland, L.; Taylor, J.A.; et al. Acute spinal cord injury is associated with prevalent cardiometabolic risk factors. *Arch. Phys. Med. Rehabil.* **2021**. [CrossRef] [PubMed]
54. Cragg, J.J.; Noonan, V.K.; Krassioukov, A.; Borisoff, J. Cardiovascular disease and spinal cord injury: Results from a national population health survey. *Neurology* **2013**, *81*, 723–728. [CrossRef] [PubMed]
55. Matos-Souza, J.R.; Pithon, K.R.; Ozahata, T.M.; Oliveira, R.T.; Teo, F.H.; Blotta, M.H.; Cliquet, A.J.; Nadruz, W.J. Subclinical atherosclerosis is related to injury level but not to inflammatory parameters in spinal cord injury subjects. *Spinal Cord* **2010**, *48*, 740–744. [CrossRef]
56. Yoon, E.S.; Heffernan, K.S.; Jae, S.Y.; Kim, H.J.; Bunsawat, K.; Fernhall, B. Metabolically healthy obesity and subclinical atherosclerosis in persons with spinal cord injury. *J. Rehabil. Med.* **2018**, *50*, 613–618. [CrossRef]
57. Bigford, G.E.; Szeto, A.; Kimball, J.; Herderick, E.E.; Mendez, A.J.; Nash, M.S. Cardiometabolic risks and atherosclerotic disease in ApoE knockout mice: Effect of spinal cord injury and Salsalate anti-inflammatory pharmacotherapy. *PLoS ONE* **2021**, *16*, e0246601. [CrossRef]
58. Chio, J.C.T.; Xu, K.J.; Popovich, P.; David, S.; Fehlings, M.G. Neuroimmunological therapies for treating spinal cord injury: Evidence and future perspectives. *Exp. Neurol.* **2021**, *341*, 113704. [CrossRef]
59. Felten, D.L.; Ackerman, K.D.; Wiegand, S.J.; Felten, S.Y. Noradrenergic sympathetic innervation of the spleen: I. Nerve fibers associate with lymphocytes and macrophages in specific compartments of the splenic white pulp. *J. Neurosci. Res.* **1987**, *18*, 28–36. [CrossRef]
60. Felten, S.Y.; Olschowka, J. Noradrenergic sympathetic innervation of the spleen: II. Tyrosine hydroxylase (TH)-positive nerve terminals form synapticlike contacts on lymphocytes in the splenic white pulp. *J. Neurosci. Res.* **1987**, *18*, 37–48. [CrossRef]

61. Coutinho, A.E.; Chapman, K.E. The anti-inflammatory and immunosuppressive effects of glucocorticoids, recent developments and mechanistic insights. *Mol. Cell. Endocrinol.* **2011**, *335*, 2–13. [CrossRef]
62. Noble, B.T.; Brennan, F.H.; Popovich, P.G. The spleen as a neuroimmune interface after spinal cord injury. *J. Neuroimmunol.* **2018**, *321*, 1–11. [CrossRef]
63. Pruss, H.; Tedeschi, A.; Thiriot, A.; Lynch, L.; Loughhead, S.M.; Stutte, S.; Mazo, I.B.; Kopp, M.A.; Brommer, B.; Blex, C.; et al. Spinal cord injury-induced immunodeficiency is mediated by a sympathetic-neuroendocrine adrenal reflex. *Nat. Neurosci.* **2017**, *20*, 1549–1559. [CrossRef]
64. Zhang, Y.; Guan, Z.; Reader, B.; Shawler, T.; Mandrekar-Colucci, S.; Huang, K.; Weil, Z.; Bratasz, A.; Wells, J.; Powell, N.D.; et al. Autonomic dysreflexia causes chronic immune suppression after spinal cord injury. *J. Neurosci.* **2013**, *33*, 12970–12981. [CrossRef]
65. Ueno, M.; Ueno-Nakamura, Y.; Niehaus, J.; Popovich, P.G.; Yoshida, Y. Silencing spinal interneurons inhibits immune suppressive autonomic reflexes caused by spinal cord injury. *Nat. Neurosci.* **2016**, *19*, 784–787. [CrossRef] [PubMed]
66. Eldahan, K.C.; Rabchevsky, A.G. Autonomic dysreflexia after spinal cord injury: Systemic pathophysiology and methods of management. *Auton. Neurosci.* **2018**, *209*, 59–70. [CrossRef]
67. Lucin, K.M.; Sanders, V.M.; Jones, T.B.; Malarkey, W.B.; Popovich, P.G. Impaired antibody synthesis after spinal cord injury is level dependent and is due to sympathetic nervous system dysregulation. *Exp. Neurol.* **2007**, *207*, 75–84. [CrossRef] [PubMed]
68. Zha, J.; Smith, A.; Andreansky, S.; Bracchi-Ricard, V.; Bethea, J.R. Chronic thoracic spinal cord injury impairs CD8+ T-cell function by up-regulating programmed cell death-1 expression. *J. Neuroinflamm.* **2014**, *11*, 65. [CrossRef]
69. Hong, J.; Chang, A.; Zavvarian, M.M.; Wang, J.; Liu, Y.; Fehlings, M.G. Level-specific differences in systemic expression of pro- and anti-inflammatory cytokines and chemokines after spinal cord injury. *Int. J. Mol. Sci.* **2018**, *19*, 2167. [CrossRef] [PubMed]
70. Gibson, A.E.; SHAPE-SCI Research Group; Buchholz, A.C.; Ginis, K.M. C-Reactive protein in adults with chronic spinal cord injury: Increased chronic inflammation in tetraplegia vs paraplegia. *Spinal Cord* **2008**, *46*, 616–621. [CrossRef] [PubMed]
71. Monahan, R.; Stein, A.; Gibbs, K.; Bank, M.; Bloom, O. Circulating T cell subsets are altered in individuals with chronic spinal cord injury. *Immunol. Res.* **2015**, *63*, 3–10. [CrossRef] [PubMed]
72. Basso, D.M. Neuroanatomical substrates of functional recovery after experimental spinal cord injury: Implications of basic science research for human spinal cord injury. *Phys. Ther.* **2000**, *80*, 808–817. [CrossRef] [PubMed]
73. Rejc, E.; Smith, A.C.; Weber, K.A.; Ugiliweneza, B.; Bert, R.J.; Negahdar, M.; Boakye, M.; Harkema, S.J.; Angeli, C.A. Spinal cord imaging markers and recovery of volitional leg movement with spinal cord epidural stimulation in individuals with clinically motor complete spinal cord injury. *Front. Syst. Neurosci.* **2020**, *14*, 559313. [CrossRef] [PubMed]
74. Kakulas, B.A. Neuropathology: The foundation for new treatments in spinal cord injury. *Spinal Cord* **2004**, *42*, 549–563. [CrossRef] [PubMed]
75. Ibanez, J.; Angeli, C.A.; Harkema, S.J.; Farina, D.; Rejc, E. Recruitment order of motor neurons promoted by epidural stimulation in individuals with spinal cord injury. *J. Appl. Physiol.* **2021**, *131*, 1100. [CrossRef]
76. Angeli, C.A.; Boakye, M.; Morton, R.A.; Vogt, J.; Benton, K.; Chen, Y.; Ferreira, C.K.; Harkema, S.J. Recovery of over-ground walking after chronic motor complete spinal cord injury. *N. Engl. J. Med.* **2018**, *379*, 1244–1250. [CrossRef]
77. Hong, J.; Chang, A.; Liu, Y.; Wang, J.; Fehlings, M.G. Incomplete spinal cord injury reverses the level-dependence of spinal cord injury immune deficiency syndrome. *Int. J. Mol. Sci.* **2019**, *20*, 3762. [CrossRef]
78. Kigerl, K.A.; Hall, J.C.; Wang, L.; Mo, X.; Yu, Z.; Popovich, P.G. Gut dysbiosis impairs recovery after spinal cord injury. *J. Exp. Med.* **2016**, *213*, 2603–2620. [CrossRef]
79. Mironets, E.; Fischer, R.; Bracchi-Ricard, V.; Saltos, T.M.; Truglio, T.S.; O'Reilly, M.L.; Swanson, K.A.; Bethea, J.R.; Tom, V.J. Attenuating neurogenic sympathetic hyperreflexia robustly improves antibacterial immunity after chronic spinal cord injury. *J. Neurosci.* **2020**, *40*, 478–492. [CrossRef]
80. Mironets, E.; Osei-Owusu, P.; Bracchi-Ricard, V.; Fischer, R.; Owens, E.A.; Ricard, J.; Wu, D.; Saltos, T.; Collyer, E.; Hou, S.; et al. Soluble TNFalpha signaling within the spinal cord contributes to the development of autonomic dysreflexia and ensuing vascular and immune dysfunction after spinal cord injury. *J. Neurosci.* **2018**, *38*, 4146–4162. [CrossRef]
81. Elefteriou, F.; Campbell, P.; Ma, Y. Control of bone remodeling by the peripheral sympathetic nervous system. *Calcif. Tissue Int.* **2014**, *94*, 140–151. [CrossRef] [PubMed]
82. Maryanovich, M.; Takeishi, S.; Frenette, P.S. Neural regulation of bone and bone marrow. *Cold Spring Harb. Perspect. Med.* **2018**, *8*, a031344. [CrossRef] [PubMed]
83. Elefteriou, F.; Ahn, J.D.; Takeda, S.; Starbuck, M.; Yang, X.; Liu, X.; Kondo, H.; Richards, W.G.; Bannon, T.W.; Noda, M.; et al. Leptin regulation of bone resorption by the sympathetic nervous system and CART. *Nature* **2005**, *434*, 514–520. [CrossRef]
84. Togari, A.; Arai, M.; Kondo, A. The role of the sympathetic nervous system in controlling bone metabolism. *Expert Opin. Ther. Targets* **2005**, *9*, 931–940. [CrossRef] [PubMed]
85. Nagao, M.; Feinstein, T.N.; Ezura, Y.; Hayata, T.; Notomi, T.; Saita, Y.; Hanyu, R.; Hemmi, H.; Izu, Y.; Takeda, S.; et al. Sympathetic control of bone mass regulated by osteopontin. *Proc. Natl. Acad. Sci. USA* **2011**, *108*, 17767–17772. [CrossRef]
86. Iversen, P.O.; Hjeltnes, N.; Holm, B.; Flatebo, T.; Strom-Gundersen, I.; Ronning, W.; Stanghelle, J.; Benestad, H.B. Depressed immunity and impaired proliferation of hematopoietic progenitor cells in patients with complete spinal cord injury. *Blood* **2000**, *96*, 2081–2083. [CrossRef]

87. Chernykh, E.R.; Shevela, E.Y.; Leplina, O.Y.; Tikhonova, M.A.; Ostanin, A.A.; Kulagin, A.D.; Pronkina, N.V.; Muradov Zh, M.; Stupak, V.V.; Kozlov, V.A. Characteristics of bone marrow cells under conditions of impaired innervation in patients with spinal trauma. *Bull. Exp. Biol. Med.* **2006**, *141*, 117–120. [CrossRef]
88. Carpenter, R.S.; Marbourg, J.M.; Brennan, F.H.; Mifflin, K.A.; Hall, J.C.E.; Jiang, R.R.; Mo, X.M.; Karunasiri, M.; Burke, M.H.; Dorrance, A.M.; et al. Spinal cord injury causes chronic bone marrow failure. *Nat. Commun.* **2020**, *11*, 3702. [CrossRef]
89. Cragg, J.J.; Noonan, V.K.; Dvorak, M.; Krassioukov, A.; Mancini, G.B.; Borisoff, J.F. Spinal cord injury and type 2 diabetes: Results from a population health survey. *Neurology* **2013**, *81*, 1864–1868. [CrossRef]
90. Gorgey, A.S.; Gater, D.R.J. Prevalence of obesity after spinal cord injury. *Top. Spinal Cord Inj. Rehabil.* **2007**, *12*, 1–7. [CrossRef]
91. Lai, Y.J.; Lin, C.L.; Chang, Y.J.; Lin, M.C.; Lee, S.T.; Sung, F.C.; Lee, W.Y.; Kao, C.H. Spinal cord injury increases the risk of type 2 diabetes: A population-based cohort study. *Spine J.* **2014**, *14*, 1957–1964. [CrossRef]
92. Farkas, G.J.; Gater, D.R. Neurogenic obesity and systemic inflammation following spinal cord injury: A review. *J. Spinal Cord Med.* **2018**, *41*, 378–387. [CrossRef] [PubMed]
93. Sun, X.; Jones, Z.B.; Chen, X.M.; Zhou, L.; So, K.F.; Ren, Y. Multiple organ dysfunction and systemic inflammation after spinal cord injury: A complex relationship. *J. Neuroinflamm.* **2016**, *13*, 260. [CrossRef]
94. Rajan, S.; McNeely, M.J.; Warms, C.; Goldstein, B. Clinical assessment and management of obesity in individuals with spinal cord injury: A review. *J. Spinal Cord Med.* **2008**, *31*, 361–372. [CrossRef] [PubMed]
95. Farkas, G.J.; Gorgey, A.S.; Dolbow, D.R.; Berg, A.S.; Gater, D.R. The influence of level of spinal cord injury on adipose tissue and its relationship to inflammatory adipokines and cardiometabolic profiles. *J. Spinal Cord Med.* **2018**, *41*, 407–415. [CrossRef]
96. Manns, P.J.; McCubbin, J.A.; Williams, D.P. Fitness, inflammation, and the metabolic syndrome in men with paraplegia. *Arch. Phys. Med. Rehabil.* **2005**, *86*, 1176–1181. [CrossRef] [PubMed]
97. Gleeson, M.; Bishop, N.C.; Stensel, D.J.; Lindley, M.R.; Mastana, S.S.; Nimmo, M.A. The anti-inflammatory effects of exercise: Mechanisms and implications for the prevention and treatment of disease. *Nat. Rev. Immunol.* **2011**, *11*, 607–615. [CrossRef] [PubMed]
98. da Silva Alves, E.; de Aquino Lemos, V.; Ruiz da Silva, F.; Lira, F.S.; Dos Santos, R.V.; Rosa, J.P.; Caperuto, E.; Tufik, S.; de Mello, M.T. Low-grade inflammation and spinal cord injury: Exercise as therapy? *Mediat. Inflamm.* **2013**, *2013*, 971841. [CrossRef] [PubMed]
99. Rosety-Rodriguez, M.; Camacho, A.; Rosety, I.; Fornieles, G.; Rosety, M.A.; Diaz, A.J.; Bernardi, M.; Rosety, M.; Ordonez, F.J. Low-grade systemic inflammation and leptin levels were improved by arm cranking exercise in adults with chronic spinal cord injury. *Arch. Phys. Med. Rehabil.* **2014**, *95*, 297–302. [CrossRef] [PubMed]
100. Griffin, L.; Decker, M.J.; Hwang, J.Y.; Wang, B.; Kitchen, K.; Ding, Z.; Ivy, J.L. Functional electrical stimulation cycling improves body composition, metabolic and neural factors in persons with spinal cord injury. *J. Electromyogr. Kinesiol.* **2009**, *19*, 614–622. [CrossRef] [PubMed]
101. Schnurr, T.M.; Jakupovic, H.; Carrasquilla, G.D.; Angquist, L.; Grarup, N.; Sorensen, T.I.A.; Tjonneland, A.; Overvad, K.; Pedersen, O.; Hansen, T.; et al. Obesity, unfavourable lifestyle and genetic risk of type 2 diabetes: A case-cohort study. *Diabetologia* **2020**, *63*, 1324–1332. [CrossRef]
102. Donath, M.Y.; Shoelson, S.E. Type 2 diabetes as an inflammatory disease. *Nat. Rev. Immunol.* **2011**, *11*, 98–107. [CrossRef]
103. Lavela, S.L.; Weaver, F.M.; Goldstein, B.; Chen, K.; Miskevics, S.; Rajan, S.; Gater, D.R.J. Diabetes mellitus in individuals with spinal cord injury or disorder. *J. Spinal Cord Med.* **2006**, *29*, 387–395. [CrossRef]
104. Berbudi, A.; Rahmadika, N.; Tjahjadi, A.I.; Ruslami, R. Type 2 Diabetes and its Impact on the immune system. *Curr. Diabetes Rev.* **2020**, *16*, 442–449. [CrossRef] [PubMed]
105. Esposito, K.; Nappo, F.; Marfella, R.; Giugliano, G.; Giugliano, F.; Ciotola, M.; Quagliaro, L.; Ceriello, A.; Giugliano, D. Inflammatory cytokine concentrations are acutely increased by hyperglycemia in humans: Role of oxidative stress. *Circulation* **2002**, *106*, 2067–2072. [CrossRef]
106. Young, D.; Hussell, T.; Dougan, G. Chronic bacterial infections: Living with unwanted guests. *Nat. Immunol.* **2002**, *3*, 1026–1032. [CrossRef]
107. Hannan, T.J.; Mysorekar, I.U.; Hung, C.S.; Isaacson-Schmid, M.L.; Hultgren, S.J. Early severe inflammatory responses to uropathogenic E. coli predispose to chronic and recurrent urinary tract infection. *PLoS Pathog.* **2010**, *6*, e1001042. [CrossRef] [PubMed]
108. Ramella-Roman, J.C.; Mathews, S.A.; Kandimalla, H.; Nabili, A.; Duncan, D.D.; D'Anna, S.A.; Shah, S.M.; Nguyen, Q.D. Measurement of oxygen saturation in the retina with a spectroscopic sensitive multi aperture camera. *Opt. Express* **2008**, *16*, 6170–6182. [CrossRef]
109. Hugenholtz, H.; Cass, D.E.; Dvorak, M.F.; Fewer, D.H.; Fox, R.J.; Izukawa, D.M.; Lexchin, J.; Tuli, S.; Bharatwal, N.; Short, C. High-dose methylprednisolone for acute closed spinal cord injury–only a treatment option. *Can. J. Neurol. Sci.* **2002**, *29*, 227–235. [CrossRef] [PubMed]
110. Cheung, V.; Hoshide, R.; Bansal, V.; Kasper, E.; Chen, C.C. Methylprednisolone in the management of spinal cord injuries: Lessons from randomized, controlled trials. *Surg. Neurol. Int.* **2015**, *6*, 142. [CrossRef] [PubMed]
111. Chikuda, H.; Yasunaga, H.; Horiguchi, H.; Takeshita, K.; Kawaguchi, H.; Matsuda, S.; Nakamura, K. Mortality and morbidity in dialysis-dependent patients undergoing spinal surgery: Analysis of a national administrative database in Japan. *J. Bone Jt. Surg. Am.* **2012**, *94*, 433–438. [CrossRef] [PubMed]

112. Liu, Z.; Yang, Y.; He, L.; Pang, M.; Luo, C.; Liu, B.; Rong, L. High-dose methylprednisolone for acute traumatic spinal cord injury: A meta-analysis. *Neurology* **2019**, *93*, e841–e850. [CrossRef]
113. Williams, D.M. Clinical pharmacology of corticosteroids. *Respir. Care* **2018**, *63*, 655–670. [CrossRef] [PubMed]
114. Buchholz, A.C.; Ginis, K.A.M.; Bray, S.R.; Craven, B.C.; Hicks, A.L.; Hayes, K.C.; Latimer, A.E.; McColl, M.A.; Potter, P.J.; Wolfe, D.L. Greater daily leisure time physical activity is associated with lower chronic disease risk in adults with spinal cord injury. *Appl. Physiol. Nutr. Metab.* **2009**, *34*, 640–647. [CrossRef] [PubMed]
115. Morton, S.C.; Shekelle, P.G.; Adams, J.L.; Bennett, C.; Dobkin, B.H.; Montgomerie, J.; Vickrey, B.G. Antimicrobial prophylaxis for urinary tract infection in persons with spinal cord dysfunction. *Arch. Phys. Med. Rehabil.* **2002**, *83*, 129–138. [CrossRef]
116. Gribble, M.J.; Puterman, M.L. Prophylaxis of urinary tract infection in persons with recent spinal cord injury: A prospective, randomized, double-blind, placebo-controlled study of trimethoprim-sulfamethoxazole. *Am. J. Med.* **1993**, *95*, 141–152. [CrossRef]
117. Biering-Sorensen, F.; Hoiby, N.; Nordenbo, A.; Ravnborg, M.; Bruun, B.; Rahm, V. Ciprofloxacin as prophylaxis for urinary tract infection: Prospective, randomized, cross-over, placebo controlled study in patients with spinal cord lesion. *J. Urol.* **1994**, *151*, 105–108. [CrossRef]
118. Fisher, H.; Oluboyede, Y.; Chadwick, T.; Abdel-Fattah, M.; Brennand, C.; Fader, M.; Harrison, S.; Hilton, P.; Larcombe, J.; Little, P.; et al. Continuous low-dose antibiotic prophylaxis for adults with repeated urinary tract infections (AnTIC): A randomised, open-label trial. *Lancet Infect. Dis.* **2018**, *18*, 957–968. [CrossRef]
119. Maynard, F.M.; Diokno, A.C. Urinary infection and complications during clean intermittent catheterization following spinal cord injury. *J. Urol.* **1984**, *132*, 943–946. [CrossRef]
120. Ploypetch, T.; Dajpratham, P.; Assanasen, S.; Thanakiatpinyo, T.; Tanvijit, P.; Karawek, J. Epidemiology of urinary tract infection among spinal cord injured patients in rehabilitation ward at Siriraj Hospital. *J. Med. Assoc. Thai.* **2013**, *96*, 99–106.
121. Salomon, J.; Denys, P.; Merle, C.; Chartier-Kastler, E.; Perronne, C.; Gaillard, J.L.; Bernard, L. Prevention of urinary tract infection in spinal cord-injured patients: Safety and efficacy of a weekly oral cyclic antibiotic (WOCA) programme with a 2 year follow-up–an observational prospective study. *J. Antimicrob. Chemother.* **2006**, *57*, 784–788. [CrossRef] [PubMed]
122. Salomon, J.; Schnitzler, A.; Ville, Y.; Laffont, I.; Perronne, C.; Denys, P.; Bernard, L. Prevention of urinary tract infection in six spinal cord-injured pregnant women who gave birth to seven children under a weekly oral cyclic antibiotic program. *Int. J. Infect. Dis.* **2009**, *13*, 399–402. [CrossRef] [PubMed]
123. Shaffer, W.O.; Baisden, J.L.; Fernand, R.; Matz, P.G. An evidence-based clinical guideline for antibiotic prophylaxis in spine surgery. *Spine J.* **2013**, *13*, 1387–1392. [CrossRef] [PubMed]
124. Abola, M.V.; Lin, C.C.; Lin, L.J.; Schreiber-Stainthorp, W.; Frempong-Boadu, A.; Buckland, A.J.; Protopsaltis, T.S. Postoperative prophylactic antibiotics in spine surgery: A propensity-matched analysis. *J. Bone Jt. Surg. Am.* **2021**, *103*, 219–226. [CrossRef] [PubMed]
125. Maciejczak, A.; Wolan-Nieroda, A.; Walaszek, M.; Kolpa, M.; Wolak, Z. Antibiotic prophylaxis in spine surgery: A comparison of single-dose and 72-hour protocols. *J. Hosp. Infect.* **2019**, *103*, 303–310. [CrossRef] [PubMed]
126. Krassioukov, A.; Warburton, D.E.; Teasell, R.; Eng, J.J. A systematic review of the management of autonomic dysreflexia after spinal cord injury. *Arch. Phys. Med. Rehabil.* **2009**, *90*, 682–695. [CrossRef] [PubMed]
127. Sharif, H.; Hou, S. Autonomic dysreflexia: A cardiovascular disorder following spinal cord injury. *Neural. Regen. Res.* **2017**, *12*, 1390–1400. [CrossRef] [PubMed]
128. Kim, J. How do I respond to autonomic dysreflexia? *Nursing* **2003**, *33*, 18. [CrossRef] [PubMed]
129. Harkema, S.J.; Wang, S.; Angeli, C.A.; Chen, Y.; Boakye, M.; Ugiliweneza, B.; Hirsch, G.A. Normalization of blood pressure with spinal cord epidural stimulation after severe spinal cord injury. *Front. Hum. Neurosci.* **2018**, *12*, 83. [CrossRef] [PubMed]
130. Harman, K.A.; DeVeau, K.M.; Squair, J.W.; West, C.R.; Krassioukov, A.V.; Magnuson, D.S.K. Effects of early exercise training on the severity of autonomic dysreflexia following incomplete spinal cord injury in rodents. *Physiol. Rep.* **2021**, *9*, e14969. [CrossRef]
131. West, C.R.; Crawford, M.A.; Laher, I.; Ramer, M.S.; Krassioukov, A.V. Passive hind-limb cycling reduces the severity of autonomic dysreflexia after experimental spinal cord injury. *Neurorehabil. Neural Repair* **2016**, *30*, 317–327. [CrossRef] [PubMed]
132. Giannantoni, A.; Di Stasi, S.M.; Stephen, R.L.; Navarra, P.; Scivoletto, G.; Mearini, E.; Porena, M. Intravesical capsaicin versus resiniferatoxin in patients with detrusor hyperreflexia: A prospective randomized study. *J. Urol.* **2002**, *167*, 1710–1714. [CrossRef]
133. Igawa, Y.; Satoh, T.; Mizusawa, H.; Seki, S.; Kato, H.; Ishizuka, O.; Nishizawa, O. The role of capsaicin-sensitive afferents in autonomic dysreflexia in patients with spinal cord injury. *BJU Int.* **2003**, *91*, 637–641. [CrossRef]
134. Rabchevsky, A.G.; Patel, S.P.; Duale, H.; Lyttle, T.S.; O'Dell, C.R.; Kitzman, P.H. Gabapentin for spasticity and autonomic dysreflexia after severe spinal cord injury. *Spinal Cord* **2011**, *49*, 99–105. [CrossRef]
135. Rabchevsky, A.G.; Patel, S.P.; Lyttle, T.S.; Eldahan, K.C.; O'Dell, C.R.; Zhang, Y.; Popovich, P.G.; Kitzman, P.H.; Donohue, K.D. Effects of gabapentin on muscle spasticity and both induced as well as spontaneous autonomic dysreflexia after complete spinal cord injury. *Front. Physiol.* **2012**, *3*, 329. [CrossRef] [PubMed]
136. Eldahan, K.C.; Williams, H.C.; Cox, D.H.; Gollihue, J.L.; Patel, S.P.; Rabchevsky, A.G. Paradoxical effects of continuous high dose gabapentin treatment on autonomic dysreflexia after complete spinal cord injury. *Exp. Neurol.* **2020**, *323*, 113083. [CrossRef]
137. Brennan, F.H.; Noble, B.T.; Wang, Y.; Guan, Z.; Davis, H.; Mo, X.; Harris, C.; Eroglu, C.; Ferguson, A.R.; Popovich, P.G. Acute post-injury blockade of alpha2delta-1 calcium channel subunits prevents pathological autonomic plasticity after spinal cord injury. *Cell Rep.* **2021**, *34*, 108667. [CrossRef]

138. Zhang, L.; Berta, T.; Xu, Z.Z.; Liu, T.; Park, J.Y.; Ji, R.R. TNF-alpha contributes to spinal cord synaptic plasticity and inflammatory pain: Distinct role of TNF receptor subtypes 1 and 2. *Pain* **2011**, *152*, 419–427. [CrossRef]
139. Taoufik, E.; Tseveleki, V.; Chu, S.Y.; Tselios, T.; Karin, M.; Lassmann, H.; Szymkowski, D.E.; Probert, L. Transmembrane tumour necrosis factor is neuroprotective and regulates experimental autoimmune encephalomyelitis via neuronal nuclear factor-kappaB. *Brain* **2011**, *134*, 2722–2735. [CrossRef] [PubMed]
140. Brambilla, R.; Ashbaugh, J.J.; Magliozzi, R.; Dellarole, A.; Karmally, S.; Szymkowski, D.E.; Bethea, J.R. Inhibition of soluble tumour necrosis factor is therapeutic in experimental autoimmune encephalomyelitis and promotes axon preservation and remyelination. *Brain* **2011**, *134*, 2736–2754. [CrossRef]
141. Novrup, H.G.; Bracchi-Ricard, V.; Ellman, D.G.; Ricard, J.; Jain, A.; Runko, E.; Lyck, L.; Yli-Karjanmaa, M.; Szymkowski, D.E.; Pearse, D.D.; et al. Central but not systemic administration of XPro1595 is therapeutic following moderate spinal cord injury in mice. *J. Neuroinflamm.* **2014**, *11*, 159. [CrossRef] [PubMed]
142. O'Reilly, M.L.; Mironets, E.; Shapiro, T.M.; Crowther, K.; Collyer, E.; Bethea, J.R.; Tom, V.J. Pharmacological inhibition of soluble tumor necrosis factor-alpha two weeks after high thoracic spinal cord injury does not affect sympathetic hyperreflexia. *J. Neurotrauma* **2021**, *38*, 2186–2191. [CrossRef]
143. Vighi, G.; Marcucci, F.; Sensi, L.; Di Cara, G.; Frati, F. Allergy and the gastrointestinal system. *Clin. Exp. Immunol.* **2008**, *153* (Suppl. 1), 3–6. [CrossRef] [PubMed]
144. Kirby, T.O.; Ochoa-Reparaz, J. The gut microbiome in multiple sclerosis: A potential therapeutic avenue. *Med. Sci.* **2018**, *6*, 69. [CrossRef] [PubMed]
145. Ochoa-Reparaz, J.; Kirby, T.O.; Kasper, L.H. The gut microbiome and multiple sclerosis. *Cold Spring Harb. Perspect. Med.* **2018**, *8*, a029017. [CrossRef]
146. Oh, D.; Cheon, K.A. Alteration of gut microbiota in autism spectrum disorder: An overview. *J. Korean Acad. Child Adolesc. Psychiatry* **2020**, *31*, 131–145. [CrossRef]
147. Limbana, T.; Khan, F.; Eskander, N. Gut microbiome and depression: How microbes affect the way we think. *Cureus* **2020**, *12*, e9966. [CrossRef]
148. Gungor, B.; Adiguzel, E.; Gursel, I.; Yilmaz, B.; Gursel, M. Intestinal Microbiota in patients with spinal cord injury. *PLoS ONE* **2016**, *11*, e0145878. [CrossRef]
149. Zhang, C.; Zhang, W.; Zhang, J.; Jing, Y.; Yang, M.; Du, L.; Gao, F.; Gong, H.; Chen, L.; Li, J.; et al. Gut microbiota dysbiosis in male patients with chronic traumatic complete spinal cord injury. *J. Transl. Med.* **2018**, *16*, 353. [CrossRef]
150. Wallace, D.J.; Sayre, N.L.; Patterson, T.T.; Nicholson, S.E.; Hilton, D.; Grandhi, R. Spinal cord injury and the human microbiome: Beyond the brain-gut axis. *Neurosurg. Focus* **2019**, *46*, E11. [CrossRef]
151. Jing, Y.; Yang, D.; Bai, F.; Zhang, C.; Qin, C.; Li, D.; Wang, L.; Yang, M.; Chen, Z.; Li, J. Melatonin treatment alleviates spinal cord injury-induced gut dysbiosis in mice. *J. Neurotrauma* **2019**, *36*, 2646–2664. [CrossRef] [PubMed]
152. Jogia, T.; Ruitenberg, M.J. Traumatic spinal cord injury and the gut microbiota: Current insights and future challenges. *Front. Immunol.* **2020**, *11*, 704. [CrossRef] [PubMed]
153. Lin, R.; Xu, J.; Ma, Q.; Chen, M.; Wang, L.; Wen, S.; Yang, C.; Ma, C.; Wang, Y.; Luo, Q.; et al. Alterations in the fecal microbiota of patients with spinal cord injury. *PLoS ONE* **2020**, *15*, e0236470. [CrossRef]
154. Schmidt, E.K.A.; Torres-Espin, A.; Raposo, P.J.F.; Madsen, K.L.; Kigerl, K.A.; Popovich, P.G.; Fenrich, K.K.; Fouad, K. Fecal transplant prevents gut dysbiosis and anxiety-like behaviour after spinal cord injury in rats. *PLoS ONE* **2020**, *15*, e0226128. [CrossRef] [PubMed]
155. Bazzocchi, G.; Turroni, S.; Bulzamini, M.C.; D'Amico, F.; Bava, A.; Castiglioni, M.; Cagnetta, V.; Losavio, E.; Cazzaniga, M.; Terenghi, L.; et al. Changes in gut microbiota in the acute phase after spinal cord injury correlate with severity of the lesion. *Sci. Rep.* **2021**, *11*, 12743. [CrossRef]
156. Jing, Y.; Yu, Y.; Bai, F.; Wang, L.; Yang, D.; Zhang, C.; Qin, C.; Yang, M.; Zhang, D.; Zhu, Y.; et al. Effect of fecal microbiota transplantation on neurological restoration in a spinal cord injury mouse model: Involvement of brain-gut axis. *Microbiome* **2021**, *9*, 59. [CrossRef] [PubMed]
157. Myers, S.A.; Gobejishvili, L.; Ohri, S.S.; Wilson, C.G.; Andres, K.R.; Riegler, A.S.; Donde, H.; Joshi-Barve, S.; Barve, S.; Whittemore, S.R. Following spinal cord injury, PDE4B drives an acute, local inflammatory response and a chronic, systemic response exacerbated by gut dysbiosis and endotoxemia. *Neurobiol. Dis.* **2019**, *124*, 353–363. [CrossRef] [PubMed]

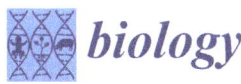

Article

The Inflammatory Response after Moderate Contusion Spinal Cord Injury: A Time Study

Minna Christiansen Lund [1,†], Ditte Gry Ellman [1,†], Maiken Nissen [1], Pernille Sveistrup Nielsen [1], Pernille Vinther Nielsen [1], Carina Jørgensen [1], Ditte Caroline Andersen [2,3,4], Han Gao [5,6], Roberta Brambilla [1,7,8], Matilda Degn [9], Bettina Hjelm Clausen [1,8] and Kate Lykke Lambertsen [1,8,10,*]

1. Department of Neurobiology Research, Institute of Molecular Medicine, University of Southern Denmark, 5000 Odense C, Denmark; minnacl@hotmail.com (M.C.L.); dellman@health.sdu.dk (D.G.E.); maiken92@live.dk (M.N.); pernillesveistrup@hotmail.com (P.S.N.); pvnielsen@health.sdu.dk (P.V.N.); carinajoergensen@hotmail.com (C.J.); rbrambilla@med.miami.edu (R.B.); bclausen@health.sdu.dk (B.H.C.)
2. Department of Clinical Research, University of Southern Denmark, 5000 Odense C, Denmark; dandersen@health.sdu.dk
3. Andersen Group, Department of Clinical Biochemistry, Odense University Hospital, 5000 Odense C, Denmark
4. Danish Center for Regenerative Medicine, Odense University Hospital, 5000 Odense C, Denmark
5. Department of Spine Surgery, Third Affiliated Hospital of Sun Yat-sen University, Guangzhou 510630, China; gaoh35@mail.sysu.edu.cn
6. Guangdong Provincial Center for Engineering and Technology Research of Minimally Invasive Spine Surgery, Guangzhou 510630, China
7. The Miami Project to Cure Paralysis, Miller School of Medicine, University of Miami, Miami, FL 33136, USA
8. Brain Research Inter-Disciplinary Guided Excellence (BRIDGE), Department of Clinical Research, University of Southern Denmark, 5000 Odense C, Denmark
9. Department of Pediatrics and Adolescent Medicine, Rigshospitalet, 2100 Copenhagen, Denmark; matildadegn@gmail.com
10. Department of Neurology, Odense University Hospital, 5000 Odense C, Denmark
* Correspondence: klambertsen@health.sdu.dk; Tel.: +45-65503806
† These authors contributed equally to this work.

Simple Summary: The neuroinflammatory response is a rather complex event in spinal cord injury (SCI) and has the capacity to exacerbate cell damage but also to contribute to the repair of the injury. This complexity is thought to depend on a variety of inflammatory mediators, of which tumor necrosis factor (TNF) plays a key role. Evidence indicates that TNF can be both protective and detrimental in SCI. In the present study, we studied the temporal and cellular expression of TNF and its receptors after SCI in mice. We found TNF to be significantly increased in both the acute and the delayed phases after SCI, alongside a robust neuroinflammatory response. As we could verify some of our results in human postmortem tissue, our results imply that diminishing the detrimental immune signaling after SCI could also enhance recovery in humans.

Abstract: Spinal cord injury (SCI) initiates detrimental cellular and molecular events that lead to acute and delayed neuroinflammation. Understanding the role of the inflammatory response in SCI requires insight into the temporal and cellular synthesis of inflammatory mediators. We subjected C57BL/6J mice to SCI and investigated inflammatory reactions. We examined activation, recruitment, and polarization of microglia and infiltrating immune cells, focusing specifically on tumor necrosis factor (TNF) and its receptors TNFR1 and TNFR2. In the acute phase, TNF expression increased in glial cells and neuron-like cells, followed by infiltrating immune cells. TNFR1 and TNFR2 levels increased in the delayed phase and were found preferentially on neurons and glial cells, respectively. The acute phase was dominated by the infiltration of granulocytes and macrophages. Microglial/macrophage expression of *Arg1* increased from 1–7 days after SCI, followed by an increase in *Itgam*, *Cx3cr1*, and *P2ry12*, which remained elevated throughout the study. By 21 and 28 days after SCI, the lesion core was populated by galectin-3+, CD68+, and CD11b+ microglia/macrophages, surrounded by a glial scar consisting of GFAP+ astrocytes. Findings were verified in postmortem tissue from individuals with SCI. Our findings support the consensus that future neuroprotective

---

Citation: Lund, M.C.; Ellman, D.G.; Nissen, M.; Nielsen, P.S.; Nielsen, P.V.; Jørgensen, C.; Andersen, D.C.; Gao, H.; Brambilla, R.; Degn, M.; et al. The Inflammatory Response after Moderate Contusion Spinal Cord Injury: A Time Study. *Biology* 2022, *11*, 939. https://doi.org/10.3390/biology11060939

Academic Editor: Huaxin Sheng

Received: 21 February 2022
Accepted: 17 June 2022
Published: 20 June 2022

Publisher's Note: MDPI stays neutral with regard to jurisdictional claims in published maps and institutional affiliations.

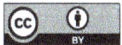

Copyright: © 2022 by the authors. Licensee MDPI, Basel, Switzerland. This article is an open access article distributed under the terms and conditions of the Creative Commons Attribution (CC BY) license (https://creativecommons.org/licenses/by/4.0/).

immunotherapies should aim to selectively neutralize detrimental immune signaling while sustaining pro-regenerative processes.

Keywords: neuroinflammation; cytokines; tumor necrosis factor; immune cells; microglia

---

1. Introduction

Spinal cord injury (SCI) is a serious neurological condition with an unknown prevalence and estimated annual incidence of between 40 and 80 cases per million of population, according to the World Health Organization. SCI often leads to irreversible motor and sensory dysfunction below the level of injury. The mechanical impact to the spinal cord initiates a primary injury, which is followed by secondary degenerative processes. The secondary degeneration occurs due to detrimental cellular and molecular events, which include glutamate excitotoxicity, edema formation, and exacerbated neuroinflammation [1]. Neuroinflammatory processes are rapidly initiated after SCI and contribute to both injury and reparative processes [2]. Although the neuroinflammatory response is most pronounced in the early phases after SCI, it continues throughout the life of the affected individual [3]. Within minutes after injury, inflammatory mediators, such as cytokines, are released by resident cells located in the injured spinal cord and take part in the recruitment, activation, and polarization of immune cells [4].

One important inflammatory cytokine is the tumor necrosis factor (TNF), which plays a role in the initiation, maintenance, and resolution of inflammation [5]. It exists in two forms: a transmembrane-bound form (tmTNF) and a soluble form (solTNF). Both types of TNF signal through one of two receptors, TNFR1 and TNFR2, however, with different binding affinities, and the robust activation of TNFR2 requires binding of tmTNF [5,6]. Furthermore, the downstream signaling pathways of the two receptors differ, and the activation of TNFR1, especially, is associated with the increased expression of pro-inflammatory cytokines and activation of programmed cell death [7], whereas TNFR2 is involved in cell survival, proliferation, and remyelination [8,9].

Several studies have examined the cellular and temporal expression of TNF and its receptors in the acute phase after SCI [10–17]. However, only a few studies focused on clarifying TNF expression in the delayed phase after SCI [11,13,18]. Besides the initial acute increase in TNF levels, these studies suggest a second increase in *Tnf* gene expression in the delayed phase after SCI. Examining TNFR1 and TNFR2 expression in the delayed phase after SCI is, to our knowledge, yet to be elucidated. As elevated TNF levels induce the expression of numerous other inflammatory cytokines [19], studies have tried to clarify the role of TNF after SCI [20–23]. Studies using conventional and cell-specific conditional TNF or TNFR-knockout mice [20,24–27], and studies using anti-TNF therapy, [21,28,29] demonstrate that TNF exhibits both neuroprotective and neurodegenerative effects after SCI. In addition, we and others have shown that interfering with solTNF-TNFR1 signaling is beneficial after SCI [22,28].

Diminishing detrimental neuroinflammatory processes, such as the excessive production of pro-inflammatory cytokines, is considered a possible therapeutic strategy in individuals with SCI; therefore, more detailed knowledge on the temporal and cellular synthesis of inflammatory mediators is required. TNF is believed to be one of the most promising neuroinflammatory targets in SCI [17]; therefore, this study investigated the temporal and cellular source of TNF and its two receptors in the acute and delayed phases after SCI using a moderate contusive SCI model in C57BL/6J mice. The findings were verified in postmortem tissue and cerebrospinal fluid (CSF), derived from individuals with SCI. In addition, we evaluated the expression profile of selected glial-derived cytokines (IL-1 β, IL-6, IL-10, and CXCL1) and examined the polarization of microglia/macrophages by investigating temporal changes in microglial/macrophage specific genes (*Itgam*, *Cx3cr1*,

Trem2, Arg1, P2ry12). Finally, we examined the activation, recruitment, and polarization of immune cells in the lesioned spinal cord.

2. Materials and Methods

2.1. CSF Collection

Human CSF samples were collected and stored at the Third Affiliated Hospital of Sun Yat-sen University in China. All individuals received a diagnosis of SCI based on clinical symptoms (ISNCSCI and ASIA score), electrophysiology, X-ray, and MRI analysis. Cases were divided into subacute (2 weeks–2 months after injury), early chronic (2–12 months after injury), and late chronic stages (>24 months after injury) (Table 1). SCI cases with complete or incomplete traumatic injury at cervical and thoracic levels were included in this study. One case had a lumbar SCI. Individuals with other neurological disorders or diabetes were excluded. CSF from healthy individuals was used as the control (Table 1), and samples were collected after overnight fasting and frozen at −80 °C. The study protocols ([2018]-02, [2018]-03, [2018]-04) were in accordance with guidelines for clinical studies approved by the Third Affiliated Hospital of Sun Yat-sen University review board.

Table 1. Gender and age distribution of SCI cases included for CSF analysis.

	Controls	Sub-Acute	Early Chronic	Late Chronic
Number of cases	5	12	10	11
Sex, n (%) men	4 (80)	11 (92)	10 (100)	11 (100)
Age, years, median (IQR)	31 (23.0; 44.5)	30.5 (28.3; 47.0)	30.0 (26.8; 36.3)	45.0 (39.0; 54.0)

2.2. Animals

Female C57BL/6J mice were purchased from Taconic A/S (Ry, Denmark) and transferred to the Biomedical Laboratory, University of Southern Denmark, where they were allowed to acclimatize for at least one week before surgery. TNF knockout ($Tnf^{-/-}$ [30]) mice were obtained by crossing heterozygous $Tnf^{+/-}$ mice, and the genotype was established using the following primers from DNA Technology A/S (Copenhagen, Denmark): *Tnf* common (5′-CCAGGAGGGAGAACAGA), *Tnf* mutant (5′-CGTTGGCTACCCGTGATATT), *Tnf* wt (5′-AGTGCCTCTTCTGCCAGTTC), *Lta*N forward (5′-GTCCAGCTCTTTTCCTCCCAAT), and *Lta*N reverse (5′-GTCCTTGAAGTCCCGGATACAC) as previously described [30,31]. All mice were group-housed with food and water ad libitum, with a 12 h light/dark cycle, and controlled temperature and humidity. Mice were cared for in accordance with the protocols and guidelines approved by the Danish Veterinary and Food Administration (J. numbers 2013–15–2934–00924 and 2019-15-0201-01615); experiments are reported in accordance with the ARRIVE guidelines, and all efforts were made to minimize pain and distress.

2.3. Induction of Spinal Cord Injury (SCI)

Mice were anesthetized with an intraperitoneal (i.p.) injection of a cocktail of ketamine (100 mg/kg, VEDCO, Saint Joseph, MO, USA) and xylazine (10 mg/kg, VEDCO). The ninth thoracic vertebra (T9) was identified based on anatomical landmarks [32], and the mice were laminectomized at T8–T10. Mice received a T9 contusion injury (75 Kdyn) using the Infinite Horizon Device (Precision Systems and Instrumentation, Brimstone, LN, USA) as previously described [28]. Sham mice were laminectomized only. After surgery, mice received a subcutaneous (s.c.) injection of isotonic saline to prevent dehydration, and for post-surgical analgesia, mice were treated with four s.c. injections of buprenorphine hydrochloride (0.001 mg/20 g body weight Temgesic, cat. no. 521634, Indivior Europe, North Chesterfield, VA, USA) at eight-hour intervals starting immediately after surgery. To prevent dehydration and infection, mice were supplemented with daily s.c. injections of isotonic saline and antibiotic gentamicin (40 mg/kg, Hexamycin, Sandoz, Copenhagen, Denmark) for the first 7 days after SCI. Mice were housed in individual cages in a recovery room at 25 °C with a 12 h light/dark cycle, until their wounds healed. Mice surviving more than 24 h after surgery were weighed at 1, 3, and 7 days after SCI and thereafter weekly.

Bladders were emptied manually twice a day for the duration of the experiments. C57BL/6J mice were allowed to survive 1, 3, 6, 12, or 24 h (acute phase, n(SCI) = 18–23/group and n(sham) = 5/group) or 3, 7, 14, 21, or 28 days (delayed phase, n(SCI) = 15/group and n(sham) = 5/group) after surgery, and naïve mice were used as the controls (n = 20). $Tnf^{-/-}$ mice were allowed to survive 1, 3, 6, 12, or 24 h after SCI (n = 2/group). In total, one C57BL/6J mouse died during surgery.

2.4. Basso Mouse Scale (BMS)

Functional recovery after SCI was determined by scoring of the hind limb locomotor performance in the open field arena using the BMS scoring system and the BMS subscore system, with the latter used to quantify finer aspects of locomotion [33]. Under observer-blinded conditions, mice were evaluated over a 4 min period 1, 3, and 7 days after SCI and weekly thereafter for up to 28 days. Before surgery, mice were handled and pre-trained in the open field to assure normal locomotion and to prevent fear and/or stress behaviors that could bias the locomotor assessment. Routinely, mice with a BMS score above 1 on the day after surgery are excluded; in the present study, however, no mice scored above 1.

2.5. Human SCI Tissue

Paraffin-embedded postmortem human spinal cord samples (Table 2) were obtained from the Miami Project Human Core Bank at the University of Miami Miller School of Medicine managed by Alexander Marcillo, M.D. and Yan Shi, M.S.

Table 2. Gender and age distribution of SCI cases included for immunofluorescent analysis.

Case	Age/Sex	Level of Injury	Cause of Injury	Post-SCI Survival Time
#1	80/F	C6–T1	Fall	15 h
#2	61/M	C1–2	Dive accident	2 weeks
#3	43/M	C7	Fall	16 days
#4	33/M	C6–7	MVA	3 weeks
#5	65/M	C4	MVA	5 weeks
#6	67/M	C5–7	Fall	6 weeks

Abbreviations: C—cervical; F—female; M—male; MVA—motor vehicle accident; T—thoracic.

2.6. Tissue Processing

Mice were deeply anesthetized with an overdose of pentobarbital (200 mg/mL) containing lidocaine (20 mg/mL) (Glostrup Apotek, Glostrup, Denmark) and transcardially perfused through the left ventricle. For reverse transcription quantitative polymerase chain reaction (RT-qPCR), in situ hybridization, protein analysis, and flow cytometry, mice were perfused with ice-cold diethyl pyrocarbonate-treated (DEPC, Sigma-Aldrich, cat. no. D5758, Soeborg, Denmark) phosphate-buffered saline (PBS, pH 7.4, Sigma-Aldrich, cat. no. P4417, Soeborg, Denmark). For immunohistochemistry and immunofluorescence staining, mice were perfused with ice-cold 4% paraformaldehyde (PFA, Sigma-Aldrich, cat. no. 158127, Soeborg, Denmark) diluted in PBS.

For RT-qPCR and protein analysis, 1 cm of spinal cord centered on the lesion area (SCI samples), or spinal cord tissue taken from the equivalent region (sham and naïve samples), was quickly removed, snap-frozen on dry ice, and stored at −80 °C until further processing.

Spinal cord segments (1 cm centered on the lesion), to be used for in situ hybridization, immunohistochemistry, and immunofluorescence staining, were quickly removed. For in situ hybridization, segments were immediately embedded in Tissue-Tek OCT compound (Leica, cat. no. 14020218926, Broendby, Denmark) and snap-frozen in gaseous CO_2. Spinal cord segments used for immunohistochemistry and immunofluorescence staining were stored in PFA for 45 min, hereafter in 20% sucrose (Sigma-Aldrich, cat. no. S7903, Soeborg, Denmark) in 0.15 M Sorensen's phosphate buffer overnight (o.n), and the next day embedded and snap-frozen in Tissue-Tek compound. Spinal cords were then cut into 20 μm thick parallel tissue sections using a cryostat, collected on SuperFrost Plus slides (Thermo Fisher

Scientific, cat. no. 10149870, Roskilde, Denmark), and stored at −20 °C (immunostaining) or −80 °C (in situ hybridization) until further processing.

For flow cytometry, spinal cord tissue containing the lesion area (1 cm centered on the lesion) and peri-lesion area (tissue 0.5 cm distal and 0.5 cm proximal to the lesion was pooled to represent peri-lesion tissue), or spinal cord tissue taken from the equivalent regions (naïve samples), was quickly removed and placed in cold RPMI (Gibco, cat. no. 21875-042, Roskilde, Denmark) containing 10% fetal bovine serum (FBS, VWR, cat. no. S1810, Soeborg, Denmark). Samples were homogenized through a 70 µm filter (AH Diagnostics, cat. no. 352350, Aarhus, Denmark) and further processed for flow cytometry.

2.7. Gene Analysis

RNA extraction: Total RNA was extracted from mice that survived 1, 3, 6, 12, and 24 h, 3, 7, 14, and 28 days after SCI, as well as from naïve controls (n = 5/group) using TRIzol Reagent (Invitrogen, cat. no. 15596018, Roskilde, Denmark) according to the manufacturer's protocol. Briefly, samples were homogenized with the appropriate amount of TRIzol Reagent, and chloroform extraction (Sigma-Aldrich cat. no. C2432, Soeborg, Denmark) was performed followed by isopropanol precipitation (Sigma-Aldrich, cat. no. I9030, Soeborg, Denmark). The RNA was washed with 75% ethanol (absolute ethanol in nuclease-free water, VWR, cat. no. 20821.365), and purified RNA was dissolved in nuclease-free water (Thermo Scientific, cat. no. R0582). Concentrations and purity were checked using a Thermo Scientific NanoDrop One spectrophotometer.

cDNA synthesis: Two µg RNA was reverse-transcribed with the High-Capacity cDNA Reverse Transcription kit from Applied Biosystems (Thermo Fisher, cat. no. 4368814, Roskilde, Denmark). A 2× reverse transcription (RT) Master mix was made, consisting of a 10X RT Buffer, 25X dNTP mix (100 mM), 10 RT Random Primers, MultiScribe Reverse Transcriptase, nuclease-free water, and equal amounts of RNA sample; the 2× RT Master mix was synthesized using an MJ Research PTC-225 Gradient Thermal Cycler from Marshall Scientific. Reverse transcription cycle conditions were as follows: 25 °C for 10 min, 37 °C for 120 min, 85 °C for 5 min, and then cooled to 4 °C. Samples were diluted to 50 ng/µL and stored at −20 °C until further processing.

RT-qPCR: Investigation of *Tnf*, *Tnfrsf1a*, *Tnfrsf1b*, *Il1b*, *Il6*, *Il10*, *Cxcl1*, Integrin subunit alpha M (*Itgam*), C-x3-c motif chemokine receptor 1 (*Cx3cr1*), triggering receptor expressed on myeloid cells 2 (*Trem2*), purinergic receptor P2Y (*P2ry12*), arginase 1 (*Arg1*), and hypoxanthine-guanin phosphoribosyltransferase 1 (*Hprt1*) mRNA expression was performed with Maxima SYBR Green (ThermoFisher Scientific, cat. no. K0223, Roskilde, Denmark) detection and carried out using a CFX Connect Real-Time PCR Detection System from Bio-Rad. Primers were designed with NCBI's nucleotide database and primer designing tool, aimed to target exon–exon junctions whenever possible, checked for self-complementarity with an Oligo calculator [34], and purchased from TAG Copenhagen (Copenhagen, Denmark). Primer sequences are listed in Table 3. The RT-qPCR reaction was performed in a 12.5 µL volume, containing 1× Maxima SYBR Green, 50 ng of template cDNA, and 600 nM forward and reverse primers. Thermal cycling conditions were as follows: 95 °C for 10 min to separate the cDNA, followed by further denaturation for 15 s, whereafter the temperature was lowered to the optimal annealing temperature for each gene (see Supplementary Table S1) for 30 s and then raised again to 72 °C for 30 s. This was caried out for 40 cycles, except for *Il10* (45 cycles, Supplementary Table S1). Finally, the samples were heated to generate a melting curve (Supplementary Table S1). A 4-fold standard curve and a calibrator were prepared from a mixture of aliquots from all experimental samples and used on every assay. "No template" and "no reverse transcriptase" controls were included as negative controls. All samples and standards were tested in triplicate, the calibrator was applied to six wells, and samples from different time points were randomly distributed across the assays. Amplification of a single desired product was confirmed by the presence of only one melting curve. Relative transcript levels were calculated using the *Pfaffl* method [35], primer efficiencies were accepted within the range of 100 ± 5% (Supplementary Table S1), and data were normalized to the reference gene *Hprt1*.

Table 3. Primers used for RT-qPCR analysis.

Gene	Primer Sequences (5′-3′)	Accession No.
Tnf	F- AGGCACTCCCCCAAAAGATG	NM_001278601.1
	R- TCACCCCGAAGTTCAGTAGACAGA	
Tnfrsf1a	F- GCCCGAAGTCTACTCCATCATTTG	NM_011609.4
	R- GGCTGGGGAGGGGGCTGGAGTTAG	
Tnfrsf1b	F- GCCCAGCCAAACTCCAAGCATC	NM_011610.3
	R- TCCTAACATCAGCAGACCCAGTG	
Il1b	F- TGCCACCTTTTGACAGTGATG	NM_008361.4
	R- CAAAGGTTTGGAAGCAGCCC	
Il6	F- AGGATACCACTCCCAACAGA	NM_001314054.1
	R- ACTCCAGGTAGCTATGGTACTC	
Il10	F- GCCAGGTGAAGACTTTCTTTCAAAC	NM_010548.2
	R- AGTCCAGCAGACTCAATACACAC	
Cxcl1	F- GCTGGGATTCACCTCAAGAAC	NM_008176.3
	R- TGTGGCTATGACTTCGGTTTG	
Itgam	F- GCCTGTCACACTGAGCAGAA	NM_008401.2
	R- TGCAACAGAGCAGTTCAGCA	
Cx3cr1	F- TCCCATCTGCTCAGGACCTC	NM_009987.4
	R- GGCCTCAGCAGAATCGTCAT	
Trem2	F- TGCTGGAGATCTCTGGGTCC	NM_031254.3
	R- AGGTCTCTTGATTCCTGGAGGT	
Arg1	F- ATGAAGAGCTGGCTGGTGTG	NM_007482.3
	R- CCAACTGCCAGACTGTGGTC	
P2ry12	F- GCCAGTGTCATTTGCTGTCAC	NM_027571.4
	R- TAGATGCCACCCCTTGCACT	
Hprt1	F- TCCTCAGACCGCTTTTTGCC	NM_013556.2
	R- TCATCATCGCTAATCACGACGC	

2.8. In Situ Hybridization for Tnf mRNA

In situ hybridization for *Tnf* mRNA was performed using a mixture of two alkaline phosphatase (AP)-labeled oligo DNA probes (3 pmol/mL) on tissue sections from C57BL/6J mice surviving 1, 3, 6, 12, and 24 h after SCI, in addition to naïve controls (*n* = 3/group). The following probes were purchased from DNA Technology (Copenhagen, Denmark): *Tnf* probes: 5′ CGTAGTCGGGGCAGCCTTGTCCCTTGAA 3′ (GC content 60.7%, Tm 67.8 °C) and 5′ CTTGACGGCAGAGAGGAGGTTGACTTTC 3′ (GC content 53.6%, Tm 62.3 °C); glyceraldehyde 3-phosphate dehydrogenase (*Gapdh*) probe: 5′ CCT-GCTTCACCACCTTCTTGATGTCA 3′ (GC content 50%, Tm = 60.2 °C). The hybridization was performed on 20 μm ethanol-fixed spinal cord sections using protocols previously described [36,37]. The hybridization signal was developed using an AP buffer containing 5-bromo-4-chloro-3-indolyl phosphate (Sigma-Aldrich, cat. no. B8503, Soeborg, Denmark) and nitroblue tetrazolium (Sigma-Aldrich, cat. no. N6876, Soeborg, Denmark). The specificity of the hybridization was documented by (1) the abolishment of the hybridization signal when hybridizing RNase A-digested sections, (2) hybridizing sections with 100-fold excess of the unlabeled probe mixture, or (3) the absence of signal in sections incubated with buffer only. Parallel sections were hybridized for the widely expressed *Gapdh* mRNA to ensure overall suitability of the tissue for hybridization.

2.9. Protein Purification

Spinal cord tissue segments from naïve mice or mice surviving 1, 3, 6, 12, or 24 h and 3, 7, 14, 21, or 28 days after SCI (*n* = 5/group) were thawed on ice, sonicated in lysis buffer (150 mM sodium chloride (Sigma-Aldrich, cat. no. 1064041000), 20 mM Tris, 1 mM Ethylene Diamine Tetra Acetate (EDTA, Sigma-Aldrich, cat. no. E9884, Soeborg,

Denmark), 1 mM ethylene glycol tetraacetic acid (EGTA, Sigma-Aldrich cat. no. E4378, Soeborg, Denmark), 1% Triton-X-100, a cocktail of phosphatase and proteinase inhibitors (Sigma-Aldrich, P5726 and Sigma-Aldrich, P0044, Soeborg, Denmark), and a cOmplete™ Mini EDTA-Free Tablet (Roche, 11836170001), pH 7.5). Samples were left shaking on ice at 4 °C for 30 min, centrifuged at $14,000 \times g$ at 4 °C for 20 min, and finally the supernatants were stored at -80 °C until further analysis. The protein concentration was determined using the Pierce BCA Protein Assay Kit (Thermo Fischer Scientific, cat. no. 23235, Roskilde, Denmark) according to the manufacturer's protocol.

2.10. Electrochemiluminescence Analysis

TNF, IL-1β, IL-6, IL-10, CXCL1, TNFR1, and TNFR2 protein levels were measured in tissue homogenates from SCI or sham mice surviving 1, 3, 6, 12, or 24 h (acute phase) and 3, 7, 14, or 28 days (delayed phase) survival, as well as from naïve controls ($n = 5$/group), using custom made MSD Mouse Pro-inflammatory V-PLEX (Mesoscale Discovery, Rockville, MD, USA, cat. no. K152BIC (acute) and K152AOH-2 (delayed)), Ultra-sensitive TNFRI (Mesoscale Discovery, cat. no. K152BIC (acute) and K1510VK-2 (delayed)), and TNFRII (Mesoscale Discovery, cat. no. K152BJC (acute) and K150ZSR-2 (delayed)) kits, as previously described [26]. Analysis of tissue derived from mice surviving 3, 7, 14, and 28 days (delayed phase) was performed separately from tissue derived from mice surviving 1, 3, 6, 12, and 24 h (acute phase) and, thus, they were analyzed as two separate experiments. Samples were diluted in Diluent 41, run in duplex on a SECTOR Imager 6000 Plate Reader (Mesoscale Discovery), and analyzed using MSD Discovery Workbench software. Samples with coefficient of variation (CV) values >25% in individual analyses were excluded. The lower limit of detection (LLOD) was a calculated concentration based on a signal 2.5 standard deviations (SD) above the blank (zero) calibrator. For protein levels below LLOD, a value of 0.5 LLOD was used for statistical analysis. LLOD values for acute experiments; IL-1β (0.19–0.22 pg/mL), IL-10 (0.81–1.34 pg/mL), CXCL1 (0.14–0.23 pg/mL), TNF (0.22–0.77 pg/mL), IL-6 (1.70–4.04 pg/mL), TNFR1 (0.57–0.61 pg/mL), and TNFR2 (15.00–35.90 pg/mL). LLOD values for delayed experiments; IL-1β (0.09 pg/mL), IL-10 (0.61 pg/mL), CXCL1 (0.13 pg/mL), TNF (0.15 pg/mL), IL-6 (1.57 pg/mL), TNFR1 (0.16 pg/mL), and TNFR2 (0.73 pg/mL).

2.11. CSF ELISA

ELISA tests on human CSF were performed at the Third Affiliated Hospital of Sun Yat-sen University in China. SolTNF (ab181421) and solTNFR1 (ab209881) were quantitatively measured using commercially available ELISA kits (Abcam, Cambridge, UK) according to the manufacturer's instructions. Before testing, CSF samples were centrifuged at $2000 \times g$ for 10 min to remove debris. Supernatants were collected for further analysis.

2.12. Immunohistochemistry for TNF

Visualizing the TNF protein in spinal cord tissue sections from C57BL/6 ($n = 3$/group) and $Tnf^{-/-}$ ($n = 2$/group) mice surviving 1, 3, 6, 12, and 24 h after SCI and naïve controls ($n = 3$) was performed using a two-step immunohistochemical protocol with an AP-conjugated secondary antibody as previously described in detail [37]. In short, sections were air-dried and fixed in 4% PFA for 10 min. Sections were then rinsed in Tris-buffered saline (TBS, pH 7.4) for 15 min, TBS + 0.1% Triton (Merck, cat. no. X100, Soeborg, Denmark) 3×15 min, and incubated with 10% FBS in TBS for 30 min at room temperature. Thereafter, sections were incubated with polyclonal rabbit anti-mouse TNF antibody (Table 4) diluted at 1:200 in 10% FBS in TBS for 1 h at room temperature, followed by 48 h at 4 °C. Next, sections were rinsed 3×15 min in TBS + 0.1% Triton and incubated with a secondary AP-conjugated antibody to rabbit IgG (Jackson ImmunoResearch, cat. no. 111–055-003, Cambridgeshire, UK) diluted at 1:200 in 10% FBS in TBS for 1 h at room temperature. The antigen–antibody complex was visualized using the AP developer used for in situ hybridization containing 1 mol/L Levamisole (Sigma-Aldrich, cat. no. PHR1798, Soeborg,

Denmark). Finally, the development was arrested in distilled water, and the sections were cover slipped in Aquatex (Sigma-Aldrich, cat. no. 1.085.620.050, Soeborg, Denmark).

Table 4. Overview of antibodies used for immunohistochemistry and immunofluorescent staining.

Antibody	Conjugated	Host (Clone)	Dilution	Source (cat. no.)
Anti-TNF	Unconjugated	Rabbit	1:200	Thermo Fischer Scientific (P-350)
Anti-TNFR1	Unconjugated	Rabbit (H-271)	1:50	Santa Cruz (sc-7895)
Anti-TNFR2	Unconjugated	Rabbit	1:200	Sigma Aldrich (HPA004796)
Anti-TNFR2	Unconjugated	Goat	1:50	R&D Systems (AF-426-PB)
Anti-MAP2	Unconjugated	Chicken	1:100	Abcam (ab5392)
Anti-CD68	Unconjugated	Rat	1:400	Bio-Rad (MCA1957)
Anti-CD68	Unconjugated	Mouse (PG-M1)	1:100	Abcam (ab783)
Anti-CD11b	Unconjugated	Rat	1:500	Bio-Rad (MCA711)
Anti-Iba1	Unconjugated	Rabbit	1:500	Wako (019–19741)
Anti-IBA1	Unconjugated	Mouse (GT10312)	1:1000	Sigma Aldrich (SAB2702364)
Anti-Galectin-3	Unconjugated	Rat (M38)	1:300	Hakon Leffler's Lab [38]
Anti-NF-L	Alexa Fluor-488	Mouse (N52)	1:50	Sigma Aldrich (MAB5266)
Anti-IL-1β	Unconjugated	Mouse (2E8)	1:50	Bio-Rad (MCA5542Z)
Anti-GFAP	Cy3	Mouse (G-A-5)	1:500	Sigma Aldrich (C9205)
Anti-GFAP	Alexa Fluor-488	Mouse (131–17719)	1:400	Invitrogen (A21294)
Anti-Rabbit	Alexa Fluor-594	Donkey	1:200	Invitrogen (A21207)
Anti-Rabbit	Alexa Fluor-488	Chicken	1:200	Invitrogen (A21441)
Anti-Rat	Alexa Fluor-594	Goat	1:200	Invitrogen (A11007)
Anti-rabbit	Alexa Fluor-594	Goat	1:200	Invitrogen (A21207)
Anti-rabbit	Alexa Fluor-488	Goat	1:200	Invitrogen (A11008)
Anti-rabbit	Alexa Fluor-568	Goat	1:200	Invitrogen (A11011)
Anti-Rat	Alexa Fluor-488	Goat	1:200	Invitrogen (A11006)
Anti-Chicken	Alexa Fluor-488	Goat	1:200	Invitrogen (A11039)
Anti-mouse	Alexa Fluor-488	Goat	1:200	Invitrogen (A11001)
Anti-mouse	Alexa Fluor-568	Goat	1:200	Invitrogen (A11004)
Anti-mouse	Alexa Fluor-555	Goat	1:200	Invitrogen (A21422)
Anti-goat	Alexa Fluor-594	Donkey	1:200	Invitrogen (A11058)

Control reactions for antibody specificity were performed on parallel sections by (1) substitution of the primary antibody with rabbit serum (Dako, cat. no. X0902, Glostrup, Denmark), (2) omission of the primary antibody in the protocol, and (3) inclusion of sections from $Tnf^{-/-}$ mice. $Tnf^{-/-}$ mice are known to be devoid of functional TNF protein [31]. Parallel sections incubated with polyclonal rabbit anti-glial fibrillary acidic protein (GFAP, Table 4) diluted at 1:4000 were included for the overall control of the immunohistochemical reaction.

2.13. Immunofluorescence Staining

Mouse tissue: Double immunofluorescence staining for TNF, TNFR1, or TNFR2 with cell-specific markers was performed on 20-μm-thick, parallel cryostat tissue sections from mice surviving 3 h, 21 days, or 28 days after SCI. Double labelling for GFAP with CD11b, CD68, or Iba1 was performed on tissue sections from mice surviving 21 or 28 days after SCI (n = 2–3/group). Sections were blocked with 10% FBS in TBS for 30 min, incubated o.n. with primary antibodies (Table 4), rinsed in TBS, and incubated with fluorescently labelled secondary antibodies for 2 h at room temperature (Table 4). For visualization of astrocytes, Cy3- or 488-conjugated anti-GFAP antibodies (Table 4) were applied for 1 h at room temperature. Sections were rinsed in TBS containing 4′,6-diamidino-2-phenylindole (DAPI, 1:1000, Sigma-Aldrich, cat. no. D9542, Soeborg, Denmark) to visualize nuclei and mounted with Aquatex.

Human tissue: Human postmortem spinal cord tissue was formalin-fixed, embedded in paraffin, and cut into 10-μm-thick sections on a microtome. Tissue sections were deparaffinized in xylene and rehydrated in graded series of ethanol (99%, 96%, 70%, 50%), immersed in water, and washed in PBS before heat-induced epitope retrieval in citrate buffer (10 mM citrate, pH 6). Next, sections were rinsed in PBS and bleached using the Autofluorescence Eliminator Reagent (Millipore, cat. no. 2160, Soeborg, Denmark) according to the manufacturer's guidelines [38]. The sections were then rinsed in PBS followed by TBS and TBS + 0.1% triton before blocking in 10% FBS in TBS for 30 min at room temperature. The sections were incubated o.n. with primary antibodies diluted in 10% FBS in TBS (Table 4). The following day, the sections were rinsed in TBS + 0.1% triton, and incubated for 2 h with secondary antibodies (Table 4) diluted in 10% FCS in TBS at room temperature, protected from light. Finally, sections were rinsed in TBS before mounting with ProLong Gold Antifade Reagent with DAPI (Sigma-Aldrich, cat. no. 10236276001, Soeborg, Denmark).

2.14. Flow Cytometry

Samples from mice surviving 3 and 24 h and 14, 21, and 28 days survival after SCI as well as naïve controls ($n = 5$/group) were processed for flow cytometry using a FACSCalibur flow cytometer and data analyzed using FACSuite software, as previously described [39]. Tissue from individual mice was processed individually, and approximately 10^6 events were acquired per sample using forward scatter (FSC) and side scatter (SSC). Microglia ($CD11b^+CD45^{dim}$), macrophages ($CD11b^+CD45^{high}Ly6C^{high}Ly6G^-$), and granulocytes ($CD11b^+CD45^{high}Ly6C^+Ly6G^+$) were identified as previously described [26]. Prior to fixation, cells were stained for live/dead cells using Fixable Viability Dye eFluoro 506 (Thermo Fischer, cat. no. 65–0866-18) diluted in PBS. Positive staining was determined based on isotype controls and the respective fluorescent minus one (FMO) control [25]. Antibodies were directly conjugated with fluorochromes (Table 5). The mean fluorescence intensity (MFI) was calculated as the geometric mean of each population in the CD45 and CD11b positive gates.

Table 5. Overview of antibodies used for flow cytometry.

Antibody	Conjugated	Host (Clone)	Dilution	Source (cat. no.)
Anti-CD45	PerCP-Cy5.5	Rat (30-F11)	1:100	BD Biosciences (561869)
Anti-CD11b	BB515	Rat (M1/70)	1:200	BD Biosciences (564454)
Anti-Ly-6C	PE-Cy7	Rat (AL-21)	1:200	BD Biosciences (560593)
Anti-Ly-6G	BV421	Rat (1A8)	1:200	BD Biosciences (562737)
IgG2b, κ	PerCP-Cy5.5	Rat (A95–1)	1:100	BD Biosciences (550764)
IgG2b, κ	BB515	Rat (A95–1)	1:200	BD biosciences (564421)
IgM, κ	PE-Cy7	Rat (clone R4–22)	1:200	BD biosciences (560572)
IgG2a, κ	BV421	Rat (clone R35–95)	1:200	BD Biosciences (562602)

2.15. Statistical Analysis

Comparisons were performed using repeated measures (RM) or regular two-way analysis of variance (ANOVA) followed by Sidak's post hoc analysis, ordinary one-way ANOVA followed by Dunnet's post hoc analysis, or by Student's t-test. Correlation analyses were performed using the nonparametric Spearman correlation test. Outliers were identified using ROUT with a False Discovery Rate (FDR) of 1%. Analyses were performed using Prism 4.0b software for Macintosh, (GraphPad Software, San Diego, CA, USA). Statistical significance was established for $p < 0.05$. Data are presented as mean ± standard error of mean (SEM), percentages, or as mean with interquartile range (IQR 25–75%).

3. Results

3.1. SCI Leads to Significant Changes in Locomotor Function

The recovery of hind limb function after a moderate contusive SCI was evaluated using the BMS score (Figure 1a) and the BMS subscore (Figure 1b). Mice exhibited immediate paraplegia with no hind limb movement after induction of SCI. Mice receiving a laminectomy (sham) only displayed minor impairment 1 day after surgery but displayed normal motor function from 3 days and onwards after surgery, as demonstrated by a normal BMS (Figure 1a) and normal BMS subscore (Figure 1b). Mice with SCI started to display improved hind limb function from day 7 and onwards but exhibited significant motor dysfunction compared to sham mice throughout the experiment (Figure 1a). Improved locomotion in SCI mice was also detected from day 14 using the BMS subscore (Figure 1b). Mice subjected to SCI experienced significant weight loss within the first 3 days after SCI, whereafter they started to regain weight (Figure 1c). Sham mice did not experience any weight loss (Figure 1c).

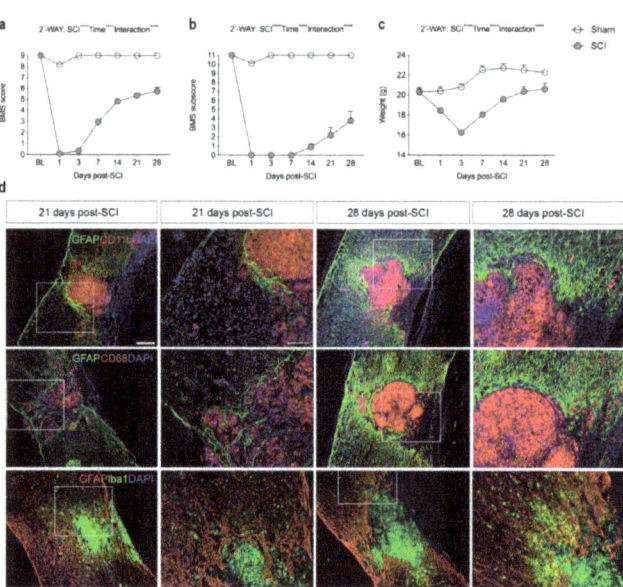

Figure 1. Analysis of locomotor function and glial reactions after SCI. (**a**) Evaluation of hind limb locomotor function. SCI and sham mice were tested 1, 3, and 7 days after surgery and weekly thereafter for 28 days. Motor behavior was scored under blinded conditions with the Basso Mouse Scale (BMS). Analysis of sham and SCI mice showed significantly lower BMS scores in SCI mice compared to sham mice (SCI: $p < 0.0001$, $F_{1,27} = 1447$; Time: $p < 0.0001$, $F_{6,134} = 253.8$; Interaction: $p < 0.0001$, $F_{6,134} = 205.4$). (**b**) Analysis of BMS subscore in SCI and sham mice demonstrating significantly lower BMS subscore in SCI mice compared to sham mice (SCI: $p < 0.0001$, $F_{1,27} = 1081$; Time: $p < 0.0001$, $F_{6,134} = 98.31$; Interaction: $p < 0.0001$, $F_{6,134} = 89.62$). (**c**) Body weight over time in SCI and sham mice (SCI: $p < 0.0001$, $F_{1,27} = 25.71$; Time: $p < 0.0001$, $F_{3.36} = 91.98$; Interaction: $p < 0.0001$, $F_{6,134} = 53.4$). Results are expressed as mean ± SEM, n-values; SCI, $n = 39$ for baseline (BL) to 3 days, $n = 29$ for 7 days, $n = 20$ for 14 and 21 days, and $n = 10$ for 28 days. Sham, $n = 20$ for baseline (BL) to 3 days, $n = 15$ for 7 days, $n = 10$ for 14 and 21 days, and $n = 5$ for 28 days. (**d**) Sections of the thoracic spinal cords were double-labeled for GFAP (green; upper and middle panels, red; lower panels) and CD11b (red; upper panel), CD68 (red; middle panel), or Iba1 (green; lower panel). DAPI was used as a nuclear marker. Scale bars: low magnification = 100 μm and high magnification = 40 μm. GFAP, glial fibrillary acidic protein; CD, cluster of differentiation; Iba1, ionized calcium binding adaptor molecule 1.

3.2. SCI Results in Glial Scar Formation

Immunofluorescent staining for the astrocyte-specific marker GFAP and microglial/macrophage-specific markers CD11b, CD68, and Iba1 at 21 and 28 days after SCI showed that activated GFAP$^+$ astrocytes formed a dense glial scar at the injury border surrounding a core lesion consisting of activated, phagocytic microglia/macrophages (Figure 1d). CD11b$^+$, CD68$^+$, and Iba1$^+$ cells were also located in the peri-lesion areas surrounding the core lesion area although not to the same extent (Figure 1d).

3.3. Tnf mRNA Synthesis Increases in the Acute Phase after SCI

We used in situ hybridization to determine the topology of cells expressing *Tnf* mRNA in the acute phase after SCI. No *Tnf* mRNA was detected under naïve conditions (Figure 2a). Already after 1 h, *Tnf* mRNA expression was detected in glial-like cells located in the white matter of the posterior funiculi (Figure 2b) and also in neuron-like cells located in the grey matter of the dorsal horn (Figure 2c). At 3 h after SCI, a high number of *Tnf* mRNA-expressing glial-like cells were scattered throughout the lesioned posterior funiculi white matter (Figure 2d) as well as in the dorsal and ventral horns (Figure 3e, shown for the ventral horn only). *Tnf* mRNA$^+$ cells in the white matter had a glial-like morphology (Figure 3f). At 6 h (Figure 2g), 12 h (Figure 2h), and 24 h (Figure 2i) after SCI, *Tnf* mRNA$^+$ glial-like cells were still found in the posterior and lateral funiculi although fewer in number than at 3 h. *Gapdh* mRNA expression was used as control, confirming the suitability of the tissue for in situ hybridization (Figure 2j). Buffer (Figure 2k) and RNase (Figure 2l) controls were devoid of signal.

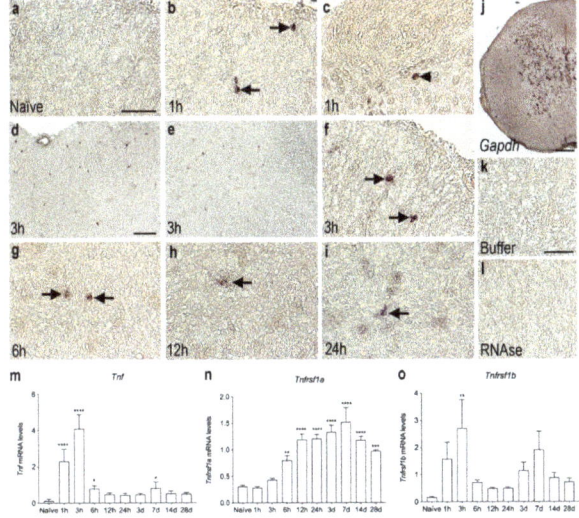

Figure 2. Cellular and temporal expression of *Tnf* mRNA in the thoracic spinal cord after SCI. (**a–i**) In situ hybridization was used to investigate the distribution of *Tnf* mRNA$^+$ cells the first 24 h after SCI. *Tnf* mRNA expression was undetectable in naïve mice (**a**). *Tnf* mRNA$^+$ cells in the white matter of the posterior funiculi (arrows in **b**) and in neuronal-like cells in the dorsal horn (arrowhead in **c**), at 1 h after SCI. *Tnf* mRNA$^+$ cells in the white matter of the posterior funiculi (**d**) and in the grey matter of the ventral horn (**e**). At 3 h, most cells displayed macrophage- or glial-like morphology (arrows in **f**). By 6 h (**g**), 12 h (**h**), and 24 h (**i**), *Tnf* mRNA$^+$ cells were mainly located in white matter areas of the damaged spinal cord (arrows). (**j**) Parallel spinal cord sections that were in situ hybridized for glyceraldehyde-3-phosphate dehydrogenase (*Gapdh*) mRNA showed a largely neuronal signal and confirmed the overall suitability of the tissue for in situ hybridization. (**k,l**) Parallel sections hybridized with buffer alone (**k**) or pretreated with RNAse A before the in situ hybridization (**l**) were devoid of signal. (**m–o**) RT-qPCR analysis of *Tnf* mRNA (**m**), *Tnfrsf1a* mRNA (**n**), and *Tnfrsf1b* mRNA (**o**) levels in naïve mice and in mice allowed 1, 3, 6, and 12 h and 1, 3, 7, 14, and 28-days survival after SCI. *Tnf* mRNA levels were significantly increased at 1, 3, and 6 h and 7 days after SCI, compared to naïve mice (Time: $p < 0.0001$, $F_{9,39} = 58.14$) (**m**). *Tnfrsf1a* mRNA levels significantly increased from 6 h to 28 days after SCI, compared to naïve mice (Time: $p < 0.0001$, $F_{9,39} = 20.01$) (**n**). *Tnfrsf1b* mRNA levels significantly increased at 3 h after SCI, compared to naïve mice (Time: $p = 0.009$, $F_{9,39} = 2.965$). Results are expressed as mean ± SEM, $n = 5$/group, * $p < 0.05$, ** $p < 0.01$, *** $p < 0.001$, **** $p < 0.0001$. Scale bars: (**a–c, f–i, k,l**) = 40 µm, (**d,e**) = 100 µm, and (**j**) = 200 µm.

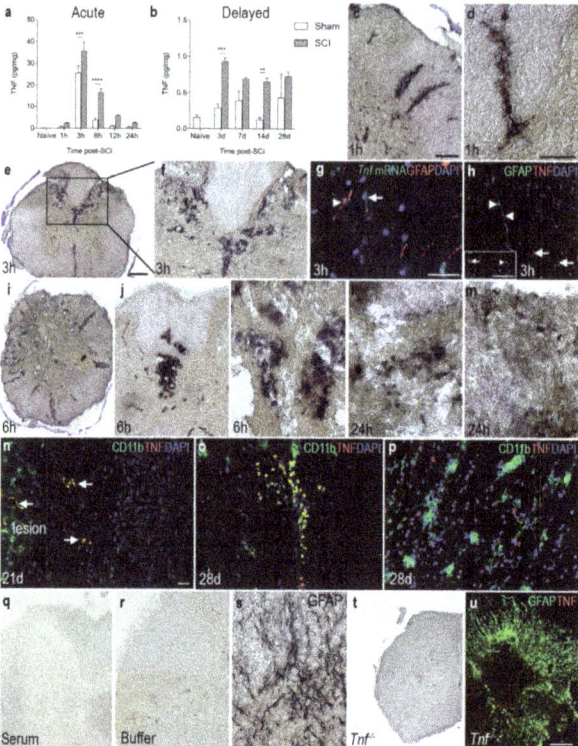

Figure 3. Overview of the spatiotemporal expression of TNF after SCI. (**a,b**) Temporal expression of TNF levels in the acute (**a**) and delayed (**b**) phase after SCI. Statistical indications represent comparisons to sham mice in the acute phase (SCI: $p < 0.0001$, $F_{1,48} = 31.7$; Time: $p < 0.0001$, $F_{5,48} = 105.4$; Interaction: $p = 0.0008$, $F_{5,48} = 5.08$) and delayed phase (Interaction: $F_{4,39} = 3.05$, $p = 0.03$; Time: $F_{4,39} = 5.22$, $p = 0.002$; SCI: $F_{1,39} = 30.74$, $p < 0.0001$) after SCI. Results are expressed as mean ± SEM, $n = 5$/group, ** $p < 0.01$, *** $p < 0.001$, **** $p < 0.0001$. (**c,d**) Representative images of TNF immunoreactivity in grey matter of the dorsal horn and the lateral funiculus (**c**), as well as the posterior funiculus (**d**) of mice that survived 1 h after SCI. (**e,f**) At 3 h, TNF immunoreactivity was high in the dorsal parts of the lesioned spinal cord. (**g**) Combined in situ hybridization for Tnf mRNA (green, arrow) and immunohistochemistry for astroglial GFAP (red, arrowhead) 3 h after SCI. (**h**) Double immunofluorescent staining for astroglial GFAP (green, arrow heads) and TNF (red, arrows) 3 h after SCI. Insert demonstrates that a minority of GFAP⁺ cells (green, arrowhead) co-expressed TNF (red, arrow). (**i–m**) Representative images of TNF immunoreactivity 6 h (**i–k**) and 24 h (**l,m**) after SCI. (**n**) Double immunofluorescent staining for TNF (red, arrow) and the microglial/macrophage marker CD11b (green) showed colocalization of TNF on CD11b⁺ cells near the lesion 21 days after SCI. (**o**) Double immunofluorescent staining for TNF (red) and the CD11b (green) showed colocalization of TNF on CD11b⁺ cells located at the peri-lesion area 28 days after SCI. DAPI (blue) was used as a nuclear marker. (**p**) TNF was also found in CD11b⁻ cells 28 days after SCI. (**q,r**) Control reactions demonstrating absence of specific staining in tissue sections incubated with rabbit IgG (**q**) or with buffer alone (**r**). (**s**) Spinal cord section stained for astrocytic GFAP as a control for the immunohistochemical reaction. (**t,u**) Thoracic spinal cord tissue sections from a $Tnf^{-/-}$ mouse 3 h after SCI, demonstrating absence of specific TNF staining. Scale bars: (**c,f,j,q**) = 40 μm, (**e,i,t,u,o**) = 100 μm, and (**d,g,h,k,l–n,p,r,s**) = 200 μm. CD, cluster of differentiation; GFAP, glial fibrillary acidic protein; TNF, tumor necrosis factor.

The in situ hybridization data were supported by RT-qPCR analysis of the temporal expression of *Tnf* mRNA in spinal cord tissue after SCI (Figure 2m). *Tnf* mRNA levels increased rapidly after SCI, with the highest expression detected at 1 and 3 h after SCI compared to naïve, and levels were still elevated at 6 h after SCI. A small, but significant, increase was also observed 7 days after SCI (Figure 2m).

The gene expression of the two TNF receptors, *Tnfrsf1a* and *Tnfrsf1b*, was also measured using RT-qPCR analysis (Figure 2n,o). *Tnfrsf1a* mRNA expression steadily increased from 6 h after SCI, reaching peak levels at 14 days after SCI, whereafter it started to decline, although it was still significantly elevated at 28 days compared to naïve (Figure 2n).

Tnfsf1b mRNA expression was significantly increased 3 h after injury and quickly decreased thereafter (Figure 2o). A second increase was observed 7 days after SCI; however, this increase did not quite reach statistical significance ($p = 0.08$).

3.4. TNF Is Increased on Glial Cells after SCI

To investigate TNF protein levels after SCI, we performed electrochemiluminescence multiplex analysis on spinal cord tissue from mice subjected to SCI and compared to naïve and sham mice (Figure 3a,b). TNF levels increased significantly over time in SCI mice compared to naïve mice. In line with our in situ hybridization and RT-qPCR analysis, TNF levels peaked 3 h after SCI and was still elevated at 6 h, compared to sham and naïve mice (Figure 3a). In the more delayed phase, TNF levels were significantly increased at 3 and 7 days after SCI, compared to sham and naïve mice (Figure 3b). Using immunohistochemistry, TNF immunoreactivity was demonstrated in scattered cells located in the dorsal horns and posterior and lateral funiculi, as well as around blood vessels 1 h after SCI (Figure 3c,d). TNF immunoreactivity was intensified in the posterior part of the damaged spinal cord 3 h after SCI (Figure 3e,f), at which time point *Tnf* mRNA (Figure 3g) and TNF protein (Figure 3h) expression was mostly confined to GFAP$^-$ cells although a few GFAP$^+$ astrocytes also co-expressed TNF (insert in Figure 3h). At 6 h after SCI, TNF immunoreactivity was localized throughout the damaged spinal cord, especially around blood vessels (Figure 3i–k). At 24 h, TNF expression was scarcely distributed throughout the spinal cord, with the overall TNF immunoreactivity decreasing at this time point compared to earlier time points (Figure 3l,m). Immunofluorescence double labeling demonstrated that TNF co-localized to CD11b$^+$ immune cells located within the lesion and in the peri-lesion area (Figure 3n) at 21 and 28 days after SCI. Serum (Figure 3q) and buffer (Figure 3r) controls were devoid of staining. Immunohistochemical staining for the abundant astroglial marker GFAP was used as a positive control for the immunohistochemical procedure (Figure 3s). Tissue sections from $Tnf^{-/-}$ mice subjected to SCI were devoid of specific TNF immunoreactivity (Figure 3t), just as double fluorescent staining for GFAP and TNF in $Tnf^{-/-}$ mice subjected to SCI were devoid of specific TNF staining (Figure 3u).

3.5. TNFR1 and TNFR2 Expression Increases in the Lesioned Spinal Cord

We analyzed the temporal and cellular expression of TNFR1 and TNFR2 in spinal cord tissue from naïve and sham mice, as well as mice that had survived 1, 3, 6, 12, and 24 h and 3, 7, 14, and 28 days after SCI (Figure 4). TNFR1 levels were found to increase significantly from 24 h after SCI and onwards (Figure 4a,b). Double immunofluorescent staining showed that TNFR1 expression was absent within the core of the lesion site, where microtubule associated protein 2$^+$ (MAP2$^+$) neurons were also absent (Figure 4c). TNFR1 expression was upregulated in areas of MAP2$^+$ degenerating neurons located in the grey matter of the peri-lesion area (Figure 4d), and its expression co-localized to ascending and descending fiber tracts more distant from the lesion area at 21 days after SCI (Figure 4e). Additionally, at 28 days, TNFR1 expression was upregulated in areas near the lesion site, alongside MAP2$^+$ degenerating neurons (Figure 4f). TNFR1 expression was found to co-localize to the soma and fibers of MAP2$^+$ cells (Figure 4g, shown for 28 days only). CD68$^+$ microglia/macrophages aligned along the damaged ascending and descending fiber tracts of the white matter, where TNFR1 expression was also localized (Figure 4h, shown for 21 days only).

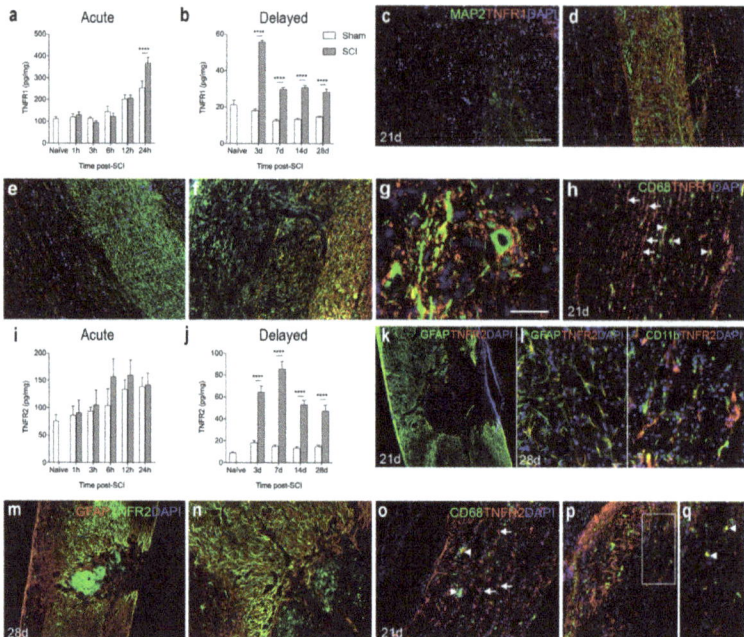

Figure 4. Spatiotemporal expression of TNF receptor 1 and 2 after SCI. (**a,b**) TNFR1 protein levels in the acute (**a**) and delayed (**b**) phases after SCI. Significant indications represent comparisons to sham mice in the acute phase (**a**, Interaction: $F_{5,48} = 4.52$, $p = 0.002$; Time: $F_{5,48} = 45.74$, $p < 0.0001$; SCI: $F_{1,48} = 2.19$, $p = 0.15$) and delayed phase (**b**, Interaction: $F_{4,40} = 49.51$, $p < 0.0001$; Time: $F_{4,40} = 52.17$, $p < 0.0001$; SCI: $F_{1,40} = 406.5$, $p < 0.0001$) after SCI. (**c–g**) Immunofluorescent double labelling for TNFR1 (red) and neuronal MAP2 (green) within the lesion site (**c**), peri-lesion area (**d,f,g**), as well as distant from the lesion site (**e**) at 21 (**c–e**) and 28 (**f,g**) days after SCI. (**h**) Immunofluorescent double labelling for TNFR1$^+$ (red) and CD68$^+$ (green) cells 21 days after SCI. (**i,j**) TNFR2 protein levels in the acute phase (**i**, Interaction: $F_{5,47} = 0.42$, $p = 0.83$; Time: $F_{5,47} = 3.89$, $p < 0.005$; SCI: $F_{1,47} = 1.75$, $p = 0.19$) and delayed phase (**j**, Interaction: $F_{4,40} = 25.04$, $p < 0.0001$; Time: $F_{4,40} = 36.07$, $p < 0.0001$; SCI: $F_{1,40} = 2702.8$, $p < 0.0001$) after SCI. (**k–n**) Immunofluorescent double labelling for TNFR2 (red: **k,l** and green: **m,n**) and GFAP$^+$ astrocytes (green: (**k,l**) and red: (**m,n**)) and CD11b$^+$ microglia/macrophages (green: (**l**)) at 21 (**k**) and 28 (**l–n**) days after SCI. (**o–q**) Immunofluorescent double labeling of TNFR2$^+$ cells (arrows in (**o**)) and CD68$^+$ microglia/macrophages (arrow heads in (**o**)). (**p**) Only a few CD68$^+$ cells co-expressed TNFR2. (**q**) represents a high magnification image of the area squared in (**p**), demonstrating TNFR2$^+$ CD68$^+$ cells located in the peri-lesion areas 21 days after SCI (arrow heads in (**q**)). DAPI was used as a nuclear marker. Scale bars: (**k,m**) = 100 µm, (**c–f,h,n–p**) = 40 µm, and (**g,l,q**) = 20 µm. Results are expressed as mean ± SEM, $n = 5$/group, **** $p < 0.0001$. GFAP, glial fibrillary acidic protein; MAP2, microtubule associated protein 2; TNFR, tumor necrosis factor receptor.

TNFR2 levels were not significantly altered in the acute phase after SCI (Figure 4i), but levels increased significantly in the more delayed phase, i.e., from 3 days after SCI and onwards (Figure 4j). Double immunofluorescence staining demonstrated that at 21 and 28 days after SCI, TNFR2 co-localized to GFAP$^+$ astrocytes forming the glial scar and CD11b$^+$ microglia (Figure 4k–n), but to some extent also to cells, possibly infiltrating macrophages, located in the core of the lesion (Figure 4m,n). At 21 days after SCI, immunofluorescent double labeling of CD68$^+$ microglia/macrophages and TNFR2 expression (Figure 4o–q) showed that TNFR2 expression was absent in most CD68$^+$ cells (Figure 4o), although a minority of the cells co-expressed TNFR2 (Figure 4p,q).

3.6. SCI Results in Increased Levels of Inflammatory Cytokines

To assess the temporal expression of selected inflammatory cytokines known to be important after SCI [4,40], we analyzed gene and protein expression levels of IL-1β, IL-6, IL-10, and CXCL1 after SCI (Figure 5). We found that *Il1b* mRNA levels increased significantly from 3–12 h after SCI, compared to naïve conditions (Figure 5a). This increase was followed by a transient increase in IL-β levels at 6 and 12 h after SCI (Figure 5b). A second increase in IL-1β levels could be detected in the delayed phase after SCI, from day 7 and onwards, with the highest expression on day 14 (Figure 5c). *Il6* mRNA levels significantly increased at 6 and 12 h after SCI (Figure 5d) and was paralleled by a transient increase in IL-6 levels (Figure 5e). A second peak in IL-6 levels was found 3 days after SCI (Figure 5f). *Il10* mRNA levels increased rapidly at 1 and 3 h after SCI whereafter they decreased again (Figure 5g). IL-10 levels transiently increased 6 h after SCI (Figure 5h) and then returned to baseline levels (Figure 5h–i). *Cxcl1* mRNA levels did not change significantly after SCI, but there was a trend towards an increase at 6 h ($p = 0.09$, Figure 5j). In contrast, CXCL1 levels increased transiently at 6 and 12 h after SCI (Figure 5k), and again from day 3 and onwards (Figure 5l).

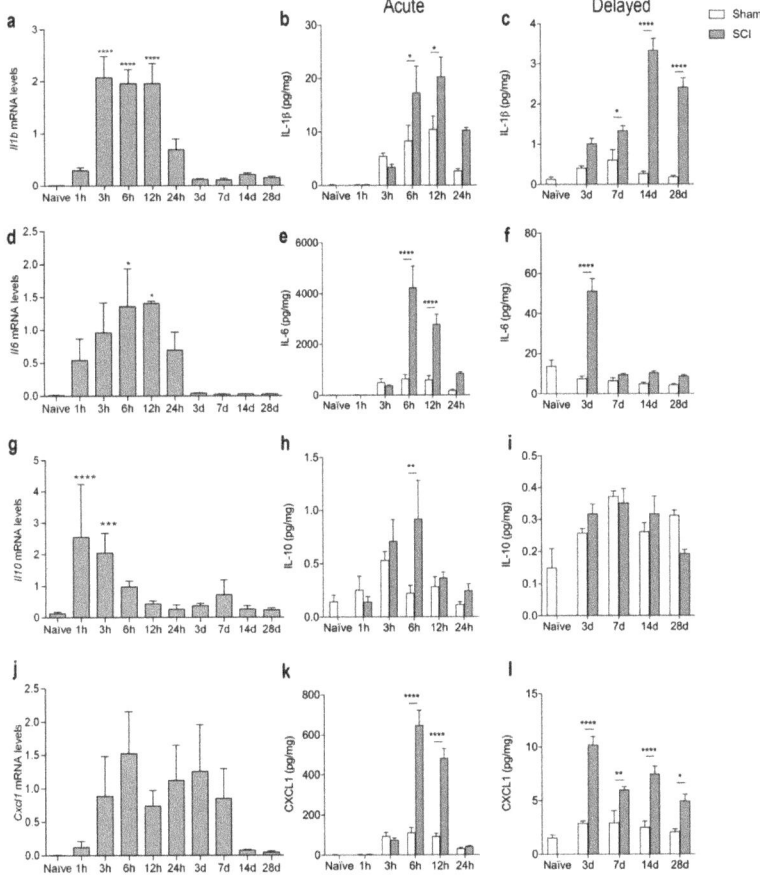

Figure 5. Temporal expression of inflammatory cytokines after SCI. (**a**–**c**) Temporal expression of *Il1b* mRNA ((**a**), $p < 0.0001$, Time: $F_{9,39} = 17.04$) and IL-1β levels in the acute phase ((**b**), Interaction: $F_{5,47} = 3.07$,

$p = 0.02$; Time: $F_{5,47} = 17.76$, $p < 0.0001$; SCI: $F_{1,47} = 10.86$, $p = 0.002$) and delayed phase ((c), Interaction: $F_{4,39} = 32.72$, $p < 0.0001$; Time: $F_{4,39} = 32.06$, $p < 0.0001$; SCI: $F_{1,39} = 175.6$, $p < 0.0001$) after SCI. (d–f) Temporal expression of *Il6* mRNA ((d), Time: $F_{9,34} = 3.33$, $p = 0.005$) and IL-6 levels in the acute phase ((e), Interaction: $F_{5,48} = 14.96$, $p < 0.0001$; Time: $F_{5,48} = 25.49$, $p < 0.0001$; SCI: $F_{1,48} = 42.99$, $p < 0.0001$) and delayed phase ((f), Interaction: $F_{4,39} = 34.84$, $p < 0.0001$; Time: $F_{4,39} = 39.20$, $p < 0.0001$; SCI: $F_{1,39} = 65.39$, $p < 0.0001$) after SCI. (g–i) Temporal expression of *Il10* mRNA ((g), Time: $F_{9,39} = 9.648$, $p < 0.0001$) and IL-10 levels in the acute phase ((h), Interaction: $F_{5,48} = 2.10$, $p = 0.08$; Time: $F_{5,48} = 4.58$, $p < 0.002$; SCI: $F_{1,48} = 4.21$, $p < 0.05$) and delayed phase ((i), Interaction: $F_{4,39} = 2.56$, $p = 0.05$; Time: $F_{4,39} = 13.23$, $p < 0.0001$; SCI: $F_{1,39} = 0.06$, $p = 0.81$) after SCI. (j–l) Temporal expression of *Cxcl1* mRNA ((j), Time: $F_{9,39} = 1.786$, $p = 0.1023$) and CXCL1 levels in the acute phase ((k), Interaction: $F_{5,48} = 39.83$, $p < 0.0001$; Time: $F_{5,48} = 69.33$, $p < 0.0001$; SCI: $F_{1,48} = 93.31$, $p < 0.0001$) and delayed phase ((l), Interaction: $F_{4,39} = 10.89$, $p < 0.0001$; Time: $F_{4,39} = 22.51$, $p < 0.0001$; SCI: $F_{1,39} = 96.25$, $p < 0.0001$) after SCI. Results are expressed as mean ± SEM, $n = 5$/group, * $p < 0.05$, ** $p < 0.01$, *** $p < 0.001$, **** $p < 0.0001$. One technical outlier was excluded in the day 28 sham group. For mRNA analysis, significant indications represent comparisons to naïve conditions and for protein analyses comparisons to sham mice.

3.7. SCI Results in Microglial Activation and Immune Cell Infiltration into Spinal Cord

We performed flow cytometry analysis to estimate microglial and infiltrating immune cell populations in the spinal cord of naïve mice and mice surviving 3 and 24 h as well as 14, 21, and 28 days after SCI (Figure 6). We gated only live cells and included $CD11b^+CD45^{dim}$ microglia and infiltrating $CD11b^+CD45^{high}$ leukocytes, which were further gated into $Ly6G^+Ly6C^+$ granulocytes and $Ly6G^-Ly6C^+$ monocytes (Figure 6a). We estimated the total number of microglia (Figure 6b–c) and infiltrating leukocytes (Figure 6d–e), as well as the number of macrophages (Figure 6f–g) and granulocytes (Figure 6h–i), in the lesion (open bars) and peri-lesion (checkered bars) areas. We found that microglial cell numbers increased significantly in the lesion compared to the peri-lesion area 3 h after SCI and stayed high in both the lesion and peri-lesion areas at 24 h (Figure 6b). In the chronic phase after SCI, microglial numbers were comparable between the lesion and peri-lesion area, except for 21 days after SCI, where microglial numbers were increased in the lesion area compared to the peri-lesion area (Figure 6c) The total number of infiltrating leukocytes increased significantly within the lesion area 24 h after SCI (Figure 6d), with both significantly increased numbers of macrophages (Figure 6f) and granulocytes (Figure 6h) located within the lesion area. In the chronic phase after SCI the number of infiltrating leukocytes (Figure 6e), including macrophages (Figure 6g) and granulocytes (Figure 6i), was comparable between the lesion and peri-lesion sites. Changes in the percentages of the cell populations after SCI can be found in Supplementary Figure S1.

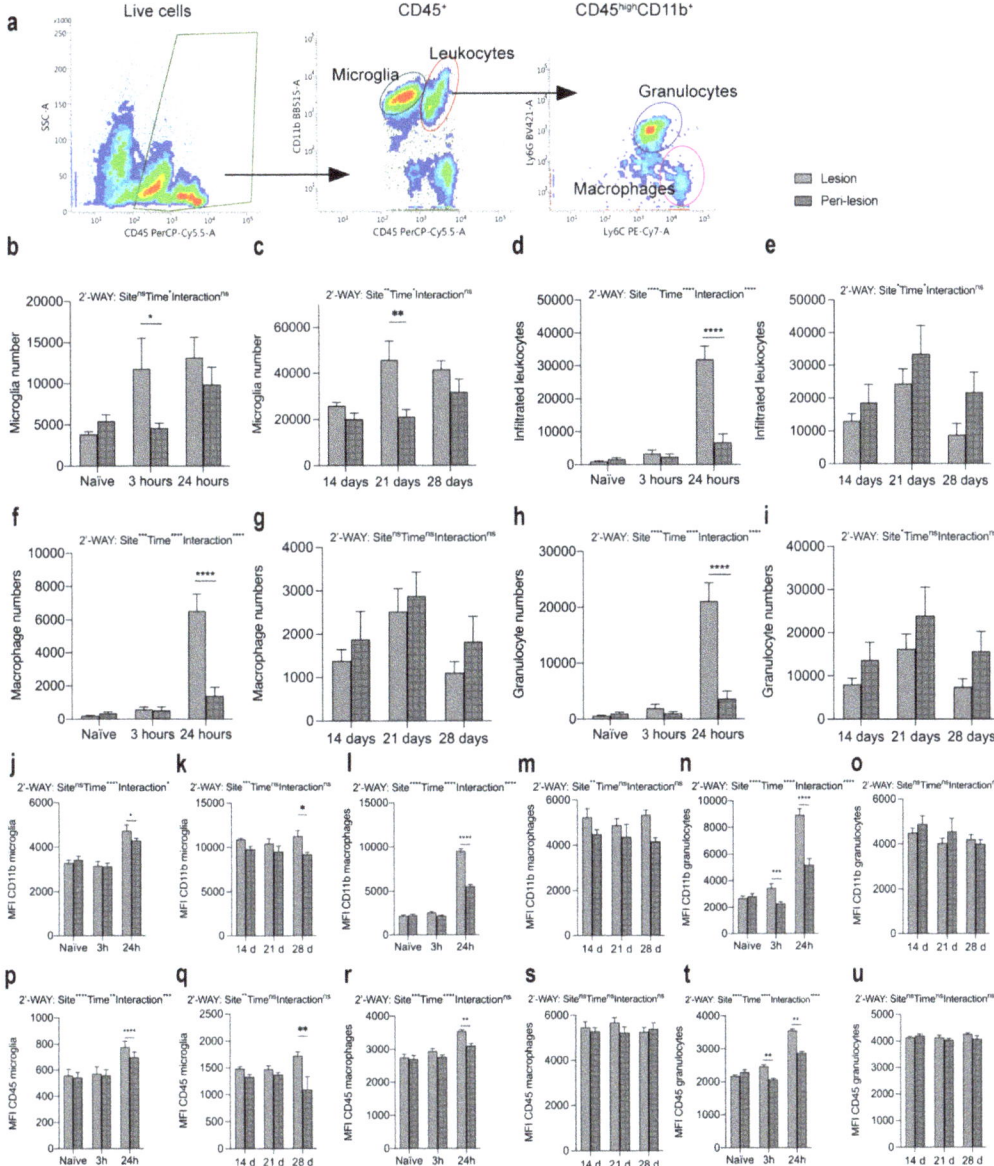

Figure 6. Changes in microglia and leukocyte populations after SCI. (**a**) Representative dot plots showing the gating strategy. Only live cells were included. (**b**,**c**) Number of microglia (CD11b$^+$CD45^{dim}) in the acute ((**b**), Interaction: $F_{2,28}$=35.16, $p < 0.0001$; Time: $F_{2,28} = 18.19$, $p < 0.0001$; Site: $F_{1,28} = 10.26$, $p = 0.003$) and chronic ((**c**), Interaction: $F_{2,22} = 2.04$, $p = 0.15$; Time: $F_{2,22} = 4.37$, $p = 0.03$; Site: $F_{1,22} = 11.14$, $p = 0.003$) phases after SCI. (**d**,**e**) Number of infiltrating leukocytes (CD11b$^+$CD45^{high}) in the acute ((**d**), Interaction: $F_{2,28} = 80.03$, $p < 0.0001$; Time: $F_{2,28} = 154.9$, $p < 0.0001$; Site: $F_{1,28} = 32.13$, $p < 0.0001$) and chronic ((**e**), Interaction: $F_{2,22} = 0.24$, $p = 0.79$; Time: $F_{2,22} = 4.09$, $p = 0.03$; Site: $F_{1,22} = 4.44$, $p < 0.05$) phases after SCI. (**f**,**g**) Number of infiltrating Ly6C$^+$Ly6G$^-$ macrophages in the acute ((**f**), Interaction: $F_{2,28} = 31.60$, $p < 0.0001$; Time: $F_{2,28} = 66.72$, $p < 0.0001$; Site: $F_{1,28} = 17.75$, $p = 0.0002$) and

chronic ((**g**), Interaction: $F_{2,22} = 0.06$, $p = 0.94$; Time: $F_{2,22} = 3.33$, $p = 0.05$; Site: $F_{1,22} = 1.54$, $p = 0.23$) phases after SCI. (**h,i**) Number of infiltrating Ly6C$^+$Ly6G$^+$ granulocytes in the acute ((**h**), Interaction: $F_{2,28} = 39.45$, $p < 0.0001$; Time: $F_{2,28} = 37.67$, $p < 0.0001$; Site: $F_{1,28} = 20.19$, $p = 0.0001$) and chronic ((**i**), Interaction: $F_{2,22} = 1.52$, $p = 0.24$; Time: $F_{2,22} = 0.73$, $p = 0.49$; Site: $F_{1,22} = 1.29$, $p = 0.27$) phases after SCI. (**j,k**) MFI for CD11b on microglia in the acute ((**j**), Interaction: $F_{2,28} = 4.19$, $p = 0.03$; Time: $F_{2,28} = 20.58$, $p < 0.0001$; Site: $F_{1,28} = 1.66$, $p = 0.21$) and chronic ((**k**), Interaction: $F_{2,22} = 0.92$, $p = 0.92$; Time: $F_{2,22} = 0.37$, $p = 0.69$; Site: $F_{1,22} = 14.62$, $p = 0.0009$) phases after SCI. (**l,m**) MFI for CD11b on macrophages in the acute ((**l**), Interaction: $F_{2,28} = 118.8$, $p < 0.0001$; Time: $F_{2,28} = 480.0$, $p < 0.0001$; Site: $F_{1,28} = 145.80$, $p < 0.0001$) and chronic ((**m**), Interaction: $F_{2,22} = 0.54$, $p = 0.59$; Time: $F_{2,22} = 0.27$, $p = 0.77$; Site: $F_{1,22} = 9,71$, $p = 0.005$) phases after SCI. (**n,o**) MFI for CD11b on granulocytes in the acute ((**n**), Interaction: $F_{2,28} = 51.38$, $p < =0.0001$; Time: $F_{2,28} = 62.49$, $p < 0.0001$; Site: $F_{1,28} = 97.29$, $p < 0.0001$) and chronic ((**o**), Interaction: $F_{2,22} = 0.76$, $p = 0.48$; Time: $F_{2,22} = 1.92$, $p = 0.17$; Site: $F_{1,22} = 0.88$, $p = 0.36$) phases after SCI. (**p,q**) MFI for CD45 on microglia in the acute ((**p**), Interaction: $F_{2,28} = 10.41$, $p = 0.0004$; Time: $F_{2,28} = 5.50$, $p < 0.01$; Site: $F_{1,28} = 27.81$, $p < 0.0001$) and chronic ((**q**), Interaction: $F_{2,22} = 3.03$, $p = 0.07$; Time: $F_{2,22} = 0.01$, $p = 0.99$; Site: $F_{1,22} = 9.55$, $p = 0.005$) phases after SCI. (**r,s**) MFI for CD45 on macrophages in the acute ((**r**), Interaction: $F_{2,28} = 3.01$, $p = 0.07$; Time: $F_{2,28} = 29.90$, $p < 0.0001$; Site: $F_{1,28} = 11.08$, $p = 0.003$) and chronic ((**s**), Interaction: $F_{2,22} = 0.73$, $p = 0.50$; Time: $F_{2,22} = 0.14$, $p = 0.87$; Site: $F_{1,22} = 0.76$, $p = 0.39$) phases after SCI. (**t,u**) MFI for CD45 on granulocytes in the acute ((**t**), Interaction: $F_{2,28} = 33.17$, $p < =0.0001$; Time: $F_{2,28} = 255.9$, $p < 0.0001$; Site: $F_{1,28} = 63.45$, $p < 0.0001$) and chronic ((**u**), Interaction: $F_{2,22} = 1.52$, $p = 0.24$; Time: $F_{2,22} = 0.73$, $p = 0.49$; Site: $F_{1,22} = 1.29$, $p = 0.27$) phases after after SCI. Open bars represent the lesion site, checkered bars represent the peri-lesion site. Results are expressed as mean ± SEM, $n = 5–11$/group, * $p < 0.05$, ** $p < 0.01$, *** $p < 0.001$, and **** $p < 0.0001$.

MFI for CD11b (Figure 6j–o) and MFI for CD45 (Figure 6p–u) were significantly increased on microglia (Figure 6j,p) and macrophages (Figure 6l,r) located within the lesion area compared to the peri-lesion area, 24 h after SCI, just as MFI for CD11b and CD45 on microglia was increased in the lesion area compared to the peri-lesion area 28 days after SCI (Figure 6k,q). In the chronic phase after SCI, MFI for CD11b and MFI for CD45 on macrophages (Figure 6m,s) did not differ between the lesion and peri-lesion areas. MFI for CD11b and CD45 on granulocytes (Figure 6h,k) were already significantly increased in the lesion area 3 h after SCI and remained increased at 24 h, compared to the peri-lesion area. No differences were observed in the chronic phase after SCI (Figure 6o,u).

We further characterized microglial/macrophage responses in the spinal cord after SCI using RT-qPCR (Figure 7a–e). We found that *Itgam* (Figure 7a) and *Cx3cr1* (Figure 7b) mRNA levels increased significantly at day 3 and remained elevated until 28 days, compared to naïve controls. *Trem2* mRNA levels increased transiently 7 days after SCI, compared to naïve conditions (Figure 7c). *Arg1* mRNA levels increased significantly 24 h after SCI and remained elevated until day 7, after which they declined (Figure 7d). The gene expression for the purinergic receptor *P2ry12* was significantly elevated 3 days after SCI and remained elevated throughout the experiment (Figure 7e).

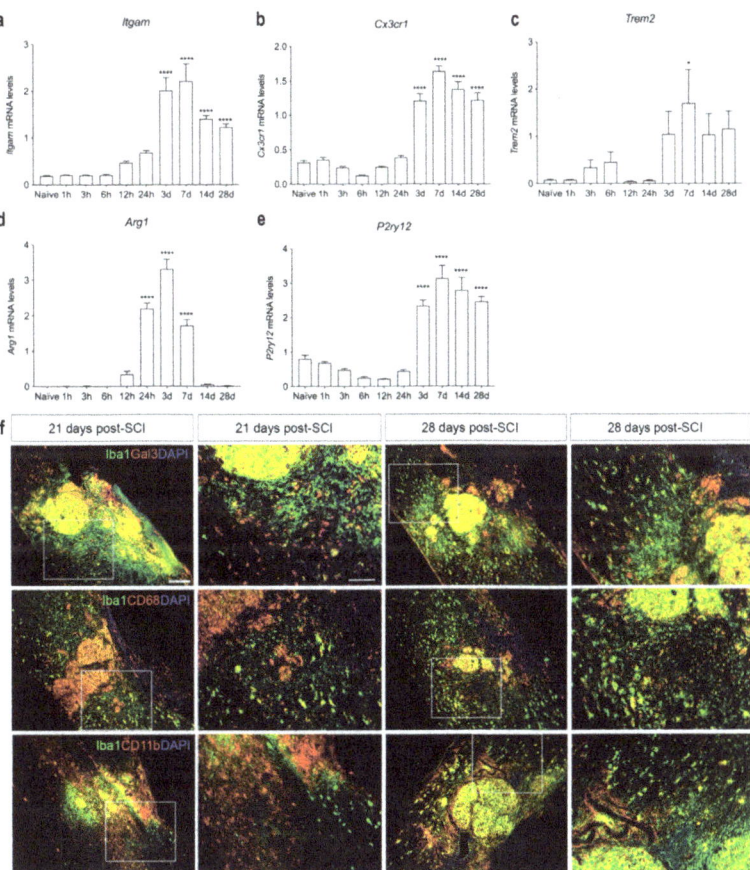

Figure 7. Characterization of microglia/macrophage reactions after SCI. (**a–e**) Temporal expression of *Itgam* ((**a**), Time: $F_{9,38} = 30.97$, $p < 0.0001$), *Cx3cr1* ((**b**), Time: $F_{9,38} = 77.32$, $p < 0.0001$), *Trem2* ((**c**), Time: $F_{9,37} = 3.218$, $p = 0.006$), *Arg1* ((**d**), Time: $F_{9,39} = 113.6$, $p < 0.001$), and *P2ry12* ((**e**), Time: $F_{9,38} = 48.17$, $p < 0.001$) mRNA levels after SCI. Results are presented as mean ± SEM, $n = 5$/group, * $p < 0.05$ and **** $p < 0.0001$. (**f**) Immunofluorescence double labeling of Iba1[+] (green) and Gal3[+] (red, upper panel), CD68[+] (red, middle panel), or CD11b[+] (red, lower panel) cells at 21 and 28 days after SCI. High magnification images represent squared areas in the low magnification images. Scale bars: low magnification = 100 μm and high magnification = 40 μm. CD, cluster of differentiation; Gal3, galectin-3; Iba1, ionized calcium binding adaptor molecule 1.

To evaluate the presence and location of activated microglia/macrophages in the injured spinal cord, we performed double immunofluorescence staining for microglial and macrophage-specific calcium-binding protein (Iba1), together with either galectin-3 (Gal3), a marker for microglial/macrophage activation [41] (upper panel in Figure 7f), the phagocytic lysosomal marker CD68 (middle panel in Figure 7f), or the general leukocyte and microglial marker CD11b (lower panel in Figure 7f) at 21 and 28 days after SCI. At both time points, Gal3, CD68, and CD11b expression was confined to CD11b[+] cells located in the core of the lesion. In the peri-lesion area, only a subpopulation of Iba1[+] cells co-expressed Gal3, CD68, or CD11b, demonstrating that different subsets of microglia express different markers in the peri-lesion area after SCI.

3.8. The Cellular Source of TNF and Its Receptors in Human Traumatic Spinal Cord Injury

Consistent with our mouse studies, we observed that TNF co-localized to a subset of Iba1$^+$ microglia/macrophages (Figure 8a,b) and to a minority of CD68$^+$ phagocytes (Figure 8c) in postmortem tissue derived from individuals with SCI. TNF did not co-localize to GFAP$^+$ astrocytes (Figure 8d). TNFR1 co-localized to NF-L$^+$ proximal dendrites (Figure 8e), and TNFR2 to GFAP$^+$ astrocytes (Figure 8f) as well as Iba1$^+$ microglia (Figure 8g), whereas TNFR2 did not co-localize to NF-L$^+$ neurons (Figure 8h). IL-1β was abundant in the lesioned spinal cord (Figure 8i,j), but only a minority was expressed by Iba1$^+$ microglia (Figure 8j). Similar to our mouse studies (Figure 7b), we observed CD68$^+$Iba1$^+$ phagocytic cells throughout the lesioned spinal cord (Figure 8k,l).

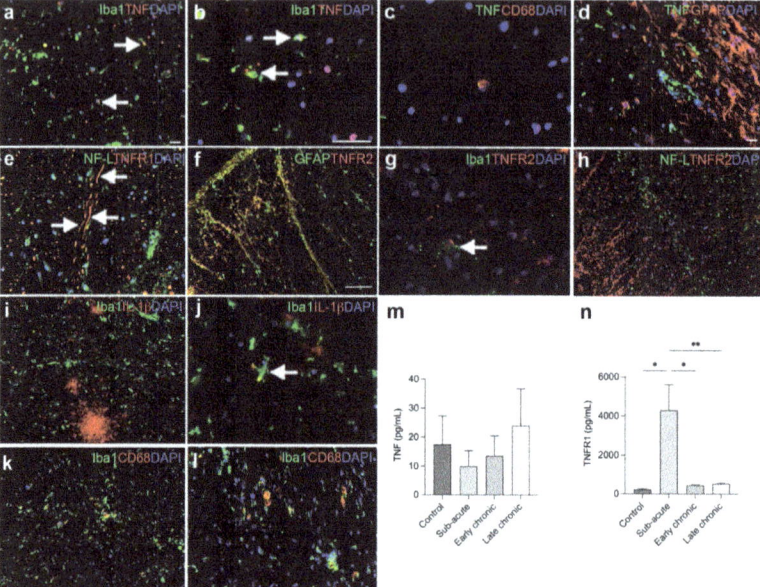

Figure 8. Characterization of TNF and TNFR in individuals with SCI. (**a,b**) Immunofluorescent double labeling of TNF (red) and Iba1 (green) expressing microglia/macrophages (arrows) in the spinal cord of an 33-year-old man with a 3-week-old C6–7 SCI. (**c**) Immunofluorescent double labeling of TNF (green) and CD68 (red) phagocytic cells in the spinal cord of an 65-year-old man with a 5-week-old C5 SCI. (**d**) Immunofluorescent double labeling of TNF$^+$ (green) cells and GFAP$^+$ astrocytes (red) in a 61-year-old man with a 2-week-old C1-2 SCI. (**e**) Immunofluorescent double labeling of TNFR1$^+$ (red) and NF-L$^+$ (green) neuronal fibers in an 67-year-old man with a 6-week-old C5-7 SCI. (**f**) Immunofluorescent double labeling of TNFR2 (red) and astroglial GFAP (green) in an 80-year-old woman with a 2-month-old C8-T1 SCI. (**g**) Immunofluorescent double labelling of TNFR2$^+$ (red) and Iba1$^+$ (green) microglia (arrow) in a 67-year-old man with a 6-week-old C5-7 SCI. (**h**) Immunofluorescent double labeling of TNFR2$^+$ (red) cells and NF-L$^+$ (green) neuronal fibers in an 33-year-old man with a 3-week-old C6-7 SCI. (**i,j**) Immunofluorescent double labeling of IL-1β (red) and Iba1 (green) in a 65-year-old man with a 5-week-old C5 SCI. IL-1β was found to co-localize to a subpopulation of Iba1$^+$ microglia (arrow in h). (**k,l**) Immunofluorescent double labeling of CD68 (red) and Iba1 (green) in a 67-year-old man with a 6-week-old C5-7 SCI (**k**) and a 33-year-old man with a 3-week-old C6-7 SCI (**l**). Scale bars: (**a,d,e,i,l**) = 20 μm; (**b,c,g,j**) = 40 μm; (**f,g,h**) = 100 μm. (**m,n**) CSF TNF (**m**) and TNFR1 (**n**), Time: $F_{3,30}$ = 10.33, p = 0.003) levels in individuals with SCI. Results are expressed as mean ± SEM, n = 5–12/group, * $p < 0.05$,** $p < 0.01$. CD, cluster of differentiation; GFAP, glial fibrillary acidic protein; Iba1, ionized calcium-binding adaptor molecule 1; IL, interleukin; NF-L, neurofilament light chain; TNF, tumor necrosis factor; TNFR, TNF receptor.

Using ELISA analysis, we observed no significant changes in CSF TNF levels between controls and individuals with sub-acute, early chronic, or late chronic SCI (Figure 8k). We observed no correlation between CSF TNF levels and age (Spearman ρ = 0.05, p = 0.84). In contrast, TNFR1 levels were significantly upregulated in individuals with SCI in the acute phase after SCI (Figure 8l). We observed no correlation between CSF TNFR1 levels and age (Spearman ρ = 0.16, p = 0.38).

4. Discussion

In the present study, we investigated neuroinflammatory responses and determined the temporal expression and cellular sources of TNF and its receptors, TNFR1 and TNFR2, in the acute and delayed phases after SCI.

It is well-known that SCI triggers a well-characterized innate cellular immune response initiated by microglia and amplified by peripheral myeloid cells, mainly neutrophils and monocytes, which migrate to the injury site [3]. By 3 days, most glial cells, including astrocytes and microglia, are at the peak of their proliferative state, resulting in the recovery of cell numbers and initiation of astroglial gliosis [42]. At the same time, monocytes differentiate into macrophages [43] and by 7 days, macrophages have reached their peak. In the present study, we found a rapid and transient increase in TNF expression between 1 and 6 h after SCI, followed by a more delayed increase between 3 and 14 days after SCI. The rapid increase in TNF levels implies that TNF is an acute driver of neuroinflammation after SCI, and this is supported by others [10,12–14,44–46]. Early after SCI, TNF was expressed within or just near the lesion, and a few *Tnf* mRNA+ cells were also detected near blood vessels, indicating that as well as modulating neuroinflammation locally, TNF also participates in signaling to the periphery [11,13]. Combined in situ hybridization and immunofluorescent staining for astrocytes co-localized *Tnf* mRNA to a few GFAP+ astrocytes 3 h after SCI, but *Tnf* mRNA+ neuron- and microglial-like cells were also present. Immunohistochemical analysis revealed that TNF was expressed by cells located in proximity to vessels, suggesting that infiltrating immune cells are major producers of TNF in the acute phase after SCI. These findings are supported by previous reports that also demonstrate TNF expression by neurons, microglia, and astrocytes, in addition to oligodendrocytes in the acute phase after SCI [12–14,17,47]. In the present study, we extend previous findings of increased *Tnf* mRNA levels in the delayed phase after SCI [13] by showing increased TNF expression from 3 to 14 days after SCI, correlating with the time points of peripheral immune cells infiltration into the injured spinal cord [40]. By 21 and 28 days after SCI, TNF was expressed mainly by CD11b+ cells, i.e., microglia and possibly infiltrating macrophages [20]. In the human spinal cord, we found TNF to be expressed mainly by Iba1+ cells, i.e., microglia and infiltrating macrophages, and to a lesser extent by CD68+ cells, presumably phagocytosing macrophages, demonstrating the translational relevance of our mouse studies. Speculation has been made as to whether the early increase in TNF expression exhibits the more detrimental role of TNF after SCI [47–49], while the secondary increase promotes neuroprotection and tissue healing [23]. However, blocking TNF with etanercept, a non-selective TNF inhibitor of both tmTNF and solTNF, 14 days after SCI did not affect functional recovery after SCI [18], and we recently showed that myeloid-derived TNF (e.g., macrophages and granulocytes), which are main contributors of TNF in the delayed phase [20], play a detrimental role in SCI [26], thus, leaving the assumption unresolved so far.

TNF mediates its signaling through its two receptors, TNFR1 and TNFR2 [50], and the upregulation of TNFR1 and TNFR2 by neurons, oligodendrocytes, and astrocytes, but not on resting microglia, have been reported in the acute phase after SCI [16]. In the present study, we demonstrated significantly increased *Tnfrsf1a* mRNA levels from 6 h after SCI, while TNFR1 levels increased significantly from 24 h and onwards after SCI. TNFR1 primarily co-localized to the soma of MAP2+ degenerating neurons located in the peri-lesion grey matter and to ascending and descending white matter fiber tracts. This was verified in human postmortem tissue, where TNFR1 co-localized to NF-L+ proximal dendrites in the injured spinal cord. TNFR1 is associated with neurodegeneration [51], and neuronal TNFR1 has been shown to enhance demyelination and exacerbate microglial inflammation [52]. Thus, our findings suggest that chronic inflammation after SCI may be sustained or promoted by increased TNFR1 expression. Additionally, TNFR2 levels increased significantly in the delayed phase after SCI. TNFR2 co-localized to GFAP$^+$ astrocytes and to CD68$^+$ and CD11b$^+$ microglia/macrophages located in the peri-lesion site at 21 and 28 days after SCI in mice. This was supported by our findings of TNFR2 expression by GFAP$^+$ astrocytes and Iba1$^+$ microglia/macrophages in the human spinal cord after SCI. The increase in TNFR2 expression by microglia is believed to be neuroprotective. In support of this, TNFR2 activation on microglia promotes the induction of anti-inflammatory pathways, and TNFR2 ablation in microglia led to the early onset of experimental autoimmune encephalomyelitis, an animal model of multiple sclerosis, with increased leukocyte infiltration, T cell activation, and demyelination [53,54]. Moreover, TNFR2 expression by astrocytes might be important for remyelination after SCI [55,56].

IL-1β, IL-6, and CXCL1 levels also increased rapidly in response to SCI. IL-1β and CXCL10 remained elevated throughout the study, whereas IL-6 returned to baseline levels 7 days after SCI. IL-10 increased only transiently 6 h after SCI. IL-10 is an anti-inflammatory cytokine [57,58] and sustained microglial activation can be inhibited by IL-10 [59]. Thus, the low IL-10 levels in the delayed phase of SCI may help sustain chronic inflammation following SCI [60], a hypothesis that is supported by findings of reduced inflammation, limited neuronal damage, and improved functional recovery following systemic administration of IL-10 in rats subjected to SCI [58,61]. IL-1β levels increased transiently from 6–12 h after SCI and again from day 7 until the end of the experiment, and IL-1β was also highly expressed in the human spinal cord after SCI. IL-1β is known to play a detrimental role in the progression of CNS injury and to contribute to maintaining microglial/macrophage activation [62–64]. IL-1knockout mice show improved locomotor activity, reduced lesion volume, and increased cell survival after SCI [64,65], and acute IL-1 receptor antagonist treatment has been shown to suppress peripheral and central inflammatory responses in SCI [66], suggesting that also IL-1 plays an important role in SCI. We suggest that the early the upregulation of IL-6 that is detected after SCI is detrimental and promotes a pro-inflammatory environment, whereas its expression in the delayed phase might be important for healing after SCI. This is based on observations showing that transiently blocking IL-6 activity in the acute phase improves functional recovery and dampens the neuroinflammatory response after SCI [67]. However, continuously blocking IL-6 signaling suppresses axonal regeneration and causes failed gliosis [68–70]. Our findings of a significant elevation in CXCL1 levels from 6 h after SCI are consistent with its well-known function as a chemokine that attracts peripheral immune cells to the injured cord [71] and identifies CXCL1 as an important player in the acute and chronic inflammatory response after SCI.

In the normal CNS, microglia display high expression of homeostatic markers, such as the purinergic receptor P2RY12 and the fractalkine receptor CX3CR1 [72]. During the first two weeks after SCI, microglia have been shown to proliferate extensively, and they accumulate around the lesion, where they position themselves at the interface between infiltrating leukocytes and astrocytes [73]. The first week after SCI, the lesion area has been shown to contain four different microglial subtypes; homeostatic microglia (predominant in the uninjured spinal cord) and inflammatory, dividing, and migrating nonhomeostatic microglia [74]. Inflammatory microglia, the predominant microglial cell type, were mostly associated with cell death and cytokine production, and were identified by low expression of *P2ry12*. Dividing microglia, mostly related to cell cycle, and migrating microglia also expressed low levels of *P2ry12*. In our study, we found that *P2ry12* levels decreased in the acute phase but restored to uninjured levels and even to increased levels 3 days after SCI. This change was paralleled by similar changes in *Cx3cr1*. *Itgam* levels increased from day 3. We also observed increased microglial numbers and increased activation within the lesion area between 3 and 24 h after SCI, with increased MFI for CD11b and CD45, along with increased levels of pro-inflammatory cytokines in the acute phase after SCI. This supports the findings of inflammatory and dividing nonhomeostatic microglia in the lesioned cord in the acute phase after SCI. Despite the presence of high numbers of cytokine-producing inflammatory and proliferating microglia in the acute phase after SCI, these are essential components of the neuroprotective scar that forms after SCI, and microglial depletion disrupts the glial scar formation, enhances immune infiltration, reduces neuronal and oligodendrocyte survival, and impairs locomotor recovery [73].

In the delayed phase after SCI, we observed that Gal3$^+$ and CD68$^+$ microglia were abundant in the peri-lesion area. CD68 expression is related to phagocytosis, and microglia-dependent pro-myelinating effects have been attributed to Gal3 expression [75], favoring a pro-regenerative phenotype that fosters myelin debris phagocytosis through TREM2 activity [76,77]. As *Trem2* expression increase only transiently 7 days after SCI in the present study, it is possible that microglia in the delayed phase after SCI remain pro-inflammatory and display reduced pro-regenerative capacity, required for proper remyelination. It is likely that the presence of increased solTNF is a key factor keeping microglia, and possibly also macrophages, in a pro-inflammatory state in the more delayed phase after SCI [20,43], i.e., from 7–10 days after injury, when myelin phagocytosing and remyelination processes are occurring [78]. This assumption is supported by previous findings in our laboratory of improved functional recovery and reduced tissue damage following topical inhibition of solTNF [28] and by recent findings using big-data integration and large-scale analytics identifying solTNF as a therapeutic target for SCI [22].

Arg1 expression after SCI (1–7 days post-SCI) has been shown to be highly specific to monocytes/macrophages (versus microglia) but displays macrophage subtype specificity [74]. As the major peripheral myeloid composition at the injury site shifts from monocytes to chemotaxis-inducing macrophages and then to inflammatory macrophages over time, there is a progressive decrease in the classic anti-inflammatory enzyme arginase 1 that is associated with increased pro-inflammatory biological processes in inflammatory macrophages. We observed a significant increase in *Arg1* expression from 24 h to 7 days after SCI, supporting findings that the lesion site becomes populated by inflammatory macrophages in the delayed phases after SCI [79]. This is also consistent with the second increase in IL-1β and TNF in the delayed phase after SCI. Thus, a future challenge is to limit the pro-inflammatory macrophage state without interfering with the beneficial effects of macrophages.

Transected axons are unable to regenerate after SCI and the glial scar, consisting of astrocytes and microglia/macrophages, is thought to be responsible for this. Therefore, manipulating the inflammatory response after SCI may help regulate the formation of the glial scar, allowing for better axonal regrow. Besides therapeutically manipulating the inflammatory response after SCI using, i.e., anti-TNF therapeutics (reviewed by [17]), transplantation with mesenchymal stem cells can inhibit excessive glial scar formation and the inflammatory response leading to improved functional outcome (reviewed by [80]). Another promising cell therapeutic approach is the use of autologous transplantation of patient-derived induced pluripotent stem cell-derived oligodendrocyte precursor cell-enriched neural stem/progenitor cells, as preclinical SCI studies have demonstrated the positive effect of these cells on robust remyelination of demyelinated axons, resulting in improved functional recovery (reviewed by [81,82]).

A limitation of the present study is that only female mice were used. The acute inflammatory profile has been demonstrated to differ between female and male mice [83,84]. Additionally, the inhibition of TNF-TNFR1 signaling has been demonstrated to be therapeutic for neuropathic pain in males but not in females [85], highlighting the importance of incorporating both male and female groups in future SCI research to account for sexual dimorphisms.

Another limitation is that only young mice were used. A recent study by Stewart et al. [83] supported the inflammation after SCI is sex-dependent both at the level of cellular recruitment and phenotype, effects of aging, however, while present, were overall less pronounced. Interestingly though, *Tnf* expression was one of the genes that differed between 4-month-old and 14-month-old SCI mice, whereas sex did not appear to affect *Tnf* expression [83]. How the temporal and cellular expression of TNF changes with age and sex after SCI remains to be elucidated.

5. Conclusions

Our study supports the consensus that neuroprotective immunotherapies aimed against the detrimental immune response, such as the signaling through TNFR1, might effectively suppress the chronic inflammation after SCI and improve recovery.

Supplementary Materials: The following supporting information can be downloaded at: https://www.mdpi.com/article/10.3390/biology11060939/s1, Figure S1: Analysis of microglia/leukocyte populations in the acute phase after SCI; Table S1: Primers for real time RT-qPCR gene amplification.

Author Contributions: Conceptualization, M.C.L., D.G.E. and K.L.L.; methodology, M.C.L., D.G.E., M.N., P.S.N., P.V.N., C.J., H.G., M.D., B.H.C. and K.L.L.; validation, M.C.L., D.G.E., M.D. and K.L.L.; formal analysis, M.C.L., D.G.E., M.N., P.S.N., H.G., M.D. and K.L.L.; investigation, M.C.L., D.G.E., H.G., M.D. and K.L.L.; resources, D.C.A. and R.B.; data curation, M.C.L. and K.L.L.; writing—original draft preparation, M.C.L. and K.L.L.; writing—review and editing, D.G.E., M.N., P.S.N., C.J., H.G., R.B., M.D., B.H.C. and K.L.L.; visualization, M.C.L. and K.L.L.; supervision, K.L.L.; project administration, K.L.L.; funding acquisition, M.C.L., H.G. and K.L.L. All authors have read and agreed to the published version of the manuscript.

Funding: This research was generously funded by the Lundbeck Foundation (R230–2016-3019), Fonden til Lægevidenskabens Fremme, Overlægerådets Legatudvalg–Odense University Hospital (M.C.L.), and the National Science Foundation for Distinguished Young Scholars of China (82001316, H.G.).

Institutional Review Board Statement: Recruitment of individuals with SCI was conducted in accordance with guidelines for clinical studies approved by the Third Affiliated Hospital of Sun Yat-sen University review board ([2018]-02, [2018]-03, [2018]-04). Postmortem human spinal cord samples were obtained from The Miami Project Human Core Bank at the University of Miami Miller School of Medicine managed by Alexander Marcillo and Yan Shi.

Informed Consent Statement: Informed consent was obtained from all subjects involved in the study.

Data Availability Statement: Requests to access datasets should be directed to klambertsen@health.sdu.dk.

Acknowledgments: We are grateful for the technical assistance provided by Ulla Damgaard Munk and proofreading by Claire Gudex.

Conflicts of Interest: The authors declare no conflict of interest and the funders had no role in the design of the study; in the collection, analyses, or interpretation of data; in the writing of the manuscript, or in the decision to publish the results.

References

1. Liu, N.K.; Xu, X.M. Neuroprotection and its molecular mechanism following spinal cord injury. *Neural Regen. Res.* **2012**, *7*, 2051–2062. [CrossRef]
2. Trivedi, A.; Olivas, A.D.; Noble-Haeusslein, L.J. Inflammation and Spinal Cord Injury: Infiltrating Leukocytes as Determinants of Injury and Repair Processes. *Clin. Neurosci. Res.* **2006**, *6*, 283–292. [CrossRef] [PubMed]
3. Beck, K.D.; Nguyen, H.X.; Galvan, M.D.; Salazar, D.L.; Woodruff, T.M.; Anderson, A.J. Quantitative analysis of cellular inflammation after traumatic spinal cord injury: Evidence for a multiphasic inflammatory response in the acute to chronic environment. *Brain* **2010**, *133*, 433–447. [CrossRef] [PubMed]
4. Bastien, D.; Lacroix, S. Cytokine pathways regulating glial and leukocyte function after spinal cord and peripheral nerve injury. *Exp. Neurol.* **2014**, *258*, 62–77. [CrossRef]
5. Fischer, R.; Kontermann, R.E.; Pfizenmaier, K. Selective Targeting of TNF Receptors as a Novel Therapeutic Approach. *Front. Cell Dev. Biol.* **2020**, *8*, 401. [CrossRef] [PubMed]
6. Atretkhany, K.N.; Gogoleva, V.S.; Drutskaya, M.S.; Nedospasov, S.A. Distinct modes of TNF signaling through its two receptors in health and disease. *J. Leukoc. Biol.* **2020**, *107*, 893–905. [CrossRef]
7. Varfolomeev, E.; Vucic, D. Intracellular regulation of TNF activity in health and disease. *Cytokine* **2018**, *101*, 26–32. [CrossRef]
8. Wajant, H.; Pfizenmaier, K.; Scheurich, P. Tumor necrosis factor signaling. *Cell Death Differ.* **2003**, *10*, 45–65. [CrossRef]

9. Brambilla, R.; Ashbaugh, J.J.; Magliozzi, R.; Dellarole, A.; Karmally, S.; Szymkowski, D.E.; Bethea, J.R. Inhibition of soluble tumour necrosis factor is therapeutic in experimental autoimmune encephalomyelitis and promotes axon preservation and remyelination. *Brain* **2011**, *134*, 2736–2754. [CrossRef]
10. Wang, C.X.; Nuttin, B.; Heremans, H.; Dom, R.; Gybels, J. Production of tumor necrosis factor in spinal cord following traumatic injury in rats. *J. Neuroimmunol.* **1996**, *69*, 151–156. [CrossRef]
11. Bartholdi, D.; Schwab, M.E. Expression of pro-inflammatory cytokine and chemokine mRNA upon experimental spinal cord injury in mouse: An in situ hybridization study. *Eur. J. Neurosci.* **1997**, *9*, 1422–1438. [CrossRef]
12. Yan, P.; Li, Q.; Kim, G.M.; Xu, J.; Hsu, C.Y.; Xu, X.M. Cellular localization of tumor necrosis factor-alpha following acute spinal cord injury in adult rats. *J. Neurotrauma* **2001**, *18*, 563–568. [CrossRef]
13. Pineau, I.; Lacroix, S. Proinflammatory cytokine synthesis in the injured mouse spinal cord: Multiphasic expression pattern and identification of the cell types involved. *J. Comp. Neurol.* **2007**, *500*, 267–285. [CrossRef]
14. Yune, T.Y.; Chang, M.J.; Kim, S.J.; Lee, Y.B.; Shin, S.W.; Rhim, H.; Kim, Y.C.; Shin, M.L.; Oh, Y.J.; Han, C.T.; et al. Increased production of tumor necrosis factor-alpha induces apoptosis after traumatic spinal cord injury in rats. *J. Neurotrauma* **2003**, *20*, 207–219. [CrossRef]
15. Yang, L.; Blumbergs, P.C.; Jones, N.R.; Manavis, J.; Sarvestani, G.T.; Ghabriel, M.N. Early expression and cellular localization of proinflammatory cytokines interleukin-1beta, interleukin-6, and tumor necrosis factor-alpha in human traumatic spinal cord injury. *Spine* **2004**, *29*, 966–971. [CrossRef]
16. Yan, P.; Liu, N.; Kim, G.M.; Xu, J.; Li, Q.; Hsu, C.Y.; Xu, X.M. Expression of the type 1 and type 2 receptors for tumor necrosis factor after traumatic spinal cord injury in adult rats. *Exp. Neurol.* **2003**, *183*, 286–297. [CrossRef]
17. Lund, M.C.; Clausen, B.H.; Brambilla, R.; Lambertsen, K.L. The Role of Tumor Necrosis Factor Following Spinal Cord Injury: A Systematic Review. *Cell. Mol. Neurobiol.* **2022**. [CrossRef]
18. Vidal, P.M.; Lemmens, E.; Geboes, L.; Vangansewinkel, T.; Nelissen, S.; Hendrix, S. Late blocking of peripheral TNF-alpha is ineffective after spinal cord injury in mice. *Immunobiology* **2013**, *218*, 281–284. [CrossRef]
19. Esposito, E.; Cuzzocrea, S. Anti-TNF therapy in the injured spinal cord. *Trends Pharmacol. Sci.* **2011**, *32*, 107–115. [CrossRef]
20. Kroner, A.; Greenhalgh, A.D.; Zarruk, J.G.; Passos Dos Santos, R.; Gaestel, M.; David, S. TNF and increased intracellular iron alter macrophage polarization to a detrimental M1 phenotype in the injured spinal cord. *Neuron* **2014**, *83*, 1098–1116. [CrossRef]
21. Genovese, T.; Mazzon, E.; Crisafulli, C.; Di Paola, R.; Muia, C.; Esposito, E.; Bramanti, P.; Cuzzocrea, S. TNF-alpha blockage in a mouse model of SCI: Evidence for improved outcome. *Shock* **2008**, *29*, 32–41. [CrossRef] [PubMed]
22. Huie, J.R.; Ferguson, A.R.; Kyritsis, N.; Pan, J.Z.; Irvine, K.A.; Nielson, J.L.; Schupp, P.G.; Oldham, M.C.; Gensel, J.C.; Lin, A.; et al. Machine intelligence identifies soluble TNFa as a therapeutic target for spinal cord injury. *Sci. Rep.* **2021**, *11*, 3442. [CrossRef] [PubMed]
23. Chi, L.Y.; Yu, J.; Zhu, H.; Li, X.G.; Zhu, S.G.; Kindy, M.S. The dual role of tumor necrosis factor-alpha in the pathophysiology of spinal cord injury. *Neurosci. Lett.* **2008**, *438*, 174–179. [CrossRef] [PubMed]
24. Kim, G.M.; Xu, J.; Song, S.K.; Yan, P.; Ku, G.; Xu, X.M.; Hsu, C.Y. Tumor necrosis factor receptor deletion reduces nuclear factor-kappaB activation, cellular inhibitor of apoptosis protein 2 expression, and functional recovery after traumatic spinal cord injury. *J. Neurosci.* **2001**, *21*, 6617–6625. [CrossRef]
25. Ellman, D.G.; Degn, M.; Lund, M.C.; Clausen, B.H.; Novrup, H.G.; Flaeng, S.B.; Jorgensen, L.H.; Suntharalingam, L.; Svenningsen, A.F.; Brambilla, R.; et al. Genetic Ablation of Soluble TNF Does Not Affect Lesion Size and Functional Recovery after Moderate Spinal Cord Injury in Mice. *Mediat. Inflamm.* **2016**, *2016*, 2684098. [CrossRef]
26. Ellman, D.G.; Lund, M.C.; Nissen, M.; Nielsen, P.S.; Sorensen, C.; Lester, E.B.; Thougaard, E.; Jorgensen, L.H.; Nedospasov, S.A.; Andersen, D.C.; et al. Conditional Ablation of Myeloid TNF Improves Functional Outcome and Decreases Lesion Size after Spinal Cord Injury in Mice. *Cells* **2020**, *9*, 2407. [CrossRef]
27. Farooque, M.; Isaksson, J.; Olsson, Y. Improved recovery after spinal cord injury in neuronal nitric oxide synthase-deficient mice but not in TNF-alpha-deficient mice. *J. Neurotrauma* **2001**, *18*, 105–114. [CrossRef]
28. Novrup, H.G.; Bracchi-Ricard, V.; Ellman, D.G.; Ricard, J.; Jain, A.; Runko, E.; Lyck, L.; Yli-Karjanmaa, M.; Szymkowski, D.E.; Pearse, D.D.; et al. Central but not systemic administration of XPro1595 is therapeutic following moderate spinal cord injury in mice. *J. Neuroinflamm.* **2014**, *11*, 159. [CrossRef]
29. Chen, K.B.; Uchida, K.; Nakajima, H.; Yayama, T.; Hirai, T.; Watanabe, S.; Guerrero, A.R.; Kobayashi, S.; Ma, W.Y.; Liu, S.Y.; et al. Tumor necrosis factor-alpha antagonist reduces apoptosis of neurons and oligodendroglia in rat spinal cord injury. *Spine* **2011**, *36*, 1350–1358. [CrossRef]
30. Pasparakis, M.; Alexopoulou, L.; Episkopou, V.; Kollias, G. Immune and inflammatory responses in TNF alpha-deficient mice: A critical requirement for TNF alpha in the formation of primary B cell follicles, follicular dendritic cell networks and germinal centers, and in the maturation of the humoral immune response. *J. Exp. Med.* **1996**, *184*, 1397–1411. [CrossRef]
31. Lambertsen, K.L.; Clausen, B.H.; Babcock, A.A.; Gregersen, R.; Fenger, C.; Nielsen, H.H.; Haugaard, L.S.; Wirenfeldt, M.; Nielsen, M.; Dagnaes-Hansen, F.; et al. Microglia protect neurons against ischemia by synthesis of tumor necrosis factor. *J. Neurosci.* **2009**, *29*, 1319–1330. [CrossRef]
32. Harrison, M.; O'Brien, A.; Adams, L.; Cowin, G.; Ruitenberg, M.J.; Sengul, G.; Watson, C. Vertebral landmarks for the identification of spinal cord segments in the mouse. *Neuroimage* **2013**, *68*, 22–29. [CrossRef]

33. Basso, D.M.; Fisher, L.C.; Anderson, A.J.; Jakeman, L.B.; McTigue, D.M.; Popovich, P.G. Basso Mouse Scale for locomotion detects differences in recovery after spinal cord injury in five common mouse strains. *J. Neurotrauma* **2006**, *23*, 635–659. [CrossRef]
34. Kibbe, W.A. OligoCalc: An online oligonucleotide properties calculator. *Nucleic Acids Res.* **2007**, *35*, W43–W46. [CrossRef]
35. Pfaffl, M.W. A new mathematical model for relative quantification in real-time RT-PCR. *Nucleic Acids Res.* **2001**, *29*, e45. [CrossRef]
36. Lambertsen, K.L.; Meldgaard, M.; Ladeby, R.; Finsen, B. A quantitative study of microglial-macrophage synthesis of tumor necrosis factor during acute and late focal cerebral ischemia in mice. *J. Cereb. Blood Flow Metab.* **2005**, *25*, 119–135. [CrossRef]
37. Lambertsen, K.L.; Gregersen, R.; Drojdahl, N.; Owens, T.; Finsen, B. A specific and sensitive method for visualization of tumor necrosis factor in the murine central nervous system. *Brain Res. Protoc.* **2001**, *7*, 175–191. [CrossRef]
38. Clausen, B.H.; Wirenfeldt, M.; Hogedal, S.S.; Frich, L.H.; Nielsen, H.H.; Schroder, H.D.; Ostergaard, K.; Finsen, B.; Kristensen, B.W.; Lambertsen, K.L. Characterization of the TNF and IL-1 systems in human brain and blood after ischemic stroke. *Acta Neuropathol. Commun.* **2020**, *8*, 81. [CrossRef]
39. Clausen, B.; Degn, M.; Martin, N.; Couch, Y.; Karimi, L.; Ormhoj, M.; Mortensen, M.L.; Gredal, H.; Gardiner, C.; Sargent, I.I.; et al. Systemically administered anti-TNF therapy ameliorates functional outcomes after focal cerebral ischemia. *J. Neuroinflamm.* **2014**, *11*, 203. [CrossRef]
40. Donnelly, D.J.; Popovich, P.G. Inflammation and its role in neuroprotection, axonal regeneration and functional recovery after spinal cord injury. *Exp. Neurol.* **2008**, *209*, 378–388. [CrossRef]
41. Tan, Y.; Zheng, Y.; Xu, D.; Sun, Z.; Yang, H.; Yin, Q. Galectin-3: A key player in microglia-mediated neuroinflammation and Alzheimer's disease. *Cell Biosci.* **2021**, *11*, 78. [CrossRef] [PubMed]
42. White, R.E.; McTigue, D.M.; Jakeman, L.B. Regional heterogeneity in astrocyte responses following contusive spinal cord injury in mice. *J. Comp. Neurol.* **2010**, *518*, 1370–1390. [CrossRef]
43. Kigerl, K.A.; Gensel, J.C.; Ankeny, D.P.; Alexander, J.K.; Donnelly, D.J.; Popovich, P.G. Identification of two distinct macrophage subsets with divergent effects causing either neurotoxicity or regeneration in the injured mouse spinal cord. *J. Neurosci.* **2009**, *29*, 13435–13444. [CrossRef] [PubMed]
44. Lee, Y.L.; Shih, K.; Bao, P.; Ghirnikar, R.S.; Eng, L.F. Cytokine chemokine expression in contused rat spinal cord. *Neurochem. Int.* **2000**, *36*, 417–425. [CrossRef]
45. Wang, C.X.; Reece, C.; Wrathall, J.R.; Shuaib, A.; Olschowka, J.A.; Hao, C. Expression of tumor necrosis factor alpha and its mRNA in the spinal cord following a weight-drop injury. *Neuroreport* **2002**, *13*, 1391–1393. [CrossRef] [PubMed]
46. Brambilla, R.; Bracchi-Ricard, V.; Hu, W.H.; Frydel, B.; Bramwell, A.; Karmally, S.; Green, E.J.; Bethea, J.R. Inhibition of astroglial nuclear factor kappaB reduces inflammation and improves functional recovery after spinal cord injury. *J. Exp. Med.* **2005**, *202*, 145–156. [CrossRef] [PubMed]
47. Simmons, R.D.; Willenborg, D.O. Direct injection of cytokines into the spinal cord causes autoimmune encephalomyelitis-like inflammation. *J. Neurol. Sci.* **1990**, *100*, 37–42. [CrossRef]
48. D'Souza, S.; Alinauskas, K.; McCrea, E.; Goodyer, C.; Antel, J.P. Differential susceptibility of human CNS-derived cell populations to TNF-dependent and independent immune-mediated injury. *J. Neurosci.* **1995**, *15*, 7293–7300. [CrossRef]
49. Akassoglou, K.; Bauer, J.; Kassiotis, G.; Pasparakis, M.; Lassmann, H.; Kollias, G.; Probert, L. Oligodendrocyte apoptosis and primary demyelination induced by local TNF/p55TNF receptor signaling in the central nervous system of transgenic mice: Models for multiple sclerosis with primary oligodendrogliopathy. *Am. J. Pathol.* **1998**, *153*, 801–813. [CrossRef]
50. McCoy, M.K.; Tansey, M.G. TNF signaling inhibition in the CNS: Implications for normal brain function and neurodegenerative disease. *J. Neuroinflamm.* **2008**, *5*, 45. [CrossRef]
51. Fischer, R.; Maier, O.; Siegemund, M.; Wajant, H.; Scheurich, P.; Pfizenmaier, K. A TNF receptor 2 selective agonist rescues human neurons from oxidative stress-induced cell death. *PLoS ONE* **2011**, *6*, e27621. [CrossRef]
52. Papazian, I.; Tsoukala, E.; Boutou, A.; Karamita, M.; Kambas, K.; Iliopoulou, L.; Fischer, R.; Kontermann, R.E.; Denis, M.C.; Kollias, G.; et al. Fundamentally different roles of neuronal TNF receptors in CNS pathology: TNFR1 and IKKbeta promote microglial responses and tissue injury in demyelination while TNFR2 protects against excitotoxicity in mice. *J. Neuroinflamm.* **2021**, *18*, 222. [CrossRef]
53. Veroni, C.; Gabriele, L.; Canini, I.; Castiello, L.; Coccia, E.; Remoli, M.E.; Columba-Cabezas, S.; Arico, E.; Aloisi, F.; Agresti, C. Activation of TNF receptor 2 in microglia promotes induction of anti-inflammatory pathways. *Mol. Cell. Neurosci.* **2010**, *45*, 234–244. [CrossRef]
54. Gao, H.; Danzi, M.C.; Choi, C.S.; Taherian, M.; Dalby-Hansen, C.; Ellman, D.G.; Madsen, P.M.; Bixby, J.L.; Lemmon, V.P.; Lambertsen, K.L.; et al. Opposing Functions of Microglial and Macrophagic TNFR2 in the Pathogenesis of Experimental Autoimmune Encephalomyelitis. *Cell Rep.* **2017**, *18*, 198–212. [CrossRef]
55. Patel, J.R.; Williams, J.L.; Muccigrosso, M.M.; Liu, L.; Sun, T.; Rubin, J.B.; Klein, R.S. Astrocyte TNFR2 is required for CXCL12-mediated regulation of oligodendrocyte progenitor proliferation and differentiation within the adult CNS. *Acta Neuropathol.* **2012**, *124*, 847–860. [CrossRef]
56. Fischer, R.; Wajant, H.; Kontermann, R.; Pfizenmaier, K.; Maier, O. Astrocyte-specific activation of TNFR2 promotes oligodendrocyte maturation by secretion of leukemia inhibitory factor. *Glia* **2014**, *62*, 272–283. [CrossRef]
57. Hellenbrand, D.J.; Reichl, K.A.; Travis, B.J.; Filipp, M.E.; Khalil, A.S.; Pulito, D.J.; Gavigan, A.V.; Maginot, E.R.; Arnold, M.T.; Adler, A.G.; et al. Sustained interleukin-10 delivery reduces inflammation and improves motor function after spinal cord injury. *J. Neuroinflamm.* **2019**, *16*, 93. [CrossRef]

58. Bethea, J.R.; Nagashima, H.; Acosta, M.C.; Briceno, C.; Gomez, F.; Marcillo, A.E.; Loor, K.; Green, J.; Dietrich, W.D. Systemically administered interleukin-10 reduces tumor necrosis factor-alpha production and significantly improves functional recovery following traumatic spinal cord injury in rats. *J. Neurotrauma* **1999**, *16*, 851–863. [CrossRef]
59. Kuno, R.; Wang, J.; Kawanokuchi, J.; Takeuchi, H.; Mizuno, T.; Suzumura, A. Autocrine activation of microglia by tumor necrosis factor-alpha. *J. Neuroimmunol.* **2005**, *162*, 89–96. [CrossRef]
60. Wang, C.X.; Olschowka, J.A.; Wrathall, J.R. Increase of interleukin-1beta mRNA and protein in the spinal cord following experimental traumatic injury in the rat. *Brain Res.* **1997**, *759*, 190–196. [CrossRef]
61. Plunkett, J.A.; Yu, C.G.; Easton, J.M.; Bethea, J.R.; Yezierski, R.P. Effects of interleukin-10 (IL-10) on pain behavior and gene expression following excitotoxic spinal cord injury in the rat. *Exp. Neurol.* **2001**, *168*, 144–154. [CrossRef] [PubMed]
62. Giulian, D.; Woodward, J.; Young, D.G.; Krebs, J.F.; Lachman, L.B. Interleukin-1 injected into mammalian brain stimulates astrogliosis and neovascularization. *J. Neurosci.* **1988**, *8*, 2485–2490. [CrossRef]
63. Bayrakli, F.; Kurtuncu, M.; Karaarslan, E.; Ozgen, S. Perineural cyst presenting like cubital tunnel syndrome. *Eur. Spine J.* **2012**, *21* (Suppl. S4), S387–S389. [CrossRef] [PubMed]
64. Sato, A.; Ohtaki, H.; Tsumuraya, T.; Song, D.; Ohara, K.; Asano, M.; Iwakura, Y.; Atsumi, T.; Shioda, S. Interleukin-1 participates in the classical and alternative activation of microglia/macrophages after spinal cord injury. *J. Neuroinflamm.* **2012**, *9*, 65. [CrossRef] [PubMed]
65. Bastien, D.; Bellver Landete, V.; Lessard, M.; Vallieres, N.; Champagne, M.; Takashima, A.; Tremblay, M.E.; Doyon, Y.; Lacroix, S. IL-1alpha Gene Deletion Protects Oligodendrocytes after Spinal Cord Injury through Upregulation of the Survival Factor Tox3. *J. Neurosci.* **2015**, *35*, 10715–10730. [CrossRef] [PubMed]
66. Yates, A.G.; Jogia, T.; Gillespie, E.R.; Couch, Y.; Ruitenberg, M.J.; Anthony, D.C. Acute IL-1RA treatment suppresses the peripheral and central inflammatory response to spinal cord injury. *J. Neuroinflamm.* **2021**, *18*, 15. [CrossRef] [PubMed]
67. Guerrero, A.R.; Uchida, K.; Nakajima, H.; Watanabe, S.; Nakamura, M.; Johnson, W.E.; Baba, H. Blockade of interleukin-6 signaling inhibits the classic pathway and promotes an alternative pathway of macrophage activation after spinal cord injury in mice. *J. Neuroinflamm.* **2012**, *9*, 40. [CrossRef]
68. Mukaino, M.; Nakamura, M.; Yamada, O.; Okada, S.; Morikawa, S.; Renault-Mihara, F.; Iwanami, A.; Ikegami, T.; Ohsugi, Y.; Tsuji, O.; et al. Anti-IL-6-receptor antibody promotes repair of spinal cord injury by inducing microglia-dominant inflammation. *Exp. Neurol.* **2010**, *224*, 403–414. [CrossRef]
69. Cafferty, W.B.; Gardiner, N.J.; Das, P.; Qiu, J.; McMahon, S.B.; Thompson, S.W. Conditioning injury-induced spinal axon regeneration fails in interleukin-6 knock-out mice. *J. Neurosci.* **2004**, *24*, 4432–4443. [CrossRef]
70. Okada, S.; Nakamura, M.; Katoh, H.; Miyao, T.; Shimazaki, T.; Ishii, K.; Yamane, J.; Yoshimura, A.; Iwamoto, Y.; Toyama, Y.; et al. Conditional ablation of Stat3 or Socs3 discloses a dual role for reactive astrocytes after spinal cord injury. *Nat. Med.* **2006**, *12*, 829–834. [CrossRef]
71. Neirinckx, V.; Coste, C.; Franzen, R.; Gothot, A.; Rogister, B.; Wislet, S. Neutrophil contribution to spinal cord injury and repair. *J. Neuroinflamm.* **2014**, *11*, 150. [CrossRef]
72. Masuda, T.; Amann, L.; Sankowski, R.; Staszewski, O.; Lenz, M.; Errico, P.D.; Snaidero, N.; Costa Jordao, M.J.; Bottcher, C.; Kierdorf, K.; et al. Novel Hexb-based tools for studying microglia in the CNS. *Nat. Immunol.* **2020**, *21*, 802–815. [CrossRef]
73. Bellver-Landete, V.; Bretheau, F.; Mailhot, B.; Vallieres, N.; Lessard, M.; Janelle, M.E.; Vernoux, N.; Tremblay, M.E.; Fuehrmann, T.; Shoichet, M.S.; et al. Microglia are an essential component of the neuroprotective scar that forms after spinal cord injury. *Nat. Commun.* **2019**, *10*, 518. [CrossRef]
74. Milich, L.M.; Choi, J.; Ryan, C.; Yahn, S.L.; Tsoulfas, P.; Lee, J.K. Single cell analysis of the cellular heterogeneity and interactions in the injured mouse spinal cord. *J. Exp. Med.* **2021**, *218*, e20210040. [CrossRef]
75. Thomas, L.; Pasquini, L.A. Galectin-3-Mediated Glial Crosstalk Drives Oligodendrocyte Differentiation and (Re)myelination. *Front. Cell. Neurosci.* **2018**, *12*, 297. [CrossRef]
76. Hoyos, H.C.; Rinaldi, M.; Mendez-Huergo, S.P.; Marder, M.; Rabinovich, G.A.; Pasquini, J.M.; Pasquini, L.A. Galectin-3 controls the response of microglial cells to limit cuprizone-induced demyelination. *Neurobiol. Dis.* **2014**, *62*, 441–455. [CrossRef]
77. Nugent, A.A.; Lin, K.; van Lengerich, B.; Lianoglou, S.; Przybyla, L.; Davis, S.S.; Llapashtica, C.; Wang, J.; Kim, D.J.; Xia, D.; et al. TREM2 Regulates Microglial Cholesterol Metabolism upon Chronic Phagocytic Challenge. *Neuron* **2020**, *105*, 837–854. [CrossRef]
78. Greenhalgh, A.D.; David, S. Differences in the phagocytic response of microglia and peripheral macrophages after spinal cord injury and its effects on cell death. *J. Neurosci.* **2014**, *34*, 6316–6322. [CrossRef]
79. Nakajima, H.; Honjoh, K.; Watanabe, S.; Kubota, A.; Matsumine, A. Distribution and polarization of microglia and macrophages at injured sites and the lumbar enlargement after spinal cord injury. *Neurosci. Lett.* **2020**, *737*, 135152. [CrossRef]
80. Pang, Q.M.; Chen, S.Y.; Xu, Q.J.; Fu, S.P.; Yang, Y.C.; Zou, W.H.; Zhang, M.; Liu, J.; Wan, W.H.; Peng, J.C.; et al. Neuroinflammation and Scarring After Spinal Cord Injury: Therapeutic Roles of MSCs on Inflammation and Glial Scar. *Front. Immunol.* **2021**, *12*, 751021. [CrossRef]
81. Khazaei, M.; Siddiqui, A.M.; Fehlings, M.G. The Potential for iPS-Derived Stem Cells as a Therapeutic Strategy for Spinal Cord Injury: Opportunities and Challenges. *J. Clin. Med.* **2014**, *4*, 37–65. [CrossRef]
82. Kawabata, S.; Takano, M.; Numasawa-Kuroiwa, Y.; Itakura, G.; Kobayashi, Y.; Nishiyama, Y.; Sugai, K.; Nishimura, S.; Iwai, H.; Isoda, M.; et al. Grafted Human iPS Cell-Derived Oligodendrocyte Precursor Cells Contribute to Robust Remyelination of Demyelinated Axons after Spinal Cord Injury. *Stem Cell Rep.* **2016**, *6*, 1–8. [CrossRef]

83. Stewart, A.N.; Lowe, J.L.; Glaser, E.P.; Mott, C.A.; Shahidehpour, R.K.; McFarlane, K.E.; Bailey, W.M.; Zhang, B.; Gensel, J.C. Acute inflammatory profiles differ with sex and age after spinal cord injury. *J. Neuroinflamm.* **2021**, *18*, 113. [CrossRef] [PubMed]
84. Stewart, A.N.; MacLean, S.M.; Stromberg, A.J.; Whelan, J.P.; Bailey, W.M.; Gensel, J.C.; Wilson, M.E. Considerations for Studying Sex as a Biological Variable in Spinal Cord Injury. *Front. Neurol.* **2020**, *11*, 802. [CrossRef]
85. Del Rivero, T.; Fischer, R.; Yang, F.; Swanson, K.A.; Bethea, J.R. Tumor necrosis factor receptor 1 inhibition is therapeutic for neuropathic pain in males but not in females. *Pain* **2019**, *160*, 922–931. [CrossRef]

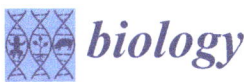

Review

Inflammation and Oxidative Stress as Common Mechanisms of Pulmonary, Autonomic and Musculoskeletal Dysfunction after Spinal Cord Injury

Cristián Rosales-Antequera [1,2], Ginés Viscor [3] and Oscar F. Araneda [2,*]

1. Physical Medicine and Rehabilitation Unit, Clínica Universidad de los Andes, Santiago 8320000, Chile; carosales@miuandes.cl
2. Integrative Laboratory of Biomechanics and Physiology of Effort, LIBFE, School of Kinesiology, Faculty of Medicine, Universidad de los Andes, Santiago 8320000, Chile
3. Physiology Section, Department of Cell Biology, Physiology and Immunology, Faculty of Biology, Universitat de Barcelona, 08028 Barcelona, Spain; gviscor@ub.edu
* Correspondence: ofaraneda@miuandes.cl

Simple Summary: When a spinal cord injury occurs, the neurons that regulate our voluntary movements, those involved in environment and somatic perception and those that regulate vegetative functions are affected. Once neuronal damage is established, the cells of other tissues are also affected in their functions, altering the interaction between organs and altering the proper functioning of the organism. Multiple studies in animal models, as well as in humans, have recognized as factors involved in organ damage the imbalance between the formation of highly reactive molecules called pro-oxidants and defensive mechanisms called antioxidants. Closely associated with this phenomenon, the inflammatory response is also pathologically activated. In this narrative review, we have analyzed the information involving these pathological processes at the level of the lung, the autonomic nervous system and the skeletal musculature after spinal cord injury. Knowing the abnormal functioning mechanisms that occur after a spinal cord injury not only offers a better understanding of the organic events but also offers future possibilities for therapeutic interventions that may benefit the thousands of patients suffering this pathology.

Abstract: One of the etiopathogenic factors frequently associated with generalized organ damage after spinal cord injury corresponds to the imbalance of the redox state and inflammation, particularly of the respiratory, autonomic and musculoskeletal systems. Our goal in this review was to gain a better understanding of this phenomenon by reviewing both animal and human studies. At the respiratory level, the presence of tissue damage is notable in situations that require increased ventilation due to lower thoracic distensibility and alveolar inflammation caused by higher levels of leptin as a result of increased fatty tissue. Increased airway reactivity, due to loss of sympathetic innervation, and levels of nitric oxide in exhaled air that are similar to those seen in asthmatic patients have also been reported. In addition, the loss of autonomic control efficiency leads to an uncontrolled release of catecholamines and glucocorticoids that induce immunosuppression, as well as a predisposition to autoimmune reactions. Simultaneously, blood pressure regulation is altered with vascular damage and atherogenesis associated with oxidative damage. At the muscular level, chronically elevated levels of prooxidants and lipoperoxidation associated with myofibrillar atrophy are described, with no reduction or reversibility of this process through antioxidant supplementation.

Keywords: spinal cord injury; pathophysiology; inflammation; oxidative stress

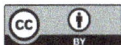

1. Introduction

Globally, the WHO estimates that between 250,000 and 500,000 people suffer from a spinal cord injury (SCI) on an annual basis, mainly associated with traffic accidents, falls or acts of violence [1].

Once the traumatic event is identified using traction and compression, ischemia-hypoxia in the areas of vascular compromise is shown involving the release of pro-inflammatory cytokines [2] and the attraction of immune cells that damage local nervous tissue via necrosis/apoptosis, both directly and through the promotion of autoimmune-type phenomena [3]. Consequently, the degree of impact on organic functions will depend on the level of the spinal cord injury. The compromise of spinal cord function has both acute and chronic effects that simultaneously alter voluntary motor control and, thus, the action of the functional bone/musculoskeletal dyad of the locomotor system, as well as the various functions of the autonomic nervous system, which have an impact on the genito-urinary control, the motility of the digestive system, the control of the respiratory system and the action of the cardiovascular system [4]. In the long term, these events promote changes in body composition [5] and increase the development of infectious [6], autoimmune processes [7], disorders of endocrine function and metabolic control that are associated with increased morbidity and mortality [8].

Secondary to the SCI, patients show alterations in the functions of different body systems. Thus, at the respiratory level, the functional residual capacity (FRC) and the forced expiratory volume in one second (FEV1) decrease, the respiratory pattern changes and the maximum inspiratory/expiratory pressure decreases [9]. Furthermore, this group has the mechanism of coughing altered by a stiffer thoracic cavity that generates greater respiratory work along with the presence of bronchial obstruction and hyperresponsiveness [10]. In addition, there are respiratory disorders during sleep, such as obstructive sleep apnea, which causes chronic intermittent hypoxia [9,11]. These effects can explain the high prevalence of symptoms like dyspnea, chronic cough, bronchial hypersecretion and an increased susceptibility to respiratory tract infections [9,12].

Another affected system in patients with SCI is the autonomic nervous system, which alters cardiovascular and respiratory regulation, leading to variable and abnormal functioning [1]. This autonomous deregulation induces neuroendocrine changes that can trigger the imbalance of the redox state and promote chronic tissue inflammation [13]. The alteration of the functioning of the autonomic nerve pathways generates a loss of efficiency in the control of the cardiovascular system, affecting both the regulation of blood pressure and heart rate [14]. It also affects the body's cooling mechanisms, apparently by the alteration of the vasomotor tone and a decrease in afferents towards the thermoregulatory centers, which generates a loss of the ability to sweat [15]. Finally, the deregulation of this system has also been associated with a case of immune deficiency [16].

Skeletal muscle is also affected prematurely after spinal cord injury, rapidly suffering significant atrophy [17]. Regarding the mechanisms involved in this process, it has been possible to identify the participation of oxidative imbalance as a key factor involved in the phenomena of muscle protein synthesis and degradation [18–20].

There is currently abundant information that involves the damage mechanisms associated with SCI, inflammation and oxidative stress. In this way, we have set ourselves the objective of describing, through a narrative review, the scientific evidence obtained from animal models and studies carried out in humans that involve these pathogenic factors with damage to the respiratory, autonomic and muscular systems typical of SCI. The selection of the chosen works was limited to original works and of review articles accessible through the PubMed search engine without publication date limits.

2. Respiratory System

Ventilatory changes: Spinal cord injury involves nerve damage that is generally described from the sensory to the muscular system. However, the muscle paralysis that the spinal cord injury generates not only involves the locomotor musculature, but rather, depending on the level of the injury, it also affects the respiratory musculature to a greater or lesser extent, which can establish changes in ventilatory pattern [21].

The respiratory musculature generates the alveolar pressure changes necessary to produce pulmonary ventilation. Thus, its involvement can lead to poor performance of the cough mechanism and atelectasis caused by deficient pulmonary ventilation [21,22].

Mateus et al. [23], through spirometry and maximal static respiratory pressure tests, assessed the muscle strength involved in forced pulmonary ventilation and its relationship with the ability to generate effective coughs in spinal cord injured patients, proving that the vital capacity correlates directly with the effectiveness of the cough, while maximal inspiratory pressure was closely related to having a higher vital capacity. It was also described with a greater involvement at higher lesion levels (C4-C5), while the tests were practically normal on patients who suffered paralysis in lower limbs (T7-L3). Therefore, the intercostal muscles, weakened, lose the possibility of reaching full lung capacity. In this way, disuse of the respiratory intercostal musculature is gradually produced, generating muscular fibrosis and a decrease of thoracic distensibility [24]. Malas et al. [25] assessed the diaphragmatic changes through ultrasonography, observing that despite the lower results obtained in the pulmonary function tests, the diaphragmatic thickness was greater in this group, which was interpreted as overcompensation, due to a greater load and respiratory rate in this muscle. The respiratory muscular weakness in spinal cord injured patients has been confirmed over the years, so that even the acceptability criteria of some functional tests such as spirometry have had to be specifically adapted to this population [26]. In fact, as early as 1980, doubts had already arisen regarding the implications and changes in the respiratory system that muscle weakness could cause. In this year, Forner et al. [27] assessed the effect of respiratory musculature paralysis on pulmonary volume, describing a drop in vital capacity and expiratory reserve volume, in addition to a decrease in peak expiratory flow. Likewise, Anke et al. [28] assessed the pulmonary function of 56 tetraplegic patients, with over six months post spinal cord injury finding a decrease in the volume of expiratory reserve and vital capacity. Baydur et al. [29] described that the forced expiratory volume, the FEV1 and the inspiratory capacity increased as the lesion was lower, reinforcing the conclusions of the previously described studies. In addition to these findings, it was observed that, in the supine position, unlike what has been described in healthy subjects, inspiratory capacity increased, which may be attributable to the compression generated by gravity in the abdominal wall, decreasing the greater distensibility of the abdomen that subjects with SCI have, thus giving them better leverage points for the action of the diaphragm. In the same line of research, Terson de Paleville et al. [30] furthered the study of the effect of the position on pulmonary volumes, describing that when the spinal cord injury was complete, the supine position benefited the forced vital capacity, while the spirometric values decreased in this position in subjects with an incomplete spinal cord injury, reinforcing the idea that the supine position on subjects with a high injury may confer some degree of mechanic muscular advantage [30].

From a different point of view, a study was conducted on the predisposing factors of the progressive loss of pulmonary function of spinal cord injured patients. Stolzmann et al. [31] evaluated 174 spinal cord injured patients, who filled out a questionnaire of respiratory health and had a follow-up with serial spirometric assessments over the course of seven years on average. This study showed that the progressive decrease of FEV1 and the FVC was linked to smoking habits, as well as other modifiable factors, more than with the gravity and the level of the spinal cord injury. In a retrospective study, the behavior of the pulmonary function of 173 spinal cord injured patients who were subjected to spirometry controls over time was described. No change in pulmonary function was observed over an average of 23 years, except for a subgroup with a higher body mass index (BMI) who decreased pulmonary volumes over time [32]. This finding is of great significance since a large percentage of spinal cord injured patients will have a forced decrease of energy consumption, which can lead to an increase in fatty tissue, followed by a decrease of muscular tissue, which leads these subjects to a chronic systematic inflammatory state, produced by the release of adipokines, like leptin [33–35]. Leptin has action at the pulmonary level, since there are receptors for this adipokine in the alveolar epithelium and in the smooth muscles of the airway [35–37]. Just as leptin has a proinflammatory role, adiponectin is also released by the fatty tissue and has an anti-inflammatory role. For this reason, Garshick et al. [35] studied the link between leptin and adiponectin with pulmonary function in spinal cord injured patients. This group of researchers found an inverse relationship between plasmatic leptin levels and FEV1 and FVC values, which might suggest that high leptin levels may also be a factor that influences the decrease in pulmonary function, specifically its vital capacity [35]. These results, which indicate an effect of chronic inflammation in spinal cord injured patients, are consistent with a previous study by the same group, in which an inverse relationship between systemic inflammation and the deterioration of pulmonary function in spinal cord injured patients had been described [38]. The decrease in vital capacity, and in nearly all inspiratory volumes, in spinal cord injured patients, coupled with the loss of thoracic cavity distensibility, is what has led to the description of a chronic restrictive ventilatory pattern in subjects with SCI that predisposes them to generate pulmonary atelectasis [21–23,37,39]. Chronic pulmonary restriction could be a problem for these subjects when they are exposed to conditions that force them to increase ventilatory capacity. From intensive care medicine, due to the possible impact of mechanical ventilation, the effect of ventilating restrictive lungs with high flow volumes has been extensively studied, since they generate an inflammatory response, either by damage through alveolar opening and closing (atelectrauma), or by overdistension (volutrauma) [40–42]. This injury is caused by the activation of alveolar macrophages due to the expression of damage associated molecular patterns (DAMPs), released by the destroyed cells of the alveolar epithelium, and such activation of the macrophages can induce further injury. In this way, an initial mechanical damage caused by ventilation with high flow volumes would stimulate local inflammatory activation, causing even more damage [43]. If we extrapolate this problem, which is pressing in the context of patients undergoing mechanical ventilation, spinal cord injured patients who have lower pulmonary distensibility and a restrictive ventilatory pattern, we could think that physical exercise, which demands an increase in pulmonary ventilation, could also induce greater inflammation and damage.

West et al. [39] observed changes in cardiopulmonary function in spinal cord injured athletes at rest and described that they maintain a restrictive pattern at rest compared to healthy athletes. Despite this, pulmonary function improves when compared to non-athletic spinal cord injured patients. The fact that persons with SCI, who participate in physical training programs, maintain restrictive ventilatory patterns reinforces the hypothesis that, during physical activity, they would be exposed to greater lung damage than healthy subjects due to the hyperventilation required by exercise. This makes it interesting to evaluate local inflammatory markers at the pulmonary level in persons with SCI during physical activity and compare them with healthy persons.

Bronchial obstruction and hyperresponsiveness: Spinal cord injured persons suffer various respiratory complications from an acute stage of injury, ranging from an increased predisposition to upper respiratory tract infections, to atelectasis and bronchospasm [44]. Chronically, persons with SCI are more exposed to respiratory disorders due to a deficit in mucociliary clearance, decreased ability to exert high expiratory flows, the repeated use of antibiotics that can change the microbiota of the respiratory tract and the generation of disorders in the autonomic nervous system, which can lead to changes in the structure and quantity of mucus, often resulting in recurrent bronchitis [45].

Almendoff et al. [46] evaluated whether there is indeed an obstructive component in spinal cord injured patients, since tetraplegic patients would have partially inhibited sympathetic innervation, being able to maintain parasympathetic innervation, promoting a basal bronchoconstrictor tone. It was observed that 48% of tetraplegic subjects obtained an improvement in both FVC and FEV1 following the use of ipratropium bromide. Later, De Luca et al. [47] added evidence that subjects with SCI, when faced with the use of beta 2 agonist inhalers, also generated an improvement in lung function, reinforcing the idea that these subjects maintain a basal obstructive component. Subsequently, Schilero et al. [10], comparing the response to ipratropium bromide between a tetraplegic group and a paraplegic group, reported that subjects with tetraplegia had a smaller basal airway caliber and a greater response to the use of this bronchodilator. These results reinforce the idea that, in high spinal cord injury, there may be an expression of the parasympathetic system without an opposing effect of the sympathetic system. Schilero et al. [48] compared the effect between albuterol and ipratropium bromide, and observed that both drugs generate a decrease in airway resistance. However, the change in resistance was more marked with ipratropium bromide than with albuterol (71% vs. 47%). These results suggest that vagal tone is the main determinant of the basal increase in bronchoconstriction.

The response to bronchodilators that has been observed in subjects with SCI may also indicate bronchial hyperresponsiveness. Triggers of bronchial hyperresponsiveness have been described, the main ones being histamine release, or some indirect external factors such as the cold and exercise [49,50]. In a study to evaluate bronchial hyperresponsiveness by Dicpinigaitis et al. [51], a group of subjects with cervical spinal cord injury were exposed to a methacholine challenge test, which demonstrated some degree of bronchial hyperresponsiveness in all participants, and furthermore, it was observed that ipratropium bromide was able to completely reverse the effect. The investigators postulated the bronchial hyperresponsiveness observed in this population most likely reflects the loss of sympathetic airway innervation and resultant unopposed cholinergic bronchoconstrictor tone which results from transection of the cervical spine. Blockade of methacholine hyperresponsiveness with ipratropium bromide suggests a muscarinic receptor-mediated phenomenon [51]. Singas et al. [52] conducted another study to see whether bronchial hyperresponsiveness could be motivated by the persons' previous or current smoking habit. For this purpose, subjects with spinal cord injury, both ex-smokers and non-smokers, were added to the evaluation and underwent a methacholine challenge test, which showed the same results in both groups. The authors thus added a new question, which was to investigate the impact that the decrease in lung volumes generates on the loss of the capacity to maintain a larger airway caliber.

The mechanisms that generate bronchial hyperresponsiveness are diverse, and recently it was described that airway inflammation may play a key role, although the acute mechanisms concerning how inflammation is linked to smooth muscle hyperresponsiveness are still unclear. However, it seems clear that, in chronic inflammation processes, airway remodeling is generated, promoting bronchial obstruction [49]. On the other hand, subjects with SCI, have characteristics that promote systemic inflammation due to their metabolic changes, propensity to be overweight and decreased muscle tissue, which may cause reduced lung function [38]. In addition, there is evidence that these characteristics are associated with an increase of IL-6 and c-reactive protein (CRP) in the blood plasma of spinal cord injured patients, since the levels of these inflammatory markers would have an inverse relationship with lung function [53]. In addition to this, it is relevant to mention the effects that inflammation causes directly in the respiratory system, such as a decrease in mucociliary clearance, changes in microbiota, increased incidence of upper respiratory tract infections and microaspirations [45,54].

To measure inflammatory markers in the airway, Radulovic et al. [55] used a noninvasive technique, assessing exhaled nitric oxide, and observed a significant increase in nitric oxide levels in tetraplegics compared to the control group, and similar to the group of asthmatic persons. While these findings are not conclusive and require further investigation, they provide indications of the presence of some local inflammatory component in the airway that may be similar to that of asthmatic persons. A summary of the topics discussed in this chapter is presented in Figure 1.

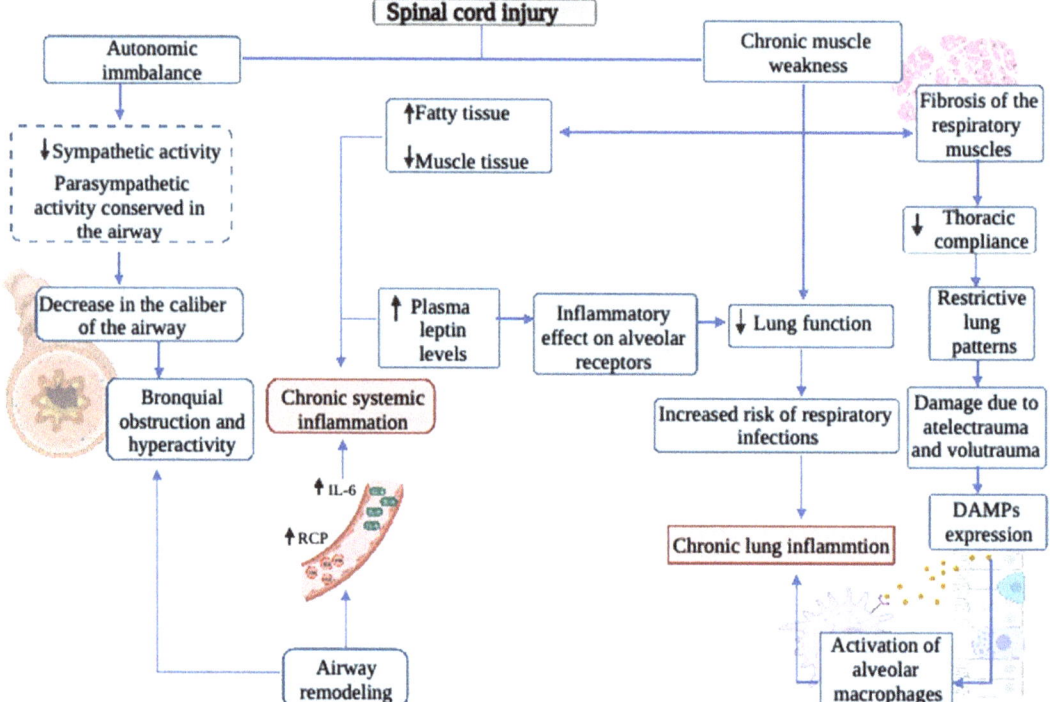

Figure 1. Overview of the role of inflammation and oxidative stress on the respiratory system in spinal cord injured patients. IL-6: Interleukin-6; CRP: C-reactive protein; DAMPs: Damage-associated molecular patterns.

3. Autonomic Nervous System

Among the neurological consequences of SCI, there is not only a serious functional compromise of the somatic nervous system, but also of the autonomic nervous system. The sympathetic nervous system, whose activity is affected when the lesion interrupts supraspinal regulatory signals, could generate problems in gastrointestinal motility, urinary continence and hemodynamic control [56,57]. The most severe expression of autonomic system disorder in subjects with SCI is autonomic dysreflexia (AD), which has its origin in the activation of dysregulated sympathetic reflexes, which can generate an exaggerated or deficient response in various functional systems, accompanied by an increase in parasympathetic tone [58]. AD can cause problems, for example, at the cardiovascular level ranging from orthostatic hypotension to severe hypertensive crises [14,54,58]. The incidence of hypertension in high spinal cord injuries is estimated to be around 46%. This incidence of hypertension is also thought to be due to increased vascular stiffness in persons with SCI [54]. The imbalance of physiological functions and loss of homeostasis caused by multiple factors, including AD, produces systemic stress that can lead to a chronic inflammatory state, which manifests as increased cardiometabolic disease and abnormal immune responses, ranging from autoimmune processes to immunosuppression [59].

Severe hypertensive conditions attributable to AD are related to the elevated and dysregulated release of catecholamines, which in the medium to long term generates endothelial damage and promotes atherogenesis, among other vascular pathologies [59–62]. Noller et al. [59] point out that the management of chronic inflammation in persons with SCI is very relevant to improve their quality of life, and for that it is necessary to understand in a deeper way the role of the autonomic nervous system. Hoekstra et al. [63]

studied the systemic inflammatory response to exercise in subjects with SCI. Subjects with a non-cervical injury generated increased catecholamine release and concurrently increased plasma IL-6 after competing in a wheelchair half-marathon event. While a direct relationship was found between the levels of catecholamines released and IL-6 levels, it is not certain that this is due to AD, since AD is more prevalent in subjects with cervical SCI. Sudden changes in arterial pressure and turbulent flows generated in the bifurcation zones of the arteries generate stress in the vascular wall. This promotes increased permeability in these areas to lipoproteins circulating in the blood [64,65]. LDL molecules penetrate such areas more easily into the vessel wall, accumulate in the tunica intima and are subsequently oxidized (oxLDL). These oxidized molecules act as patterns associated with molecular damage (DAMPs), generate endothelial damage and activate proinflammatory processes through pattern recognition receptors (PRRs) [64,66]. Damaged and activated endothelial cells express adhesion molecules and cytokines such as E-selectin, P-selectin, VCAM-1 and ICAM-1, which attract monocytes to the site of the atherosclerotic lesion and promote their conversion to macrophages [67,68]. These activated cells phagocytize cholesterol esters and form foam cells, stimulating an inflammatory reaction with migration of vascular smooth muscle cells that stabilize the atheroma plaque with fibrotic tissue. Simultaneously to the innate inflammatory response, an adaptive response involving different types of T and B cells is triggered against the atheroma plaque and renders it unstable [64,68]. On the other hand, oxidative stress plays a fundamental role in the atherosclerotic process. Thus, the vascular wall has oxidative systems such as xanthine oxidase, mitochondrial respiratory chain enzymes, lipoxygenases, NOX and antioxidant systems, including superoxide dismutase (SOD), catalase and glutathione peroxidase [64,69,70]. Activation of LOX-1, a macrophage receptor that is triggered by oxLDL, induces endothelial oxidative stress by increasing NOX activity which increases hydrogen peroxide and superoxide levels [64,71,72]. Oxidative stress activates NF-κB through transduction pathways via PI3K and MAPK activation, which initiates apoptotic signal transduction and produces cell damage. In addition, oxidative stress reduces PPARγ activity and adiponectin levels. Both stimulate the AMPK protein, which is an inhibitor of NOX activity. Thus, oxidative stress inhibits this AMPK, and the action of NOX is promoted, which ultimately would further increase the release of NFkB [64].

At the cardiovascular level, the consequences of a spinal cord injury involve a significant morbidity and mortality impact. In general, plasma levels of catecholamines are usually low; however, there are situations in which loss of supraspinal control leads to a deregulated release of catecholamines. In addition, a hyperresponsiveness of alpha-adrenergic receptors is observed, which may be caused by both receptor hypersensitivity and a deficit of noradrenaline reuptake by the sympathetic neuron [73,74]. An altered lipid profile has also been observed in subjects with SCI, with elevated LDL and decreased HDL values. This increases the risk of heart disease and systemic atherosclerosis, which may be determined by low physical activity, inadequate diet and uncontrolled sympathetic activity [73].

Furthermore, the action of the autonomic nervous system on the promotion of inflammation may derive not only from the effects at the cardiovascular level, but also from its direct or indirect effect on the immune system. The specific mechanisms leading to immunosuppression in subjects with SCI are currently unknown, but different factors that may influence immune function have been observed. In a study conducted on laboratory rats, it was observed that the frequency of AD episodes increased as time since the injury passed, along with increased immunosuppression, probably due to the uncontrolled release of catecholamines and glucocorticoids [58]. Postganglionic noradrenergic fibers release catecholamines that target organs and lymphoid cells, causing a rapid increase of these cells in the blood. However, a chronic release of catecholamines, in the long term, produces the opposite effect, leading to leukopenia. Regarding the specific effect on the different types of immune response, the chronic increase of circulating catecholamines could have an inhibitory effect on the production of cytokines for the TH1 type immune response, but not so on the TH2 response [74,75]. It has also been observed that the relationship between elevated catecholamines and immune dysfunction occurs when the level of the lesion interrupts supraspinal control of the sympathetic innervation of the spleen, producing an increase of local catecholamines in this organ, even though the total circulating catecholamines in these subjects is lower, possibly due to an alteration of the innervation of the adrenal gland [56,75,76].

Likewise, just as immunosuppression has been described in subjects with spinal cord injury, there are also cases of long-term autoimmunity induced by spinal cord injury [77–79]. Thus, it has been described that spinal cord injury can expose CNS antigens to the circulation, which could provoke the activation of lymphocytes, which have specific receptors for these antigens. Activation of B cells can lead to the production of autoantibodies that ultimately lead to an autoimmune response and generate inflammation and neurotoxicity, resulting in poor recovery [79–82]. In an animal model, it was observed that rodents with B lymphocyte deficiency had a better motor recovery than control rodents, which suggests that there may be a relationship between these cells and the autoimmune response [83,84].

In a comparative study conducted by Saltzman et al. [85] on humans with and without SCI, the differential expression of a network of genes in peripheral blood was observed, to which a role in the structure and maturation of lymphoid tissue was attributed. Some of these genes were involved in inflammatory processes and in the regulation of B lymphocyte function. The importance of this network is that three molecules (BCMA, APRIL and BAFF) were encoded with a known role in producing autoimmune conditions [85,86]. BCMA is a receptor of the tumor necrosis factor (TNF) family that has been shown to mediate B cell survival and activation processes [85,87]. In addition, it is associated with an increase in the population of self-reactive cells [85,88–90]. Conversely, APRIL and BAFF are members of the TNF ligand superfamily, located in the germinal center of lymphoid organs, where they promote the survival, activation, maturation and differentiation of antibody-producing and memory B cells [85,91]. BAFF and APRIL can bind to BCMA and thus activate the NF-kB pathway, which triggers survival reactions for B cells [85]. Herman et al. [92] deepened the study previously carried out by Saltzman by increasing the number of people evaluated and confirmed changes in gene expression in subjects with spinal cord injury associated with lymphoid organs. In addition, it was observed that there was an increase in the expression of these genes as the lesion was higher than the T5 level.

Toll like receptors (TLRs) are innate pathogen recognition receptors present on immune cells that stimulate this process. TLR activation activates inflammatory mediators [93]. In the study conducted by Herman et al. [92], it was also observed that these TLRs were overexpressed in subjects with spinal cord injury above T5, which may promote an uncontrolled inflammatory response as has been studied in patients with sepsis who also present such TLR overexpression. TLR modulating agents are currently being studied in clinical trials for the management of autoimmune diseases and inflammatory responses and could be an alternative to be evaluated in subjects with SCI [92,94]. See the mechanisms overview in Figure 2.

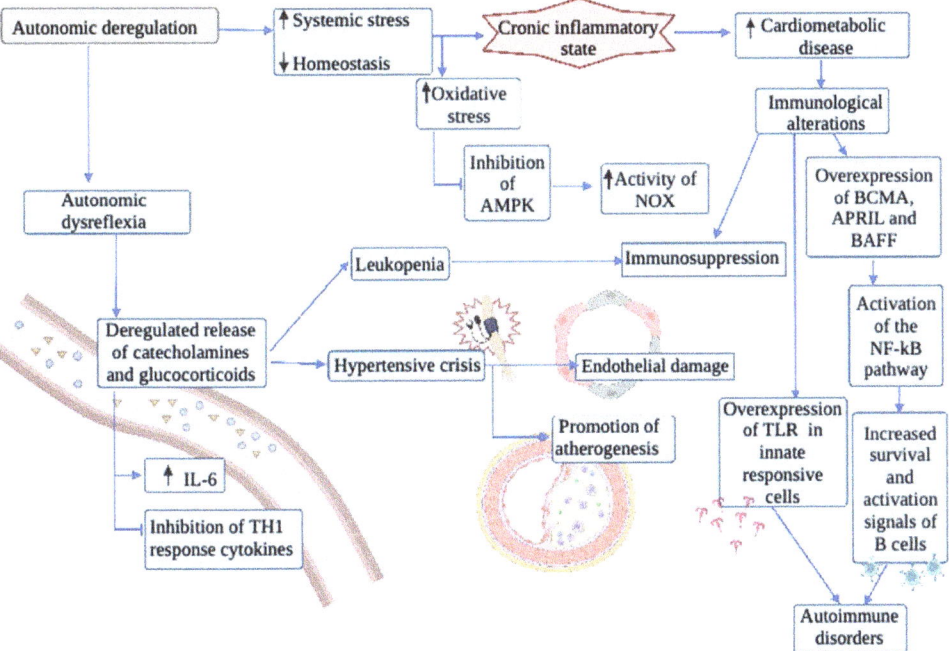

Figure 2. Overview of the role of inflammation and oxidative stress on the autonomic nervous system in patients with spinal cord injury. IL-6: Interleukin-6; AMPK: AMP-activated protein kinase; BCMA: B-cell maturation antigen; APRIL: A proliferation-inducing ligand; BAFF: B-cell–activating factor; NF-kB: Nuclear factor kappa B; TLR: Toll like receptors; NOX: NADPH oxidase.

4. Muscular System

Among the multiple consequences produced by SCI, immobility, disuse and muscular atrophy have an impact on the functioning of the locomotor system, which includes both bone tissue and skeletal muscle [95]. This deterioration is caused by both the denervation of the muscle resulting from acute spinal damage, and by the secondary damage resulting from the inflammatory reaction caused by neuronal death [96,97]. In addition, from the time of injury and in the long term, there is a decrease in blood flow to the regions below the lesion [98,99]. The muscle tissue in these patients shows a decrease in the radius of the fibers, loss of nuclei that alters regenerative capacity and a decreased number of mitochondria and their functionality [100,101]. In addition, within months, the change from type I fibers begins to occur until, within years, type IIx fibers predominate [17]. Associated with this process, increases in mediators that favor muscle protein degradation, such as myostastin [102], interleukin 6 [103,104] and TNF alpha [105,106] have been observed.

While the trophic effect of muscle innervation has been known since ancient times, the precise understanding of the mechanisms of chronic muscle involvement caused by SCI, resulting in continuous atrophy, possibly associated with oxidative damage, is still unclear [107]. Muscle atrophy is caused by an imbalance between proteolysis and protein synthesis. This process can be explained by muscle disuse, advanced age or exposure to microgravity conditions, resulting in loss of strength and a decrease in muscle mass [108–110]. In the study of this phenomenon, in an animal model, Kondo et al. [111] related oxidative damage to muscle atrophy caused by immobilization, observing an increase in thiobarbituric acid reactive substance (TBARS) and glutathione disulfide (GSSG) levels. Furthermore, in this study, a decrease in atrophy was found after vitamin E supplementation, thus attributing a large part of the origin of this phenomenon to oxidative stress. The main source of ROS production related to atrophy produced by immobilization has also been studied. Thus, Gram et al. [112] investigated how mitochondrial function and reactive oxygen species emission behaved in a group of young and older men subjected to two weeks of one-leg immobilization. First, it was observed that immobilization increased H_2O_2 production along with decreasing ATP formation by this organelle. Moreover, this effect on mitochondrial functioning was reversible after a six-week program of aerobic training on a cycloergometer [112]. Second, Liu et al. [113] suggest that the main source of ROS production associated with muscle atrophy is the NADPH oxidase 4 (NOX4), located in the sarcoplasmic reticulum. In addition, they investigated the role of calstabin 1 in this process, since it has been described that this protein favors the closure of the ryanodine receptor when muscle contraction ends; therefore, a dissociation between both proteins would decrease muscle strength. Thus, they designed a study in rats evaluating NOX4 expression after spinal cord injury at the T4 level. The results showed that an overexpression of NOX4 leads to an increase in the oxidation state, causing a prooxidant environment that dissociates calstabin 1 from the receptor of ryanodine 1, which could be one of the mechanisms of alteration of muscle contraction.

Hyperactivity of the renin-angiotensin system (RAS) is another phenomenon that has been widely studied, which is involved in several chronic pathologies, such as cardiac dysfunction. In this sense, Kadoguchi et al. [114] suggested that, if an increase in angiotensin II could produce systemic and cardiac altering effects, perhaps it could also have some implication on skeletal muscle function. Thus, in a study first carried out in an animal model, it was shown that rats administered with angiotensin II showed a greater loss of muscle mass and a decrease in the cross-sectional area of muscle fibers if compared to control rats. In addition, an increase in MuRF-1 and atrogyn-1, both part of the ubiquitin-proteosome degradative system, was observed [115]. In addition, although a decrease in the oxidative enzymatic activity of citrate synthase and mitochondrial complexes 1 and 3 was observed, superoxide generation from NADPH oxidase increased. Kadoguchi et al. [110] hypothesized that, if NOX2 is the main source of superoxide generation, and that there was an overexpression of a gene for NOX2 against muscle damage, angiotensin II could then play a role in NOX activity, thereby promoting the generation of muscle atrophy. To test their hypothesis, they studied an animal model in mice with a control group and a NOX2-deficient group, and angiotensin II was administered to both groups. Deletion of NOX2 prevented angiotensin II induced skeletal muscle atrophy by improving the balance between protein synthesis and degradation. In addition, they observed a decrease in the phosphorylation of AKT, which is a necessary signaling pathway in the process of protein synthesis. The authors noted that, therefore, NOX2 may be a therapeutic target for angiotensin II induced skeletal muscle atrophy.

In another area, Savikj et al. [116] conducted a study to assess whether spinal cord injury induces an oxidative imbalance leading to muscle damage. Regarding this study, they developed a comparative study in humans with complete spinal cord injury versus a healthy control group by obtaining muscle biopsies in the first, third and twelfth month after spinal cord injury. In this study, it was observed that in the skeletal muscle of spinal cord injured patients, there is an overexpression of xanthine oxidase in the first three months, and in a more chronic way at 12 months, increased levels of 4-HNE and a decrease in the content of superoxide dismutase 2 (SOD2). In addition, there is evidence linking oxidative stress with the activation of proteases at the skeletal muscle level, attributing to the mitochondria the main responsibility for the production of ROS in muscle atrophy [107,117,118]. Thus, Min et al. [107] evaluated the effect of mitochondrial ROS on muscle atrophy using a rat animal model focused on the administration of a mitochondrial antioxidant called SS-31, which is selective for the mitochondrial membrane. In this study, it was observed that immobilization compared to a control group of non-immobilized rats generated atrophy, increased ROS and the activation of proteolysis. When SS-31 was administered, ROS levels decreased, as did muscle atrophy and protein degradation [107]. To evaluate the effect of supplementation on muscle atrophy, Arc-Chagnaud et al. [119] conducted a study using a mixture of antioxidants and anti-inflammatory drugs (741 mg of polyphenols, 138 mg of vitamin E, 80 µg of selenium and 2.1 g of omega-3). Moreover, they observed the effect of physical deconditioning on muscle atrophy, using a 60-day head-down bed rest (HDBR) model in healthy volunteers. Out of the 20 subjects assessed by induced rest, only half received a mixture of antioxidants and anti-inflammatory drugs. The results showed that, after two months, all participants suffered loss of muscle mass. The authors highlighted the complexity of oxidative pathways that make it difficult to understand how oxidative stress influences muscle atrophy and questioned the effect of a nutritional intervention with antioxidants in preventing muscle deconditioning in long-duration space missions. However, it should be noted that the results of this study are in contrast with the results obtained by Min et al. [107] and Kondo et al. [111], who used antioxidants, which raises the question of how oxidative stress influences muscle atrophy. Figure 3 shows a summary of the mechanisms described in the paragraph above.

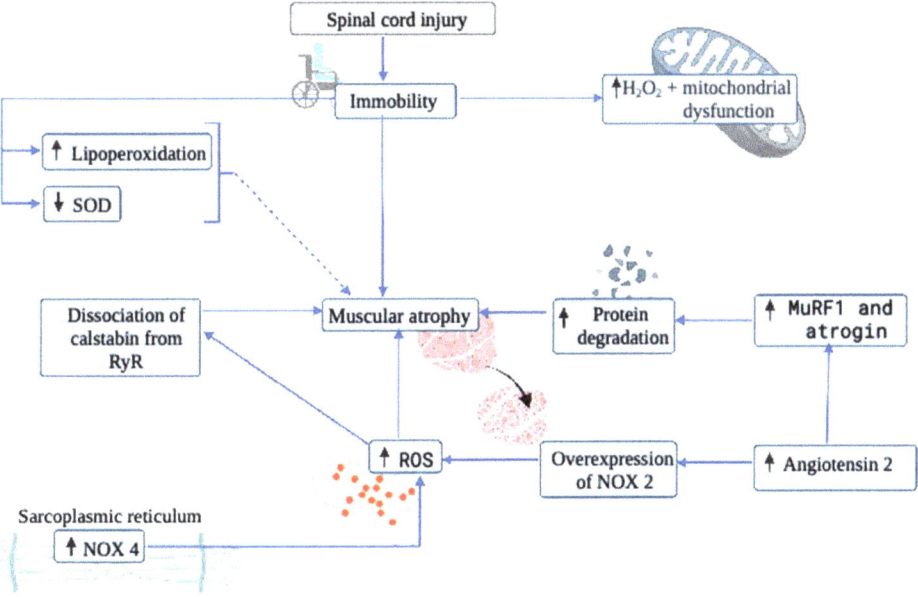

Figure 3. Overview of the role of inflammation and oxidative stress on muscle tissue in spinal cord injured patients. SOD: Superoxide dismutase; NOX4: NADPH oxidase 4; NOX2: NADPH oxidase 2; ROS: Reactive oxygen species; MuRF1: Muscle RING-finger protein-1.

5. Conclusions

At the time a spinal cord injury is produced, a loss of motor capacity is evident, and a period of vital risk related to neurological compromise, instability of cardio-respiratory function and the development of infections is established. After this period, ranging from weeks to months, new relationships between different organs are established, now affecting functions that were initially unharmed. Thus, bone and muscle mass decreases, the respiratory system suffers restricted and inefficient ventilatory activity due to the affectation of its musculature, while the abnormal functioning of the autonomic nervous system will affect the action of various organs. In this review, we have described that the development of alterations in the redox state and the manifestation of increased inflammatory activity—that affects both individual tissues and at systemic level—is a common mechanism for the malfunctioning of these different but closely functionally integrated systems. The boundaries between the two processes are also blurred and one often promotes the emergence of the other. They are also involved in pathological processes as diverse as muscle atrophy and fibrosis secondary to disuse, as well as autoimmune diseases. Finally, it is interesting to note that, although much research is still pending (since there are many different events underlying these phenomena), application of antioxidant and anti-inflammatory therapies have been proposed either theoretically and through experimental studies [120–123] to delay or reverse the complications of this clinical condition. These lines of research offer a novel attractive approach that can have a significant impact on the quality of life of these patients.

Author Contributions: C.R.-A., G.V. and O.F.A. worked on the design, methodology, and drafting of the manuscript. All authors have read and agreed to the published version of the manuscript.

Funding: This research received no external funding.

Institutional Review Board Statement: Not applicable.

Informed Consent Statement: Not applicable.

Data Availability Statement: Not applicable.

Conflicts of Interest: The authors declare no conflict of interest.

References

1. WHO. Spinal Cord Injury. 2013. Available online: https://www.who.int/news-room/fact-sheets/detail/spinal-cord-injury (accessed on 1 February 2020).
2. Bastien, D.; Lacroix, S. Cytokine pathways regulating glial and leukocyte function after spinal cord and peripheral nerve injury. *Exp. Neurol.* **2014**, *258*, 62–77. [CrossRef] [PubMed]
3. McDonald, J.W.; Sadowsky, C. Spinal-cord injury. *Lancet* **2002**, *359*, 417–425. [CrossRef]
4. Krassioukov, A. Autonomic function following cervical spinal cord injury. *Respir. Physiol. Neurobiol.* **2009**, *169*, 157–164. [CrossRef] [PubMed]
5. Raguindin, P.F.; Bertolo, A.; Zeh, R.M.; Fränkl, G.; Itodo, O.A.; Capossela, S.; Bally, L.; Minder, B.; Brach, M.; Eriks-Hoogland, I.; et al. Body Composition According to Spinal Cord Injury Level: A Systematic Review and Meta-Analysis. *J. Clin. Med.* **2021**, *10*, 3911. [CrossRef]
6. Dinh, A.; Bouchand, F.; Davido, B.; Duran, C.; Denys, P.; Lortat-Jacob, A.; Rottman, M.; Salomon, J.; Bernard, L. Management of established pressure ulcer infections in spinal cord injury patients. *Med. Mal. Infect.* **2019**, *49*, 9–16. [CrossRef]
7. Popovich, P.G.; Stokes, B.T.; Whitacre, C.C. Concept of autoimmunity following spinal cord injury: Possible roles for T lymphocytes in the traumatized central nervous system. *J. Neurosci. Res.* **1996**, *45*, 349–363. [CrossRef]
8. Gorgey, A.S.; Dolbow, D.R.; Dolbow, J.D.; Khalil, R.K.; Castillo, C.; Gater, D.R. Effects of spinal cord injury on body composition and metabolic profile—Part I. *J. Spinal. Cord. Med.* **2014**, *37*, 693–702. [CrossRef]
9. Schilero, G.J.; Spungen, A.M.; Bauman, W.A.; Radulovic, M.; Lesser, M. Pulmonary function and spinal cord injury. *Respir. Physiol. Neurobiol.* **2009**, *166*, 129–141. [CrossRef]
10. Schilero, G.J.; Grimm, D.R.; Bauman, W.A.; Lenner, R.; Lesser, M. Assessment of airway caliber and bronchodilator responsiveness in subjects with spinal cord injury. *Chest* **2005**, *127*, 149–155. [CrossRef]
11. Bernardi, M.; Fedullo, A.L.; Di Giacinto, B.; Squeo, M.R.; Aiello, P.; Dante, D.; Romano, S.; Magaudda, L.; Peluso, I.; Palmery, M.; et al. Cardiovascular Risk Factors and Haematological Indexes of Inflammation in Paralympic Athletes with Different Motor Impairments. *Oxid. Med. Cell Longev.* **2019**, *2019*, 6798140. [CrossRef]
12. Schilero, G.J.; Bauman, W.A.; Radulovic, M. Traumatic Spinal Cord Injury: Pulmonary Physiologic Principles and Management. *Clin. Chest. Med.* **2018**, *39*, 411–425. [CrossRef] [PubMed]
13. Martínez Rodríguez, L.; Pérez, A.M.; del Mar López Rodríguez, M. Heart rate variability biofeedback. *THERAPEÍA* **2019**, *11*, 95–119.
14. Phillips, A.A.; Krassioukov, A.V. Contemporary Cardiovascular Concerns after Spinal Cord Injury: Mechanisms, Maladaptations, and Management. *J. Neurotrauma.* **2015**, *32*, 1927–1942. [CrossRef] [PubMed]
15. Griggs, K.E.; Price, M.J.; Goosey-Tolfrey, V.L. Cooling athletes with a spinal cord injury. *Sports Med.* **2015**, *45*, 9–21. [CrossRef] [PubMed]
16. Mironets, E.; Fischer, R.; Bracchi-Ricard, V.; Saltos, T.M.; Truglio, T.S.; O'Reilly, M.L.; Swanson, K.A.; Bethea, J.R.; Tom, V.J. Attenuating Neurogenic Sympathetic Hyperreflexia Robustly Improves Antibacterial Immunity After Chronic Spinal Cord Injury. *J. Neurosci.* **2020**, *40*, 478–492. [CrossRef]
17. Biering-Sørensen, B.; Kristensen, I.B.; Kjaer, M.; Biering-Sørensen, F. Muscle after spinal cord injury. *Muscle Nerve.* **2009**, *40*, 499–519. [CrossRef]
18. Yarar-Fisher, C.; Bickel, C.S.; Kelly, N.A.; Stec, M.J.; Windham, S.T.; McLain, A.B.; Oster, R.A.; Bamman, M.M. Heightened TWEAK-NF-κB signaling and inflammation-associated fibrosis in paralyzed muscles of men with chronic spinal cord injury. *Am. J. Physiol. Endocrinol. Metab.* **2016**, *310*, E754–E761. [CrossRef]

19. Antonioni, A.; Fantini, C.; Dimauro, I.; Caporossi, D. Redox homeostasis in sport: Do athletes really need antioxidant support? *Res. Sports Med.* **2019**, *27*, 147–165. [CrossRef]
20. Powers, S.K.; Smuder, A.J.; Criswell, D.S. Mechanistic links between oxidative stress and disuse muscle atrophy. *Antioxid. Redox. Signal.* **2011**, *15*, 2519–2528. [CrossRef]
21. Brown, R.; Di Marco, A.F.; Hoit, J.D.; Garshick, E. Respiratory dysfunction and management in spinal cord injury. *Respir. Care* **2006**, *51*, 853–868.
22. Berlowitz, D.J.; Wadsworth, B.; Ross, J. Respiratory problems and management in people with spinal cord injury. *Breathe* **2016**, *12*, 328–340. [CrossRef] [PubMed]
23. Mateus, S.R.M.; Beraldo, P.S.S.; Horan, T.A. Maximal static mouth respiratory pressure in spinal cord injured patients: Correlation with motor level. *Spinal. Cord.* **2007**, *45*, 569–575. [CrossRef] [PubMed]
24. Kang, S.W.; Shin, J.C.; Park, C.I.; Moon, J.H.; Rha, D.W.; Cho, D.H. Relationship between inspiratory muscle strength and cough capacity in cervical spinal cord injured patients. *Spinal. Cord.* **2006**, *44*, 242–248. [CrossRef] [PubMed]
25. Malas, F.Ü.; Köseoğlu, F.; Kara, M.; Ece, H.; Aytekin, M.; Öztürk, G.T.; Özçakar, L.; Ulaşlı, A.M. Diaphragm ultrasonography and pulmonary function tests in patients with spinal cord injury. *Spinal. Cord.* **2019**, *57*, 679–683. [CrossRef]
26. Kelley, A.; Garshick, E.; Gross, E.R.; Lieberman, S.L.; Tun, C.G.; Brown, R. Spirometry testing standards in spinal cord injury. *Chest* **2003**, *123*, 725–730. [CrossRef]
27. Forner, J.V. Lung volumes and mechanics of breathing in tetraplegics. *Paraplegia* **1980**, *18*, 258–266. [CrossRef]
28. Anke, A.; Aksnes, A.K.; Stanghelle, J.K.; Hjeltnes, N. Lung volumes in tetraplegic patients according to cervical spinal cord injury level. *Scand. J. Rehabil. Med.* **1993**, *25*, 73–77.
29. Baydur, A.; Adkins, R.H.; Milic-Emili, J. Lung mechanics in individuals with spinal cord injury: Effects of injury level and posture. *J. Appl. Physiol.* **2001**, *90*, 405–411. [CrossRef]
30. Terson de Paleville, D.G.; Sayenko, D.G.; Aslan, S.C.; Folz, R.J.; McKay, W.B.; Ovechkin, A.V. Respiratory motor function in seated and supine positions in individuals with chronic spinal cord injury. *Respir. Physiol. Neurobiol.* **2014**, *203*, 9–14. [CrossRef]
31. Stolzmann, K.L.; Gagnon, D.R.; Brown, R.; Tun, C.G.; Garshick, E. Longitudinal change in FEV1 and FVC in chronic spinal cord injury. *Am. J. Respir. Crit. Care Med.* **2008**, *177*, 781–786. [CrossRef]
32. Van Silfhout, L.; Peters, A.E.J.; Berlowitz, D.J.; Schembri, R.; Thijssen, D.; Graco, M. Long-term change in respiratory function following spinal cord injury. *Spinal. Cord.* **2016**, *54*, 714–719. [CrossRef] [PubMed]
33. Shojaei, M.H.; Alavinia, S.M.; Craven, B.C. Management of obesity after spinal cord injury: A systematic review. *J. Spinal. Cord. Med.* **2017**, *40*, 783–794. [CrossRef] [PubMed]
34. Farkas, G.J.; Gater, D.R. Neurogenic obesity and systemic inflammation following spinal cord injury: A review. *J. Spinal. Cord. Med.* **2018**, *41*, 378–387. [CrossRef] [PubMed]
35. Garshick, E.; Walia, P.; Goldstein, R.L.; Teylan, M.; Lazzari, A.A.; Tun, C.G.; Hart, J.E. Plasma Leptin and Reduced FEV1 and FVC in Chronic Spinal Cord Injury. *PM&R* **2018**, *10*, 276–285.
36. Bruno, A.; Chanez, P.; Chiappara, G.; Siena, L.; Giammanco, S.; Gjomarkaj, M.; Bonsignore, G.; Bousquet, J.; Vignola, A.M. Does leptin play a cytokine-like role within the airways of COPD patients? *Eur. Respir. J.* **2005**, *26*, 398–405. [CrossRef]
37. Vernooy, J.H.; Ubags, N.D.; Brusselle, G.G.; Tavernier, J.; Suratt, B.T.; Joos, G.F.; Wouters, E.F.; Bracke, K.R. Leptin as regulator of pulmonary immune responses: Involvement in respiratory diseases. *Pulm. Pharmacol. Ther.* **2013**, *26*, 464–472. [CrossRef]
38. Garshick, E.; Stolzmann, K.L.; Gagnon, D.R.; Morse, L.R.; Brown, R. Systemic inflammation and reduced pulmonary function in chronic spinal cord injury. *PM&R* **2011**, *3*, 433–439.
39. West, C.R.; Campbell, I.G.; Shave, R.E.; Romer, L.M. Resting cardiopulmonary function in Paralympic athletes with cervical spinal cord injury. *Med. Sci. Sports Exerc.* **2012**, *44*, 323–329. [CrossRef]
40. Hickling, K.G.; Walsh, J.; Henderson, S.; Jackson, R. Low mortality rate in adult respiratory distress syndrome using low-volume, pressure-limited ventilation with permissive hypercapnia: A prospective study. *Crit. Care Med.* **1994**, *22*, 1568–1578. [CrossRef]
41. Hickling, K.G.; Henderson, S.J.; Jackson, R. Low mortality associated with low volume pressure limited ventilation with permissive hypercapnia in severe adult respiratory distress syndrome. *Intensive. Care Med.* **1990**, *16*, 372–377. [CrossRef]
42. Carrasco Loza, R.; Villamizar Rodríguez, G.; Medel Fernández, N. Ventilator-Induced Lung Injury (VILI) in acute respiratory distress syndrome (ARDS): Volutrauma and Molecular Effects. *Open. Respir. Med. J.* **2015**, *9*, 112–119. [CrossRef] [PubMed]
43. Whitsett, J.A.; Alenghat, T. Respiratory epithelial cells orchestrate pulmonary innate immunity. *Nat. Immunol.* **2015**, *16*, 27–35. [CrossRef] [PubMed]
44. Yong, T.; Lili, Y.; Wen, Y.; Xinwei, W.; Xuhui, Z. Pulmonary edema and hemorrhage, possible causes of pulmonary infection and respiratory failure in the early stage of lower spinal cord injury. *Med. Hypotheses.* **2012**, *79*, 299–301. [CrossRef] [PubMed]
45. Burns, S.P. Acute Respiratory Infections in Persons with Spinal Cord Injury. *Phys. Med. Rehabil. Clin. N. Am.* **2007**, *18*, 203–216. [CrossRef]
46. Almenoff, P.L.; Alexander, L.R.; Spungen, A.M.; Lesser, M.D.; Bauman, W.A. Bronchodilatory effects of ipratropium bromide in patients with tetraplegia. *Paraplegia* **1995**, *33*, 274–277. [CrossRef]
47. DeLuca, R.V.; Grimm, D.R.; Lesser, M.; Bauman, W.A.; Almenoff, P.L. Effects of a β2-agonist on airway hyperreactivity in subjects with cervical spinal cord injury. *Chest* **1999**, *115*, 1533–1538. [CrossRef]
48. Schilero, G.J.; Hobson, J.C.; Singh, K.; Spungen, A.M.; Bauman, W.A.; Radulovic, M. Bronchodilator effects of ipratropium bromide and albuterol sulfate among subjects with tetraplegia. *J. Spinal. Cord Med.* **2018**, *41*, 42–47. [CrossRef]

49. Cockcroft, D.W.; Davis, B.E. Mechanisms of airway hyperresponsiveness. *J. Allergy. Clin. Immunol.* **2006**, *118*, 551–559. [CrossRef]
50. Araneda, O.F.; Carbonell, T.; Tuesta, M. Update on the Mechanisms of Pulmonary Inflammation and Oxidative Imbalance Induced by Exercise. *Oxid. Med. Cell Longev.* **2016**, *2016*, 4868536. [CrossRef]
51. Dicpinigaitis, P.V.; Spungen, A.M.; Bauman, W.A.; Absgarten, A.; Almenoff, P.L. Bronchial hyperresponsiveness after cervical spinal cord injury. *Chest* **1994**, *105*, 1073–1076. [CrossRef]
52. Singas, E.; Lesser, M.; Spungen, A.M.; Bauman, W.A.; Almenoff, P.L. Airway hyperresponsiveness to methacholine in subjects with spinal cord injury. *Chest* **1996**, *110*, 911–915. [CrossRef] [PubMed]
53. Hart, J.E.; Morse, L.; Tun, C.G.; Brown, R.; Garshick, E. Cross-sectional associations of pulmonary function with systemic inflammation and oxidative stress in individuals with chronic spinal cord injury. *J. Spinal. Cord. Med.* **2016**, *39*, 344–352. [CrossRef] [PubMed]
54. Bauman, W.; Korsten, M.; Radulovic, M.; Schilero, G.; Wech, J.; Spungen, A. 31st G. Heiner sell lectureship: Secondary medical consequences of spinal cord injury. *Top. Spinal. Cord. Inj. Rehabil.* **2012**, *18*, 354–378. [CrossRef]
55. Radulovic, M.; Schilero, G.J.; Wecht, J.M.; La Fountaine, M.; Rosado-Rivera, D.; Bauman, W.A. Exhaled nitric oxide levels are elevated in persons with tetraplegia and comparable to that in mild asthmatics. *Lung* **2010**, *188*, 259–262. [CrossRef] [PubMed]
56. Teasell, R.W.; Arnold, J.M.; Krassioukov, A.; Delaney, G.A. Cardiovascular consequences of loss of supraspinal control of the sympathetic nervous system after spinal cord injury. *Arch. Phys. Med. Rehabil.* **2000**, *81*, 506–516. [CrossRef]
57. Hou, S.; Rabchevsky, A.G. Autonomic consequences of spinal cord injury. *Compr. Physiol.* **2014**, *4*, 1419–1453.
58. Zhang, Y.; Guan, Z.; Reader, B.; Shawler, T.; Mandrekar-Colucci, S.; Huang, K.; Weil, Z.; Bratasz, A.; Wells, J.; Powell, N.D.; et al. Autonomic dysreflexia causes chronic immune suppression after spinal cord injury. *J. Neurosci.* **2013**, *33*, 12970–12981. [CrossRef]
59. Noller, C.M.; Groah, S.L.; Nash, M.S. Inflammatory stress effects on health and function after spinal cord injury. *Top. Spinal. Cord. Inj. Rehabil.* **2017**, *23*, 207–217. [CrossRef]
60. Cowan, R.E.; Nash, M.S. Cardiovascular disease, SCI and exercise: Unique risks and focused countermeasures. *Disabil. Rehabil.* **2010**, *32*, 2228–2236. [CrossRef]
61. Madden, K.S.; Sanders, V.M.; Felten, D.L. Catecholamine influences and sympathetic neural modulation of immune responsiveness. *Annu. Rev. Pharmacol. Toxicol.* **1995**, *35*, 417–448. [CrossRef]
62. Köseoğlu, B.F.; Safer, V.B.; Öken Akselim, S. Cardiovascular disease risk in people with spinal cord injury: Is there a possible association between reduced lung function and increased risk of diabetes and hypertension. *Spinal. Cord.* **2017**, *55*, 87–93. [CrossRef] [PubMed]
63. Hoekstra, S.P.; Leicht, C.A.; Kamijo, Y.-I.; Kinoshita, T.; Stephenson, B.T.; Goosey-Tolfrey, V.L.; Bishop, N.C.; Tajima, F. The inflammatory response to a wheelchair half-marathon in people with a spinal cord injury—The role of autonomic function. *J. Sports Sci.* **2019**, *37*, 1717–1724. [CrossRef] [PubMed]
64. Marchio, P.; Guerra-Ojeda, S.; Vila, J.M.; Aldasoro, M.; Victor, V.M.; Mauricio, M.D. Targeting Early Atherosclerosis: A Focus on Oxidative Stress and Inflammation. *Oxid. Med. Cell Longev.* **2019**, *2019*, 8563845. [CrossRef] [PubMed]
65. Davies, P.F. Hemodynamic shear stress and the endothelium in cardiovascular pathophysiology. *Nat. Clin. Pract. Cardiovasc. Med.* **2009**, *6*, 16–26. [CrossRef] [PubMed]
66. Miteva, K.; Madonna, R.; De Caterina, R.; Van Linthout, S. Innate and adaptive immunity in atherosclerosis. *Vascul. Pharmacol.* **2018**, *Online ahead of print*. [CrossRef]
67. Kattoor, A.J.; Kanuri, S.H.; Mehta, J.L. Role of Ox-LDL and LOX-1 in Atherogenesis. *Curr. Med. Chem.* **2019**, *26*, 1693–1700. [CrossRef]
68. Hopkins, P.N. Molecular biology of atherosclerosis. *Physiol. Rev.* **2013**, *93*, 1317–1542. [CrossRef]
69. Landmesser, U.; Spiekermann, S.; Preuss, C.; Sorrentino, S.; Fischer, D.; Manes, C.; Mueller, M.; Drexler, H. Angiotensin II induces endothelial xanthine oxidase activation: Role for endothelial dysfunction in patients with coronary disease. *Arterioscler Thromb Vasc. Biol.* **2007**, *27*, 943–948. [CrossRef]
70. Förstermann, U.; Xia, N.; Li, H. Roles of Vascular Oxidative Stress and Nitric Oxide in the Pathogenesis of Atherosclerosis. *Circ. Res.* **2017**, *120*, 713–735. [CrossRef]
71. Chang, X.; Zhao, Z.; Zhang, W.; Liu, D.; Ma, C.; Zhang, T.; Meng, Q.; Yan, P.; Zou, L.; Zhang, M. Natural Antioxidants Improve the Vulnerability of Cardiomyocytes and Vascular Endothelial Cells under Stress Conditions: A Focus on Mitochondrial Quality Control. *Oxid. Med. Cell. Longev.* **2021**, *2021*, 6620677. [CrossRef]
72. Chen, X.P.; Xun, K.L.; Wu, Q.; Zhang, T.T.; Shi, J.S.; Du, G.H. Oxidized low density lipoprotein receptor-1 mediates oxidized low density lipoprotein-induced apoptosis in human umbilical vein endothelial cells: Role of reactive oxygen species. *Vascul. Pharmacol.* **2007**, *47*, 1–9. [CrossRef] [PubMed]
73. Popa, C.; Popa, F.; Grigorean, V.T.; Onose, G.; Sandu, A.M.; Popescu, M.; Burnei, G.; Strambu, V.; Sinescu, C. Vascular dysfunctions following spinal cord injury. *J. Med. Life.* **2010**, *3*, 275–285. [PubMed]
74. Meisel, C.; Schwab, J.M.; Prass, K.; Meisel, A.; Dirnagl, U. Central nervous system injury-induced immune deficiency syndrome. *Nat. Rev. Neurosci.* **2005**, *6*, 775–786. [CrossRef] [PubMed]
75. Allison, D.J.; Ditor, D.S. Immune dysfunction and chronic inflammation following spinal cord injury. *Spinal. Cord.* **2015**, *53*, 14–18. [CrossRef] [PubMed]

76. Schmid, A.; Huonker, M.; Stahl, F.; Barturen, J.-M.; König, D.; Heim, M.; Lehmann, M.; Keul, J. Free plasma catecholamines in spinal cord injured persons with different injury levels at rest and during exercise. *J. Auton. Nerv. Syst.* **1998**, *68*, 96–100. [CrossRef]
77. Schwab, J.M.; Zhang, Y.; Kopp, M.A.; Brommer, B.; Popovich, P.G. The paradox of chronic neuroinflammation, systemic immune suppression, autoimmunity after traumatic chronic spinal cord injury. *Exp. Neurol.* **2014**, *258*, 121–129. [CrossRef]
78. Riegger, T.; Conrad, S.; Liu, K.; Schluesener, H.J.; Adibzahdeh, M.; Schwab, J.M. Spinal cord injury-induced immune de- pression syndrome (SCI-IDS). *Eur. J. Neurosci.* **2007**, *25*, 1743–1747. [CrossRef]
79. Ankeny, D.P.; Lucin, K.M.; Sanders, V.M.; McGaughy, V.M.; Popovich, P.G. Spinal cord injury triggers systemic autoimmunity: Evidence for chronic B lymphocyte activation and lupus-like autoantibody synthesis. *J. Neurochem.* **2006**, *99*, 1073–1087. [CrossRef]
80. Hailer, N.P. Immunosuppression after traumatic or ischemic CNS damage: It is neuroprotective and illuminates the role of microglial cells. *Prog. Neurobiol.* **2008**, *84*, 211–233. [CrossRef]
81. Hayes, K.C.; Hull, T.C.; Delaney, G.A.; Potter, P.J.; Sequeira, K.A.; Campbell, K.; Popovich, P.G. Elevated serum titers of proinflammatory cytokines and CNS autoantibodies in patients with chronic spinal cord injury. *J. Neurotrauma.* **2002**, *19*, 753–761. [CrossRef]
82. Kil, K.; Zang, Y.C.; Yang, D.; Markowski, J.; Fuoco, G.S.; Vendetti, G.C.; Rivera, V.M.; Zhang, J.Z. T cell responses to myelin basic protein in patients with spinal cord injury and multiple sclerosis. *J. Neuroimmunol.* **1999**, *9*, 201–207. [CrossRef]
83. Ankeney, D.P.; Guan, Z.; Popovich, P.G. B cells produce pathogenic antibodies and impair recovery after spinal cord injury in mice. *J. Clin. Invest.* **2009**, *119*, 2990–2999. [CrossRef] [PubMed]
84. Ankeny, D.P.; Popovich, P.G. B cells and autoantibodies: Complex roles in CNS injury. *Trends Immunol.* **2010**, *31*, 332–338. [CrossRef] [PubMed]
85. Saltzman, J.W.; Battaglino, R.A.; Salles, L.; Jha, P.; Sudhakar, S.; Garshick, E.; Stott, H.L.; Zafonte, R.; Morse, L.R. B-cell maturation antigen, a proliferation-inducing ligand, and B-cell activating factor are candidate mediators of spinal cord injury-induced autoimmunity. *J. Neurotrauma.* **2013**, *30*, 434–440. [CrossRef] [PubMed]
86. Mackay, F.; Silveira, P.A.; Brink, R. B cells and the BAFF/APRIL axis: Fast-forward on autoimmunity and signaling. *Curr. Opin. Immunol.* **2007**, *19*, 327–336. [CrossRef]
87. Rickert, R.C.; Jellusova, J.; Miletic, A.V. Signaling by the tumor necrosis factor receptor superfamily in B-cell biology and disease. *Immunol. Rev.* **2011**, *244*, 115–133. [CrossRef]
88. Mackay, F.; Woodcock, S.A.; Lawton, P.; Ambrose, C.; Baetscher, M.; Schneider, P.; Tschopp, J.; Browning, J.L. Mice transgenic for BAFF develop lymphocytic disorders along with autoimmune manifestations. *J. Exp. Med.* **1999**, *190*, 1697–1710. [CrossRef]
89. Vadacca, M.; Margiotta, D.; Sambataro, D.; Buzzulini, F.; Lo Vullo, M.; Rigon, A.; Afeltra, A. Pathway in Sjö"gren syndrome and systemic lupus erythematosus: Relationship with chronic inflammation and disease activity. *Reumatismo* **2010**, *62*, 259–265.
90. Mackay, F.; Schneider, P. Cracking the BAFF code. *Nat. Rev. Immunol.* **2009**, *9*, 491–502. [CrossRef]
91. Dekaban, G.A.; Thawer, S. Pathogenic antibodies are ac- tive participants in spinal cord injury. *J. Clin. Invest.* **2009**, *119*, 2881–2884. [CrossRef]
92. Herman, P.E.; Bloom, O. Altered leukocyte gene expression after traumatic spinal cord injury: Clinical implications. *Neural. Regen. Res.* **2018**, *13*, 1524–1529. [PubMed]
93. Foster, S.L.; Medzhitov, R. Gene-specific control of the TLR-in- duced inflammatory response. *Clin. Immunol.* **2009**, *130*, 7–15. [CrossRef] [PubMed]
94. Gao, W.; Xiong, Y.; Li, Q.; Yang, H. Inhibition of toll-like receptor signaling as a promising therapy for inflammatory diseases: A jour- ney from molecular to nano therapeutics. *Front Physiol.* **2017**, *8*, 508. [CrossRef] [PubMed]
95. Clark, J.; Findlay, D. Musculoskeletal Health in the Context of Spinal Cord Injury. *Curr. Osteoporos. Rep.* **2017**, *15*, 433–442. [CrossRef] [PubMed]
96. Ahuja, C.S.; Wilson, J.R.; Nori, S.; Kotter, M.R.N.; Druschel, C.; Curt, A.; Fehlings, M.G. Traumatic spinal cord injury. *Nat. Rev. Dis. Prim.* **2017**, *3*, 17018. [CrossRef]
97. Powers, S.K.; Smuder, A.J.; Judge, A.R. Oxidative stress and disuse muscle atrophy: Cause or consequence? *Curr. Opin. Clin. Nutr. Metab. Care* **2012**, *15*, 240–245. [CrossRef]
98. Menéndez, H.; Ferrero, C.; Martín-Hernández, J.; Figueroa, A.; Marín, P.; Herrero, A. Chronic effects of simultaneous electromyostimulation and vibration on leg blood flow in spinal cord injury. *Spinal. Cord.* **2016**, *54*, 1169–1175. [CrossRef]
99. West, C.R.; Alyahya, A.; Laher, I.; Krassioukov, A. Peripheral vascular function in spinal cord injury: A systematic review. *Spinal. Cord.* **2013**, *51*, 10–19. [CrossRef]
100. Gorgey, A.; Witt, O.; O'Brien, L.; Cardozo, C.; Chen, Q.; Lesnefsky, E.; Graham, Z. Mitochondrial health and muscle plasticity after spinal cord injury. *Eur. J. Appl. Physiol.* **2019**, *119*, 315–331. [CrossRef]
101. Hyatt, H.; Deminice, R.; Yoshihara, T.; Powers, S.K. Mitochondrial dysfunction induces muscle atrophy during prolonged inactivity: A review of the causes and effects. *Arch. Biochem. Biophys.* **2019**, *662*, 49–60. [CrossRef]
102. Invernizzi, M.; Carda, S.; Rizzi, M.; Grana, E.; Squarzanti, D.F.; Cisari, C.; Molinari, C.; Renò, F. Evaluation of serum myostatin and sclerostin levels in chronic spinal cord injured patients. *Spinal. Cord.* **2015**, *53*, 615–620. [CrossRef] [PubMed]
103. Bank, M.; Stein, A.; Sison, C.; Glazer, A.; Jassal, N.; McCarthy, D.; Shatzer, M.; Hahn, B.; Chugh, R.; Davies, P.; et al. Elevated circulating levels of the pro-inflammatory cytokine macrophage migration inhibitory factor in individuals with acute spinal cord injury. *Arch. Phys. Med. Rehabil.* **2015**, *96*, 633–644. [CrossRef] [PubMed]

104. Belizário, J.; Fontes-Oliveira, C.; Borges, J.; Kashiabara, J.; Vannier, E. Skeletal muscle wasting and renewal: A pivotal role of myokine IL-6. *Springerplus* **2016**, *5*, 619. [CrossRef] [PubMed]
105. Yune, T.; Chang, M.; Kim, S.; Lee, Y.; Shin, S.; Rhim, H.; Kim, Y.; Shin, M.; Oh, Y.; Han, C.; et al. Increased production of tumor necrosis factor-alpha induces apoptosis after traumatic spinal cord injury in rats. *J. Neurotrauma.* **2003**, *20*, 207–219. [CrossRef]
106. Phillips, T.; Leeuwenburgh, C. Muscle fiber specific apoptosis and TNF-alpha signaling in sarcopenia are attenuated by life-long calorie restriction. *FASEB J.* **2005**, *19*, 668–670. [CrossRef]
107. Min, K.; Smuder, A.J.; Kwon, O.S.; Kavazis, A.N.; Szeto, H.H.; Powers, S.K. Mitochondrial-targeted antioxidants protect skeletal muscle against immobilization-induced muscle atrophy. *J. Appl. Physiol.* **2011**, *111*, 1459–1466. [CrossRef]
108. Powers, S.K.; Kavazis, A.N.; McClung, J.M. Oxidative stress and disuse muscle atrophy. *J. Appl. Physiol.* **2007**, *102*, 2389–2397. [CrossRef]
109. Barker, T.; Traber, M.G. From animals to humans: Evidence linking oxidative stress as a causative factor in muscle atrophy. *J. Physiol.* **2007**, *583*, 421–422. [CrossRef]
110. Kadoguchi, T.; Takada, S.; Yokota, T.; Furihata, T.; Matsumoto, J.; Tsuda, M.; Mizushima, W.; Fukushima, A.; Okita, K.; Kinugawa, S. Deletion of NAD(P)H Oxidase 2 Prevents Angiotensin II-Induced Skeletal Muscle Atrophy. *Biomed. Res. Int.* **2018**, *2018*, 3194917. [CrossRef]
111. Kondo, H.; Miura, M.; Itokawa, Y. Oxidative stress in skeletal muscle atrophied by immobilization. *Acta. Physiol. Scand.* **1991**, *142*, 527–528. [CrossRef]
112. Gram, M.; Vigelsø, A.; Yokota, T.; Helge, J.W.; Dela, F.; Hey-Mogensen, M. Skeletal muscle mitochondrial H2O2 emission increases with immobilization and decreases after aerobic training in young and older men. *J. Physiol.* **2015**, *593*, 4011–4027. [CrossRef] [PubMed]
113. Liu, X.H.; Harlow, L.; Graham, Z.A.; Bauman, W.A.; Cardozo, C. Spinal Cord Injury Leads to Hyperoxidation and Nitrosylation of Skeletal Muscle Ryanodine Receptor-1 Associated with Upregulation of Nicotinamide Adenine Dinucleotide Phosphate Oxidase 4. *J. Neurotrauma.* **2017**, *34*, 2069–2074. [CrossRef] [PubMed]
114. Kadoguchi, T.; Kinugawa, S.; Takada, S.; Fukushima, A.; Furihata, T.; Homma, T.; Masaki, Y.; Mizushima, W.; Nishikawa, M.; Takahashi, M.; et al. Angiotensin II can directly induce mitochondrial dysfunction, decrease oxidative fibre number and induce atrophy in mouse hindlimb skeletal muscle. *Exp. Physiol.* **2015**, *100*, 312–322. [CrossRef] [PubMed]
115. Kitajima, Y.; Yoshioka, K.; Suzuki, N. The ubiquitin-proteasome system in regulation of the skeletal muscle homeostasis and atrophy: From basic science to disorders. *J. Physiol. Sci.* **2020**, *70*, 40. [CrossRef]
116. Savikj, M.; Kostovski, E.; Lundell, L.S.; Iversen, P.O.; Massart, J.; Widegren, U. Altered oxidative stress and antioxidant defence in skeletal muscle during the first year following spinal cord injury. *Physiol. Rep.* **2019**, *7*, e14218. [CrossRef]
117. Smuder, A.J.; Kavazis, A.N.; Min, K.; Powers, S.K. Exercise protects against doxorubicin-induced oxidative stress and proteolysis in skeletal muscle. *J. Appl. Physiol.* **2011**, *110*, 935–942. [CrossRef]
118. Whidden, M.A.; Smuder, A.J.; Wu, M.; Hudson, M.B.; Bradley Nelson, W.; Powers, S.K. Oxidative stress is required for mechanical ventilation-induced protease activation in the diaphragm. *J. Appl. Physiol.* **2010**, *108*, 1376–1382. [CrossRef]
119. Arc-Chagnaud, C.; Py, G.; Fovet, T.; Roumanille, R.; Demangel, R.; Pagano, A.F.; Delobel, P.; Blanc, S.; Jasmin, B.J.; Blottner, D.; et al. Evaluation of an Antioxidant and Anti-inflammatory Cocktail Against Human Hypoactivity-Induced Skeletal Muscle Deconditioning. *Front Physiol.* **2020**, *11*, 71. [CrossRef]
120. Coyoy-Salgado, A.; Segura-Uribe, J.J.; Guerra-Araiza, C.; Orozco-Suárez, S.; Salgado-Ceballos, H.; Feria-Romero, I.A.; Gallardo, J.M.; Orozco-Barrios, C.E. The Importance of Natural Antioxidants in the Treatment of Spinal Cord Injury in Animal Models: An Overview. *Oxid. Med. Cell Longev.* **2019**, *2019*, 3642491. [CrossRef]
121. Zhang, P.; Hölscher, C.; Ma, X. Therapeutic potential of flavonoids in spinal cord injury. *Rev. Neurosci.* **2017**, *28*, 87–101. [CrossRef]
122. Pannu, R.; Barbosa, E.; Singh, A.K.; Singh, I. Attenuation of acute inflammatory response by atorvastatin after spinal cord injury in rats. *J. Neurosci. Res.* **2005**, *79*, 340–350. [CrossRef] [PubMed]
123. Kawabe, J.; Koda, M.; Hashimoto, M.; Fujiyoshi, T.; Furuya, T.; Endo, T.; Okawa, A.; Yamazaki, M. Neuroprotective effects of granulocyte colony-stimulating factor and relationship to promotion of angiogenesis after spinal cord injury in rats: Laboratory investigation. *J. Neurosurg. Spine* **2011**, *15*, 414–421. [CrossRef] [PubMed]

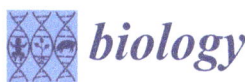

Article

Development of a Spinal Cord Injury Model Permissive to Study the Cardiovascular Effects of Rehabilitation Approaches Designed to Induce Neuroplasticity

Liisa Wainman [1,2], Erin L. Erskine [1,2], Mehdi Ahmadian [1,2,3], Thomas Matthew Hanna [1,4] and Christopher R. West [1,2,5,*]

[1] Centre for Chronic Disease Prevention and Management, Faculty of Medicine, University of British Columbia, Kelowna, BC V1V 1V7, Canada; lwain27@student.ubc.ca (L.W.); erin.erskine@ubc.ca (E.L.E.); mahmadia@student.ubc.ca (M.A.); tmhanna7@student.ubc.ca (T.M.H.)
[2] International Collaboration of Repair Discoveries (ICORD), University of British Columbia, Vancouver, BC V5Z 1M9, Canada
[3] School of Kinesiology, Faculty of Education, University of British Columbia, Vancouver, BC V6T 1Z1, Canada
[4] Department of Biology, Faculty of Science, University of British Columbia Okanagan, Kelowna, BC V1V 1V7, Canada
[5] Department of Cell and Physiological Sciences, Faculty of Medicine, University of British Columbia, Vancouver, BC V6T 1Z3, Canada
* Correspondence: chris.west@ubc.ca

Simple Summary: People living with high-level spinal cord injury experience worse cardiovascular health than the general population. In most spinal cord injuries, there are some remaining functioning pathways leading from the brain through the spinal cord to the organs and muscles, but not enough to sustain normal levels of function. Recently, therapies that aim to increase the strength of connections in these remaining pathways have shown great potential in restoring walking, hand, and breathing function in the spinal cord injured population. In order to test these therapies for their effects on cardiovascular function, we developed a new type of spinal cord injury rat model that spares enough pathways for these therapies to act upon but still produces measurable reductions in heart and blood vessel function that can be targeted with interventions/treatments.

Abstract: As primary medical care for spinal cord injury (SCI) has improved over the last decades there are more individuals living with neurologically incomplete (vs. complete) cervical injuries. For these individuals, a number of promising therapies are being actively researched in pre-clinical settings that seek to strengthen the remaining spinal pathways with a view to improve motor function. To date, few, if any, of these interventions have been tested for their effectiveness to improve autonomic and cardiovascular (CV) function. As a first step to testing such therapies, we aimed to develop a model that has sufficient sparing of descending sympathetic pathways for these interventions to target yet induces robust CV impairment. Twenty-six Wistar rats were assigned to SCI (n = 13) or naïve (n = 13) groups. Animals were injured at the T3 spinal segment with 300 kdyn of force. Fourteen days post-SCI, left ventricular (LV) and arterial catheterization was performed to assess in vivo cardiac and hemodynamic function. Spinal cord lesion characteristics along with sparing in catecholaminergic and serotonergic projections were determined via immunohistochemistry. SCI produced a decrease in mean arterial pressure of 17 ± 3 mmHg ($p < 0.001$) and left ventricular contractility (end-systolic elastance) of 0.7 ± 0.1 mmHg/μL ($p < 0.001$). Our novel SCI model produced significant decreases in cardiac and hemodynamic function while preserving $33 \pm 9\%$ of white matter at the injury epicenter, which we believe makes it a useful pre-clinical model of SCI to study rehabilitation approaches designed to induce neuroplasticity.

Keywords: cardiovascular; contusion; neuroplasticity

Citation: Wainman, L.; Erskine, E.L.; Ahmadian, M.; Hanna, T.M.; West, C.R. Development of a Spinal Cord Injury Model Permissive to Study the Cardiovascular Effects of Rehabilitation Approaches Designed to Induce Neuroplasticity. *Biology* **2021**, *10*, 1006. https://doi.org/10.3390/biology10101006

Academic Editors: Cédric G. Geoffroy and Warren Alilain

Received: 1 August 2021
Accepted: 29 September 2021
Published: 7 October 2021

Publisher's Note: MDPI stays neutral with regard to jurisdictional claims in published maps and institutional affiliations.

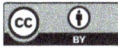

Copyright: © 2021 by the authors. Licensee MDPI, Basel, Switzerland. This article is an open access article distributed under the terms and conditions of the Creative Commons Attribution (CC BY) license (https://creativecommons.org/licenses/by/4.0/).

1. Introduction

Spinal cord injury (SCI) is a debilitating condition which, in addition to inducing sensorimotor dysfunction, also impairs autonomic function. Cardiovascular disease (CVD) has emerged as the primary cause of morbidity and mortality for individuals living with SCI [1]. SCI-induced dysregulation of the cardiovascular (CV) system occurs primarily as a result of altered descending control of sympathetic preganglionic neurons (SPNs). In turn, such reduced medullary input to SPNs causes a host of CV complications including resting hypotension, orthostatic hypotension (OH; sudden decrease in BP upon changing posture), autonomic dysreflexia (AD; sudden episodic hypertension accompanied by reflex bradycardia), and left-ventricular systolic function, which precipitate the early development of CVD [2].

In addition to changes in CV control, the sympathetic nervous system undergoes remarkable plasticity. These changes include decreased synaptic density accompanied by an increase in the number of inhibitory synapses rostral to the injury [3]. Caudal to the lesion, increased synaptogenesis [4] and changes in SPN morphology occurs, including increased arborization of SPNs [5] and axonal sprouting [6]. Historically, such sympathetic neuroplasticity has largely been considered detrimental due to the association of such plasticity with the expression of autonomic dysreflexia, immune suppression and neuropathic pain following SCI [7–9].

In the wider field of SCI, a number of recent promising interventions have been proposed that seeks to either leverage plasticity for functional benefit or alter such plasticity to offset functional decline. For example, the delivery of acute intermittent hypoxia (AIH) has been shown to enhance synaptic input onto spinal motor neurons and increase spinal excitability, both of which increase synaptic strength [10,11] and subsequently improve motor output in the acute [12,13] and chronic settings post-SCI [14,15]. Activity based therapy (ABT) is another intervention that has been demonstrated to facilitate the recovery of specific tasks (i.e., swimming) [16,17], hind-limb [18,19], and forelimb function [20,21]. These functional benefits are associated with increased spinal brain-derived neurotrophic factor (BDNF) levels and synaptic plasticity [22]. In all the aforementioned studies, the benefits of these therapies have been demonstrated in incomplete models of cervical and/or lower-thoracic (i.e., T9/10) SCI, wherein the injury is either not severe enough to induce CV dysfunction (i.e., the incomplete cervical models) or below the spinal level at which innervation to the key vascular beds and heart occurs (i.e., the low thoracic T9/T10 models).

For the CV system, a number of rat models have been developed to study the CV consequences of SCI, as well as the efficacy of various therapeutics. Two of the models that have received most traction are the T3/T4 complete transection model or a very severe midline contusion injury [23,24], though others also exist [25]. Both transection and severe contusion injuries (i.e., 400 kdyn contusion model) have been effective in producing changes to the CV function that mimic those observed clinically with high-lesion SCI, such as the presence of pronounced hypotension, reduced systolic cardiac function, and the presence of autonomic dysreflexia and orthostatic intolerance [23,26–29]. However, because these models either severed all pathways (in the case of transection injuries) or preserved such few medullary sympathetic pathways (i.e., <5% in the case of severe contusion) they are likely to be inappropriate to test the application of interventions designed to strengthen spinal sympathetic pathways. Indeed, in the few studies that have investigated the effect of ABT on CV function using such models post-SCI it has been shown that ABT was ineffective in restoring blood pressure control and systolic cardiac function, presumably because there were not sufficient bulbo-spinal sympathetic pathways left for ABT to target [27]. Instead, any benefits of ABT in these settings appear to be limited to the peripheral circulation and/or muscle.

Here, we present an in vivo and histological validation of a new moderately severe mid-line contusion injury model at the T3 level that we believe demonstrates an excellent balance between sparing sufficient bulbo-spinal sympathetic pathways that can be targeted with therapies, yet still induces a consistent and measurable decline in CV function that mimics that which occurs clinically. We propose that this model also more accurately reflects the changing demographic observed clinically, where the number of individuals with neurologically incomplete high-level injuries now outnumber those with neurologically complete injuries.

2. Materials and Methods

2.1. Ethical Approval

All procedures were conducted in accordance with the Canadian Council for Animal Care. Ethical approval was also obtained from the University of British Columbia (ACC-A18-0344).

2.2. Experimental Design

A total of 26 male Wistar rats (Charles River Laboratories, 11 ± 1 week old) were assigned to either SCI (n = 13) or naive (n = 13) groups. Study endpoint was conducted at 2 weeks post-SCI. This timeframe was selected as reductions in BP fully manifest by day 6 [29] and cardiac dysfunction is present immediately following injury [30,31] and persists into the chronic phase (i.e., 12 weeks post-SCI) [31,32]. Following in vivo measures, 5 SCI animals were randomly selected for standard spinal cord immunohistochemistry quantification of the injury site, and the 3 animals had their spinal cords harvested and cut in the longitudinal axis to visualize descending catecholaminergic and serotonergic bulbo-spinal projections, both of which are known to play a key role in CV control in the chronic phase post-SCI [24,33].

2.3. Spinal Cord Injury Surgery

Rats were prepared for spinal cord contusion surgery as described in previous studies [24,26,34,35]. The surgical preparation is depicted in Figure 1A. Briefly, on the day of SCI animals were anesthetized (5% isoflurane chamber induction, maintenance on 1.5–2% isoflurane; Piramal Critical Care, Bethlehem, PA, USA) and administered enrofloxacin (10 mg/kg; Bayer Animal Health, Shawnee, KS, USA), buprenorphine (0.5 mg/kg; Ceva Animal Health, Cambridge, ON, Canada) and warmed lactated ringer's solution (5 mL subcutaneously; Baxter Corporation, Portland, OR, USA). A dorsal midline incision was made and paraspinal musculature was bluntly dissected to expose C8–T5 spinous processes. A T3 laminectomy was performed exposing the T3 dura. Rodents were then transported and mounted on a plastic staging platform where the T2 and T4 spinous processes were stabilized with curved tip clamps. Using a high-definition camera secured to the mounting frame, the custom impactor tip (3 mm; Infinite Horizons (IH) Impactor; Precision Systems and Instrumentation, Fairfax Station, VA, USA) was adjusted to track midline over the T3 dura. The impactor tip was dropped on the cord with 300 kdyn of predefined force (316 ± 14 kdyn force, 1673 ± 128 mm displacement, 124 ± 5 mm/s velocity). The muscle and the skin incisions were closed with 4-0 coated vicryl (Ethicon, Somerville, MA, USA). Velocity, force of impact, and distance travelled by the impactor were recorded. Animals were recovered in an incubator for 30 min at 37 °C 50% humidity and received a subsequent 5 mL lactated ringer's solution before they were returned to their home cages.

2.4. Post-Surgical Care

For 4 days post injury, animals were administered subcutaneous lactated ringers (3× per day, 5 mL), buprenorphine (3× per day, 0.02 mg/kg) and enrofloxacin (1× per day, 10 mg/kg). Bladders were manually voided 4× per day until spontaneous voiding was regained (4–6 days post-injury). Animals were pair-housed on oat bedding with rubber matting to prevent the ingestion of woodchips due to opioid-induced pica and to aid in mobility. Animals were provided a supportive diet consisting of Hydrogel (ClearH$_2$O), fruit, spinach, and cereal until mobility was regained and pica subsided.

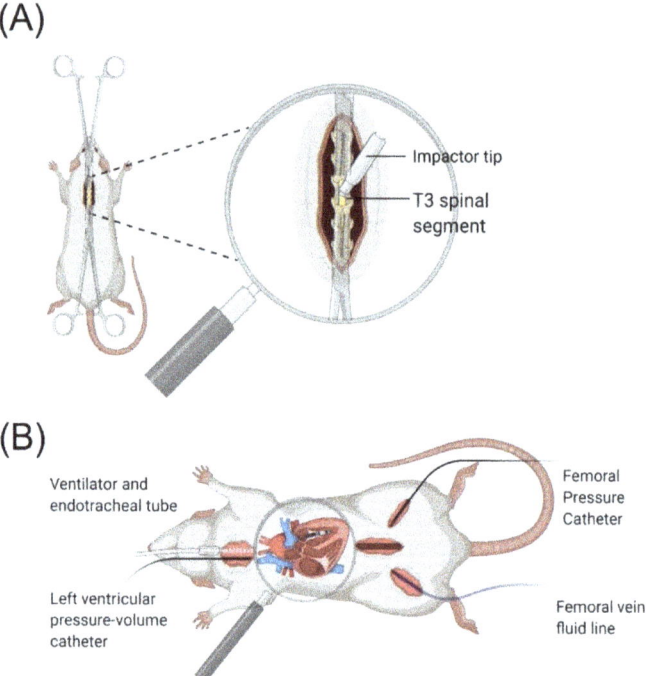

Figure 1. (**A**) Rodent SCI surgery setup depicting laminectomy and contusion injury method. (**B**) In vivo terminal preparation consisting of an endotracheal tube and ventilator, left ventricular pressure-volume catheter, femoral artery pressure catheter, and femoral venous line.

2.5. Outcome Surgery

At 14 days post-SCI, echocardiography was performed to assess left ventricular (LV) structure, cardiac catheterization was performed to model LV pressure-volume relationships and assess LV contractility, arterial catheterization was performed to assess blood pressure and a venous line was placed for intravenous fluid administration to maintain acid-base balance (Figure 1B).

For the terminal in vivo assessments, animals were anesthetized with intraperitoneal urethane (1.6 ± 0.4 mg/kg; Sigma-Aldrich, St. Louis, MO, USA). Animals were instrumented with a rectal thermometer and all procedures were performed on a heating pad (RightTemp; Kent Scientific, Torrington, CT, USA) to maintain core body temperature at 37 ± 0.5 °C. Transthoracic echocardiography was used to obtain B-mode parasternal long axis images to measure LV volumes (Vevo 3100; VisualSonics, Toronto, ON, Canada). Next, the rat was placed supine, and a midline incision was performed from mandible to manubrium. Sternohyoid muscle was bluntly dissected then trachea and right common carotid artery (CCA) isolated. A tracheostomy was performed, an endotracheal tube was secured, and the animal was ventilated on 100% O_2 (VentElite; Harvard Apparatus, Holliston, MA, USA) using a standard tidal volume and breathing frequency calculation based off the animal's mass [36]. The CCA was pierced, and a 1.9-French pressure-volume (PV) admittance catheter (Transonic Scisense, Ithaca, NY, US) advanced into the LV [36]. Bilateral incisions along the inguinal ligament were performed and the femoral artery and vein were isolated. A 1.6-French pressure catheter (Transonic Scisense, Ithaca, NY, USA) was placed into the left femoral artery and advanced into the abdominal aorta for collection of hemodynamic data. The right femoral vein was cannulated with a fluid delivery line (PE50 tubing) for constant infusion of lactated ringer's solution throughout the experiment (1.7 mL/kg/h; Pump 11 Elite, Harvard Apparatus, Holliston, MA, USA). Finally, a ventral laparotomy was performed and inferior vena cava isolated to perform inferior vena cava occlusions (IVCOs) which enables venous return to be reduced and the slope of the end-systolic pressure-volume relationship to be obtained. The slope of this relationship is end-systolic elastance and is the reference standard for load-independent LV contractility [36].

Following the completion of instrumentation, the animal was allowed to stabilize for 15 min prior to the collection of a 5 min baseline for the assessment of hemodynamics and cardiac function. An IVCO was then performed to assess end-systolic elastance.

2.6. Ethanasia and Tissue Processing

Following the completion of all in vivo measures, 8 animals were selected at random for immunohistological preparation. Rats were perfused transcardially with 200–300 mL of 0.1 M phosphate-buffered saline (PBS; Sigma-Aldrich, St. Louis, MA, USA) and fixed with 400–500 mL 4% paraformaldehyde (PF; Sigma-Aldrich, St. Louis, MA, USA). Lesion sites (±4 mm from epicenter; T1–T5 segments) were dissected following perfusion and stored in PF for no more than 48 h followed by at least 24 h in 10% sucrose before being flash frozen in Shandon Cryomatrix (Thermo Scientific, Cat: 67-690-06, Waltham, MA, USA) and stored at −80 °C.

2.7. Data Analysis

Echocardiography indices were obtained from an average of 3 end-systolic and end-diastolic images from each animal and used to correct PV estimates of volumes.

All PV indices were analyzed using the PV loop analysis software in Labchart8 (AD Instruments). The following measures of LV systolic function were averaged across the final 60 s of baseline data: stroke volume (SV; calculated as end diastolic volume [EDV]-end systolic volume [ESV]), ejection fraction (EF; calculated as SV/EDV×100%), end-systolic pressure (Pes), the maximal rate of rise of the LV pressure (dP/dt_{max}), dP/dt_{max} normalized to end-diastolic volume ($dP/dt_{max}-EDV$), stroke work (SW; area inside the PV loop), stroke work index (SWI; SWI = SW/g), cardiac output (CO = SV·HR), cardiac index (CI; CI = CO/g), The following indexes of diastolic function were also measured from the same loops: end-diastolic pressure (Ped), maximal rate of fall of the LV pressure waveform (dP/dt_{min}), and the time constant of LV pressure decay during isovolumetric relaxation. Hemodynamic indices systolic blood pressure (SBP), diastolic blood pressure (DBP), pulse pressure (PP) (calculated as PP = SBP−DBP), heart rate (HR), mean arterial pressure (MAP; calculated as MAP = 1/3SBP + 2/3 DBP) and systemic vascular resistance (SVR; SVR = MAP/CO) were extracted from the same 60 s.

Load-independent indices of LV contractility were calculated from one IVC occlusion. One 10-s section of the IVC occlusion was selected and loops that occurred during an expiration were removed to prevent respiratory-induced changes in intrathoracic pressure right-shifting the PV loop. Preload-recruitable stroke work (PRSW) was evaluated as the slope of the linear regression of SW and EDV. End-systolic elastance (Ees) was taken as the slope of the end-systolic pressure-volume relationship. dP/dt_{max}-EDV was calculated as the slope of the linear regression of dP/dt_{max} to EDV.

Arterial elastance (Ea) was calculated as Ea = Pes/SV. Ea/Ees was calculated as the quotient of Ea divided by Ees.

2.8. Immunohistochemistry

Spinal cords were cut using a cryostat (Leica, CM3050s, Wetzlar, Germany) in either the transverse (n = 5) or longitudinal (n = 3) plane. Transverse sections were cut at 10 μm thickness with an inter-section distance of 1 mm. Longitudinal sections (n = 3) were cut at 10 μm thickness and with an inter-section distance of 600 μm.

Slides were thawed and dried at room temperature for 20 min then a hydrophobic barrier was drawn. Slides were rehydrated with 3 10-min washes in PBS followed by incubation in blocking solution (10% normal donkey serum) in PBS-Tx-Azd for 45 min. Slide were then incubated with primary antibodies over night. The next day the tissue was washed three times (15 min each) with PBS, incubated with secondary antibodies for 2 h, and then washed with PBS three times (15 min each). Finally, the slides were cover-slipped using ProLong Gold antifade mounting medium (Invitrogen, LSP36930, Waltham, MA, USA).

For transverse sections primary antibodies were used as follows; mouse GFAP (Glial fibrillary acidic protein; 1:1000, Sigma; G3893, Waltham, MA, USA), chicken polyclonal MBP (Myelin basic protein; 1:1000, Aves Labs; MBP), guineapig NeuN (Neuronal nuclei; 1:500, Sigma; ABN90P, St. Louis, MA, USA). The following secondaries were used; donkey anti-mouse Cy3 (1:800, Jackson Immunoresearch; 705-166-147, West Grove, PA, USA), donkey anti-chicken pAb Alexa647 (1:800, Jackson Immunoresearch; 7056-606-148, West Grove, PA, USA), donkey anti-guineapig DyLight405 (1:800, Jackson Immunoresearch; 711-475-152, West Grove, PA, USA).

For longitudinal slides primary antibodies were used as follows; sheep TH (tyrosine hydroxylase; 1:200, EMD Milipore; AB1542, Burlington, VT, USA), rabbit 5-HT (5-hydroxytryptamine; 1:2000, Immunostar; 20080. Hudson, NY, US). The following secondaries were used; Donkey anti-sheep Cy3 (1:200, Jackson Immunoresearch; 713-166-147, West Grove, PA, USA) and donkey anti-rabbit DyLight488 (1:1000, Abcam; ab96899, Cambridge, UK).

Immunofluorescence imaging was performed using an Axio Imager M2 microscope (Zeiss, Oberkochen, Germany) with an Axiocam 705 mono camera (Zeiss, Oberkochen, Germany) using ZEN 2 Blue software (Zeiss, Oberkochen, Germany). Images were digitally processed using Zen 2 Blue software (Zeiss, Oberkochen, Germany).

Analysis was performed in ImageJ (ImageJ, Rockville, MD, USA). Lesion area and white matter sparing were quantified every 400 μm from 2.0 mm rostral to 2.0 mm caudal to the injury epicenter. The injury epicenter section was based on the section with the least intact GFAP signal. Lesion area was manually outlined based on the following definition: GFAP-negative or GFAP-positive area with disrupted or abnormal cytoarchitecture. Care was taken to avoid inclusion of any artifacts. Myelin preservation (i.e., white matter sparing) was estimated by manually outlining MBP-positive area with normal or near-normal cytoarchitecture. Lesion volume was then calculated according to the following formula: Volume = Σ (area · section thickness · number of sections between samples) [24].

For longitudinal sections, images were imported into ImageJ (ImageJ, Rockville, MD, USA) and converted to 8-bit. The backgrounds were then subtracted, and for each stain, the images were set to a threshold only including pixels with intensity values from 20–255. The analyzed regions were selected by tracing the epicenter and selecting 2 × 1 mm rectangles 0.5 mm rostral and caudal to the border of the lesion. After measuring the positive pixel density of the enclosed areas, the density of the caudal area was divided by the density of the rostral area to calculate the percent difference. The relative density of an anterior, posterior and central section of the cord for each animal was calculated and expressed as means and standard deviations calculated from 3 animals.

2.9. Statistics

Between-group differences in all in vivo physiological outcomes were analyzed using an independent samples t-test in SPSS (IBM SPSS Statistics, Chicago, IL, USA). Data are expressed as means ± standard deviation. Statistical significance was set at $p < 0.05$. Graphical representations of in vivo data were produced in MATLAB (MathWorks, Natick, MA, USA) and Prism (GraphPad Prism, San Diego, CA, USA). Histological images were produced in Zen Image Processing (Zeiss, Oberkochen, Germany).

3. Results

At study termination SCI rats were significantly lighter than naïve animals ($p = 0.014$; Figure 2) but there was no significant difference in body mass of SCI animals at day 14 post-injury vs. pre-injury ($p = 0.154$).

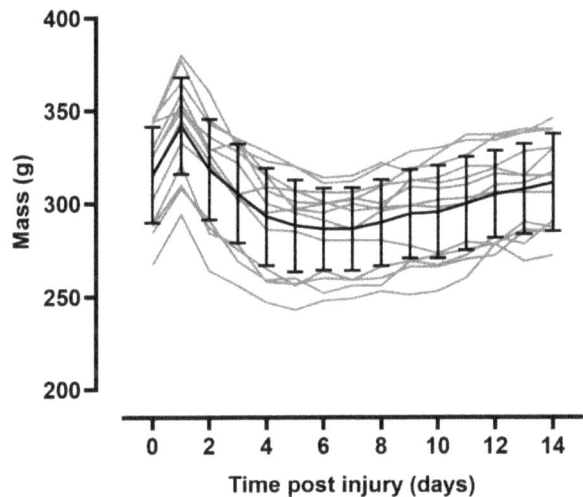

Figure 2. Body mass with time pre/post-injury. Note there were no significant differences in body mass across the 14-day study period. Black lines indicate mean mass ± SD, grey lines represent individual animals body mass.

3.1. Resting Hemodynamics Are Impaired in T3 300 kdyn SCI Rats

Hemodynamic indices are presented in Table 1 and Figure 3. SBP, DBP, PP and MAP were all significantly reduced among SCI compared to naïve rats (all $p < 0.001$). HR was significantly higher among SCI rats compared to naïve rats ($p = 0.008$). Systemic vascular resistance (SVR) was also reduced in SCI rats compared to naïve ($p = 0.038$).

Table 1. Anthropometric, hemodynamic and pressure-volume data for 2-week post T3 300 kdyn SCI and naïve rats.

	Naïve			SCI			p-Value
			Hemodynamic Data				
SBP (mmHg)	121	±	7	96	±	11	<0.001
DBP (mmHg)	70	±	7	58	±	9	<0.001
MAP (mmHg)	88	±	7	70	±	9	<0.001
PP (mmHg)	50	±	4	38	±	6	<0.001
HR (BPM)	413	±	38	462	±	48	0.008
SVR (mmHg·min^{-1}μL^{-1}) *	0.89	±	0.20	0.74	±	0.12	0.038
			Pressure-Volume Data				
ESV (μL)	66	±	18	59	±	11	0.256
EDV (μL)	311	±	47	261	±	23	0.002
Systolic Function							
SW (mmHg·mL)	33	±	7	21	±	4	<0.001
SWI (mmHg·mL^{-1}100 g^{-1})	10.90	±	2.53	7.52	±	1.64	<0.001
CO (mL/min)	102	±	20	93	±	12	0.201
CI (mL·min^{-1}100 g^{-1})	33.69	±	7.72	35.22	±	7.32	0.610
SV (μL)	245	±	33	202	±	24	0.001
Pes (mmHg)	98	±	11	75	±	10	<0.001
EF (%)	79	±	4	77	±	5	0.272
dP/dt$_{max}$ (mmHg/s)	10316	±	809	6084	±	755	<0.001

Table 1. Cont.

	Naïve			SCI			p-Value
Ees (mmHg/µL) **	1.59	±	0.23	0.89	±	0.24	<0.001
Ea (mmHg/µL)	0.41	±	0.09	0.38	±	0.07	0.296
Ea/Ees **	0.26	±	0.06	0.44	±	0.23	0.021
PRSW (mmHg) *	131	±	30	94	±	17	0.001
+dP/dt$_{max}$–EDV (mmHg·s^{-1} µL^{-1}) *	34	±	7	27	±	4	<0.001
Diastolic Function							
dP/dt$_{min}$ (mmHg/s)	−5890	±	449	−4021	±	630	<0.001
Ped (mmHg)	3	±	2	4	±	4	0.231
τ (ms)	7.32	±	0.77	8.03	±	3	0.416

Data are presented as means ± SD. *p*-values represent significant difference following independent samples t test. SBP, systolic blood pressure; DBP, diastolic blood pressure; MAP, mean arterial pressure; PP, pulse pressure; HR, heart rate; SVR, systemic vascular resistance; ESV, end-systolic volume; EDV, end-diastolic volume; SW, stroke work; SWI, stroke work index; CO, cardiac output; CI, cardiac index; SV, stroke volume; Pes, end-systolic pressure; EF, ejection fraction; dP/dt$_{max}$, maximum rate of rise of left ventricular pressure; Ees, end-systolic pressure-volume relationship; Ea, arterial elastance; PRSW, preload-recruitable stroke work; dP/dt$_{min}$, maximum rate of decay of left ventricular pressure; Ped, end-diastolic pressure; τ time constant of left ventricular pressure decay. * denotes naïve n = 12, SCI n = 12, ** denotes naïve n = 12, SCI n = 9 due to difficulties in performing IVC occlusions in some animals.

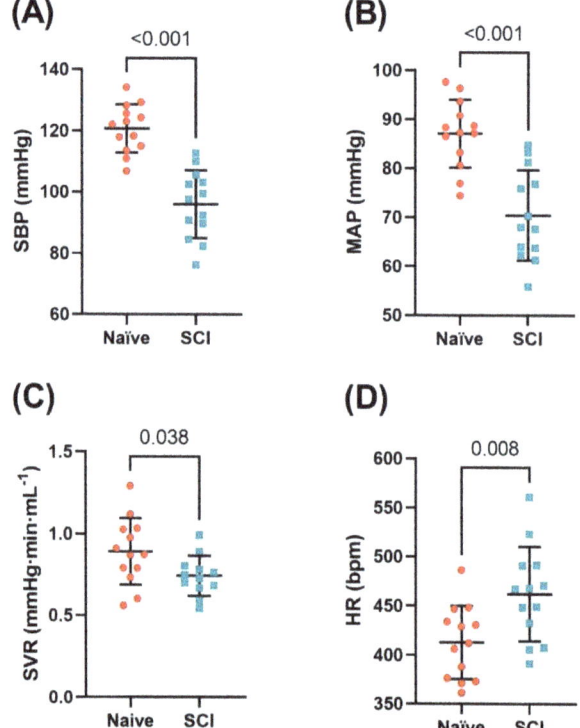

Figure 3. Comparison of resting hemodynamic indices of naïve (n = 13) and spinal cord injured (SCI) rats (n = 13) two weeks post-injury. Bars represent the means and standard deviations overlaid with individual data. (**A**) Systolic blood pressure (SBP) was significantly lower in SCI compared to naïve animals (25 ± 4 mmHg, $p < 0.001$). (**B**) Mean arterial pressure (MAP) was significantly lower among SCI compared to naïve animals (17 ± 3 mmHg, $p < 0.001$). (**C**) Systemic vascular resistance (SVR) was significantly lower among SCI compared to naïve animals (0.11 ± 0.08 mmHg·min^{-1} µL^{-1}, $p = 0.034$). (**D**): Heart rate (HR) was significantly higher among SCI compared to naïve animals (49 ± 17 beats per minute, BPM; $p = 0.008$).

3.2. Left Ventricular Systolic Function Is Impaired in T3 300 kdyn SCI Rats

LV measures of systolic and diastolic function are reported in Table 1 and select indices are displayed in Figure 4. Among SCI rats, a decrease in EDV ($p = 0.002$) and SV ($p = 0.001$) was observed compared to naïve rats, in the absence of changes to ESV ($p = 0.256$) and EF ($p = 0.272$). SW and SWI were significantly lower among SCI rats compared to naïve (both $p < 0.001$). Conversely, there was no difference in CO or CI between groups ($p = 0.201$; $p = -0.610$, respectively). Pes, Pmax and the maximum rate of rise of LV pressure (dP/dt_{max}) were lower among SCI compared to naïve rats (all $p < 0.001$). Measures of load-independent function, Ees ($p < 0.001$), dP/dt_{max}−EDV ($p < 0.001$), and PRSW ($p = 0.001$) were significantly lower in SCI compared to naïve rats. Ea was not significantly different between groups ($p = 0.296$), however Ea/Ees was significantly higher in SCI rats compared to naïve.

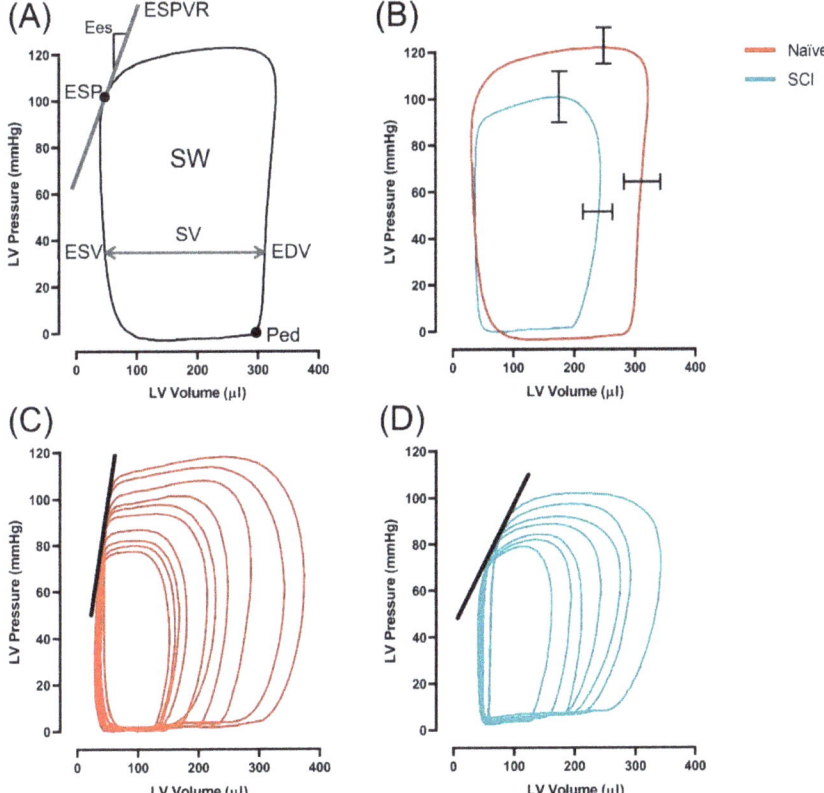

Figure 4. At 2 weeks post-SCI, animals underwent left ventricular catheterization to assess cardiac function. Pressure-volume analysis revealed reduced pressure, volume, and contractile function among SCI compared to naïve rats. (**A**) An example pressure-volume loop labelled with relevant indices acquired from pressure-volume analysis (ESV; end-systolic volume, EDV; end-diastolic volume, Pes; end-systolic pressure, Ped; end-diastolic pressure, SV; stroke volume, SW; stroke work (area of the pressure volume loop), ESPVR; end systolic pressure volume relationship, Ees slope of ESPVR). (**B**) Example basal pressure volume loop from SCI and naïve rats, overlaid with SEM bars, demonstrating diminished LV maximum pressure (22 ± 4 mmHg; $p < 0.001$) and EDV (50 ± 15 ul; $p = 0.002$) in SCI compared to naïve animals. C-D: Example inferior vena cava occlusions from naïve (**C**) and SCI (**D**) groups demonstrating reduced Ees among SCI compared to naïve animals (0.7 ± 0.1 mmHg/ul; $p < 0.001$).

For diastolic function, dP/dt$_{min}$ was significantly lower among SCI rats compared to naïve ($p > 0.001$) in the absence of differences in end diastolic pressure ($p = 0.231$) and time constant of LV pressure decay (tau, $p = 0.416$).

3.3. Moderately-Severe T3 Midline Injury Interrupts Descending Pathways

Following moderately-severe T3 SCI the lesion area was 1.75 ± 0.40 mm^2 leaving $21 \pm 6\%$ tissue sparing. Lesion volume was 4.26 ± 1.28 mm^3. White matter sparing at the epicenter was $33 \pm 9\%$ (Figure 5). The density of 5-HT$^+$ fibres caudal to the epicenter was reduced to $9 \pm 2\%$ of rostral density (Figure 6). The density of TH$^+$ fibres caudal to the epicenter were reduced to $18 \pm 9\%$ of the rostral density (Figure 6).

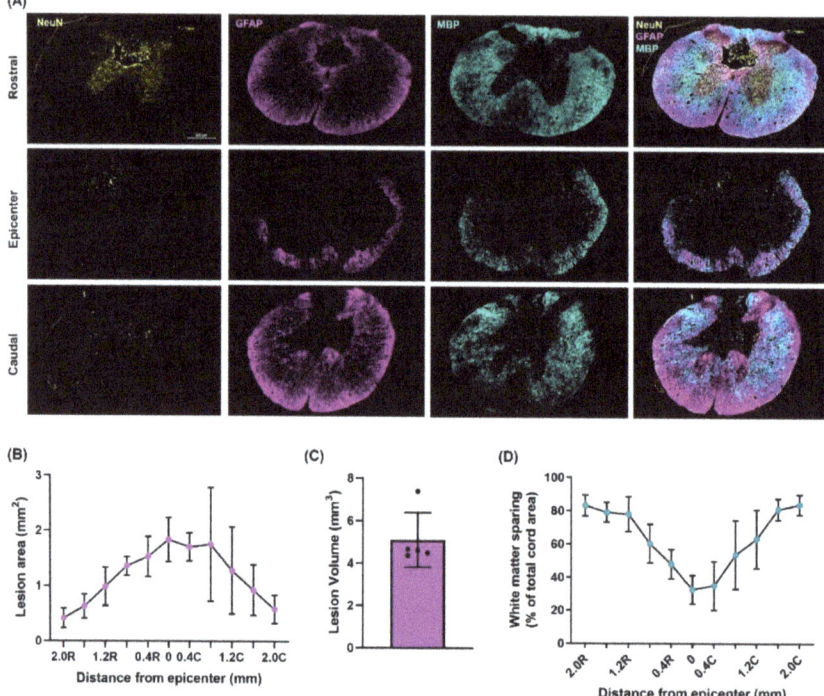

Figure 5. Lesion site characterization. (**A**) Representative immunohistological images of the rostral (top), epicenter (middle), and caudal (bottom) sections. Stains from left to right are Neuronal Nuclei (NeuN), Glial Fibrillary Protein (GFAP), Myelin Basic Protein (MBP), and the merged stain. Data were quantified every 400 μm from the lesion epicenter to a distance of 2 mm rostrally and caudally (n = 5). (**B**) The GFAP signal was used to quantify lesion area which reached an area of 1.75 ± 0.40 mm^2 at the epicenter. Data points and bars represent the mean and standard deviations, respectively. (**C**) Lesion volume was calculated as Volume = Σ (area · section thickness · number of sections between samples) [24] and was found to be 4.26 ± 1.28 mm^3. Bars represent the means and standard deviations overlaid with individual data. (**D**) White matter sparing was quantified using the MBP signal and reached a minimum sparing at the epicenter of $33 \pm 9\%$. Data points and bars represent the mean and standard deviations, respectively.

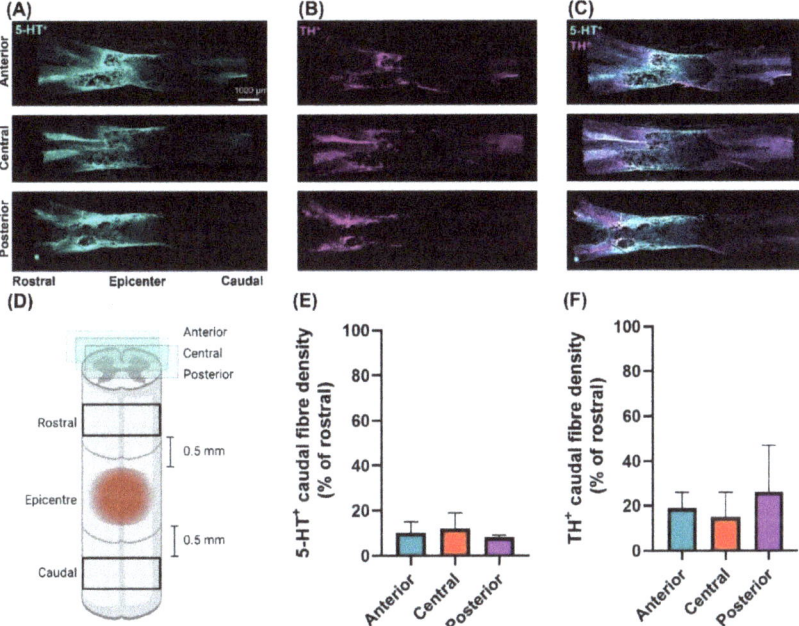

Figure 6. Representative immunohistological images of longitudinal spinal cord sections, anterior (top), central (middle), and posterior (bottom) (**A–C**). Stains from left to right are 5-HT$^+$, TH$^+$ and merged. Each quantified section was 500 μm removed from the one previous (**D**) Schematic depicting the anatomical location of where densities of 5-HT$^+$ and TH$^+$ were measured 0.5 mm rostral and caudal to the epicenter with the area of study being 2 mm wide by 1 mm tall. The associated density plots comparing the caudal to the rostral stain density across anterior, central and posterior sections for 5-HT$^+$ (**E**) TH$^+$ (**F**). Caudal sparing was quantified as 9 ± 2% and 18 ± 9% relative to rostral for 5-HT$^+$ and TH$^+$, respectively (n = 3). Data are presented as means ± standard error.

4. Discussion

We have developed a novel moderately severe high-thoracic midline contusion SCI model that produces robust and clinically relevant impairment in cardiac and hemodynamic function whilst preserving 33 ± 9% of white matter at the injury epicenter. Though our model also robustly reduces the density of 5-HT$^+$ and TH$^+$ fibres at and below the injury epicenter, we were able to clearly visualize both TH$^+$ and 5-HT$^+$ fibres projecting through and below the injury site. As such we believe this model provides a nice balance between producing a clinically relevant decline in CV function yet sparing sufficient bulbospinal sympathetic and serotonergic pathways that can be targeted with therapies designed to induce/alter spinal neuroplasticity with a view to improving CV function.

4.1. Resting Hemodynamics Are Impaired in T3 300 kdyn SCI Rats

Reduced SBP and MAP have been demonstrated in a variety of high-thoracic contusion, clip compression and transection SCI models. Though it is difficult to compare BP across studies due to heterogeneity in measurement technique and rodent strain, the magnitude of decline in SBP and MAP is typically in the 15–25 mmHg range with complete transection or severe contusion at the T2–T4 spinal level [24,26,27,32,34,37]. We found a similar 25 mmHg decline in the present study despite our model being less severe and exhibiting more sparing at the injury epicenter (see below) than those typically used to induce CV dysfunction. It has been recently shown that the major "hot-spot" for blood pressure control are the splanchnic projecting SPNs that exit the cord at the T11–T13 level [28].

SPNs in this region of the cord are under the control of both descending bulbo-spinal catecholaminergic and serotonergic [33] pathways originating in the RVLM and Raphe, respectively. Histological analyses of TH$^+$ and 5-HT$^+$ fibres in longitudinal sections of the spinal cord revealed our injury significantly reduces the density of both sets of fibers at and below (vs. above) the injury site. In turn, this loss of catecholaminergic and serotonergic excitatory input to SPNs reduces vascular tone, leading to splanchnic pooling and hypotension [38]. Persistent hypotension is of clinical importance as it contributes to the disproportionate burden of ischemic stroke heart disease observed in SCI [2]. Notably, a 20 mmHg decline in SBP and MAP is typical of that observed in individuals with chronic high-level SCI [39,40], thus increasing the potential for translation of findings using this model. Importantly, whilst TH$^+$ and 5-HT$^+$ fibre density was reduced post-SCI we were able to clearly visualize both TH$^+$ and 5-HT$^+$ fibres traversing the injury site. We believe the presence of such fibres, whilst insufficient to offset hypotension, can act as a target for neurotherapeutic interventions that aim to strengthen synaptic input.

4.2. Left Ventricular Systolic Function Is Impaired in T3 300 kdyn SCI Rats

Another major finding of the present was that almost all pressure- and volume-related indices of resting LV function were significantly decreased in SCI vs. naïve rats, with the exception of ESV and EF. We have previously reported similar findings in more severe models of SCI (i.e., T3 400 kdyn contusion with 5 s dwell, or T3 complete transection) [24,26,27,34,37], but not in less-severe models of SCI (T3 200 kdyn contusion, 5 s dwell) [34]. Reductions in volumetric function post-SCI also occurs clinically with high-level SCI. Although there was no difference in ESV, SV was lower in SCI rats likely due to reduced preload (i.e., EDV). Interestingly, this decrease in SV was compensated by increases in HR resulting in no statistical difference in CO between groups. A SCI-induced increase in HR has also been demonstrated in other studies with injuries at the T3–T5 spinal level, and has been hypothesized to result from increased sympathetic activity above the level of injury [41] as this injury model spares some sympathetic input to T1 level SPNs. It is equally possible, however, that SCI induces changes in cardiovagal balance such that HR can increase via vagal withdrawal sufficiently to normalize CO. Whilst the reduction in resting pressure and volume indices of LV systolic function are likely due to reduced catecholaminergic and serotonergic input to the SPNs in the T2–T5 level of the spinal cord [42], these indices are also critically dependent on changes in pre-load and afterload, both of which are impacted by SCI, as evidenced by reduced EDV and systemic blood pressure in this present study. Unlike resting pressure-volume indices, $dP/dt_{max}-EDV$, PRSW and Ees obtained from IVC occlusions are largely insensitive to changes in load or rate [43] and as such are considered the reference metrics for LV systolic function [36]. We found all 3 metrics were significantly reduced in SCI vs. naïve rats, presumably due to the reduced density of 5-HT$^+$ and TH$^+$ fibres at and below the injury epicenter. The magnitude of reduction in these indices of contractility is similar to that observed in our more severe injury models [26,27,32,35] despite our current model sparing more white matter and there being a clear visualization of both TH$^+$ and 5-HT$^+$ fibres traversing the injury site. The reduction in Ees precipitated an increase in the Ea/Ees ratio, implying this SCI model impairs cardiac efficiency.

4.3. T3 Moderately-Severe Contusion Injury Interrupts Descending Pathways

Moderately-severe T3 spinal cord contusion injury resulted in substantial white matter damage at the epicenter and a lesion that extended at least 2 mm rostral and caudally encompassing the T2 spinal level thus interrupting supraspinal control to SPNs critical for CV regulation at the spinal levels described above. These histological findings are supported by the reduced density of 5-HT$^+$ and TH$^+$ fibres below the lesion suggesting that serotonergic and catecholaminergic input to SPNs is reduced by this model of SCI. Serotonergic [44,45] and catecholaminergic [46,47] bulbo-spinal fibres densely innervate areas of the cord associated with input to SPNs. Loss of supraspinal 5-HT$^+$ fibres play a key role in inducing CV dysregulation including contributing to the development of AD and hypotension observed post-SCI [33,48]. Other models of SCI which have explored the relationship between 5-HT$^+$ preservation and CV function post-SCI include complete crush [25], and partial transection [49] models of SCI at the T4 level. Neither crush injury nor partial transection reported reduced MAP despite showing reduced/absent density of serotonergic fibres caudal to the injury. While these SCI models were performed at a more caudal spinal level, CV dysfunction is seen in severe injuries as low as T6. This observation suggests, perhaps, that the mechanism of injury is not severe enough to sever sufficient pathways to impair CV function, given that it is necessary to decrease white matter sparing substantially to induce a decline in CV function post-SCI [24]. Other models of SCI which demonstrated motor recovery following ABT utilized a T10 contusive injury which resulted in 8–22% white matter sparing at the epicenter [17] or T10 hemisection models with approximately 35% white matter sparing [18]. Such levels of 'required' sparing suggests that our model maintains sufficient pathways for successful application of therapies to induce neuroplasticity.

4.4. Comparison to Other Rodent Models of CV Instability

A number of rodent models of CV dysfunction have now been proposed in the literature and we have summarized the findings and gaps in knowledge from these models in Table 2. To aid in this comparison, we selected a number of key findings that we believe are critical for an animal model to exhibit when studying the efficacy of interventions aimed at inducing neuroplasticity. Our selected indices included reduced blood pressure, cardiac pressures and cardiac volumes, as well as sufficient tissue and white matter sparing at the epicentre and the presence of catecholaminergic and serotonergic fibres traversing the injury site. In the studies conducted to date that we are aware of, whilst almost all of the high-thoracic models induce reductions in blood pressure and/or heart function it is likely that only the current T3 contusion model has sufficient tissue sparing and catecholaminergic/serotonergic projections for such therapies to work. As such we believe our model achieves a feat not previously achieved in prior models; that is, modest tissue sparing at the injury epicenter yet a severe reduction in cardiac and hemodynamic function.

Table 2. Comparisons with previous models of SCI that have been used to induce cardiovascular dysfunction.

	Injury Model					
	T3 300 kdyn Contusion	T2 400 kdyn Contusion	T2 200 kdyn Contusion	T2-3 Transection	T4 Complete Crush	T10 400 kdyn Contusion
↓ Blood pressure	✓	✓	✓	✓	✗	✗
↓ Cardiac pressures	✓	✓	?	✓	?	?
↓ Cardiac output	✗	✓	✗	✓	?	?
>15% tissue sparing	✓	✗	✗	✗	?	?
>20% white matter Preservation	✓	✗	✗	✗	?	✗
Preserved sub-lesional serotonergic/ catecholaminergic pathways	✓	✗	✓	?	✗	N/A
References		[24,26,27,34]	[24,34]	[23,30,32]	[25]	[50,51]

An additional benefit of this model is that animal health was greatly improved over our typical experience with more severe contusion and transection injury models. Notably, animals regained spontaneous voiding within 5 days post-injury compared to the typical 10 days seen among transected rats [52], returned to pre-injury health scores and pre-surgical body mass by 14 days-post injury and mortality was remarkably low with 93% of all animals surviving the initial injury surgery and no mortality across the 14-day period. We believe this model, therefore, improves upon animal welfare and decreases the burden of care on researchers.

4.5. Limitations

This model has yet to be tested in female rats to account for sex differences in autonomic function. Although we know that cardiac dysfunction manifests within the first 4 h post-SCI [31], and there are similar impairments at 3 and 7 days [53], 5 weeks [34], and 12 weeks post-SCI [32] the time course of CV function beyond 12 weeks in contusive models of SCI has not yet been characterized.

5. Conclusions

Here, we have presented a high-thoracic contusion model of SCI which demonstrated marked CV decline and modest tissue sparing at the epicenter, a feat not achieved by previous SCI models. Given the recent impetus of the field to move towards interventions that aim to enhance neuroplasticity (i.e., ABT and/or AIH) we believe this model will be useful to test the efficacy of these interventions to improve CV and autonomic function.

Author Contributions: Conceptualization, L.W. and C.R.W.; Data curation, L.W.; formal analysis, L.W., E.L.E. and T.M.H., Funding acquisition, C.R.W., Investigation, L.W. and M.A., methodology, L.W., M.A., E.L.E., T.M.H. and C.R.W.; Project administration, E.L.E.; Resources, E.L.E., Supervision, C.R.W.; visualization, L.W., E.L.E. and T.M.H. writing—original draft preparation, L.W.; writing—review and editing, L.W., E.L.E., T.M.H. and C.R.W. All authors have read and agreed to the published version of the manuscript.

Funding: This research was funded by Praxis as a part of the Blusson Integrated Cares Partnership, number GR004076. Research in the lab of Christopher West is funded by an infrastructure grant from the Canadian Foundation for Innovation and BC Knowledge Development Fund: grant number 34803.

Institutional Review Board Statement: The study was conducted according to the guidelines of the Declaration of Helsinki and approved by the clinical Research Ethics Board of the University of British Columbia (ACC-A18-0344; 24 January 2019).

Informed Consent Statement: Not applicable.

Data Availability Statement: Data available upon request.

Acknowledgments: The authors thank Ryan L. Hoiland and Liam C. Stewart for their excellent technical assistance.

Conflicts of Interest: The authors declare no conflict of interest.

References

1. Garshick, E.; Kelley, A.; A Cohen, S.; Garrison, A.; Tun, C.G.; Gagnon, D.; Brown, R. A prospective assessment of mortality in chronic spinal cord injury. *Spinal Cord* **2005**, *43*, 408–416. [CrossRef]
2. Cragg, J.J.; Noonan, V.K.; Krassioukov, A.; Borisoff, J. Cardiovascular disease and spinal cord injury: Results from a national population health survey. *Neurology* **2013**, *81*, 723–728. [CrossRef] [PubMed]
3. Llewellyn-Smith, I.J.; Weaver, L.C. Changes in synaptic inputs to sympathetic preganglionic neurons after spinal cord injury. *J. Comp. Neurol.* **2001**, *435*, 226–240. [CrossRef] [PubMed]
4. Brennan, F.H.; Noble, B.T.; Wang, Y.; Guan, Z.; Davis, H.; Mo, X.; Harris, C.; Eroglu, C.; Ferguson, A.R.; Popovich, P.G. Acute post-injury blockade of α2δ-1 calcium channel subunits prevents pathological autonomic plasticity after spinal cord injury. *Cell Rep.* **2021**, *34*, 108667. [CrossRef] [PubMed]
5. Krenz, N.R.; Weaver, L.C. Changes in the morphology of sympathetic preganglionic neurons parallel the development of autonomic dysreflexia after spinal cord injury in rats. *Neurosci. Lett.* **1998**, *243*, 61–64. [CrossRef]
6. Weaver, L.C.; Verghese, P.; Bruce, J.; Fehlings, M.; Krenz, N.; Marsh, D. Autonomic dysreflexia and primary afferent sprouting after clip-compression injury of the rat spinal cord. *J. Neurotrauma* **2001**, *18*, 1107–1119. [CrossRef] [PubMed]
7. Hou, S.; Duale, H.; Cameron, A.A.; Abshire, S.M.; Lyttle, T.S.; Rabchevsky, A.G. Plasticity of lumbosacral propriospinal neurons is associated with the development of autonomic dysreflexia after thoracic spinal cord transection. *J. Comp. Neurol.* **2008**, *509*, 382–399. [CrossRef]
8. Prüss, H.; Tedeschi, A.; Thiriot, A.; Lynch, L.; Loughhead, S.M.; Stutte, S.; Mazo, I.B.; Kopp, M.A.; Brommer, B.; Blex, C.; et al. Spinal cord injury-induced immunodeficiency is mediated by a sympathetic-neuroendocrine adrenal reflex. *Nat. Neurosci.* **2017**, *20*, 1549–1559. [CrossRef]
9. Christensen, M.D.; Hulsebosch, C.E. Chronic central pain after spinal cord injury. *J. Neurotrauma* **1997**, *14*, 517–537. [CrossRef]

10. Christiansen, L.; Urbin, M.A.; Mitchell, G.S.; Perez, M.A. Acute intermittent hypoxia enhances corticospinal synaptic plasticity in humans. *eLife* **2018**, *7*, e34304. [CrossRef]
11. DeVinney, M.J.; Huxtable, A.G.; Nichols, N.L.; Mitchell, G.S. Hypoxia-induced phrenic long-term facilitation: Emergent properties. *Ann. N. Y. Acad. Sci.* **2013**, *1279*, 143–153. [CrossRef]
12. Baker-Herman, T.L.; Fuller, D.D.; Bavis, R.W.; Zabka, A.G.; Golder, F.J.; Doperalski, N.J.; Johnson, R.A.; Watters, J.J.; Mitchell, G.S. BDNF is necessary and sufficient for spinal respiratory plasticity following intermittent hypoxia. *Nat. Neurosci.* **2003**, *7*, 48–55. [CrossRef]
13. Golder, F.J. Spinal synaptic enhancement with acute intermittent hypoxia improves respiratory function after chronic cervical spinal cord injury. *J. Neurosci.* **2005**, *25*, 2925–2932. [CrossRef]
14. Lovett-Barr, M.R.; Satriotomo, I.; Muir, G.D.; Wilkerson, J.E.R.; Hoffman, M.S.; Vinit, S.; Mitchell, G.S. Repetitive intermittent hypoxia induces respiratory and somatic motor recovery after chronic cervical spinal injury. *J. Neurosci.* **2012**, *32*, 3591–3600. [CrossRef]
15. Prosser-Loose, E.J.; Hassan, A.; Mitchell, G.S.; Muir, G.D. Delayed Intervention with intermittent hypoxia and task training improves forelimb function in a rat model of cervical spinal injury. *J. Neurotrauma* **2015**, *32*, 1403–1412. [CrossRef]
16. Magnuson, D.S.K.; Smith, R.R.; Brown, E.H.; Enzmann, G.; Angeli, C.; Quesada, P.M.; Burke, D. Swimming as a model of task-specific locomotor retraining after spinal cord injury in the rat. *Neurorehabilit. Neural Repair* **2009**, *23*, 535–545. [CrossRef]
17. Smith, R.R.; Shum-Siu, A.; Baltzley, R.; Bunger, M.; Baldini, A.; Burke, D.A.; Magnuson, D.S. Effects of swimming on functional recovery after incomplete spinal cord injury in rats. *J. Neurotrauma* **2006**, *23*, 908–919. [CrossRef]
18. Shah, P.K.; Garcia-Alias, G.; Choe, J.; Gad, P.; Gerasimenko, Y.; Tillakaratne, N.; Zhong, H.; Roy, R.R.; Edgerton, V.R. Use of quadrupedal step training to re-engage spinal interneuronal networks and improve locomotor function after spinal cord injury. *Brain* **2013**, *136*, 3362–3377. [CrossRef] [PubMed]
19. Brown, A.K.; Woller, S.A.; Moreno, G.; Grau, J.W.; Hook, M.A. Exercise therapy and recovery after SCI: Evidence that shows early intervention improves recovery of function. *Spinal Cord* **2011**, *49*, 623–628. [CrossRef] [PubMed]
20. Sandrow-Feinberg, H.R.; Izzi, J.; Shumsky, J.S.; Zhukareva, V.; Houle, J.D. Forced exercise as a rehabilitation strategy after unilateral cervical spinal cord contusion injury. *J. Neurotrauma* **2009**, *26*, 721–731. [CrossRef] [PubMed]
21. Fenrich, K.K.; Hallworth, B.W.; Vavrek, R.; Raposo, P.J.; Misiaszek, J.E.; Bennett, D.J.; Fouad, K.; Torres-Espin, A. Self-directed rehabilitation training intensity thresholds for efficient recovery of skilled forelimb function in rats with cervical spinal cord injury. *Exp. Neurol.* **2020**, *339*, 113543. [CrossRef] [PubMed]
22. Ying, Z.; Roy, R.R.; Edgerton, V.R.; Gómez-Pinilla, F. Exercise restores levels of neurotrophins and synaptic plasticity following spinal cord injury. *Exp. Neurol.* **2005**, *193*, 411–419. [CrossRef]
23. West, C.; Crawford, M.; Poormasjedi-Meibod, M.-S.; Currie, K.D.; Fallavollita, A.; Yuen, V.; McNeill, J.H.; Krassioukov, A.V. Passive hind-limb cycling improves cardiac function and reduces cardiovascular disease risk in experimental spinal cord injury. *J. Physiol.* **2014**, *592*, 1771–1783. [CrossRef]
24. Squair, J.W.; West, C.R.; Popok, D.; Assinck, P.; Liu, J.; Tetzlaff, W.; Krassioukov, A.V. High thoracic contusion model for the investigation of cardiovascular function after spinal cord injury. *J. Neurotrauma* **2017**, *34*, 671–684. [CrossRef]
25. Trueblood, C.T.; Iredia, I.W.; Collyer, E.S.; Tom, V.J.; Hou, S. Development of cardiovascular dysfunction in a rat spinal cord crush model and responses to serotonergic interventions. *J. Neurotrauma* **2019**, *36*, 1478–1486. [CrossRef] [PubMed]
26. Squair, J.W.; Deveau, K.M.; Harman, K.A.; Poormasjedi-Meibod, M.-S.; Hayes, B.; Liu, J.; Magnuson, D.S.; Krassioukov, A.V.; West, C.R. Spinal cord injury causes systolic dysfunction and cardiomyocyte atrophy. *J. Neurotrauma* **2018**, *35*, 424–434. [CrossRef] [PubMed]
27. DeVeau, K.M.; Harman, K.A.; Squair, J.W.; Krassioukov, A.V.; Magnuson, D.S.K.; West, C.R. A comparison of passive hindlimb cycling and active upper-limb exercise provides new insights into systolic dysfunction after spinal cord injury. *Am. J. Physiol. Circ. Physiol.* **2017**, *313*, H861–H870. [CrossRef]
28. Squair, J.W.; Gautier, M.; Mahe, L.; Soriano, J.E.; Rowald, A.; Bichat, A.; Cho, N.; Anderson, M.A.; James, N.D.; Gandar, J.; et al. Neuroprosthetic baroreflex controls haemodynamics after spinal cord injury. *Nature* **2021**, *590*, 308–314. [CrossRef]
29. West, C.R.; Popok, D.; Crawford, M.A.; Krassioukov, A.V. Characterizing the temporal development of cardiovascular dysfunction in response to spinal cord injury. *J. Neurotrauma* **2015**, *32*, 922–930. [CrossRef]
30. Fossey, M.; Squair, J.; Poormasjedi-Meibod, M.; Hayes, B.; Erskine, E.; Ahmadian, M.; West, C. Impaired cardiac function following experimental spinal cord injury occurs due to the loss of descending sympathetic control and precedes structural remodeling. *FASEB J.* **2021**, *35*. [CrossRef]
31. Williams, A.M.; Manouchehri, N.; Erskine, E.; Tauh, K.; So, K.; Shortt, K.; Webster, M.; Fisk, S.; Billingsley, A.; Munro, A.; et al. Cardio-centric hemodynamic management improves spinal cord oxygenation and mitigates hemorrhage in acute spinal cord injury. *Nat. Commun.* **2020**, *11*, 1–12. [CrossRef] [PubMed]
32. Poormasjedi-Meibod, M.-S.; Mansouri, M.; Fossey, M.; Squair, J.W.; Liu, J.; McNeill, J.H.; West, C.R. Experimental spinal cord injury causes left-ventricular atrophy and is associated with an upregulation of proteolytic pathways. *J. Neurotrauma* **2019**, *36*, 950–961. [CrossRef] [PubMed]
33. Hou, S.; Saltos, T.M.; Mironets, E.; Trueblood, C.T.; Connors, T.M.; Tom, V.J. Grafting embryonic raphe neurons reestablishes serotonergic regulation of sympathetic activity to improve cardiovascular function after spinal cord injury. *J. Neurosci.* **2020**, *40*, 1248–1264. [CrossRef]

34. Squair, J.W.; Liu, J.; Tetzlaff, W.; Krassioukov, A.V.; West, C.R. Spinal cord injury-induced cardiomyocyte atrophy and impaired cardiac function are severity dependent. *Exp. Physiol.* **2018**, *103*, 179–189. [CrossRef] [PubMed]
35. DeVeau, K.M.; Martin, E.K.; King, N.T.; Shum-Siu, A.; Keller, B.B.; West, C.R.; Magnuson, D.S. Challenging cardiac function post-spinal cord injury with dobutamine. *Auton. Neurosci.* **2018**, *209*, 19–24. [CrossRef] [PubMed]
36. Pacher, P.; Nagayama, T.; Mukhopadhyay, P.; Bátkai, S.; Kass, D.A. Measurement of cardiac function using pressure–volume conductance catheter technique in mice and rats. *Nat. Protoc.* **2008**, *3*, 1422–1434. [CrossRef]
37. Inskip, J.A.; Ramer, L.M.; Ramer, M.S.; Krassioukov, A.V.; Claydon, V.E. Spectral analyses of cardiovascular control in rodents with spinal cord injury. *J. Neurotrauma* **2012**, *29*, 1638–1649. [CrossRef]
38. Claydon, V.; Steeves, J.D.; Krassioukov, A. Orthostatic hypotension following spinal cord injury: Understanding clinical pathophysiology. *Spinal Cord* **2006**, *44*, 341–351. [CrossRef]
39. West, C.R.; Wong, S.C.; Krassioukov, A.V. Autonomic cardiovascular control in paralympic athletes with spinal cord injury. *Med. Sci. Sports Exerc.* **2014**, *46*, 60–68. [CrossRef]
40. Hubli, M.; Krassioukov, A.V. Ambulatory blood pressure monitoring in spinal cord injury: Clinical practicability. *J. Neurotrauma* **2014**, *31*, 789–797. [CrossRef]
41. Lujan, H.L.; Dicarlo, S.E. T5 spinal cord transection increases susceptibility to reperfusion-induced ventricular tachycardia by enhancing sympathetic activity in conscious rats. *Am. J. Physiol. Circ. Physiol.* **2007**, *293*, H3333–H3339. [CrossRef]
42. Strack, A.; Sawyer, W.; Hughes, J.; Platt, K.; Loewy, A. A general pattern of CNS innervation of the sympathetic outflow demonstrated by transneuronal pseudorabies viral infections. *Brain Res.* **1989**, *491*, 156–162. [CrossRef]
43. Suga, H.; Sagawa, K.; Shoukas, A.A. Load independence of the instantaneous pressure-volume ratio of the canine left ventricle and effects of epinephrine and heart rate on the ratio. *Circ. Res.* **1973**, *32*, 314–322. [CrossRef]
44. Minson, J.; Chalmers, J.; Drolet, G.; Kapoor, V.; Llewellyn-Smith, I.; Mills, E.; Morris, M.; Pilowsky, P. Central serotonergic mechanisms in cardiovascular regulation. *Cardiovasc. Drugs Ther.* **1990**, *4*, 27–32. [CrossRef] [PubMed]
45. Chalmers, J.P.; Pilowsky, P.M.; Minson, J.B.; Kapoor, V.; Mills, E.; West, M.J. Central serotonergic mechanisms in hypertension. *Am. J. Hypertens.* **1988**, *1*, 79–83. [CrossRef] [PubMed]
46. Sawchenko, P.E.; Bohn, M.C. Glucocorticoid receptor-immunoreactivity in C1, C2, and C3 adrenergic neurons that project to the hypothalamus or to the spinal cord in the rat. *J. Comp. Neurol.* **1989**, *285*, 107–116. [CrossRef]
47. Bruinstroop, E.; Cano, G.; Vanderhorst, V.G.; Cavalcante, J.C.; Wirth, J.; Sena-Esteves, M.; Saper, C.B. Spinal projections of the A5, A6 (locus coeruleus), and A7 noradrenergic cell groups in rats. *J. Comp. Neurol.* **2012**, *520*, 1985–2001. [CrossRef] [PubMed]
48. Cormier, C.M.; Mukhida, K.; Walker, G.; Marsh, D.R. Development of autonomic dysreflexia after spinal cord injury is associated with a lack of serotonergic axons in the intermediolateral cell column. *J. Neurotrauma* **2010**, *27*, 1805–1818. [CrossRef]
49. Hou, S.; Lu, P.; Blesch, A. Characterization of supraspinal vasomotor pathways and autonomic dysreflexia after spinal cord injury in F344 rats. *Auton. Neurosci.* **2013**, *176*, 54–63. [CrossRef]
50. Harman, K.A.; DeVeau, K.M.; Squair, J.W.; West, C.R.; Krassioukov, A.V.; Magnuson, D.S.K. Effects of early exercise training on the severity of autonomic dysreflexia following incomplete spinal cord injury in rodents. *Physiol. Rep.* **2021**, *9*, e14969. [CrossRef]
51. Harman, K.A.; States, G.; Wade, A.; Stepp, C.; Wainwright, G.; Deveau, K.; King, N.; Shum-Siu, A.; Magnuson, D.S.K. Temporal analysis of cardiovascular control and function following incomplete T3 and T10 spinal cord injury in rodents. *Physiol. Rep.* **2018**, *6*, e13634. [CrossRef] [PubMed]
52. Ramsey, J.B.; Ramer, L.M.; Inskip, J.A.; Alan, N.; Ramer, M.S.; Krassioukov, A.V. Care of rats with complete high-thoracic Spinal cord injury. *J. Neurotrauma* **2010**, *27*, 1709–1722. [CrossRef] [PubMed]
53. Fossey, M.; Poormasjedi-Meibod, M.; Hayes, B.; Erskine, E.L.; Azad, R.K.; Granville, D.J.; Ramer, M.S.; West, C.R. A reduction in cardiac function precedes structural adaptations in experimental spinal cord injury. *FASEB J.* **2019**, *33*, 831.7. [CrossRef]

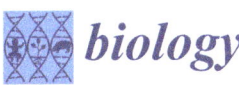

Article

Osteopenia in a Mouse Model of Spinal Cord Injury: Effects of Age, Sex and Motor Function

Michelle A. Hook [1,*], Alyssa Falck [2], Ravali Dundumulla [1], Mabel Terminel [1], Rachel Cunningham [1], Arthur Sefiani [1], Kayla Callaway [1], Dana Gaddy [2] and Cédric G. Geoffroy [1]

[1] Department of Neuroscience and Experimental Therapeutics, College of Medicine, Texas A&M Health Science Center, Bryan, TX 77807, USA; ravalidundumulla@gmail.com (R.D.); mabelt19@gmail.com (M.T.); rcunnink@gmail.com (R.C.); sefiani@tamu.edu (A.S.); kjcallaway33@tamu.edu (K.C.); geoffroy@tamu.edu (C.G.G.)

[2] Veterinary Integrative Biosciences, College of Veterinary Medicine and Biomedical Sciences, College Station, TX 77843, USA; afalck@cvm.tamu.edu (A.F.); dgaddy@cvm.tamu.edu (D.G.)

* Correspondence: michellehook@tamu.edu; Tel.: +1-979-436-0568

Citation: Hook, M.A.; Falck, A.; Dundumulla, R.; Terminel, M.; Cunningham, R.; Sefiani, A.; Callaway, K.; Gaddy, D.; Geoffroy, C.G. Osteopenia in a Mouse Model of Spinal Cord Injury: Effects of Age, Sex and Motor Function. *Biology* 2022, 11, 189. https://doi.org/10.3390/biology11020189

Academic Editor: Huaxin Sheng

Received: 29 November 2021
Accepted: 22 January 2022
Published: 26 January 2022

Publisher's Note: MDPI stays neutral with regard to jurisdictional claims in published maps and institutional affiliations.

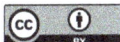

Copyright: © 2022 by the authors. Licensee MDPI, Basel, Switzerland. This article is an open access article distributed under the terms and conditions of the Creative Commons Attribution (CC BY) license (https://creativecommons.org/licenses/by/4.0/).

Simple Summary: In the first two years following spinal cord injury, people lose up to 50% of bone below the injury. This injury-induced bone loss significantly affects rehabilitation and leaves people vulnerable to fractures and post-fracture complications, including lung and urinary tract infections, blood clots in the veins, and depression. Unfortunately, little is known about the factors driving this bone loss. In fact, even though we know that injury, age, and sex independently increase bone loss, there have been no studies looking at the cumulative effects of these variables. People with spinal injury are aging, and the age at which injuries occur is increasing. It is essential to know whether these factors together will further compromise bone. To examine this, we assessed bone loss in young and old, male and female mice after spinal injury. As expected, we found that aging alone decreased motor activity and bone volume. Spinal injury also reduced bone volume, but it did not worsen the effects of age. Instead, injury effects appeared related to reduced rearing activity. The data suggest that although partial weight-bearing does not reduce bone loss after spinal cord injury, therapies that put full weight on the legs may be clinically effective.

Abstract: After spinal cord injury (SCI), 80% of individuals are diagnosed with osteopenia or osteoporosis. The dramatic loss of bone after SCI increases the potential for fractures 100-fold, with post-fracture complications occurring in 54% of cases. With the age of new SCI injuries increasing, we hypothesized that a SCI-induced reduction in weight bearing could further exacerbate age-induced bone loss. To test this, young (2–3 months) and old (20–30 months) male and female mice were given a moderate spinal contusion injury (T9–T10), and recovery was assessed for 28 days (BMS, rearing counts, distance traveled). Tibial trabecular bone volume was measured after 28 days with ex vivo microCT. While BMS scores did not differ across groups, older subjects travelled less in the open field and there was a decrease in rearing with age and SCI. As expected, aging decreased trabecular bone volume and cortical thickness in both old male and female mice. SCI alone also reduced trabecular bone volume in young mice, but did not have an additional effect beyond the age-dependent decrease in trabecular and cortical bone volume seen in both sexes. Interestingly, both rearing and total activity correlated with decreased bone volume. These data underscore the importance of load and use on bone mass. While partial weight-bearing does not stabilize/reverse bone loss in humans, our data suggest that therapies that simulate complete loading may be effective after SCI.

Keywords: spinal cord injury; osteopenia; bone loss; recovery of function

1. Introduction

In the first two years following a spinal cord injury (SCI), there is a 30–50% decrease in bone mineral density in the lower limbs [1–4]. This demineralization occurs primarily in the trabecular bone found in the distal and proximal epiphysis and metaphysis of the femur and tibia, respectively [5–7]. Albeit more slowly, decreases in cortical bone mineralization and thinning of the cortical bone walls also occur [3,8–10], rendering the lower limbs susceptible to fracture. More than 30% of adults living with SCI sustain fragility fractures of the lower extremities [11–16], an incidence two-fold greater than in the able-bodied population, with most fractures occurring during normal daily living activities (i.e., transferring to and from a wheelchair, dressing, and bathing [17]). These fractures not only compromise rehabilitation, they also increase morbidity, mortality, and healthcare costs. Alarmingly, post fracture complications also occur in 50% of SCI patients [15,18,19]. These complications include, but are not limited to, respiratory and urinary tract infections, venous thromboembolic events, fracture non-union or mal-union, and depression. Bone loss after SCI significantly reduces a person's quality of life and compromises physical well-being.

Numerous factors have been implicated in SCI-induced bone loss. First, there is loss of signaling from muscle to bone. There is rapid loss of muscle after SCI: with muscle weights reduced by 40–60% in young male rats just two weeks after a spinal cord transection [20]. Normally, during muscle contractions and weight bearing, muscles release signaling molecules including myokines that modulate the activity of osteoblasts and osteoclasts, thereby affecting bone formation and resorption respectively [21–23]. For example, the recently discovered myokine irisin is reported to increase osteoblast differentiation and suppress osteoclast activity [24–26], although evidence suggests that its effects may be dose and duration of exposure dependent [27]. Second, the disruption of sympathetic neuronal signaling with SCI is posited to affect bone health by, e.g., allowing intravenous shunts to open throughout bone, reducing blood flow through the tissue. The resulting vascular stasis leads to decreased gas and nutrient exchange, and promotion of local hyper-pressure which triggers osteoclast formation [28]. Dysfunction of the pituitary-hypothalamic axis [29–31], increased adiposity in the bone marrow and muscle [22,32–35], as well as insulin resistance [22], inflammation [36], and deficiencies of Vitamin D [37] also contribute to bone loss after SCI. The multifactorial effects of SCI ultimately result in bone formation being uncoupled from bone resorption, with a reduction in bone mass and decreased skeletal integrity.

Along with SCI, aging and time post-injury exponentially increase fracture risk [38,39]. In the able-bodied population, bone mass peaks at about 25–30 years and then begins to decline [40,41]. In fact, by 50–59 years of age, it is estimated that 5.1% of individuals in this age group have osteoporosis, and an additional 40.2% have low bone mass [42]. Pre-existing low bone mass and osteoporosis subsequently render older individuals vulnerable to SCI, with an increasing incidence of injuries due to falls occurring in people older than 60 years [43–48]. Superimposing SCI onto an already compromised system further compounds the risk for fracture and related complications.

Similarly, changes in levels of sex hormones with age affect bone loss. After 50 years of age, the incidence of osteoporosis and low bone mass is more than three times greater in females than in males [49,50], an effect attributed to the rapid loss of estrogen during menopause [51–53]. The effects of estrogen on bone are particularly relevant for SCI. Amenorrhea and perimenopause symptoms are frequently observed in the acute phase of SCI in both humans and animal models [54–56]. SCI coupled with an acute decrease in estrogen levels, and prolonged decreases with aging, would significantly compromise bone health. While the majority of traumatic SCIs occur in males, this demographic is changing particularly in older age groups [45–47,57]. It is essential that we develop strategies to reduce the loss of bone seen in the early stages of SCI and facilitate the rebuilding of bone in chronic stages for all age and sex groups.

Surprisingly, however, despite significant effects of SCI, age, and sex on bone loss, there have been no studies looking at the interactive effects on bone in an SCI model. To address this, the current study assessed bone loss in young and old, male and female mice after a moderate spinal contusion injury. We recorded locomotor function, activity levels in an open field, and rearing for one month post injury. At the end of recovery, cancellous and compact bone was compared across groups. Commensurate with clinical findings, we found significant effects of age and sex on bone loss, as well as age-dependent positive correlations between bone loss and rearing activity.

2. Methods

2.1. Subjects

Both young (2–3 months) and old (20–30 months) male and female C57BL/6 mice served as subjects. In total, 15 young males (4 shams, 11 SCI), 15 young females (7 shams, 8 SCI), 9 old males (4 shams, 5 SCI), and 16 old females (8 sham, 8 SCI) were available in our Texas A&M Health Science Center animal facility for transfer to this animal use protocol and assessment in this study. The mice were housed with littermates in ventilated cages and maintained on a 12 h light-dark cycle, with access to both food and water ad libitum. Mixed groups of aged and sex-matched SCI and sham mice were housed together, with their positions on the cage racks randomized across groups. All testing and surgeries occurred during the light cycle. Following a contusion injury, subjects' bladders were expressed manually every morning between 7:00 and 9:00 a.m. and evening between 4:30 and 6:30 p.m. This schedule was maintained until subjects regained bladder function (operationally defined as voiding on own for three consecutive days). All of the experiments reported here were reviewed and approved by the Institutional Animal Care Committee at Texas A&M and were consistent with the NIH guidelines for animal care and use.

2.2. Spinal Contusion Injury

The mice were given a moderate spinal contusion injury (50 kdyne, T9–T10, Infinite Horizons Impactor), or served as sham-injured controls. Briefly, under deep anesthesia with isoflurane (2% gas, Piramal Pharma Solutions, Telangana, India), a small skin incision was made over the spinal cord column covering lamina T7–T12. The spinous process of T9 was located, and the T9–T10 vertebrae were removed (laminectomy). For the spinal contusion injury, the vertebral column was fixed within the IH device, using two Adson forceps, and a controlled impact was delivered to the exposed cord with a stainless steel impactor tip. The mouse was visually inspected for evidence of bruising of the cord, and then the muscles were sutured and the skin closed with Dermabond. All mice received daily injections of saline (0.9%) and buprenorphine (0.05 mg/kg, Par Pharmaceutical Chestnut Ridge, Chestnut Ridge, NY, USA) for 3 days and penicillin (5 mg/kg/day, Bayer Healthcare LLC, Animal Health Division Shawnee Mission, Shawnee, KS, USA) for 7 days. Mice were monitored daily, with their bladder expressed manually twice every day until the mice were able to urinate without assistance or till the end of the experiment. As the focus of this experiment was on spinal cord injury effects, rather than other stressors associated with handling, anesthesia or peripheral injury that could affect bone health [58,59], sham-injured mice served as controls. Sham mice underwent all of the same surgical and general husbandry procedures as the spinal contusion mice with the exception of the controlled impact to the exposed spinal cord, enabling the assessment of the contusion effects on bone and activity independent of general surgery/recovery.

2.3. Assessment of Motor Recovery

Locomotor function was assessed for 28 days post injury using the Basso Mouse Scale (BMS [60]). This test measures hindlimb motor movement with scores ranging from slight ankle movement (BMS = 1) to occasional plantar weight supported stepping (BMS = 4) and coordinated walking (BMS = 9). BMS scores were collected on the day following injury, and then every other day from days 1–13 post injury, and every 3rd day from day 16 until day 28 post-injury. Mice were placed in the open enclosure (120 cm long, 60 cm wide, 23 cm deep) and observed for 4 min. Experimenters were kept blind to subject's experimental treatment. Subjects were excluded from the experiment if BMS scores were >3 on the day following injury.

Motor recovery was also assessed with a rearing test. The mice were placed in a high-ceiling Plexiglas chamber (27 cm long, 15 cm wide, 17 cm high) for 5 min, in a quiet dark room (with red light), and videotaped. The number of rears performed in the 5-min session was determined from post hoc video analyses. Rearing activity was assessed prior to surgery, and then every 7th day until day 28 post-injury.

Open field activity levels were also assayed in automated activity chambers (43 cm long, 43 cm wide, 15 cm deep, Hamilton-Kinder LLC, Chula Vista, CA, USA). Activity was detected as infrared beam crosses (2.5 cm spacing). Each mouse was placed in the center of an open field chamber and allowed to explore the apparatus freely for 10 min. The distance traveled within the study time-period was recorded. Open field activity was assessed prior to surgery and every 7 days until day 28.

At the end of the recovery period, the mice were deeply anesthetized (100 mg/kg of beuthanasia, intraparietal) and perfused intracardially with PBS and 4% paraformaldehyde. Following perfusion, a 1 cm segment centered at the lesion site was extracted and prepared for cryostat sectioning. Sagittal sections (25 µm) were collected and stained as follows. Sections were washed (3× with 0.4% Triton X-100 in 1× PBS), then blocked using 5% normal horse serum (VWR 102643-676, Radnor, PA, USA), diluted in 0.4% Triton X-100 in 1× PBS, for 1 h. Sections were then incubated with primary anti-glial fibrillary acidic protein (GFAP) antibody (1:500, Cat. No. 13-0300, ThermoFisher Scientific, Waltham, MA, USA), diluted in 1× PBS with 0.4% Triton X-100 (PBS-TX), at 25 °C overnight. The sections were then washed 3 times in PBS-TX before being incubated with Alexa Fluor Plus 488 secondary antibody (1:1000, Cat. No. A32814, ThermoFisher Scientific) in PBS-TX for 1 h and DAPI (1 µg/mL, Cat. No. 62248, ThermoFisher Scientific) for 5 min. After being washed once more (PBS), the slices were mounted onto Superfrost Plus slides and coverslipped (Cat. No. F6182, Sigma, St. Loius, MO, USA). Sections were imaged at 10× on a Zeiss Axio Observer 7 fluorescent microscope. The contour (polygonal) tool in Zen 3.2 (Carl Zeiss AG, Oberkochen, Germany) software was used to trace and measure lesion size, tracing the glial scar border labeled with GFAP surrounding a DAPI+ inner region. Three spinal cord sections per mouse were imaged and analyzed.

2.4. Tibial MicroCT Analysis

Tibiae were harvested at sacrifice and fixed in neutral buffered formalin prior to evaluation of trabecular bone volume and architecture as well as cortical bone geometry by micro-computed tomography (µCT50, Scanco Medical, Brüttisellen, Switzerland). Briefly, the proximal tibia and tibial midshaft regions were scanned as 12 µm isotropic voxel size using 55 kVp, 114 mA, and 200-ms. Bone volume fraction (BV/TV, %), trabecular thickness (Tb.Th, mm), trabecular separation (Tb.Sp, mm), trabecular number (Tb.N, 1/mm), connectivity density (ConnD $1/mm^3$), and volumetric bone mineral density (BMD, mg/mm^3) were calculated using previously published methods [61]. The cancellous bone region was obtained using a semi-automated contouring program that separated cancellous from cortical bone. At the midshaft, of the tibia, total cross sectional area (CSA, mm^2), cortical thickness (Ct.Th, mm), periosteal perimeter (mm), and endosteal perimeter (mm) were assessed in a 1 mm long region. Bone was segmented from soft tissue using the same threshold for all groups, 245 mg HA/cm^3 for trabecular and 682 mg HA/cm^3 for cortical bone. All microCT scanning and analyses were compliant with published American Society for Bone and Mineral Research (ASBMR) guidelines for rodents [62]. For the assessment of bone, the investigators were kept blind to all subject's experimental treatment. Age, sex, and injury condition were revealed at the end of all assessments.

2.5. Statistical Analyses

Three-way repeated measure ANCOVAs were used to compare locomotor recovery, open field activity and rearing across groups. In these analyses, Day 1 BMS scores served as covariates in tests of locomotor function, and pre-injury assessments of rearing and open field activity were covariates in these respective analyses. In all tests, day post injury served as the repeated measure. Significant main effects ($p < 0.05$) of age, sex, or injury were further analyzed with independent t-tests to examine temporal effects on behavior.

Three-way ANOVAs were also used to compare trabecular bone volume and architecture, and cortical bone geometry across groups, followed by post hoc independent t-tests comparing the means of groups that differed by only one factor (age, sex, or injury). Differences were considered significant when $p < 0.05$. All data analyses were performed using SPSS version 27.0 (SPSS, Inc., Chicago IL, USA).

3. Results

3.1. The Effects of SCI on Motor Recovery Are Task Dependent

All sham-operated subjects had the maximum BMS score of 9 across days. SCI significantly decreased locomotor function. Further examining the SCI subjects only, a three-way ANCOVA revealed no effect of sex (F $(1,27) < 0.01$, $p > 0.05$) or age (F $(1,27) < 0.01$, $p > 0.05$) on the recovery of locomotor function (Figure 1A). All groups recovered plantar weight supported stepping by Day 14 post injury. Analyses of the lesion size at 28 days post injury also revealed no significant differences between groups (F $(3,17) = 1.51$, $p > 0.05$, Figure 1B,C).

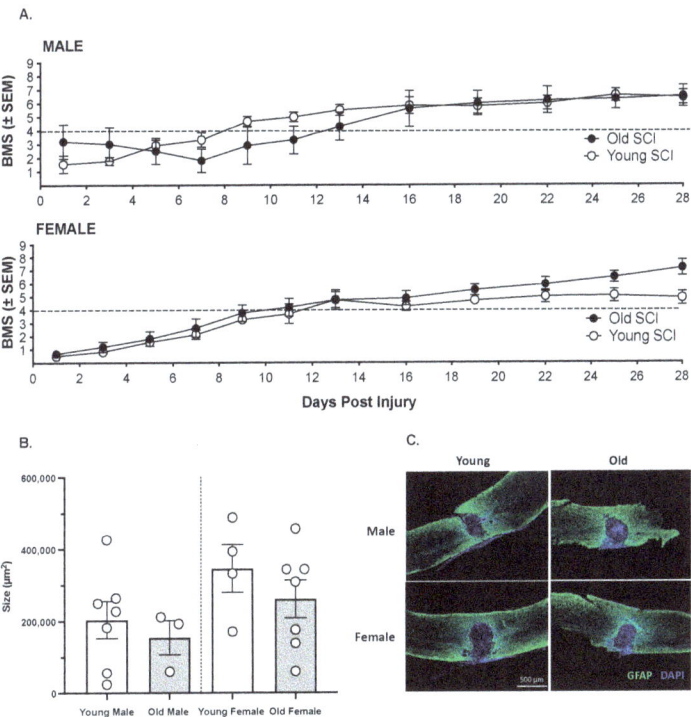

Figure 1. (**A**). Irrespective of age or sex all mice recovered locomotor function, assessed with the BMS scale, over 28 days post injury. There were no significant differences in recovery across groups. The Mean ± SEM for each group is shown across days, and the dashed line represents the score for plantar, weight supported stepping. (**B**). Similarly, age and sex did not affect lesion size at 28 days post injury. The white circles represent individual subjects. (**C**). Representative images of the lesion, visualized with GFAP and DAPI staining, from each demographic are shown. For BBB analyses (**A**), n = 5 old males, 11 young males, 8 old females, 8 young females. For lesion analyses (**B**), n = 3 old males, 6 young males, 7 old females, 4 young females.

Open field activity, however, was affected by injury, sex, and age (Figure 2). Not surprisingly, subjects given a sham injury displayed increased open field activity relative to SCI subjects (F (1,46) = 12.48, $p < 0.001$). This effect was largely driven by reduced activity in all groups during the early phase of SCI. There was an effect of surgery on activity on Day 7 post injury ($t = -3.64$, $p < 0.001$), but no differences were observed across groups on Days 14–21 ($t < -1.09$, $p > 0.05$, on all days). Statistical comparisons were not performed for Day 28, because the data for young females were corrupted and could not be included. As can be seen in Figure 2, however, there were no differences in open field activity for sham and contused mice in the remaining groups on Day 28. Similarly, the females displayed increased open field activity relative to males on Day 7 post injury ($t = 2.45$, $p < 0.02$), but at no other timepoint. Irrespective of the timepoint post injury, young mice displayed greater open field activity than old mice ($t > 2.04$, $p < 0.05$ for all comparisons).

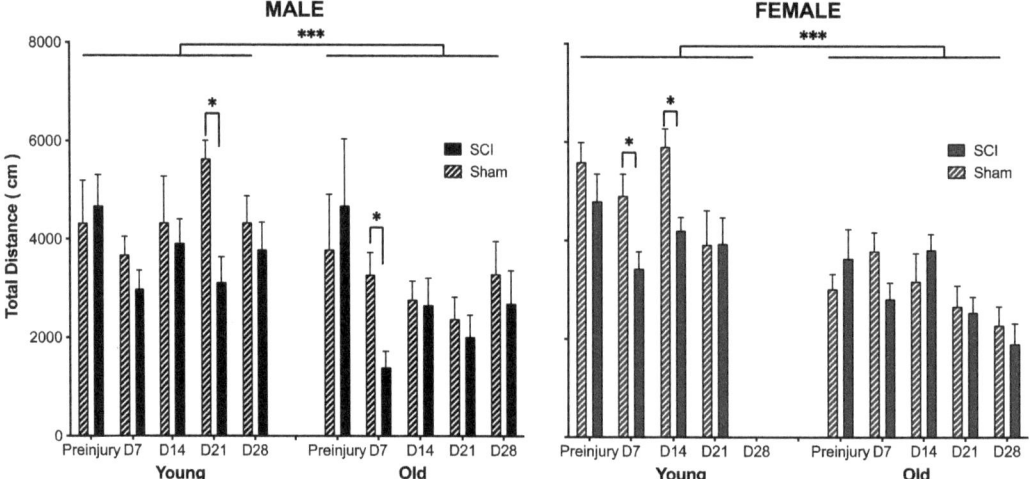

Figure 2. Age, sex and SCI affected open field activity. The young mice displayed greater activity in the open field than the old mice, with females also displaying increased activity relative to males. Not surprisingly, there was a main effect of SCI on activity. SCI reduced activity relative to sham controls, particularly in the early stage of injury (Day 7), irrespective of the demographic observed. Days (D) post injury are denoted on the x-axis, with the mean (±SEM) distance traveled in 10 min depicted on the y-axis. n = 4 sham and 5 SCI old males; 4 sham and 11 SCI young males; 8 sham and 7 SCI old females; 7 sham and 8 SCI young females. *** $p < 0.0001$ and * $p < 0.01$.

As shown in Figure 3, there was also a significant main effect of injury (F (1,46) = 63.99, $p < 0.001$) and age (F (1,46) = 21.33, $p < 0.001$), but no effect of sex (F (1,46) < 1.0, $p > 0.05$) on rearing. There was also a significant interaction between injury and age (F (1,46) = 16.95, $p < 0.001$). Rearing was decreased in SCI subjects at all timepoints post injury, relative to sham controls ($t > 2.58$, $p < 0.01$ in all comparisons). Similarly, young subjects reared more than old subjects at all days post injury ($t > 3.14$, $p < 0.005$, for all comparisons). It is also noted that the sham subjects decreased rearing across testing days, likely reflecting decreased exploration as the experimental testing chamber became more familiar across sessions.

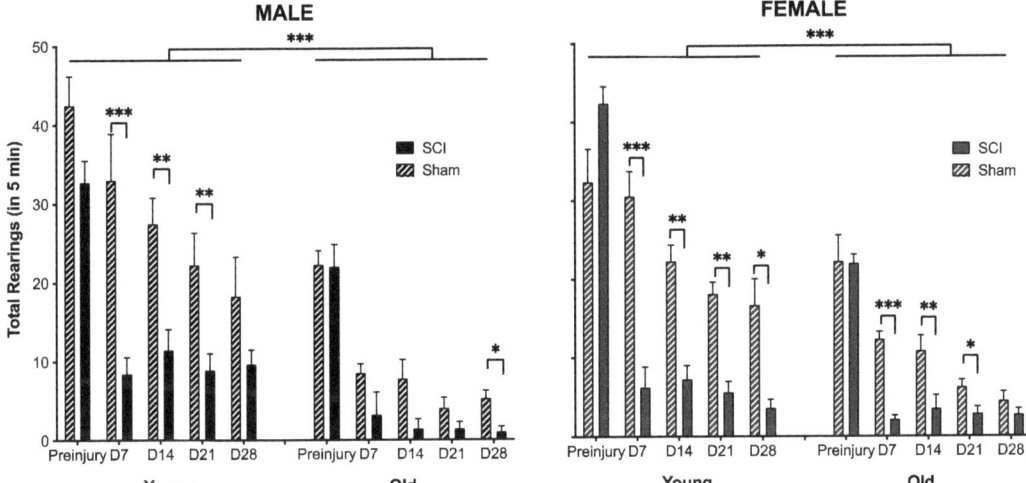

Figure 3. Age and SCI affected rearing activity. The young mice reared more than the old mice and SCI reduced rearing activity relative to sham controls, irrespective of the demographic observed. There was no effect of sex on rearing behavior. Days (D) post injury are denoted on the x-axis, with the mean (±SEM) number of rears in 5 min shown on the y axis. n = 4 sham and 5 SCI old males; 4 sham and 11 SCI young males; 8 sham and 7 SCI old females; 7 sham and 8 SCI young females. *** $p < 0.0001$, ** $p < 0.001$, * $p < 0.01$.

3.2. SCI Significantly Increases Bone Loss

A three-way ANOVA revealed main effects of age (F (1,46) = 88.7, $p < 0.0001$), sex (F (1,46) = 26.36, $p < 0.0001$) and injury (F (1,46) = 9.12, $p < 0.005$) on trabecular bone volume (Figure 4A,B), as well as a significant interaction between injury and age (F (1,46) = 6.14, $p < 0.05$). Irrespective of sex and injury, old mice had lower trabecular bone volume than young mice ($t > 3.75$, $p < 0.0005$ for all comparisons). The young females also had lower trabecular bone remaining compared with the young males ($t = 3.36, 3.95$, for Sham and SCI subjects respectively, $p < 0.002$). There was no difference between trabecular bone volume for old sham males compared with old sham females ($t = 0.40$, $p > 0.05$), but the old male mice with SCI did have more trabecular bone volume than their female counterparts ($t = 2.95$, $p < 0.01$). Significant effects of SCI on bone volume were only evident in the young mice ($t = 2.94, 2.80$, for males and females respectively, $p < 0.01$). There was no effect of SCI on bone volume in the old male and female subjects.

There were also main effects of age (F (1,19) = 144.50, $p < 0.0001$) and sex (F (1,27) = 17.02, $p < 0.001$) on trabecular number (Figure 4C), and significant interactions between sex and age (F (1,19) = 14.20, $p < 0.005$) as well as injury and age (F (1,19) = 5.12, $p < 0.05$). Again, irrespective of sex and injury, old mice had lower trabecular bone numbers than young mice ($t > 3.91$, $p < 0.0009$ for all comparisons). The young females also had lower numbers of trabeculae than the young males ($t = 3.33, 5.03$, for Sham and SCI subjects respectively, $p < 0.002$). There was no difference between trabecular number for old sham males compared with old sham females ($t = 0.14$, $p > 0.05$), but the old SCI male mice did have greater trabecular numbers than old female SCI mice ($t = 2.11$, $p < 0.01$). Significant effects of SCI on trabecular number were only evident in the young female mice ($t = 2.10$, $p < 0.05$). There was no effect of SCI on trabecular number in the young male, old male or old female subjects.

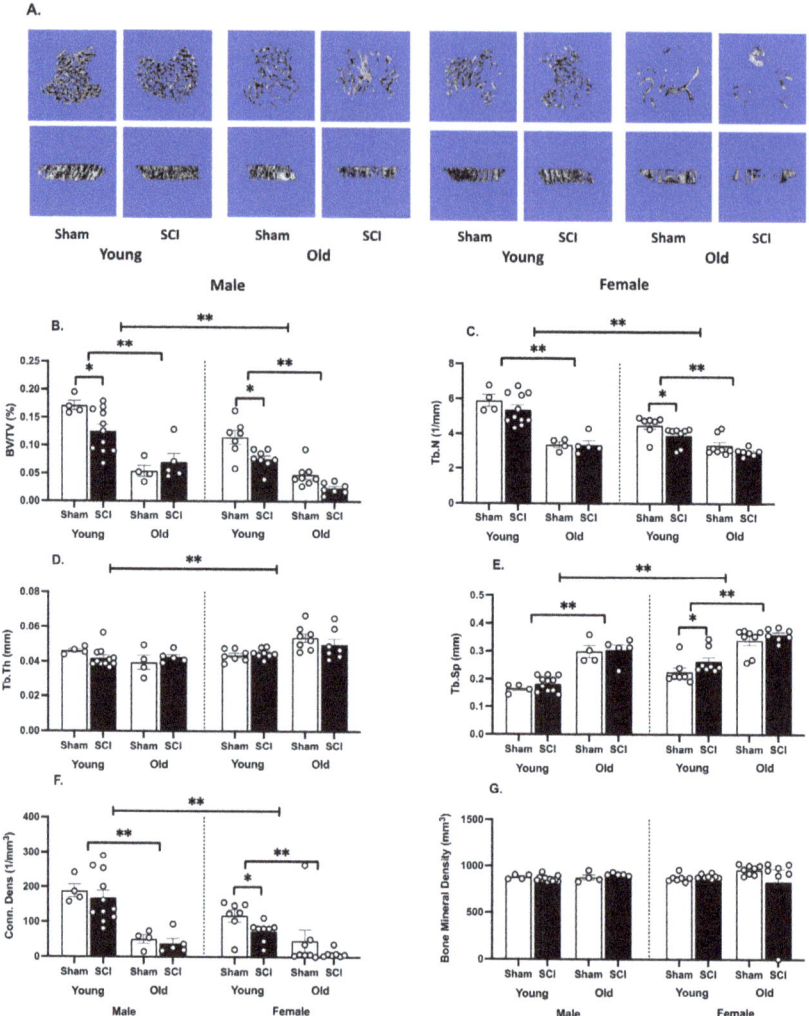

Figure 4. SCI, age, and sex affected trabecular bone. (**A**). Coronal (**top** panels) and lateral (**bottom** panels) view of microCT 3D reconstructions of 200 contiguous slices of the tibial metaphysis from a representative mouse in each group. (**B**). Females has less trabecular volume than males and, irrespective of sex, trabecular volume decreased with age. For the young subjects, SCI also decreased trabecular volume. (**C**). Females also had a reduced number of trabeculae, and the number of spicules was lower in older subjects regardless of sex. In young females there was also a decrease in trabecular number with age. (**D**). There was a main effect of sex on trabecular thickness, with females showing increased thickness relative to males. Age and sex did not affect this parameter. (**E**). Sex, age and SCI affected trabecular spacing. Spacing increased in females, relative to males, and in older subjects relative to young. SCI increased trabecular spacing in the young females. (**F**). Connective density was also greater in males relative to females, and in young compared to old mice. SCI decreased connective density in young females. (**G**). There was no effect of sex, age or SCI on bone mineral density. Means ± SEMs are plotted for each group. Individual subjects are shown with the round, white symbols. n = 4 sham and 5 SCI old males; 4 sham and 11 SCI young males; 8 sham and 7 SCI old females; 7 sham and 8 SCI young females. ** $p < 0.01$, * $p < 0.05$.

There was a main effect of sex only on trabecular thickness (F (1,17) = 19.03, $p < 0.001$, Figure 4D), with significant interactions between sex and age (F (1,17) = 15.61, $p < 0.001$) as well as sex, injury, and age (F (1,17) = 9.77, $p < 0.01$). The sex effect was driven by the old subjects. Old female mice, with and without SCI, had greater trabecular thickness than the old male mice ($t = 5.49, 2.40$, for Sham and SCI subjects respectively, $p < 0.05$).

Consistent with the other trabecular parameters, for trabecular spacing, there were main effects of age (F (1,19) = 136.90, $p < 0.0001$) and sex (F (1,27) = 27.38, $p < 0.0001$), but no effects of injury or significant interactions (Figure 4E). All young mice had less trabecular spacing than their sex and injury-matched conspecifics ($t > 5.41, p < 0.0001$ for all comparisons). Young sham males also had less trabecular spacing than the young sham females ($t = 2.56, p < 0.05$), and both the young and old male SCI mice had less spacing than the young and old female SCI mice, respectively ($t = 4.65, 2.72, p < 0.01$ for both analyses).

There were also main effects of age (F (1,19) = 126.90, $p < 0.0001$) and sex (F (1,27) = 5.44, $p < 0.05$), and no effects of injury on connective density (Figure 4F). There was also a significant interaction between injury and age on this parameter (F (1,19) = 6.80, $p < 0.05$). All young mice had greater connective density than their sex and injury matched conspecifics ($t > 4.12, p < 0.0005$ for all comparisons). Sex effects were seen in the SCI subjects only ($t = 3.32, 2.27$, for young and old SCI subjects respectively, $p < 0.05$). Specifically, an effect of injury was seen in the young females ($t = 2.16, p < 0.05$), with SCI decreasing connective density. No effects of sex, age, or SCI were seen on volumetric bone mineral density (Figure 4G).

For cortical bone measurements (Figure 5), only age affected cortical thickness and periosteal perimeter measures (F (1,45) = 45.40, $p < 0.001$; F (1,18) = 14.77, $p < 0.005$, Figure 5C,D, respectively). Young mice had greater cortical thickness than the old mice matched for sex and injury ($t > 2.16, p < 0.05$ for all comparisons), and smaller periosteal perimeters for all groups except the sham males ($t > 2.42, p < 0.05$ for all comparisons). Both age and sex also affected endosteal perimeters (F (1,18) = 28.91, $p < 0.0001$; F (1,27) = 4.86, $p < 0.05$, respectively, Figure 5E). Post hoc comparisons showed that young mice had greater cortical thickness than the old mice matched for sex and injury for all comparisons, except for the sham males ($t > 2.91, p < 0.01$ for all comparisons). There were no effects of SCI on cortical bone at one month post injury.

3.3. Open Field Activity and Rearing Were Significantly Correlated with Decreases in Tibial Trabecular Bone Volume

Pearson's product-moment correlations were used to examine the relationship between trabecular bone volume and motor activity in the SCI subjects only. With no change in motor function, sham subjects were not included in these analyses. There was no correlation between BMS scores collected on Day 28 and trabecular bone volume ($r = -0.14, p > 0.05$, Figure 6A,B). However, both open field activity and rearing behavior were significantly correlated with trabecular bone volume ($r = 0.44, 0.54$ respectively, $p < 0.01$, Figure 6C,E). The correlation between open field activity and bone volume was driven by the young male subjects ($r = 0.74, p < 0.005$). Correlations between bone volume and activity were not significant for any other group. The correlation between rearing and bone volume was powered by the young subjects ($r = 0.54, p < 0.01$, Figure 6D,F), although at an individual group level the only correlation that was significant was for the old females ($r = 0.74, p < 0.05$).

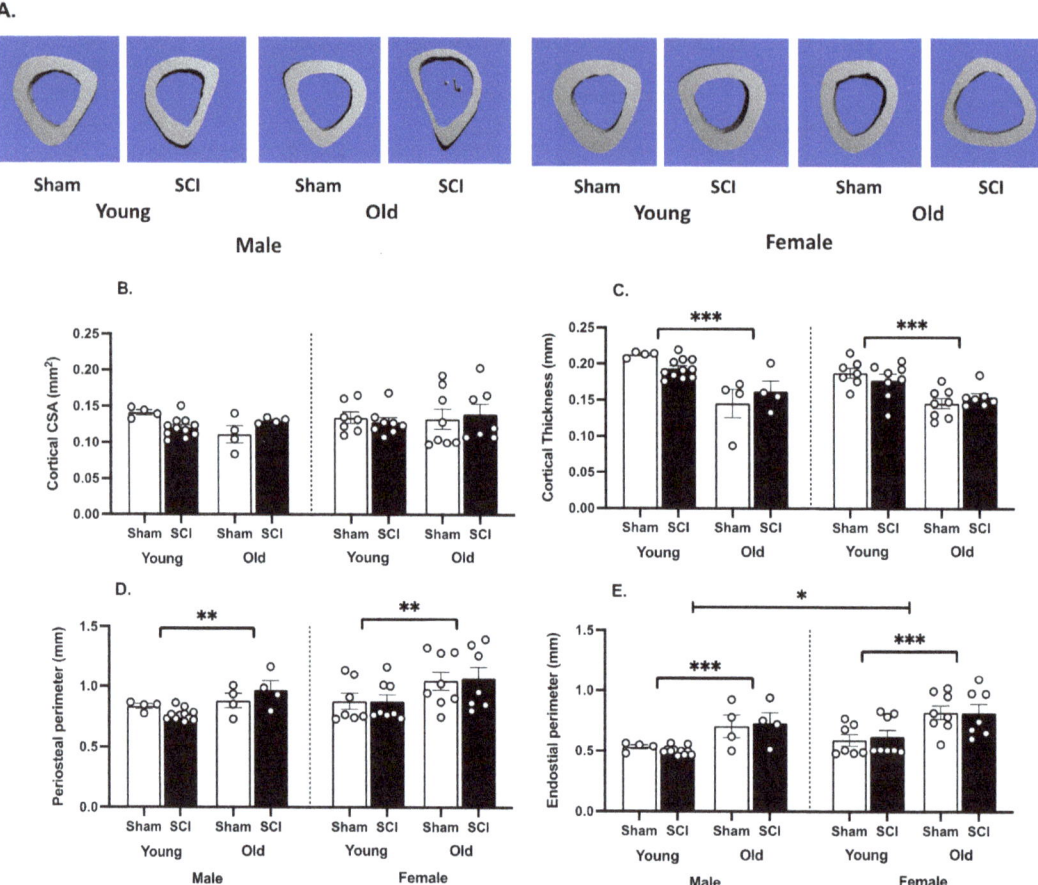

Figure 5. SCI did not affect cortical bone structure after only one month. (**A**). Coronal views of microCT 3D reconstructions of the 50 contiguous slices of the tibial mid-diaphysis from a representative mouse in each group. (**B**). There was also no effect of age or sex on cortical bone cross sectional area. (**C**). Age did, however, decrease cortical thickness and (**D**). increased the periosteal perimeter. (**E**). Both age and sex also affected the endosteal perimeter. The endosteal perimeter increased with age, and was larger in females than males. Means ± SEMs are plotted for each group. Individual subjects are shown with the round, white symbols. n = 4 sham and 5 SCI old males; 4 sham and 11 SCI young males; 8 sham and 7 SCI old females; 7 sham and 8 SCI young females. *** $p < 0.001$, ** $p < 0.01$, * $p < 0.05$.

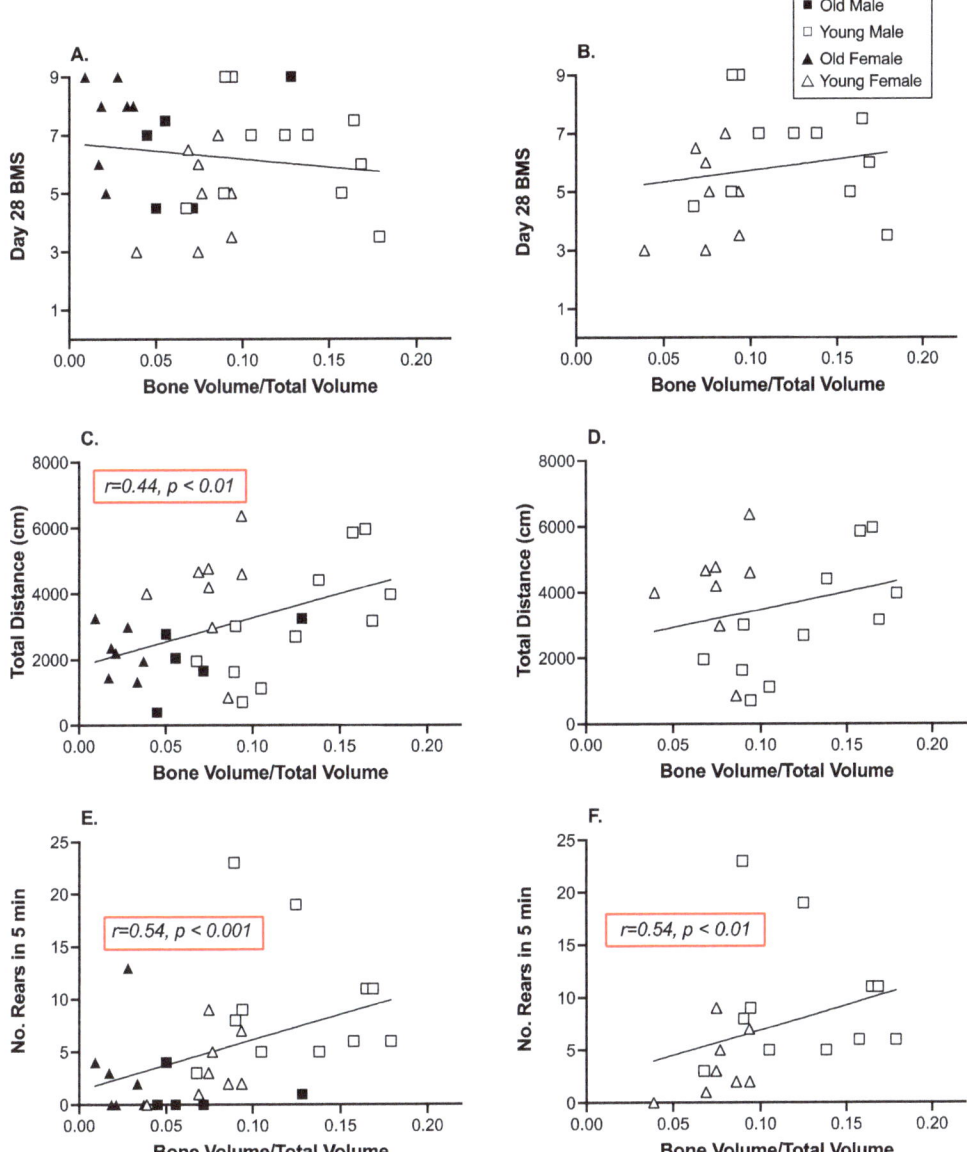

Figure 6. There was no correlation between trabecular bone volume and locomotor function *per se*, but open field activity and rearing were associated with increased bone volume. (**A**). BMS scores collected on Day 28 were not correlated with bone volume across all SCI mice or (**B**). in young SCI mice only. (**C**). There was a strong correlation between open field activity (on Day 21 post injury) and tibia bone volume. (**D**). The correlation between open field activity was not seen in the young mice per se, but was clear for young male mice alone. (**E**). Rearing was also strongly correlated with tibia trabecular bone volume. (**F**). This effect was also clear in the young SCI subjects alone and particularly in the young female subjects. n = 5 SCI old and 11 SCI young males; 7 SCI old and 8 SCI young females.

4. Discussion

Despite the recovery of plantar weight-supported stepping, SCI resulted in decreased tibial trabecular bone volumes in mice one month after injury. The effects of SCI on bone loss were only seen in young mice, irrespective of sex, but this was likely influenced in part by dramatically lower bone volumes seen in older subjects with and without injury producing a floor effect. Trabecular bone volumes were 2–3 fold lower in old mice compared with their young, sex-matched conspecifics. Interestingly, the relationship between trabecular bone volume and activity was also contingent on age. Trabecular bone volume was significantly correlated with open field activity in young males only, and bone volume correlated with rearing in the young, but not old, mice. These data suggest that load and use may reduce bone loss after SCI, but that the effectiveness of physical therapy may be contingent on patient demographics.

The lack of effects of locomotor function on bone volume in the mice, concur with our previous findings in a rat contusion SCI model and with human data. In a previous study of young male rats with a moderate contusion injury we found that recovery of locomotor function did not reduce bone loss after SCI. Despite the recovery of plantar stepping, rats with SCI had lower cancellous bone volume, lower bone formation rate, lower osteoid surface, and higher osteoclast surface at one-month post-injury than age-matched controls [36]. In the current study, there was also no correlation between trabecular bone function and recovered locomotor function, assessed with the BMS scale. Most studies with humans have also shown that standing or walking with assistance is not sufficient to improve bone parameters after SCI (for review see [19]). Instead, the efficacy of activity-based interventions appears contingent on the duration of training and the mechanical strain induced with muscle loading [19]. In the clinical studies, for example, improvements in bone parameters were seen when the number of weekly training sessions were increased, as well as with increased compressive loads during activity (for review see [19]). In the current study, the mice recovered plantar-weight supported stepping, but the SCI might still affect the amount of locomotion that they engage in. For example, both rodents and humans have an increased incidence of depression after SCI [63–71], which could reduce motivation to move in the home cage. Rather than locomotor function per se, focusing on activities that place high compressive loads on the bone or increasing the duration of physical activity may be important for re-establishing bone formation after SCI.

Supporting this premise, in the present study we found that increased tibial trabecular bone volume was associated with increased activity levels in an open field and increased rearing. Our interpretation of these data is limited, as activity in the open field is not a complete representation of activity in the home cage and correlations do not denote causation. Nonetheless, these data do suggest that increasing locomotor activity or the load placed on the hindlimbs, below the level of injury, in rearing might protect against bone loss, or increase bone formation, in the mouse SCI model. Notably, the data also suggest that the effects of physical activity may be contingent on the targeted demographic. While tibial trabecular bone volume correlated with increased open field activity and increased rearing in young mice, there was no clear relationship between these variables in the older subjects. Research on the effects of age and physical therapy in older people with SCI is extremely limited, with most studies focused on young adults. There are only two published case reports on older adults with chronic SCI, that were trained three times a week with functional electrical stimulation leg cycle ergometry. For the older adults, training increased lean mass, decreased % body fat, and increased scores on quality-of-life questionnaires. However, it did not improve bone mineral density [72,73]. A recent prospective study of factors associated with a change in bone density in chronic SCI [74], also included participants with a mean age of 55.1 ± 14.4 (SD) years (ranging from 24.7–87.1 years). Interestingly, this large study with 152 participants, found that wheelchair users lost more bone mineral density at the knee than walkers per year, an effect that was independent of age. These data stress the importance of post-injury exercise and potential benefits irrespective of age. However, it is likely that the intensity of the activity and the duration would need to be significantly higher to yield benefits in older, compared to young, adults with SCI [75]. Indeed, even in the able-bodied population, traditional exercise programs seem to be less osteogenic in mature compared to young adults [76]. There appears to be a decline in the sensitivity of bone to mechanical loading with aging. In fact, aging is also associated with declines in the number and function of bone forming osteoblasts, and the differentiation of these cells from multipotent mesenchymal stem cells [77–82].

Sex also affects bone loss in the general population, with osteoporosis significantly increased in post-menopausal women. While changes in hormone levels link sex to age in most human studies of bone loss, rats and mice do not experience the abrupt loss of estrogen at menopause, nor do androgen levels seem to decrease with age in male mice [83–85]. SCI, however, does produce transient changes in testosterone and estrogen in rodent models, which could differentially affect bone loss [55,86–90]. In the current study, we observed significant effects of sex on trabecular bone volume and number, as well as spacing, thickness, and connective density, irrespective of injury. Young females had lower bone volumes than males, likely corresponding to their lower body weight per se. Indeed, young adult men have almost 25% greater whole body bone mineral content compared with women [91], a difference that can be largely predicted simply based on average height differences between the sexes [92]. Young men also develop greater tibia trabecular bone volume in late puberty, primarily with greater trabecular thickness and trabecular number [93–95]. Intriguingly, in humans, these sex differences are only seen in the periphery, and not at central sites [92,96,97]. Our findings in the mouse model concur with the sex differences seen in humans. In the older subjects, however, sex effects were only observed after SCI. After SCI, the older males had increased trabecular bone volume and numbers remaining, increased thickness, and decreased spacing between trabecules compared with the old females, likely due to the fact that so little trabecular bone remained in the aged females to be impacted by SCI (Figure 4A). Interestingly, changes in the trabecular bone with SCI were not related to activity in the older subjects. As can be seen in Figures 3 and 4, rearing and open field activity did not differ between males and females with or without SCI at the older age.

Overall, the data collected in the mouse model of SCI suggest that while simple locomotion is not the key to improving bone integrity after SCI, activities that place high compressive load on the hindlimbs and increased duration of training might improve skeletal integrity. While our data suggest that the benefits of training may be restricted to young adult subjects, there is data to indicate that older adults also benefit from physical rehabilitation in terms of general and potentially bone health in the clinical setting [74]. One limitation of the current study, however, is that our assessments were limited to the acute and subacute stages of SCI. The proposed requisites of training would present challenges in early stages of SCI, as normal weight bearing is often not possible. However, other ways of loading the bone, including electrical stimulation of the muscles, have been explored. In rat models of SCI (complete thoracic transections), electrical stimulation has been shown to reduce bone resorption rates, increase multiple measures of trabecular bone mass, restore cortical mechanical strength, and alter gene expression in bone marrow progenitor cells [98,99]. Specifically, Qin and colleagues found that electrical stimulation increased gene expression for signaling pathways responsible for osteoblast differentiation and function, as well as for the regulation of osteoclasts by cells of the osteoblast lineage. While caution would be required, these data suggest that interventions in the acute phase of injury might reduce the dramatic loss of bone inherent to this stage of SCI. Notably early electrical stimulation could also be applied irrespective of injury severity.

Conceptually, exoskeleton training could also be used in combination with electrical stimulation to increase physical activity and place gravitational load on the lower limbs. A number of bionic exoskeletons are now FDA approved for assisting walking after SCI, including Ekso™, Rewalk™, and Indego® systems, as well as the implanted neuroprostheses, Parastep® 1, which uses functional neuromuscular stimulation (FNS) to generate a majority of the muscular torque required to move and stabilize the lower extremities. These exoskeletal ambulation devices can significantly improve cardiovascular and psychological health [100–104]. However, unfortunately, there is no evidence to suggest that use of these devices can protect against or reverse SCI-induced bone loss. As part of a multicenter study evaluating the effectiveness of the Parastep® 1, Needham-Shropshire et al. [105] assessed bone mineral density in the proximal femur. Sixteen people, at least six months post SCI, completed 32 sessions (three sessions per week over 11 weeks) of Parastep® 1 ambulation training and an additional eight weeks of FNS training There were no changes in bone mineral density in the proximal femur. Similarly, Thoumie et al. [106] reported no beneficial effects of training, with the RGO-II hybrid orthosis, on bone. The lack of effects seen with exoskeleton training could stem from limitations in the duration of walking, which is significantly constrained by fatigue. Indeed, more recently, Karelis et al. [107] reported a tendency for an increase (14.5%) in the bone mineral density of the tibia with use of the battery-powered, motor driven Ekso robotic exoskeleton system, at least three times per week for up to 60 min of free overground walking. Powered exoskeletons that enable increased time spent walking may impact bone. Delayed onset of rehabilitative training might also limit the effectiveness of exoskeleton training. In the Parastep evaluation, training was not initiated until at least six months post injury. Based on the findings of the present study in mice, however, the lower gravitational loads placed on the leg bones when using orthotic devices may be the most critical limitation for osteogenic efficacy. The orthotic components of ambulatory systems are designed to protect the insensate joints and osteoporotic bones of users from possible damage with loads applied during walking [108]. Moreover, ground-reaction forces increase as walking speed increases [109]. Slower walking in orthotic devices would place less compressive force on the bone, and potentially limit the effects of training on osteogenesis. According to Frost's mechanostat theory [110], there is an optimal range of mechanical loading essential for osteogenesis. The range of mechanical loading that is required to reduce or reverse bone loss after SCI needs to be determined [19].

Currently, there are no clinical guidelines for the prevention or reversal of SCI-induced bone loss. Moreover, interventions that are effective for other forms of osteoporosis have limited efficacy after SCI. While this is not surprising, given the multifaceted etiology of bone loss after SCI, the dramatic bone loss seen after SCI significantly affects psychological and physical well-being. Further exploration of the critical factors contributing to acute bone loss and the development of strategies to improve long-term bone health is an urgent and unmet need for people living with spinal cord injury.

5. Conclusions

In sum, commensurate with both preclinical and clinical data, spinal cord injury led to a significant loss of trabecular bone volume below the level of injury. The effects of SCI on bone were only significant in young mice, with the dramatically lower bone volumes seen in older subjects likely masking any effects of injury. Intriguingly, tibial trabecular bone volume in the young SCI mice was significantly correlated with rearing activity. Increased rearing, which would place a high compressive load on the hindlimbs, positively correlated with increased bone volume. These data suggest that while the effectiveness of physical therapy may be contingent on patient demographics, interventions initiated early after SCI that place high compressive load on the hindlimbs may reduce bone loss.

Author Contributions: Conceptualization, M.A.H., C.G.G. and D.G.; methodology, M.A.H., C.G.G. and D.G.; formal analysis, M.A.H. and D.G.; investigation, M.T., A.F., R.D., R.C., A.S. and K.C.; resources, M.A.H., C.G.G. and D.G.; data curation, M.A.H., R.D., A.F. and D.G.; writing—original draft preparation, M.A.H.; writing—review & editing, M.A.H., C.G.G. and D.G.; visualization, M.A.H.; supervision, M.A.H., C.G.G. and D.G.; project administration, M.A.H., C.G.G. and D.G.; funding acquisition, M.A.H., C.G.G. and D.G. All authors have read and agreed to the published version of the manuscript.

Funding: This research was generously funded by a grant from the Texas A&M Triads for Transformation to M.A.H., C.G.G., and D.G., as well as the Craig H. Neilsen foundation to M.A.H.

Institutional Review Board Statement: The study was conducted and approved by the Institutional Animal Care Committee at Texas A&M University (IACUC 2017-0156 on 19 June 2017). All of the experiments reported here were reviewed and approved by the and were consistent with the NIH guidelines for animal care and use.

Informed Consent Statement: Not applicable.

Data Availability Statement: The data presented in this study are available on request from the corresponding author.

Acknowledgments: The authors would like to thank additional laboratory members for their support in these studies, including Kiralyn Brakel, Josephina Rau, Sanskruthi Guduri and Annebel Hemphill.

Conflicts of Interest: The authors declare no conflict of interest.

References

1. Garland, D.E.; Adkins, R.H.; Stewart, C.A.; Ashford, R.; Vigil, D. Regional osteoporosis in women who have a complete spinal cord injury. *J. Bone Jt. Surg Am.* **2001**, *83*, 1195–1200. [CrossRef] [PubMed]
2. Garland, D.E.; Stewart, C.A.; Adkins, R.H.; Hu, S.S.; Rosen, C.; Liotta, F.J.; Weinstein, D.A. Osteoporosis after spinal cord injury. *J. Orthop. Res.* **1992**, *10*, 371–378. [CrossRef] [PubMed]
3. de Bruin, E.D.; Dietz, V.; Dambacher, M.A.; Stussi, E. Longitudinal changes in bone in men with spinal cord injury. *Clin. Rehabil.* **2000**, *14*, 145–152. [CrossRef] [PubMed]
4. Giangregorio, L.; McCartney, N. Bone loss and muscle atrophy in spinal cord injury: Epidemiology, fracture prediction, and rehabilitation strategies. *J. Spinal Cord. Med.* **2006**, *29*, 489–500. [CrossRef] [PubMed]
5. Biering-Sorensen, F.; Bohr, H.H.; Schaadt, O.P. Longitudinal study of bone mineral content in the lumbar spine, the forearm and the lower extremities after spinal cord injury. *Eur. J. Clin. Invest.* **1990**, *20*, 330–335. [CrossRef]
6. Modlesky, C.M.; Majumdar, S.; Narasimhan, A.; Dudley, G.A. Trabecular bone microarchitecture is deteriorated in men with spinal cord injury. *J. Bone Miner. Res.* **2004**, *19*, 48–55. [CrossRef] [PubMed]
7. Shields, R.K.; Dudley-Javoroski, S. Musculoskeletal plasticity after acute spinal cord injury: Effects of long-term neuromuscular electrical stimulation training. *J. Neurophysiol.* **2006**, *95*, 2380–2390. [CrossRef]
8. Modlesky, C.M.; Slade, J.M.; Bickel, C.S.; Meyer, R.A.; Dudley, G.A. Deteriorated geometric structure and strength of the midfemur in men with complete spinal cord injury. *Bone* **2005**, *36*, 331–339. [CrossRef]
9. Eser, P.; Frotzler, A.; Zehnder, Y.; Wick, L.; Knecht, H.; Denoth, J.; Schiessl, H. Relationship between the duration of paralysis and bone structure: A pQCT study of spinal cord injured individuals. *Bone* **2004**, *34*, 869–880. [CrossRef]
10. Coupaud, S.; McLean, A.N.; Purcell, M.; Fraser, M.H.; Allan, D.B. Decreases in bone mineral density at cortical and trabecular sites in the tibia and femur during the first year of spinal cord injury. *Bone* **2015**, *74*, 69–75. [CrossRef]
11. Ragnarsson, K.T.; Sell, G.H. Lower extremity fractures after spinal cord injury: A retrospective study. *Arch. Phys. Med. Rehabil.* **1981**, *62*, 418–423. [PubMed]
12. Vestergaard, P.; Krogh, K.; Rejnmark, L.; Mosekilde, L. Fracture rates and risk factors for fractures in patients with spinal cord injury. *Spinal Cord.* **1998**, *36*, 790–796. [CrossRef] [PubMed]
13. Lazo, M.G.; Shirazi, P.; Sam, M.; Giobbie-Hurder, A.; Blacconiere, M.J.; Muppidi, M. Osteoporosis and risk of fracture in men with spinal cord injury. *Spinal Cord.* **2001**, *39*, 208–214. [CrossRef] [PubMed]
14. Carbone, L.D.; Chin, A.S.; Burns, S.P.; Svircev, J.N.; Hoenig, H.; Heggeness, M.; Bailey, L.; Weaver, F. Mortality after lower extremity fractures in men with spinal cord injury. *J. Bone Miner. Res.* **2014**, *29*, 432–439. [CrossRef] [PubMed]
15. Gifre, L.; Vidal, J.; Carrasco, J.; Portell, E.; Puig, J.; Monegal, A.; Guanabens, N.; Peris, P. Incidence of skeletal fractures after traumatic spinal cord injury: A 10-year follow-up study. *Clin. Rehabil.* **2014**, *28*, 361–369. [CrossRef]
16. Edwards, W.B.; Schnitzer, T.J. Bone Imaging and Fracture Risk after Spinal Cord. Injury. *Curr. Osteoporos. Rep.* **2015**, *13*, 310–317. [CrossRef]
17. Keating, J.F.; Kerr, M.; Delargy, M. Minimal trauma causing fractures in patients with spinal cord injury. *Disabil. Rehabil.* **1992**, *14*, 108–109. [CrossRef]
18. Morse, L.R.; Giangregorio, L.; Battaglino, R.A.; Holland, R.; Craven, B.C.; Stolzmann, K.L.; Lazzari, A.A.; Sabharwal, S.; Garshick, E. VA-based survey of osteoporosis management in spinal cord injury. *PM R* **2009**, *1*, 240–244. [CrossRef]
19. Abdelrahman, S.; Ireland, A.; Winter, E.M.; Purcell, M.; Coupaud, S. Osteoporosis after spinal cord injury: Aetiology, effects and therapeutic approaches. *J. Musculoskelet. Neuronal. Interact.* **2021**, *21*, 26–50.
20. Zeman, R.J.; Zhao, J.; Zhang, Y.; Zhao, W.; Wen, X.; Wu, Y.; Pan, J.; Bauman, W.A.; Cardozo, C. Differential skeletal muscle gene expression after upper or lower motor neuron transection. *Pflug. Arch.* **2009**, *458*, 525–535. [CrossRef]
21. Dudley-Javoroski, S.; Shields, R.K. Muscle and bone plasticity after spinal cord injury: Review of adaptations to disuse and to electrical muscle stimulation. *J. Rehabil. Res. Dev.* **2008**, *45*, 283–296. [CrossRef] [PubMed]

22. Qin, W.; Bauman, W.A.; Cardozo, C. Bone and muscle loss after spinal cord injury: Organ interactions. *Ann. N. Y. Acad. Sci.* **2010**, *1211*, 66–84. [CrossRef] [PubMed]
23. Clark, J.M.; Findlay, D.M. Musculoskeletal Health in the Context of Spinal Cord. Injury. *Curr. Osteoporos. Rep.* **2017**, *15*, 433–442. [CrossRef] [PubMed]
24. Colaianni, G.; Cuscito, C.; Mongelli, T.; Oranger, A.; Mori, G.; Brunetti, G.; Colucci, S.; Cinti, S.; Grano, M. Irisin enhances osteoblast differentiation in vitro. *Int. J. Endocrinol.* **2014**, *2014*, 902186. [CrossRef] [PubMed]
25. Colaianni, G.; Grano, M. Role of Irisin on the bone-muscle functional unit. *Bonekey Rep.* **2015**, *4*, 765. [CrossRef]
26. Kawao, N.; Moritake, A.; Tatsumi, K.; Kaji, H. Roles of Irisin in the Linkage from Muscle to Bone During Mechanical Unloading in Mice. *Calcif. Tissue Int.* **2018**, *103*, 24–34. [CrossRef]
27. Estell, E.G.; Le, P.T.; Vegting, Y.; Kim, H.; Wrann, C.; Bouxsein, M.L.; Nagano, K.; Baron, R.; Spiegelman, B.M.; Rosen, C.J. Irisin directly stimulates osteoclastogenesis and bone resorption in vitro and in vivo. *Elife* **2020**, *9*, e58172. [CrossRef]
28. Shams, R.; Drasites, K.P.; Zaman, V.; Matzelle, D.; Shields, D.C.; Garner, D.P.; Sole, C.J.; Haque, A.; Banik, N.L. The Pathophysiology of Osteoporosis after Spinal Cord. Injury. *Int. J. Mol. Sci.* **2021**, *22*, 3057. [CrossRef]
29. Huang, T.S.; Wang, Y.H.; Lee, S.H.; Lai, J.S. Impaired hypothalamus-pituitary-adrenal axis in men with spinal Cord. injuries. *Am. J. Phys. Med. Rehabil.* **1998**, *77*, 108–112. [CrossRef]
30. Jiang, S.D.; Jiang, L.S.; Dai, L.Y. Mechanisms of osteoporosis in spinal cord injury. *Clin. Endocrinol.* **2006**, *65*, 555–565. [CrossRef]
31. del Rivero, T.; Bethea, J.R. The effects of spinal cord injury on bone loss and dysregulation of the calcium/parathyroid hormone loop in mice. *Osteoporos. Sarcopenia* **2016**, *2*, 164–169. [CrossRef] [PubMed]
32. Minaire, P.; Edouard, C.; Arlot, M.; Meunier, P.J. Marrow changes in paraplegic patients. *Calcif. Tissue Int.* **1984**, *36*, 338–340. [CrossRef] [PubMed]
33. Elder, C.P.; Apple, D.F.; Bickel, C.S.; Meyer, R.A.; Dudley, G.A. Intramuscular fat and glucose tolerance after spinal cord injury—A cross-sectional study. *Spinal Cord.* **2004**, *42*, 711–716. [CrossRef] [PubMed]
34. Gorgey, A.S.; Dudley, G.A. Skeletal muscle atrophy and increased intramuscular fat after incomplete spinal cord injury. *Spinal Cord.* **2007**, *45*, 304–309. [CrossRef] [PubMed]
35. Yan, J.; Li, B.; Chen, J.W.; Jiang, S.D.; Jiang, L.S. Spinal cord injury causes bone loss through peroxisome proliferator-activated receptor-gamma and Wnt signalling. *J. Cell Mol. Med.* **2012**, *16*, 2968–2977. [CrossRef] [PubMed]
36. Metzger, C.E.; Gong, S.; Aceves, M.; Bloomfield, S.A.; Hook, M.A. Osteocytes reflect a pro-inflammatory state following spinal cord injury in a rodent model. *Bone* **2019**, *120*, 465–475. [CrossRef]
37. Bauman, W.A.; Cardozo, C.P. Osteoporosis in individuals with spinal cord injury. *PM R* **2015**, *7*, 188–201, quiz 201. [CrossRef]
38. Maimoun, L.; Ben Bouallegue, F.; Gelis, A.; Aouinti, S.; Mura, T.; Philibert, P.; Souberbielle, J.C.; Piketty, M.; Garnero, P.; Mariano-Goulart, D.; et al. Periostin and sclerostin levels in individuals with spinal cord injury and their relationship with bone mass, bone turnover, fracture and osteoporosis status. *Bone* **2019**, *127*, 612–619. [CrossRef]
39. Zleik, N.; Weaver, F.; Harmon, R.L.; Le, B.; Radhakrishnan, R.; Jirau-Rosaly, W.D.; Craven, B.C.; Raiford, M.; Hill, J.N.; Etingen, B.; et al. Prevention and management of osteoporosis and osteoporotic fractures in persons with a spinal cord injury or disorder: A systematic scoping review. *J. Spinal Cord. Med.* **2019**, *42*, 735–759. [CrossRef]
40. Exton-Smith, A.N.; Millard, P.H.; Payne, P.R.; Wheeler, E.F. Pattern of development and loss of bone with age. *Lancet* **1969**, *2*, 1154–1157. [CrossRef]
41. Firooznia, H.; Golimbu, C.; Rafii, M.; Schwartz, M.S.; Alterman, E.R. Quantitative computed tomography assessment of spinal trabecular bone. I. Age-related regression in normal men and women. *J. Comput. Tomogr.* **1984**, *8*, 91–97. [CrossRef]
42. Wright, N.C.; Looker, A.C.; Saag, K.G.; Curtis, J.R.; Delzell, E.S.; Randall, S.; Dawson-Hughes, B. The recent prevalence of osteoporosis and low bone mass in the United States based on bone mineral density at the femoral neck or lumbar spine. *J. Bone Miner. Res.* **2014**, *29*, 2520–2526. [CrossRef] [PubMed]
43. van den Berg, M.E.; Castellote, J.M.; Mahillo-Fernandez, I.; de Pedro-Cuesta, J. Incidence of spinal cord injury worldwide: A systematic review. *Neuroepidemiology* **2010**, *34*, 184–192. [CrossRef] [PubMed]
44. Knutsdottir, S.; Thorisdottir, H.; Sigvaldason, K.; Jonsson, H., Jr.; Bjornsson, A.; Ingvarsson, P. Epidemiology of traumatic spinal Cord. injuries in Iceland from 1975 to 2009. *Spinal Cord.* **2012**, *50*, 123–126. [CrossRef]
45. DeVivo, M.J.; Chen, Y. Trends in new injuries, prevalent cases, and aging with spinal cord injury. *Arch. Phys. Med. Rehabil.* **2011**, *92*, 332–338. [CrossRef]
46. Nijendijk, J.H.; Post, M.W.; van Asbeck, F.W. Epidemiology of traumatic spinal Cord. injuries in The Netherlands in 2010. *Spinal Cord.* **2014**, *52*, 258–263. [CrossRef]
47. McCaughey, E.J.; Purcell, M.; McLean, A.N.; Fraser, M.H.; Bewick, A.; Borotkanics, R.J.; Allan, D.B. Changing demographics of spinal cord injury over a 20-year period: A longitudinal population-based study in Scotland. *Spinal Cord.* **2016**, *54*, 270–276. [CrossRef]
48. Barbara-Bataller, E.; Mendez-Suarez, J.L.; Aleman-Sanchez, C.; Sanchez-Enriquez, J.; Sosa-Henriquez, M. Change in the profile of traumatic spinal cord injury over 15 years in Spain. *Scand. J. Trauma Resusc. Emerg. Med.* **2018**, *26*, 27. [CrossRef]
49. Hernlund, E.; Svedbom, A.; Ivergard, M.; Compston, J.; Cooper, C.; Stenmark, J.; McCloskey, E.V.; Jonsson, B.; Kanis, J.A. Osteoporosis in the European Union: Medical management, epidemiology and economic burden. A report prepared in collaboration with the International Osteoporosis Foundation (IOF) and the European Federation of Pharmaceutical Industry Associations (EFPIA). *Arch. Osteoporos.* **2013**, *8*, 136. [CrossRef]

50. Alswat, K.A. Gender Disparities in Osteoporosis. *J. Clin. Med. Res.* **2017**, *9*, 382–387. [CrossRef]
51. Krolner, B.; Tondevold, E.; Toft, B.; Berthelsen, B.; Nielsen, S.P. Bone mass of the axial and the appendicular skeleton in women with Colles' fracture: Its relation to physical activity. *Clin. Physiol.* **1982**, *2*, 147–157. [CrossRef] [PubMed]
52. Nilas, L.; Christiansen, C. Rates of bone loss in normal women: Evidence of accelerated trabecular bone loss after the menopause. *Eur. J. Clin. Invest.* **1988**, *18*, 529–534. [CrossRef] [PubMed]
53. Stepan, J.J.; Tesarova, A.; Havranek, T.; Jodl, J.; Formankova, J.; Pacovsky, V. Age and sex dependency of the biochemical indices of bone remodelling. *Clin. Chim Acta* **1985**, *151*, 273–283. [CrossRef]
54. Dannels, A.; Charlifue, S. The perimenopause experience for women with spinal Cord. injuries. *SCI. Nurs.* **2004**, *21*, 9–13.
55. Hubscher, C.H.; Armstrong, J.E.; Johnson, J.R. Effects of spinal cord injury on the rat estrous cycle. *Brain Res.* **2006**, *1100*, 118–124. [CrossRef]
56. Rutberg, L.; Friden, B.; Karlsson, A.K. Amenorrhoea in newly spinal Cord. injured women: An effect of hyperprolactinaemia? *Spinal Cord.* **2008**, *46*, 189–191. [CrossRef]
57. Furlan, J.C.; Krassioukov, A.V.; Fehlings, M.G. The effects of gender on clinical and neurological outcomes after acute cervical spinal cord injury. *J. Neurotrauma* **2005**, *22*, 368–381. [CrossRef]
58. Ng, J.S.; Chin, K.Y. Potential mechanisms linking psychological stress to bone health. *Int. J. Med. Sci.* **2021**, *18*, 604–614. [CrossRef]
59. Baker-LePain, J.C.; Nakamura, M.C.; Lane, N.E. Effects of inflammation on bone: An update. *Curr. Opin. Rheumatol.* **2011**, *23*, 389–395. [CrossRef]
60. Basso, D.M.; Fisher, L.C.; Anderson, A.J.; Jakeman, L.B.; McTigue, D.M.; Popovich, P.G. Basso Mouse Scale for locomotion detects differences in recovery after spinal cord injury in five common mouse strains. *J. Neurotrauma* **2006**, *23*, 635–659. [CrossRef]
61. Perrien, D.S.; Akel, N.S.; Edwards, P.K.; Carver, A.A.; Bendre, M.S.; Swain, F.L.; Skinner, R.A.; Hogue, W.R.; Nicks, K.M.; Pierson, T.M.; et al. Inhibin A is an endocrine stimulator of bone mass and strength. *Endocrinology* **2007**, *148*, 1654–1665. [CrossRef] [PubMed]
62. Bouxsein, M.L.; Boyd, S.K.; Christiansen, B.A.; Guldberg, R.E.; Jepsen, K.J.; Muller, R. Guidelines for assessment of bone microstructure in rodents using micro-computed tomography. *J. Bone Miner. Res.* **2010**, *25*, 1468–1486. [CrossRef] [PubMed]
63. Maldonado-Bouchard, S.; Peters, K.; Woller, S.A.; Madahian, B.; Faghihi, U.; Patel, S.; Bake, S.; Hook, M.A. Inflammation is increased with anxiety- and depression-like signs in a rat model of spinal cord injury. *Brain Behav. Immun.* **2016**, *51*, 176–195. [CrossRef]
64. Luedtke, K.; Bouchard, S.M.; Woller, S.A.; Funk, M.K.; Aceves, M.; Hook, M.A. Assessment of depression in a rodent model of spinal cord injury. *J. Neurotrauma* **2014**, *31*, 1107–1121. [CrossRef]
65. Brakel, K.; Aceves, A.R.; Aceves, M.; Hierholzer, A.; Nguyen, Q.N.; Hook, M.A. Depression-like behavior corresponds with cardiac changes in a rodent model of spinal cord injury. *Exp. Neurol.* **2019**, *320*, 112969. [CrossRef] [PubMed]
66. Brakel, K.; Aceves, M.; Garza, A.; Yoo, C.; Escobedo, G.; Jr Panchani, N.; Shapiro, L.; Hook, M. Inflammation increases the development of depression behaviors in male rats after spinal cord injury. *Brain Behav Immun Health* **2021**, *14*, 100258. [CrossRef]
67. Wu, J.; Zhao, Z.; Sabirzhanov, B.; Stoica, B.A.; Kumar, A.; Luo, T.; Skovira, J.; Faden, A.I. Spinal cord injury causes brain inflammation associated with cognitive and affective changes: Role of cell cycle pathways. *J. Neurosci. Off. J. Soc. Neurosci.* **2014**, *34*, 10989–11006. [CrossRef]
68. Williams, R.; Murray, A. Prevalence of depression after spinal cord injury: A meta-analysis. *Arch. Phys. Med. Rehabil.* **2015**, *96*, 133–140. [CrossRef]
69. Farrell, K.; Houle, J.D. Systemic Inhibition of Soluble Tumor Necrosis Factor with XPro1595 Exacerbates a Post-Spinal Cord. Injury Depressive Phenotype in Female Rats. *J. Neurotrauma* **2019**, *36*, 2964–2976. [CrossRef]
70. do Espirito Santo, C.C.; da Silva Fiorin, F.; Ilha, J.; Duarte, M.; Duarte, T.; Santos, A.R.S. Spinal cord injury by clip-compression induces anxiety and depression-like behaviours in female rats: The role of the inflammatory response. *Brain Behav. Immun.* **2019**, *78*, 91–104. [CrossRef]
71. Elliott, T.R.; Frank, R.G. Depression following spinal cord injury. *Arch. Phys. Med. Rehabil.* **1996**, *77*, 816–823. [CrossRef]
72. Dolbow, D.R.; Gorgey, A.S.; Cifu, D.X.; Moore, J.R.; Gater, D.R. Feasibility of home-based functional electrical stimulation cycling: Case report. *Spinal Cord.* **2012**, *50*, 170–171. [CrossRef] [PubMed]
73. Dolbow, D.R.; Gorgey, A.S.; Ketchum, J.M.; Moore, J.R.; Hackett, L.A.; Gater, D.R. Exercise adherence during home-based functional electrical stimulation cycling by individuals with spinal cord injury. *Am. J. Phys. Med. Rehabil.* **2012**, *91*, 922–930. [CrossRef] [PubMed]
74. Morse, L.R.; Nguyen, N.; Battaglino, R.A.; Guarino, A.J.; Gagnon, D.R.; Zafonte, R.; Garshick, E. Wheelchair use and lipophilic statin medications may influence bone loss in chronic spinal cord injury: Findings from the FRASCI-bone loss study. *Osteoporos. Int.* **2016**, *27*, 3503–3511. [CrossRef]
75. Turner, C.H.; Takano, Y.; Owan, I. Aging changes mechanical loading thresholds for bone formation in rats. *J. Bone Miner. Res.* **1995**, *10*, 1544–1549. [CrossRef]
76. Hughes, J.M.; Charkoudian, N.; Barnes, J.N.; Morgan, B.J. Revisiting the Debate: Does Exercise Build Strong Bones in the Mature and Senescent Skeleton? *Front. Physiol.* **2016**, *7*, 369. [CrossRef]
77. Tsuji, T.; Hughes, F.J.; McCulloch, C.A.; Melcher, A.H. Effects of donor age on osteogenic cells of rat bone marrow in vitro. *Mech. Ageing Dev.* **1990**, *51*, 121–132. [CrossRef]

78. Quarto, R.; Thomas, D.; Liang, C.T. Bone progenitor cell deficits and the age-associated decline in bone repair capacity. *Calcif. Tissue Int.* **1995**, *56*, 123–129. [CrossRef]
79. Majors, A.K.; Boehm, C.A.; Nitto, H.; Midura, R.J.; Muschler, G.F. Characterization of human bone marrow stromal cells with respect to osteoblastic differentiation. *J. Orthop. Res.* **1997**, *15*, 546–557. [CrossRef]
80. Nishida, S.; Endo, N.; Yamagiwa, H.; Tanizawa, T.; Takahashi, H.E. Number of osteoprogenitor cells in human bone marrow markedly decreases after skeletal maturation. *J. Bone Miner. Metab* **1999**, *17*, 171–177. [CrossRef]
81. Muschler, G.F.; Nitto, H.; Boehm, C.A.; Easley, K.A. Age- and gender-related changes in the cellularity of human bone marrow and the prevalence of osteoblastic progenitors. *J. Orthop. Res.* **2001**, *19*, 117–125. [CrossRef]
82. Yeh, L.C.; Wilkerson, M.; Lee, J.C.; Adamo, M.L. IGF-1 Receptor Insufficiency Leads to Age-Dependent Attenuation of Osteoblast Differentiation. *Endocrinology* **2015**, *156*, 2872–2879. [CrossRef] [PubMed]
83. Fuller, K.N.Z.; Thyfault, J.P. Barriers in translating preclinical rodent exercise metabolism findings to human health. *J. Appl. Physiol.* **2021**, *130*, 182–192. [CrossRef] [PubMed]
84. Finch, C.E.; Felicio, L.S.; Mobbs, C.V.; Nelson, J.F. Ovarian and steroidal influences on neuroendocrine aging processes in female rodents. *Endocr. Rev.* **1984**, *5*, 467–497. [CrossRef]
85. Almeida, M.; Han, L.; Martin-Millan, M.; Plotkin, L.I.; Stewart, S.A.; Roberson, P.K.; Kousteni, S.; O'Brien, C.A.; Bellido, T.; Parfitt, A.M.; et al. Skeletal involution by age-associated oxidative stress and its acceleration by loss of sex steroids. *J. Biol. Chem.* **2007**, *282*, 27285–27297. [CrossRef]
86. Gelderd, J.B.; Peppler, R.D. Effect of spinal Cord. transection on the reproductive system in the female rat. *Neuroendocrinology* **1979**, *29*, 293–299. [CrossRef]
87. Shah, P.K.; Song, J.; Kim, S.; Zhong, H.; Roy, R.R.; Edgerton, V.R. Rodent estrous cycle response to incomplete spinal cord injury, surgical interventions, and locomotor training. *Behav. NeuroSci.* **2011**, *125*, 996–1002. [CrossRef]
88. Yarrow, J.F.; Phillips, E.G.; Conover, C.F.; Bassett, T.E.; Chen, C.; Teurlings, T.; Vasconez, A.; Alerte, J.; Prock, H.; Jiron, J.M.; et al. Testosterone Plus Finasteride Prevents Bone Loss without Prostate Growth in a Rodent Spinal Cord. Injury Model. *J. Neurotrauma* **2017**, *34*, 2972–2981. [CrossRef]
89. Yarrow, J.F.; Ye, F.; Balaez, A.; Mantione, J.M.; Otzel, D.M.; Chen, C.; Beggs, L.A.; Baligand, C.; Keener, J.E.; Lim, W.; et al. Bone loss in a new rodent model combining spinal cord injury and cast immobilization. *J. Musculoskelet. Neuronal. Interact.* **2014**, *14*, 255–266.
90. Stewart, A.N.; MacLean, S.M.; Stromberg, A.J.; Whelan, J.P.; Bailey, W.M.; Gensel, J.C.; Wilson, M.E. Considerations for Studying Sex as a Biological Variable in Spinal Cord. Injury. *Front. Neurol.* **2020**, *11*, 802. [CrossRef]
91. Boot, A.M.; de Ridder, M.A.; van der Sluis, I.M.; van Slobbe, I.; Krenning, E.P.; Keizer-Schrama, S.M. Peak bone mineral density, lean body mass and fractures. *Bone* **2010**, *46*, 336–341. [CrossRef] [PubMed]
92. Almeida, M.; Laurent, M.R.; Dubois, V.; Claessens, F.; O'Brien, C.A.; Bouillon, R.; Vanderschueren, D.; Manolagas, S.C. Estrogens and Androgens in Skeletal Physiology and Pathophysiology. *Physiol. Rev.* **2017**, *97*, 135–187. [CrossRef] [PubMed]
93. Burghardt, A.J.; Kazakia, G.J.; Ramachandran, S.; Link, T.M.; Majumdar, S. Age- and gender-related differences in the geometric properties and biomechanical significance of intracortical porosity in the distal radius and tibia. *J. Bone Miner. Res.* **2010**, *25*, 983–993. [PubMed]
94. Dalzell, N.; Kaptoge, S.; Morris, N.; Berthier, A.; Koller, B.; Braak, L.; van Rietbergen, B.; Reeve, J. Bone micro-architecture and determinants of strength in the radius and tibia: Age-related changes in a population-based study of normal adults measured with high-resolution pQCT. *Osteoporos. Int.* **2009**, *20*, 1683–1694. [CrossRef]
95. Khosla, S.; Riggs, B.L.; Atkinson, E.J.; Oberg, A.L.; McDaniel, L.J.; Holets, M.; Peterson, J.M.; Melton, L.J., 3rd. Effects of sex and age on bone microstructure at the ultradistal radius: A population-based noninvasive in vivo assessment. *J. Bone Miner. Res.* **2006**, *21*, 124–131. [CrossRef] [PubMed]
96. Macdonald, H.M.; Nishiyama, K.K.; Kang, J.; Hanley, D.A.; Boyd, S.K. Age-related patterns of trabecular and cortical bone loss differ between sexes and skeletal sites: A population-based HR-pQCT study. *J. Bone Miner. Res.* **2011**, *26*, 50–62. [CrossRef]
97. Nieves, J.W.; Formica, C.; Ruffing, J.; Zion, M.; Garrett, P.; Lindsay, R.; Cosman, F. Males have larger skeletal size and bone mass than females, despite comparable body size. *J. Bone Miner. Res.* **2005**, *20*, 529–535. [CrossRef]
98. Qin, W.; Sun, L.; Cao, J.; Peng, Y.; Collier, L.; Wu, Y.; Creasey, G.; Li, J.; Qin, Y.; Jarvis, J.; et al. The central nervous system (CNS)-independent anti-bone-resorptive activity of muscle contraction and the underlying molecular and cellular signatures. *J. Biol. Chem.* **2013**, *288*, 13511–13521. [CrossRef]
99. Zhao, W.; Peng, Y.; Hu, Y.; Guo, X.E.; Li, J.; Cao, J.; Pan, J.; Feng, J.Q.; Cardozo, C.; Jarvis, J.; et al. Electrical stimulation of hindlimb skeletal muscle has beneficial effects on sublesional bone in a rat model of spinal cord injury. *Bone* **2021**, *144*, 115825. [CrossRef]
100. Baunsgaard, C.B.; Nissen, U.V.; Brust, A.K.; Frotzler, A.; Ribeill, C.; Kalke, Y.B.; Leon, N.; Gomez, B.; Samuelsson, K.; Antepohl, W.; et al. Exoskeleton gait training after spinal cord injury: An exploratory study on secondary health conditions. *J. Rehabil. Med.* **2018**, *50*, 806–813. [CrossRef]
101. Juszczak, M.; Gallo, E.; Bushnik, T. Examining the Effects of a Powered Exoskeleton on Quality of Life and Secondary Impairments in People Living With Spinal Cord Injury. *Top. Spinal Cord. Inj. Rehabil.* **2018**, *24*, 336–342. [CrossRef] [PubMed]
102. Park, J.H.; Kim, H.S.; Jang, S.H.; Hyun, D.J.; Park, S.I.; Yoon, J.; Lim, H.; Kim, M.J. Cardiorespiratory Responses to 10 Weeks of Exoskeleton-Assisted Overground Walking Training in Chronic Nonambulatory Patients with Spinal Cord. Injury. *Sensors* **2021**, *21*, 5022. [CrossRef] [PubMed]

103. Asselin, P.; Cirnigliaro, C.M.; Kornfeld, S.; Knezevic, S.; Lackow, R.; Elliott, M.; Bauman, W.A.; Spungen, A.M. Effect of Exoskeletal-Assisted Walking on Soft Tissue Body Composition in Persons With Spinal Cord. Injury. *Arch. Phys. Med. Rehabil.* **2021**, *102*, 196–202. [CrossRef]
104. Xiang, X.N.; Zong, H.Y.; Ou, Y.; Yu, X.; Cheng, H.; Du, C.P.; He, H.C. Exoskeleton-assisted walking improves pulmonary function and walking parameters among individuals with spinal cord injury: A randomized controlled pilot study. *J. Neuroeng. Rehabil.* **2021**, *18*, 86. [CrossRef] [PubMed]
105. Needham-Shropshire, B.M.; Broton, J.G.; Klose, K.J.; Lebwohl, N.; Guest, R.S.; Jacobs, P.L. Evaluation of a training program for persons with SCI. paraplegia using the Parastep 1 ambulation system: Part 3. Lack of effect on bone mineral density. *Arch. Phys. Med. Rehabil.* **1997**, *78*, 799–803. [CrossRef]
106. Thoumie, P.; Le Claire, G.; Beillot, J.; Dassonville, J.; Chevalier, T.; Perrouin-Verbe, B.; Bedoiseau, M.; Busnel, M.; Cormerais, A.; Courtillon, A.; et al. Restoration of functional gait in paraplegic patients with the RGO-II hybrid orthosis. A multicenter controlled study. II: Physiological evaluation. *Paraplegia* **1995**, *33*, 654–659. [CrossRef] [PubMed]
107. Karelis, A.D.; Carvalho, L.P.; Castillo, M.J.; Gagnon, D.H.; Aubertin-Leheudre, M. Effect on body composition and bone mineral density of walking with a robotic exoskeleton in adults with chronic spinal cord injury. *J. Rehabil. Med.* **2017**, *49*, 84–87. [CrossRef] [PubMed]
108. Sheffler, L.R.; Chae, J. Neuromuscular electrical stimulation in neurorehabilitation. *Muscle Nerve* **2007**, *35*, 562–590. [CrossRef]
109. Feskanich, D.; Willett, W.; Colditz, G. Walking and leisure-time activity and risk of hip fracture in postmenopausal women. *JAMA* **2002**, *288*, 2300–2306. [CrossRef]
110. Frost, H.M. Bone "mass" and the "mechanostat": A proposal. *Anat. Rec.* **1987**, *219*, 1–9. [CrossRef]

Article

Evaluation of the Cardiometabolic Disorders after Spinal Cord Injury in Mice

Adel B. Ghnenis [1], Calvin Jones [1], Arthur Sefiani [1], Ashley J. Douthitt [1], Andrea J. Reyna [2], Joseph M. Rutkowski [2] and Cédric G. Geoffroy [1,*]

[1] Department of Neuroscience and Experimental Therapeutics, College of Medicine, Texas A&M Health Science Center, Bryan, TX 77807, USA; abghneni@med.umich.edu (A.B.G.); bonesjones64@tamu.edu (C.J.); sefiani@tamu.edu (A.S.); ashleydouthitt@tamu.edu (A.J.D.)
[2] Department of Medical Physiology, College of Medicine, Texas A&M Health Science Center, Bryan, TX 77807, USA; areyna94@tamu.edu (A.J.R.); rutkowski@tamu.edu (J.M.R.)
* Correspondence: geoffroy@tamu.edu; Tel.: +1-979-436-9023

Simple Summary: The present study demonstrates severity-dependent effects of a thoracic T8 injury on cardiometabolic dysfunctions in adult mice. While these chronic cardiometabolic issues can be multifactorial, the data indicate that systemic inflammatory response is likely to be involved. These findings are supportive of the role of systemic inflammation following SCI being critical in identifying therapeutic targets and predicting long-term outcomes.

Abstract: Changes in cardiometabolic functions contribute to increased morbidity and mortality after chronic spinal cord injury. Despite many advancements in discovering SCI-induced pathologies, the cardiometabolic risks and divergences in severity-related responses have yet to be elucidated. Here, we examined the effects of SCI severity on functional recovery and cardiometabolic functions following moderate (50 kdyn) and severe (75 kdyn) contusions in the thoracic-8 (T8) vertebrae in mice using imaging, morphometric, and molecular analyses. Both severities reduced hindlimbs motor functions, body weight (g), and total body fat (%) at all-time points up to 20 weeks post-injury (PI), while only severe SCI reduced the total body lean (%). Severe SCI increased liver echogenicity starting from 12 weeks PI, with an increase in liver fibrosis in both moderate and severe SCI. Severe SCI mice showed a significant reduction in left ventricular internal diameters and LV volume at 20 weeks PI, associated with increased LV ejection fraction as well as cardiac fibrosis. These cardiometabolic dysfunctions were accompanied by changes in the inflammation profile, varying with the severity of the injury, but not in the lipid profile nor cardiac or hepatic tyrosine hydroxylase innervation changes, suggesting that systemic inflammation may be involved in these SCI-induced health complications.

Keywords: spinal cord injury severity; cardiometabolic disease; liver and cardiac dysfunctions; fibrosis

1. Introduction

It is estimated that there are 245,000 to 353,000 persons suffering from SCI in the United States, with approximately 17,500 new cases each year [1]. These injured individuals are known to face lifelong locomotor disabilities, resulting from the injury to the central nervous system leading to neural cells loss, axon degeneration, and other cellular events at the injury site [2,3]. What is less known is that people living with SCI experience numerous detrimental medical complications that have great influence on their quality of life, including diabetes and cardiovascular disease [4,5]. Individuals with chronic SCI are prone to cardiometabolic disease [6–9]. In the general population, risk factors, such as metabolic syndrome (MS), obesity, glucose intolerance, hypertension, high blood triglycerides levels, and decreased high-density lipoprotein (HDL) [10,11], increase the prevalence of cardiovascular disease (CVD) [12,13]. In the general population, more than a third of US individuals suffer from MS [14,15]. MS symptoms are more prevalent in SCI patients than in the general population. In a recent study, it was estimated that more than 50% of SCI patients have symptoms of MS [16]. Increased lipid profile, an important biomarker for MS, induces insulin resistance, systemic inflammation, and oxidative stress [17]. The high prevalence of MS and decreased physical activity affect the balance between energy intake and energy expenditure and predispose these individuals to MS. In this regard, individuals suffering from SCI have reduced physical activity, systemic inflammation, and changes in the distribution pattern of adipose tissue in the body, which can all participate in the development of MS in these population [18,19].

SCI not only effects motor and sensory function within the central nervous system, but also disrupts the peripheral neural circuitry and signals to vital organs in the body, resulting in severe long-term complications outside of the central nervous system [4]. A large body of evidence indicates that SCI has major effects on body composition and metabolism [20–22], which can lead to a variety of risk factors including obesity [7,23,24], lower limbs skeletal muscle atrophy [25,26], decreased daily energy expenditure [13], changes in glucose-insulin homeostasis [21,22,27], and cardiovascular disease [28]. Assessment of body composition following SCI is critical to predict the development of cardiometabolic diseases, but is not commonly accessible in clinical evaluations [29,30]. Data from both humans and experimental animals indicate that in the early stages of SCI, body weight is decreased due to the reduction in lean body mass and fat depots [31,32]. These changes depend on the injury severity, level of injury, and duration of the injury [22,33].

The liver is a key organ regulating many metabolic processes in the body, and plays a vital role in body energy metabolism [34]. Under normal physiological conditions, digested food components such as glucose, amino acids, and fatty acids are transported to the liver. The liver metabolizes glucose into pyruvate for ATP production and produces the substrates required to synthesize fatty acids through lipogenesis. These fatty acids can be stored as lipid droplets and membrane structures in the hepatocytes or secreted into blood circulation. During starvation, liver gluconeogenesis induces glucose production and promotes lipolysis. These metabolic pathways are highly regulated through neuronal (the sympathetic and parasympathetic system) and hormonal (insulin and glucagon) pathways [35]. Therefore, liver dysfunction may lead to many complications including type 2 diabetes, insulin resistance, and nonalcoholic fatty liver diseases (NAFLD) [36]. Although SCI increases the prevalence of MS, only a few human studies have examined liver function following SCI. Using ultrasound imaging, Sipski et al. reported that approximately 80% of chronic SCI patients exhibited liver abnormality [37]. A recent study by Rankin et al. used magnetic resonance imaging (MRI) to demonstrate increased liver adiposity during chronic SCI which impacts the metabolic profile, highlighting the critical need to measure liver adiposity following SCI [38]. In a rat SCI model, Sauerbeck et al. reported hepatic changes including increased lipid infiltration and inflammation in the liver as early as 3 weeks PI [39]. The systemic inflammation and increased inflammatory cytokines in the liver following SCI may significantly induce liver dysfunction [40,41]. Understanding the progression of metabolic diseases could help identify points of intervention to increase the life expectancy and quality of life of individuals with SCI.

CVD is the leading cause of mortality among SCI individuals [42]. Depending on the severity and injury level, SCI may disrupt the innervation to the heart, causing cardiovascular autonomic dysfunction, leading to blood pressure and heart rate dysregulation [43–46]. In humans, patients with cervical and high-thoracic level injuries are more likely to develop CVD [47], probably due to the change in sympathetic nervous activity. For this reason, most of the data from experimental animals are focused on the SCI above the sixth thoracic vertebra (T6) [48]. This includes T5 complete transection in rats [49,50] and T3 moderate or severe contusion in rats [51,52] which can lead to significant changes in cardiovascular function. While thoracic and lumbar SCI represent 50% of the injuries and 40% the clinical studies which assessed the effects of low-thoracic/lumbar SCI on CVD in humans [47], the effects of low-thoracic/lumbar SCI in pre-clinical models have not been assessed. Additionally, very few studies have assessed the cardiovascular (and metabolic) dysfunctions at chronic time points in animal models. In the present study, we focused on evaluating the impact of thoracic-8 vertebrae (T8) SCI contusions on the cardiometabolic function following long term injury. The aim is to examine the changes in cardiometabolic functions following SCI without altering the sympathetic control of the heart at chronic time points in mice. Male mice received T8 contusions at two severity levels and were monitored by echocardiography, EchoMRI, GTT, body weight, behavior assessments of functional regeneration, and histological evaluation of the liver, heart, and spinal cord after 20 weeks. Results revealed new aspects of cardiometabolic alterations that occur after SCI, revealing the critical role that SCI severity plays on CVD.

2. Materials and Methods

2.1. Animal Care and Procedure for SCI

All experimental animal procedures were approved by the Texas A&M University Institutional Animal Use and Care Committee (IACUC). C57BL/6 mice were purchased from Taconic and bred in our vivarium. Six-month-old male mice were randomly assigned to one of three treatment groups: sham, moderate (50 kdyn), or severe (75 kdyn) SCI. Each cage housed up to 5 mice, which were housed in a climate-controlled facility in ventilated cages with a 12-h light/dark cycle. All mice were fed a control diet with ad libitum access to water. SCI was induced by contusion to the spinal cord as previously described [53]. Briefly, mice were anesthetized by 3% induction and maintained on 1.5% of isoflurane inhalation and the surgical site at thoracic T8 was shaved and sterilized by isopropyl alcohol. The surgical site was incised, and a partial dorsal laminectomy was performed at T8-9 to expose the spinal cord without penetrating the dura. SCI was induced using the NYU-MASCIS weight-drop impactor [54] at 50 kdyn for moderate and at 75 kdyn for severe SCI (2-sec dwell time). The back muscles were sutured, and the skin was closed with surgical glue. Sham mice received only a laminectomy identical to the other groups without a contusion. After surgery, all mice received saline solution and buprenorphine (0.05 mg/kg, Par Pharmaceutical Chestnut Ridge, Chestnut Ridge, NY, USA) daily for 3 days for hydration and pain, respectively, and penicillin (5 mg/kg/day, Bayer Healthcare LLC, Animal Health Division Shawnee Mission, Shawnee, KS, USA) once daily for 7 days to prevent secondary infection. Mice were monitored daily, with their bladder expressed manually twice every day until the mice were able to urinate without assistance or till the end of the experiment.

2.2. Behavioral Assessment

Motor functional recovery of hindlimbs was assessed by the Basso Mouse Scale (BMS) and rotarod tests. BMS test was performed as previously described [55,56]; mice were observed for 5 min by two observers blinded to injury type groups. Many features were noted, including ankle movements, stepping pattern, coordination, paw placement, trunk instability, and tail position, with a minimum score of 0 (no movement) to a maximum score of 9 (normal locomotion). Both observers agreed on each of the final scores for each mouse and the average score of all mice within a group is considered the final score for that group.

Rotarod testing was performed as previously described [55], with one individual blinded to injury type performed the test. Mice are placed on a rod (Ugo Basile, Gemonio, Germany) rotating at increasing speeds from 5 to 50 rpm in 3-min intervals with constant acceleration. The latency to fall (in seconds) was averaged between two trials per session. Mice are first acclimated to the test for two sessions for five days the week before injury, and one additional session one day before injury (baseline). Both BMS and rotarod tests were performed at baseline and then at day 3, 7, 14, 21, 28, and then every two weeks up to 140 days PI.

2.3. Body Composition Analysis

All mouse body compositions (fat tissue % and lean tissue %) were determined by an EchoMRI-100 quantitative magnetic resonance whole body composition analyzer (EchoMRI-100H, Echo Medical Systems, Houston, TX) as previously described [57]. Each mouse was weighed and scanned without anesthesia. Mice were scanned at baseline prior to injury and then at 4-, 8-, 12-, 16-, and 20-weeks PI. The body weight of each mouse was collected using a digital scale at 7, 14, 21, and 28 days and then monthly thereon until the end of the experiment.

2.4. Liver Ultrasound Image Acquisition and Analysis

Mice liver parenchyma was assessed for changes in structures before and after SCI using ultrasound imaging as described previously [58] with modifications as described below. Briefly, mice were anesthetized with 3% isoflurane and maintained with 1.5% isoflurane. Heart rate and temperature were monitored throughout the procedure. The abdominal cavity was shaved before applying Nair to remove the remaining hair. Ultrasound gel was then placed on the mouse's abdomen as a final step before the probe was applied to image the liver and kidney. The images were taken using a VisualSonics 3100 high frequency machine along with MX 550 D transducer probe. For consistency, two-dimensional B-mode images were acquired with the following acquisition settings (frequency = 40 MHz, frame rate = 165 fps, gain = 35 dB, depth = 15 mm, width = 14.08 mm, dynamic range = 60 dB). Images captured the entirety of both organs separately. After imaging, mice were allowed to recover in a cage and observed for signs of pain or discomfort. The echogenicity of the liver was examined and analyzed using ImageJ software as previously described [58] with modifications described below. Three regions of interest (ROI) plane were selected manually surrounding the portal vein excluding the hepatic vessels and imaging artifacts (area circle size 1 cm^2). The mean gray value of each of the three circles was calculated at three different areas for each ROI plane, averaged, and analyzed for each mouse. The same procedure was applied to the kidney images (around the cortex area), except for the circle area size of 0.5 cm^2, which was used as an internal control. The intensity of liver images was normalized to the kidney images for each mouse. Data are presented as a hepatic to renal (H/R) ratio.

2.5. Echocardiography Analysis

Mice were scanned with echocardiogram to assess cardiac structure and function at different time points as previously described [59]. Mice were imaged under anesthesia with isoflurane (induction at 3% and then maintained on 1.5%) with a heart rate of 400 to 500 beats per minutes. Chest hair was removed, and warm ultrasound transmission gel was applied. Parasternal short axis view of the heart with M-mode echocardiograph was acquired using VisualSonics 3100 high frequency machine along with MX 550 D transducer probe with 40 MHz center frequency. Parasternal long axis B-mode ultrasound was used as a reference image for the M-mode acquisition of the short axis. To ensure comparison between all measurements, focus was emphasized on the midventricular level of the heart, by identifying the papillary muscles. Left ventricle measurements were performed using the auto LV analysis tool by tracing the internal diameters of the ventricle, averaged from three consecutive cycles for each animal [59–63]. To limit noise caused by respiratory movements, images were acquired when the mice was not actively breathing, as assessed with the respiratory rate provided with the ultrasound system. The functional parameters and anatomical measurements of LV that were assessed include (left ventricle internal diameter (LVID), left ventricular (LV) mass, left ventricular posterior wall thickness (LVPW), left ventricular anterior wall thickness (LVAW), cardiac output (CO), stroke volume (SV), ejection fraction (EF), and fractional shortening (FS) as previously described [59–61].

2.6. Glucose Metabolism

Intraperitoneal glucose tolerance test (IPGTT) was performed before SCI surgery and at 14 weeks and 20 weeks PI as previously described [59]. Briefly, after mice fasted for 16 h, a baseline fasting blood glucose level was recorded before each mouse received intraperitoneal administration of 20% (2 g/kg) glucose solution (Sigma, Kawasaki, Japan). Blood glucose levels were recorded 15, 30, 60, and 90 min after administration. Blood glucose levels were quantified using a glucose meter (Bayer Contour Next EZ blood glucose meter, Bayer HealthCare, IN, USA) by taking a blood sample (<5 µL) from a small incision made at the tip of the tail using clean surgical scissors. Area under the curve (AUC) for blood glucose levels in each mouse during IPGTT was calculated using GraphPad Prism (Prism 9.0, GraphPad Software, San Diego, CA, USA).

2.7. Triglyceride, Cholesterol, and Insulin Analysis

Liver samples were analyzed for triglyceride content and concentration. Liver medial lobe samples were collected fresh from each mouse right before perfusion. Samples were then immediately flash frozen using liquid nitrogen and stored at $-80\ ^\circ$C until testing. Approximately 0.25 g of liver tissue were homogenized in 2:1 chloroform methanol, mixed with 1 mol/L $CaCl_2$, and centrifuged for 15 min at 13,000 rpm at 4 $^\circ$C as previously described [64]. Then, 400 µL of the lower lipid phase was removed and placed in a fume hood to allow for evaporation. Once evaporated, the samples were reconstituted in isopropanol and directly analyzed using Infinity^{TM} Triglycerides Liquid Stable Reagent (Cat. No. TR22421, ThermoFisher Scientific, Waltham, MA, USA) according to the manufacturer's instructions. The resulting assay values were then normalized to the liver tissue mass to produce absorbed triglyceride content (µg/mg).

Plasma samples were analyzed for triglyceride content, cholesterol, and insulin concentrations. Blood samples were collected from the submandibular vein at 18 weeks post SCI and centrifuged at 14,000 rpm for 15 min at 4 $^\circ$C to separate the plasma. Plasma triglyceride concentrations (mg/dL) were analyzed using Infinity^{TM} Triglycerides Liquid Stable Reagent according to the manufacturer's instructions. Free cholesterol concentration (µM) was determined using Invitogen^{TM} Amplex® Red Cholesterol Assay Kit (Cat. No. A12216, ThermoFisher Scientific) per the manufacturer's instructions. Lastly, plasma insulin concentrations (ng/mL) were assessed using Ultra-Sensitive Mouse Insulin ELISA Kit (Cat. No. 90080, Crystal Chem, Elk Grove Village, IL, USA) according to the manufacturer's instructions.

2.8. Histological Analysis of Heart and Liver Tissues

Mice were perfused. Heart and liver tissues were removed and fixed in 4% paraformaldehyde (PFA) in 1× PBS for 24 h before incubating in 15% then 30% sucrose solution for 24 h each. Heart samples were then cut in the middle across the transverse plane. The lower parts of the hearts (containing the apex) were embedded. Left lobe liver sections were embedded such that the tissue closest to the portal triad would be sectioned. Both heart and liver tissues were placed in OCT compound (Cat. No. 625501-01, Sakura Finetek, Torrance, CA, USA, Inc., Torrance, CA, USA) for embedding. Heart cross sections from the middle point of the heart and left lobe of liver transverse sections were cut at 8 µm thickness with 50 µm between each section using a cryostat (Leica Biosystems CM3050 S). Sections were stained with Masson's trichrome staining (Sigma-Aldrich, HT15-1KT) according to the manufacturer's instructions to examine perivascular accumulation of collagen in the tissue. Analysis and quantification of fibrotic areas were performed as previously described [65] where 3–4 sections per tissue were imaged at 20× on a Zeiss Axio Observer 7 fluorescent microscope. Quantification of the left ventricle and liver sections was performed using ImageJ software (NIH, Bethesda, MD, USA). Briefly, the total area for each image was computed and the color-based threshold tool was used to highlight the fibrotic (blue) regions of tissue in each image. To ensure standardization, the hues were set at 130 and 190 for each fibrotic image.

LV thickness was measured using Zen Lite software. For each mouse, 3–4 representative heart sections were chosen. For each section, the LVAW and LVPW thickness was measured by drawing three lines spanning the entire wall thickness and then averaging the length of three drawn lines. The precise locations of these lines were chosen to measure the thickness at the best tissue structural integrity (i.e., no tears resulting from mounting) and avoiding the regions surrounding the papillary muscles.

2.9. Tyrosine Hydroxylase (TH) Immunofluorescence Staining of the Heart and Liver

To assess if the T8 contusion SCI affected innervation of the heart and liver, both heart and liver sections were stained for Tyrosine Hydroxylase (TH). Three consecutive transverse heart and left lobe liver sections from each mouse were cut at 10 µm thickness and directly mounted onto Superfrost® Plus MicroSlides (Cat. No. 48311-703, VWR, Radnor, PA, USA). Sections were washed 3 times using 1× PBS and blocked for 1 h using 5% normal horse serum diluted in 0.4% Triton X-100 in 1× PBS. Sections were incubated overnight at room temperature in TH antibody (1:500, Cat. No. AB152, Millipore Sigma, Burlington, MA, USA) diluted with 2% normal horse serum in 0.4% Triton X-100 in 1× PBS. After washing, secondary antibody Alexa Fluor Plus 488 (1:500, Cat. No. A32814, ThermoFisher Scientific) diluted with 2% normal horse serum in 0.4% Triton X-100 in 1× PBS was applied to the sections for 2 h at room temperature. Sections were then incubated in DAPI (1:2000, Cat. No. 62248, ThermoFisher Scientific) and washed 3 times using 1× PBS and cover slipped for examination under the microscope. Images were taken at 20× magnification on a Zeiss Axio Observer 7 fluorescent microscope. Each image was acquired as a z-stack and the maximum projection was used for quantification. For heart sections, 3 images for each region of the LV anterior wall (LVAW), LV posterior wall (LVPW), and LV lateral wall were quantified for TH staining using Quantitative Pathology and Bioimage Analysis software (QuPath v0.3.0, Scotland). In brief, pixel classifiers were programmed to distinguish between positive, negative, and background staining. Total positive and negative areas (μm^2) were generated and the ratio of the two provided a percentage of TH positive staining within each section. For each mouse, an average TH positive staining was calculated by averaging the percent positive of the LVAW, LVPW, and lateral wall portions for all three heart sections. The average percent positive for the three sections was then averaged to produce the final TH percent positive value for each mouse.

Quantification of TH staining within the liver sections was done using QuPath v0.3.0. Three liver sections were quantified per animal. For each liver section, 3 vessels between 100 µm and 200 µm were chosen for a complete and accurate analysis. A brush tracer tool with a standardized diameter of 26 µm was used to create an annotation around the outer edge of the vasculature. The border region was then filled in to include the entire vessel within the annotation. For each liver section, an average TH positive staining percentage was calculated from the analysis of the three annotated vessels. An average TH positive staining was calculated by averaging the percent positive for all three vessels per sections, followed by averaging the percent positive for the three liver sections to produce the final TH percent positive value for each mouse.

2.10. Histological Analysis of SC Injury

To examine the degree of injury caused by the impactor, spinal cords were harvested from contused mice at 20 weeks PI. Mice were anesthetized with intraperitoneal injection of 100 µL of Sodium pentobarbital (Fatal-Plus®) before being euthanized via perfusion with 4% paraformaldehyde (PFA) in 1x phosphate buffer solution (PBS) (Cat. No. 14200075, Life Technologies, Carlsbad, CA, USA). Samples were soaked in 15% and 30% sucrose overnight prior to embedding in OCT compound (Cat. No. 625501-01, Sakura Finetek USA, Inc., Torrance, CA, USA), followed by longitudinal sectioning at a thickness of 25 µm using a cryostat (Leica Biosystems CM3050 S). Fixed sections of spinal cord tissue were washed (3× with 0.4% Triton X-100 in 1x PBS), then blocked using 5% normal horse serum (VWR 102643-676, diluted in 0.4% Triton X-100 in 1× PBS) for 1 hour. Sections were incubated with primary anti-glial fibrillary acidic protein (GFAP) antibody (1:500, Cat. No. 13-0300, ThermoFisher Scientific) diluted in 0.4% Triton X-100 in 1× PBS and incubated at 25 °C overnight. The sections were then washed before being incubated with Alexa Fluor Plus 488 secondary antibody (1:1000, Cat. No. A32814, ThermoFisher Scientific) in 0.4% Triton X-100 in 1× PBS for 1 hour and DAPI (1 µg/mL, Cat. No. 62248, ThermoFisher Scientific) for 5 min. After being washed once more, the slices were mounted, and cover slipped (Cat. No. F6182, Sigma) before being imaged at 20× on a Zeiss Axio Observer 7 fluorescent microscope. The contour (polygonal) tool in the Zen 3.2 (Carl Zeiss AG, Jena, Germany) software was used to trace and measure lesion and cavity size. The lesion size was measured by tracing the glial scar border labeled with GFAP surrounding a DAPI+ inner region. Cavity size was measured by measuring the region within the spinal cord without any visible nuclei yet surrounded by GFAP labeled glial scar. Three spinal cord sections per animal were imaged and analyzed.

2.11. Blood Cytokines Measurements

Plasma concentrations of IFN-γ, IL-10, IL-17A/CTLA8, IL-6, TNF-α, and IL-1β were measured using MILLIPLEX® Mouse Cytokine/Chemokine Magnetic Bead Panel (MCYTOMAG-70K-Millipore Sigma, Burlington, MA) according to the manufacturer's instructions. Briefly, approximately 100 µL of blood samples were collected from the submandibular facial vein using a sterile lancet in BD Microtainer® blood collection tubes (cat# BD 365985). Blood samples were collected before SCI surgery and immediately prior to necropsy. Samples were centrifuged at 15,000× g for 15 min to separate the plasma. Plasma samples were stored at −80 °C until the assay was conducted. Plasma samples were diluted 2-fold in Assay Buffer provided in the kit per the manufacturer's recommendation. Samples, quality controls, and standards were aliquoted into the provided 96-well plate in duplicate followed by the antibody-immobilized beads. After a 16-h incubation at 4 °C and respective wash steps, detection antibodies and Streptavidin-Phycoerythrin were added. Washing was conducted using a hand-held magnet. After the completion of the protocol, the plate was analyzed using a Luminex® 200™ (cat# LX200-XPON3.1) multiplex analyzer with the xPONENT 3.1 software. The data represent the average mean fluorescent intensity values from the duplicates. The values at the chronic 5-month timepoint were divided by the baseline values to determine the "fold change from baseline" value plotted.

2.12. Statistical Analysis

Two-way ANOVA test was followed by Tukey's multiple comparison post hoc analysis to assess the differences between the groups. All analyses were performed using GraphPad Prism (Prism 9.0, GraphPad Software, San Diego, CA, USA). Differences were considered significant at $p \leq 0.05$, tendencies at $p \leq 0.10$. Data are presented as means ± SEM.

3. Results

3.1. Experimental Design and Data Collection

To examine the impact of SCI severity after T8 contusion on the cardiometabolic functions, six month old male mice (corresponding to ~25 years old in humans, when the first peak of SCI is observed [66]) were randomly sorted into sham, moderate SCI (50 kdyn), or severe SCI (75 kdyn) groups. There was n = 6 for sham, n = 8 for moderate SCI, and n = 9 for severe SCI at the beginning of the experiment. Mice were tested for parameters of body weight, EchoMRI, echocardiography and liver ultrasound imaging, IPGTT, and BMS and Rotarod scores as described in the experimental shown in Figure 1 and Table 1.

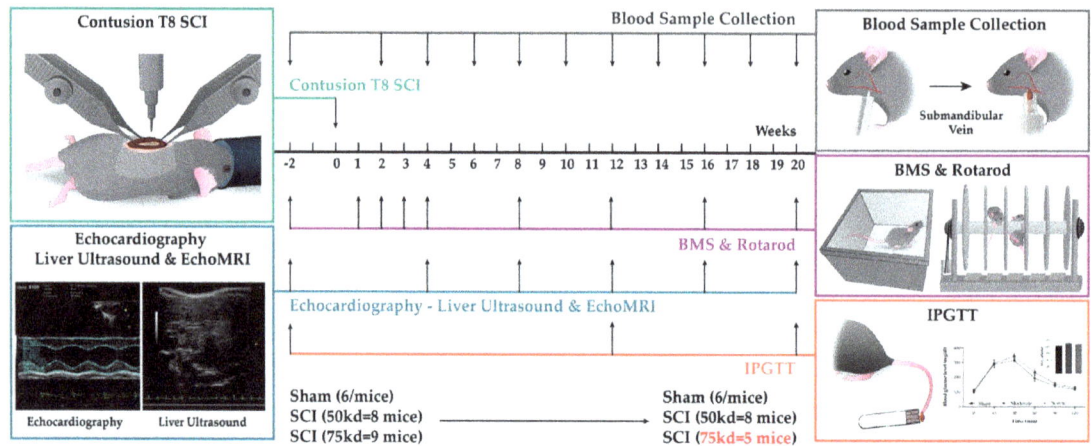

Figure 1. Schematic diagram of the experimental design. Six-month-old male mice were used to measure a baseline for Echo MRI, echocardiography (Echo), liver ultrasound, intraperitoneal glucose tolerance test (IPGTT), and body weight (BW). At day 0, T8 contusion SCI was induced, and the same measurements were performed at 4-, 8-, 12-, 16-, and 20-weeks post-injury. IPGTT was performed only at the 12 and 20-week time point. Blood plasma was collected twice monthly. For behavioral assessments, BMS and rotarod tests were performed pre-injury and again at days 2 then week 1, 2, 3, 4, 6, 8, 10, 12, 14, 16, 18, and 20 post-injury. At week 20 post-SCI, animals were sacrificed, blood plasma was collected, and tissues (hearts, livers, and spinal cords) were harvested for histological analyses.

Table 1. Summary of number of treatment groups; the experiments were performed up to 20 weeks post SCI.

	Number of Mice			Set of Experiments				
Mice Group	Sham	50 kd	75 kd	BMS & Rotarod	Echocardiography & Liver Ultrasound	EchoMRI	Blood Samples	IPGTT
Pre SCI	6	8	9	+	+	+	+	+
W1	6	8	9	+	-	-	-	-
W2	6	8	9	+	-	-	+	-
W3	6	8	9	+	-	-	-	-
W4	6	8	9	+	+	+	+	+
W5	6	8	9	-	-	-	-	-
W6	6	8	9	-	-	-	+	-
W7	6	8	9	-	-	-	-	-
W8	6	8	8	+	+	+	+	+
W9	6	8	8	-	-	-	-	-
W10	6	8	6	-	-	-	+	-
W11	6	8	6	-	-	-	-	-
W12	6	8	6	+	+	+	+	+
W13	6	8	6	-	-	-	-	-
W14	6	8	6	-	-	-	+	-
W15	6	8	6	-	-	-	-	-
W16	6	8	6	+	+	+	+	+
W17	6	8	6	-	-	-	-	-
W18	6	8	5	-	-	-	+	-
W19	6	8	5	-	-	-	-	-
W20	6	8	5	+	+	+	+	+

+: Yes, -: No.

3.2. Sustained Reduction of Motor Function after Chronic SCI

Motor functional recovery was assessed following SCI by BMS and Rotarod at multiple timepoints. BMS scores are shown in Figure 2A. Sham mice were not affected by the sham surgical procedure without contusion. For mice that received moderate SCI, the BMS scores dropped to 1.06 ± 0.32 at day 2 after SCI and gradually recovered up to a score of 3.25 ± 0.55 at the end time point (20 weeks). For mice that received severe SCI, BMS scores dropped near to 0.55 ± 0.43 at day 2 after SCI and gradually recovered up to a score of 2.6 ± 1.05 at the end time point. Interestingly, some differences emerged between moderate and severe SCI mice, where severely injured mice showed a significantly decreased recovery timeline compared to moderately injured mice. Rotarod assessment was also performed to determine the extent of hindlimb function on mice (Figure 2B). Mice from both injuries exhibited a significant decrease on time on the rotarod after SCI compared to sham controls. No significant differences were observed between severe and moderate injured mice. There was significant attrition in SCI severe group. Indeed, while all the sham and moderately injured mice survived the 20 weeks timepoint, 45% of the severely injured mice died prior to the study endpoint of 20 weeks (only 5/9 survived, Figure 2C).

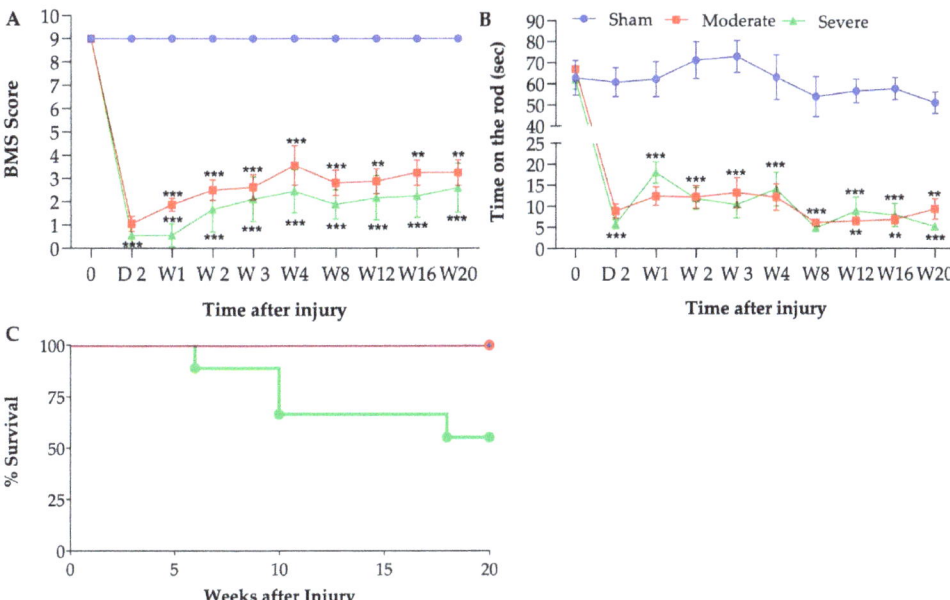

Figure 2. Behavioral testing after SCI. BMS scores (**A**), Rotarod score (**B**). Behavioral tests performed at baseline before injury and on days 2, 7, 14, 21, 28, and then monthly PI. (**C**) Percent survival during the experiment. Repeated measures two-way ANOVA: Tukey's multiple comparisons test was used to determine the differences between the groups. Data presented as means $\pm$ SEM, n = 5–9 per group. * $p \leq 0.03$, ** $p \leq 0.002$, *** $p \leq 0.001$.

3.3. Severity-Dependent Reduction of Body Weight and Body Composition

As expected, both moderate and severe groups lost weight within the first week post SCI (Figure 3A). While this loss stabilized in the moderate group, the weight dropped further by week 2 in the severely injured group. Both groups slowly regained some weight over the 20-week period, without reaching their baseline levels. Both groups were significantly lower than the sham group. While not statistically different, the moderate group tend to recover weight better than the severe group. Fat and lean body composition were measured using EchoMRI. By 4 weeks PI, the percentages of body fat and body lean were significantly reduced in the severe group compared to the sham group (Figure 3B,C). Similarly, the moderate group presented a significantly reduced percentage of body fat compared to sham (Figure 3B), while the percentage of lean body mass was also reduced without reaching statistical difference (Figure 3C).

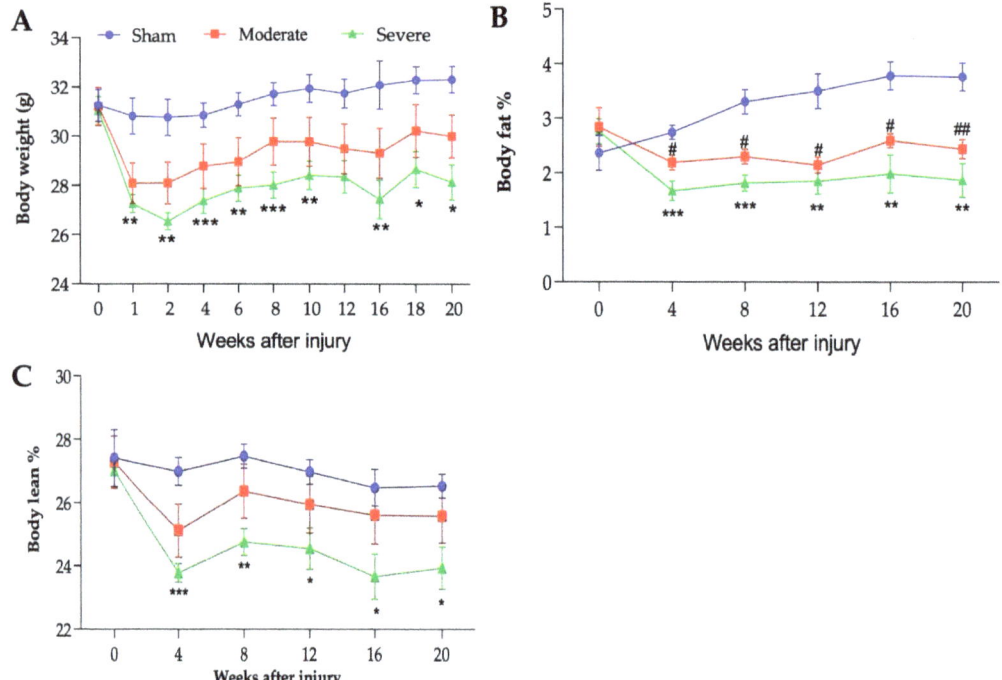

Figure 3. Injury-severity dependent body composition changes. (A) Body weight (g), (B) percentage of body fat, and (C) percentage of lean body mass. Statistical analysis was performed using repeated measures two-way ANOVA; Tukey's multiple comparisons test was used to determine the differences between the groups. Data presented as mean ± SEM, n = 6 (sham), 8 (moderate), and 5–9 (severe). * $p \leq 0.03$, ** $p \leq 0.002$, *** $p \leq 0.001$ difference between sham and severe groups and # $p \leq 0.03$, ## $p \leq 0.002$ difference between sham and moderate groups.

3.4. Severe SCI Induced Stronger Liver Pathology

Liver ultrasound analysis was performed prior to SCI and at 4-, 8-, 12-, 16-, and 20-weeks PI to examine the liver shape and structure (Figure 4A). By 12 weeks PI, the severe group tended to be increased in the liver echogenicity, although not reaching statistical levels compared to the sham and moderate injured groups (Figure 4B). Histological analysis of the liver at 20 weeks exhibited a significant increase in fibrotic tissues in severely injured mice and a non-significant upward increase in moderate group, compared to the sham animals (Figure 4C,D).

3.5. Severe SCI Induced Cardiac Dysfunction

Echocardiography was performed to assess cardiac structure and function following SCI. In the severe SCI group, LVID during systole (LVID;s) was reduced at 16 weeks PI and reached statistical significance at 20 weeks PI (Figure 5A). No significant reduction in LVID during diastole (LVID;d) was observed (Figure 5B). The reduction of LVID;s was associated with the reduction in LV volume (Figure 5C) and no significant difference in LV volume was observed in LVID;d (Figure 5D). Interestingly, both ejection fractioning

(EF) and fractional shortening (FS) trended upward at 16 weeks and significantly increased at 20 weeks PI in the severely injured group compared to the sham and moderate group (Figure 5E,F, respectively). Masson's trichrome staining of the left ventricular sections showed significant change in collagen accumulation in severe SCI and an upward trend in the moderate group compared to their sham controls (Figure 6A,B). While there were no significant differences in other cardiac parameters such as LV mass, SV, CO, HR, and LVPW and LVAW thickness using echocardiography scanning (Table 2), histological analysis of the LVPW and LVAW thicknesses revealed a significant increase in LVPW and LVAW thickness compared to moderate and sham groups, respectively (Figure 6C).

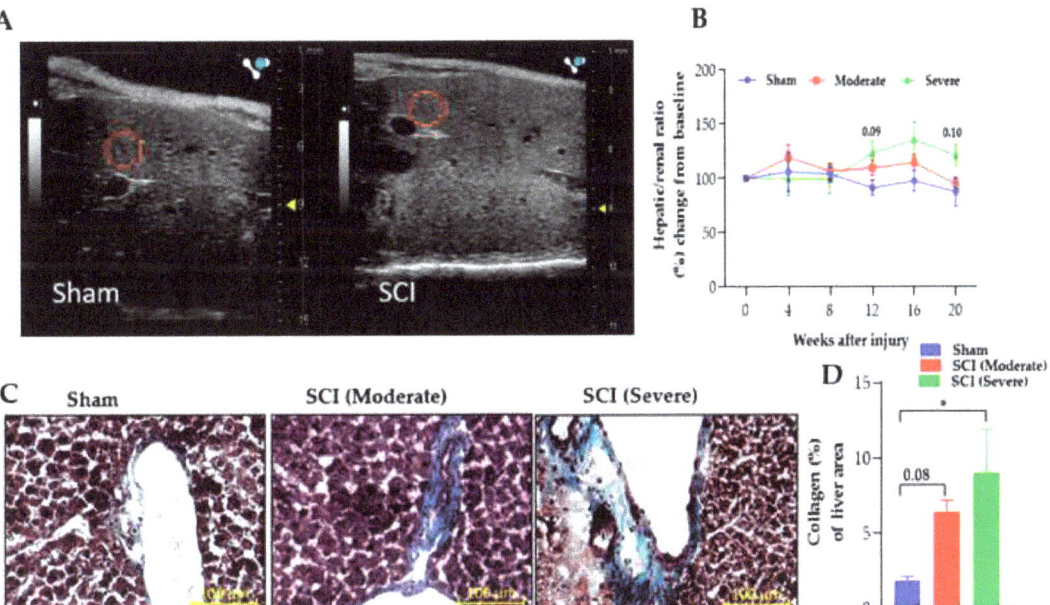

Figure 4. **Injury-severity dependent reduction in liver function**. SCI induced liver intensity and fibrosis. (**A**) Representative images of liver show echogenicity of the liver parenchyma increased in the severe group compared to sham group using ultrasound imaging at 20 weeks PI of sham and severe SCI. Red circles located on the liver images represent areas of interest that were quantified. (**B**) Severe SCI increased liver intensity after 12 weeks PI compared to sham group. Kidney tissue was used as the internal control with data represented as a ratio of hepatic/renal percent change from baseline measurements. (**C**) Representative liver sections stained with Masson's trichrome of sham, moderate-SCI, and severe-SCI at 20 weeks PI. (**D**) Quantification of collagen contents (blue) in the liver. SCI significantly increased fibrotic tissue in severe injured group and there is a trend towards an increase in the moderate group compared to the sham control. Scale bar = 100μm. Values presented as mean ± S.E.M of 3–4 sections/mouse; n = 6 (sham), 8 (moderate), and 5–9 (severe). Data analyzed by two-way ANOVA. Tukey's multiple comparisons test was used to determine the differences between the groups; one-way ANOVA for D. * $p \leq 0.03$, ** $p \leq 0.002$, *** $p \leq 0.001$.

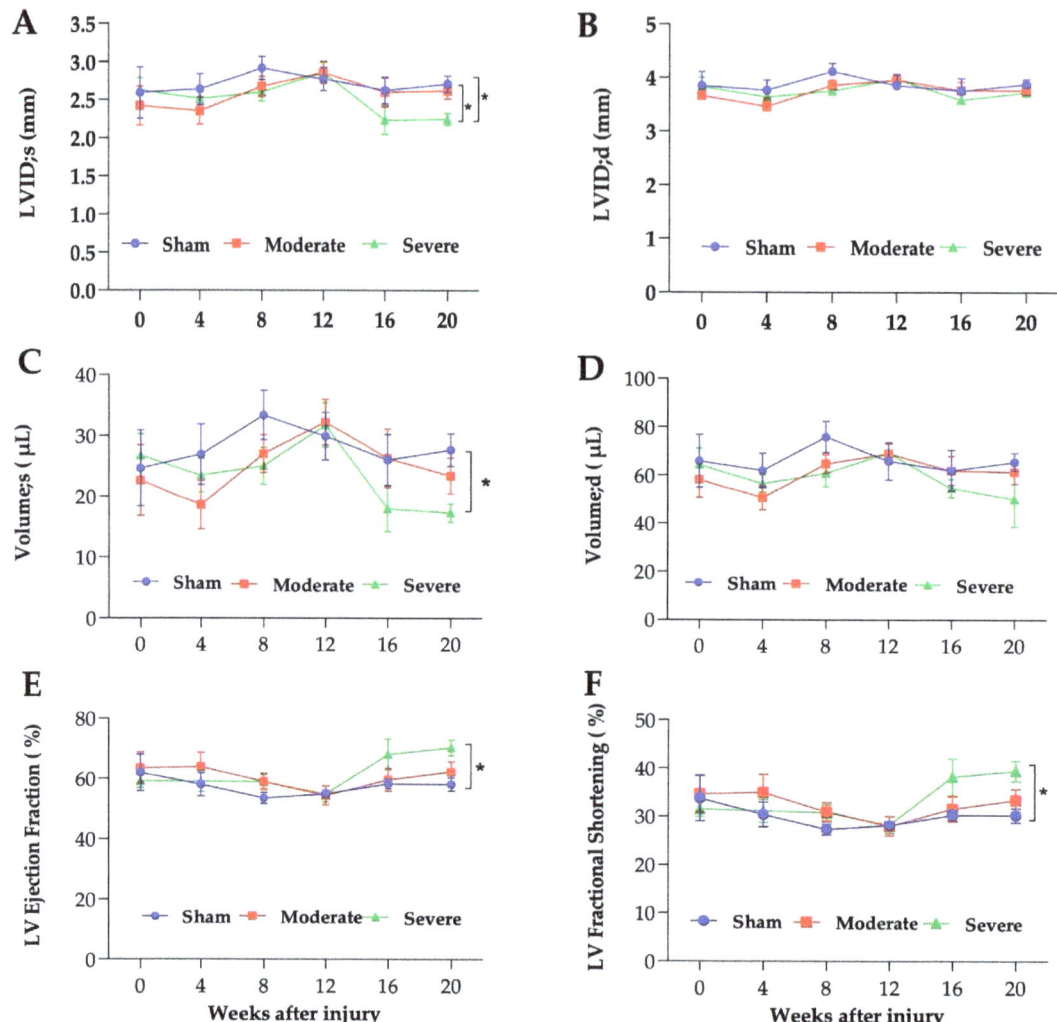

Figure 5. *Injury-severity dependent development of cardiac dysfunction*. Echocardiography assessment. (**A**) Left ventricular internal diameter during systole (LVID;s) and (**B**) during diastole (LVID;d). (**C**) LV volume during systole and (**D**) LV volume during diastole. (**E**) Ejection fraction (EF) and (**F**) fractional shortening (FS). n = 6 (sham), 8 (moderate), and 5–9 (severe). Data analyzed by two-way ANOVA. Tukey's multiple comparisons test was used to determine the differences between the groups. Data presented as mean ± SEM, * $p \leq 0.03$, ** $p \leq 0.002$, *** $p \leq 0.001$.

3.6. No Changes in Glucose or Lipids Metabolism after Chronic SCI in Mice

Using IPGTT, we did not observe any significant changes in glucose metabolism up to 20 weeks PI. This is consistent with previous reports which state that SCI induces slight change in serum glucose at 23 days PI [67]. IPGTTs were performed prior to injury, then at 14- and 20-weeks PI. Results showed that the glucose concentrations and area under the curve (AUC) were similar between the groups pre-injury (Figure 7A). No significant differences were observed in glucose concentration and AUC at 14- and 20-weeks PI between any of the groups (Figure 7B,C). Fasting glucose concentrations were also similar between all groups up to 20 weeks PI (Figure 7D).

Table 2. Parameters of echocardiography results of sham, moderate, and severe SCI at different time points. Data are means ± S.E.M; n = 5–9 per group. Parameters of cardiac structure and function in mice before SCI and at 4-, 8-, 12-, 16-, and 20-weeks post-SCI of sham, moderate (50-kdyn), and severe (75-kdyn) mice. HR, heart rate; SV, stroke volume; CO, cardiac output; LV Mass, left ventricular mass; LVAW;s, LV anterior wall thickness at the end of systole; LVAW;d, LV anterior wall thickness at the end of diastole; LVPW;s, LV posterior wall thickness at the end of systole; LVPW;d, LV posterior wall thickness at the end of diastole; LVID;d, LV anterior diameter at the end of diastole.

Parameters Time	Surgery	HR (BPM)	SV (µL)	CO (mL/min)	LV Mass (mg)	LVAW;s (mm)	LVAW;d (mm)	LVPW;s (mm)	LVPW;d (mm)
Baseline	Sham	494 ± 31.8	38.6 ± 3.1	18.8 ± 1.2	128 ± 13.2	1.5 ± 0.1	1.0 ± 0.1	1.4 ± 0.1	1.1 ± 0.1
	Moderate	449 ± 14.7	35.5 ± 2.8	15.8 ± 1.1	134 ± 16.6	1.4 ± 0.1	0.9 ± 0.5	1.7 ± 0.1	1.3 ± 0.2
	Severe	447 ± 15.2	38.1 ± 3.2	17.1 ± 1.6	117 ± 4.8	1.3 ± 0.0	0.94 ± 0.0	1.4 ± 0.1	1.0 ± 0.1
4 weeks	Sham	493 ± 21.8	35 ± 3.2	17.1 ± 1.3	119.4 ± 5.5	1.3 ± 0.1	0.94 ± 0.0	1.46 ± 0.1	1.1 ± 0.1
	Moderate	482 ± 12.5	32 ± 3.3	15.5 ± 1.7	121 ± 10.2	1.4 ± 0.1	0.97 ± 0.0	1.6 ± 0.1	1.2 ± 0.1
	Severe	497 ± 12.4	32.9 ± 2.1	16.4 ± 1.3	134 ± 17.8	1.45 ± 0.1	1.1 ± 0.1	1.56 ± 0.1	1.1 ± 0.1
8 weeks	Sham	451 ± 21.1	40.2 ± 2.8	17.9 ± 0.7	103.3 ± 5.9	1.25 ± 0.1	0.9 ± 0.01	1.1 ± 0.0	0.8 ± 0.0
	Moderate	478 ± 20.1	37.7 ± 1.1	17.9 ± 0.6	119.2 ± 12.1	1.5 ± 0.1	1.0 ± 0.1	1.3 ± 0.1	0.87 ± 0.1
	Severe	472 ± 16.2	35.8 ± 3.2	16.9 ± 1.7	113.3 ± 18.8	1.4 ± 0.1	0.9 ± 0.0	1.4 ± 0.1	0.98 ± 0.1
12 weeks	Sham	498 ± 16.3	36 ± 3.9	17.8 ± 1.8	143 ± 16.6	1.4 ± 0.1	1.0 ± 0.1	1.5 ± 0.1	1.16 ± 0.2
	Moderate	492 ± 17.7	36.7 ± 1.5	18 ± 1.0	110.4 ± 7.5	1.3 ± 0.5	0.9 ± 0.0	1.2 ± 0.1	0.89 ± 0.1
	Severe	519 ± 15.7	37..5 ± 0.5	19.4 ± 0.5	110.6 ± 7.6	1.3 ± 0.1	0.9 ± 0.0	1.25 ± 0.1	0.89 ± 0.1
16 weeks	Sham	501 ± 24.7	35.9 ± 4.5	17.9 ± 2.3	118.7 ± 9.1	1.3 ± 0.1	0.9 ± 0.0	1.5 ± 0.1	1.1 ± 0.1
	Moderate	476 ± 17.5	35.6 ± 2.0	16.9 ± 1.1	116.2 ± 7.8	1.4 ± 0.1	1.0 ± 0.1	1.3 ± 0.0	0.96 ± 0.0
	Severe	503 ± 3.5	36.5 ± 2.6	18.4 ± 1.3	131.6 ± 20.4	1.4 ± 0.1	0.96 ± 0.0	1.8 ± 0.2	1.2 ± 0.2
20 weeks	Sham	449 ± 10	37.8 ± 1.7	17 ± 0.8	142.4 ± 22.2	1.5 ± 0.0	1.1 ± 0.1	1.4 ± 0.1	1.1 ± 0.2
	Moderate	480 ± 6.7	37.9 ± 3.3	18.1 ± 1.4	119.3 ± 6.9	1.5 ± 0.1	1.0 ± 0.0	1.4 ± 0.1	1.0 ± 0.1
	Severe	477 ± 17.5	42.6 ± 5.8	20 ± 2.4	119.6 ± 5.9	1.5 ± 0.1	1.0 ± 0.0	1.5 ± 0.1	1.0 ± 0.1

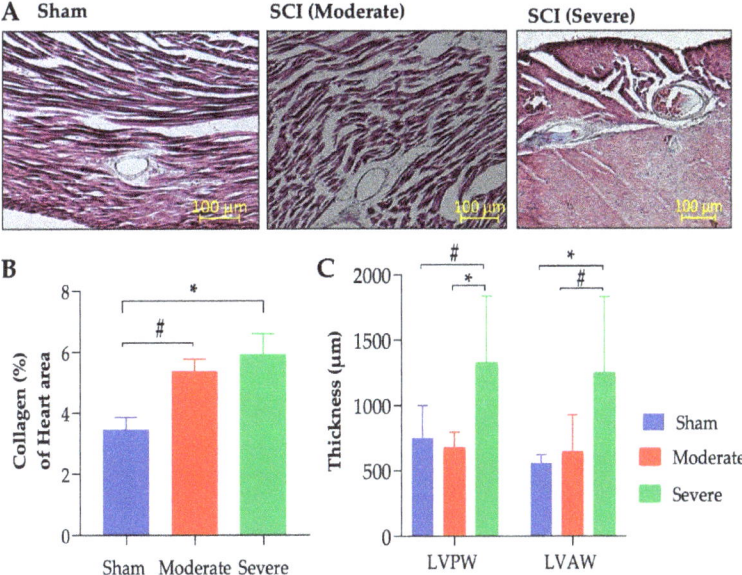

Figure 6. Injury-severity dependent increase in cardiac remodeling. (**A**) Representative 40× sections of Masson's trichrome of sham, moderate-SCI, and severe-SCI after 20 weeks PI. (**B**) Quantification

of collagen contents (blue) in the LV tissue. SCI significantly increased fibrotic tissue in the severe injured group and there is a trend to increase in the moderate group compared to the sham control. (**C**). LVPW and LVAW thickness. Scale bar = 100 µm. Values presented as mean ± S.E.M of 3–4 sections/mouse; n = 6 (sham), 8 (moderate), and 5–9 (severe). Data analyzed by ANOVA. * $p < 0.05$ and # $p < 0.1$.

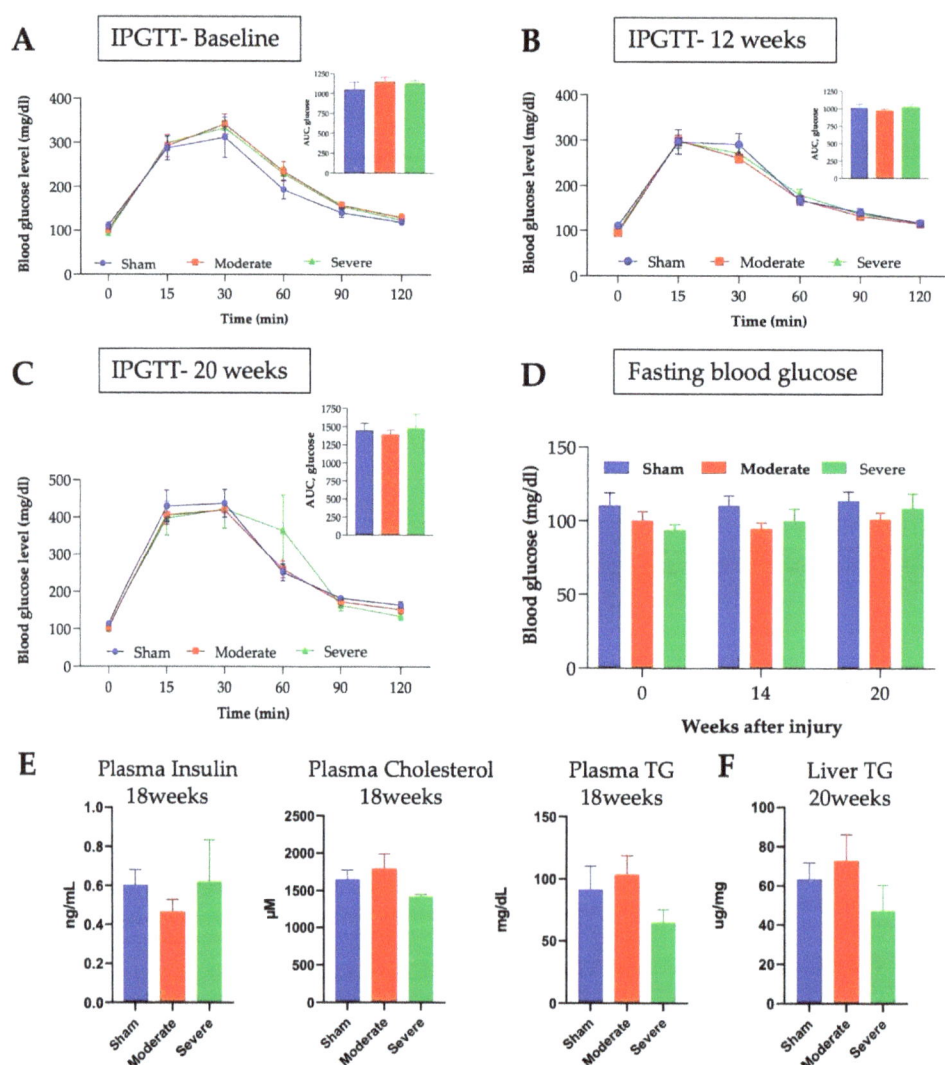

Figure 7. No changes in glucose metabolism after SCI regardless of the injury severity. IPGTT was performed pre-injury (**A**), at 12 weeks (**B**), and at 20 weeks PI (**C**). (**D**) Fasting blood glucose concentrations at different time points. No differences are observed for any of these measures. Plasma insulin, cholesterol, and triglyceride levels (**E**) were tested at 18 weeks PI. Liver triglyceride content (**F**) was assessed after euthanasia at 20 weeks PI. Values presented as mean ± S.E.M. N = 6 (sham), 8 (moderate), and 5–9 (severe). Data analyzed by two-way ANOVA or one-way ANOVA (**D–F**). * $p < 0.05$.

Complementary to the lack of a significant difference in glucose metabolism, no significant changes in plasma insulin levels between the sham, moderate, or severe SCI models were found at 18 weeks PI (Figure 7E). The 18 weeks PI results show that there was also no significant difference in plasma cholesterol concentrations (Figure 7E). Although there was no statistically significant change in triglyceride levels both in the plasma (Figure 7E) and the liver (Figure 7F), there was a trend of decrease in the severely injured model ($p = 0.13$ between moderate and severe SCI for plasma TG levels). A decrease in triglyceride levels coincided with our EchoMRI findings showing a much lower compositional fat % in severely injured mice. Of note, no difference in temperature was observed at 20 weeks in between the groups (not shown).

3.7. Severe SCI Induced Changes in SC Injury

The lesion and cavity size at the spinal cord injury sites were analyzed to compare the size of the injury following different severities (Figure 8A,B). There is an upward trend in the lesion size $p = 0.06$ (Figure 8C) and cavity size $p = 0.2$ (Figure 8D) and a significant increase in total injury size $p = 0.02$ with increasing severity. The severe group is 40% more likely to have a cavity at the injury site relative to the moderate group. There is a significant negative correlation between total injury size and BMS score $p = 0.04$ (Figure 8E) and a non-significant negative correlation between total injury size and Rotarod performance $p = 0.06$ (Figure 8F). Interestingly, we observed a trend for a positive correlation between total injury size and LVAW;s, not reaching statistical difference $p = 0.09$ (Figure 8G), but suggesting that mice with the most severe injuries might develop more cardiac dysfunctions.

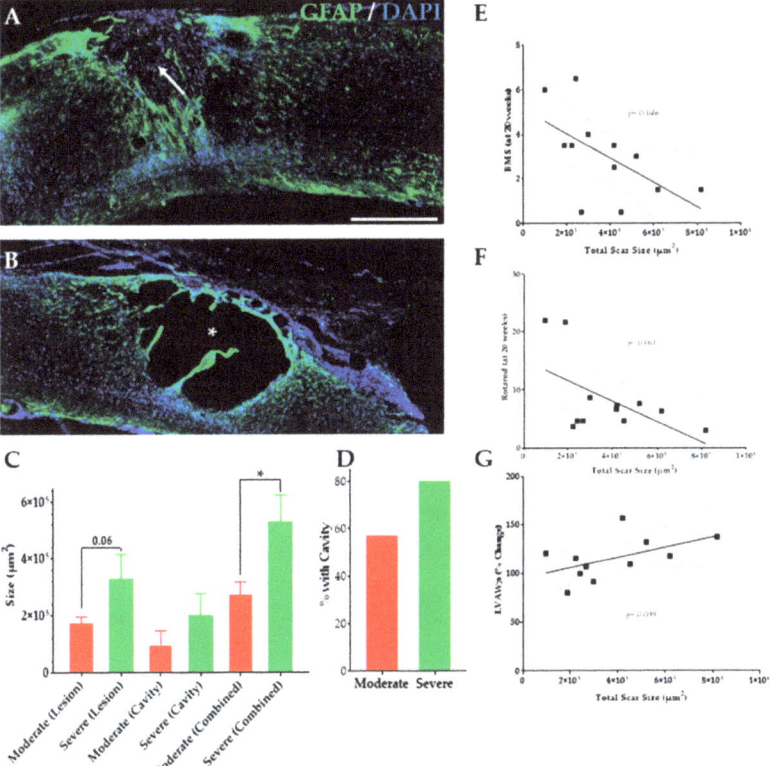

Figure 8. Lesion size and relation to behavior and changes in cardiovascular measures. Sample image of spinal cord (severe group) stained with GFAP (green) and DAPI (blue) showing (**A**) a lesion

(white arrow) and (**B**) a cavity (white asterisk) site. (**C**) The average lesion, cavity, and total injury size at 5 months post SCI. (**D**) The percent of mice with cavities at the site of injury. Linear trends of the (**E**) BMS score at 20 weeks PI, (**F**) rotarod performance (time on the rod in seconds) at 20 weeks PI, and (**G**) percent change in LVAW;s in relation to the total injury size of moderate and severe groups. Student's T-test comparing the means of 2 groups. Linear regression analysis to determine correlation between variables. Data presented as means ± SEM, n = 8 (moderate), and 5 (severe). Linear regression trend line ± 95% confidence interval. Scale bar = 500 µm. * $p < 0.05$.

3.8. SCI and Plasma Cytokines

To assess the effects of chronic SCI on cytokine expression, the relative plasma concentrations of IFN-γ, IL-10, IL-6, TNF-α, and IL-1β were measured. We observed an increase in IL-1β concentration in the severe SCI group $p = 0.05$ (Figure 9C). No significant differences were observed between any cohort for the other cytokines, although there was a trend for a decrease in IL-10 (Figure 9B) and an increase in IL-6 (Figure 9A) in the severely injured mice.

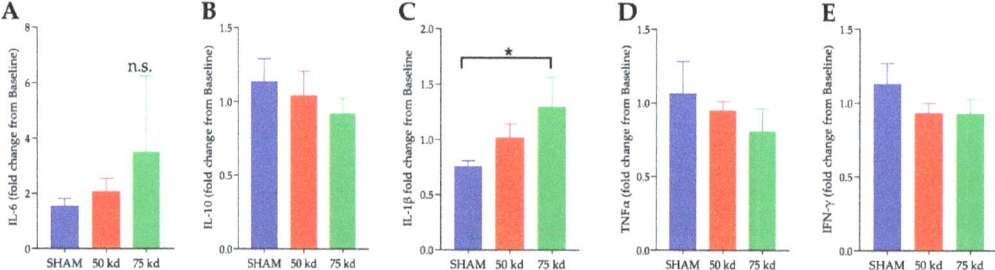

Figure 9. Injury-severity dependent increase in pro-inflammatory molecule. Plasma cytokines of (**A**) IL-6, (**B**) IL-10, (**C**) IL-1β, (**D**) TNF-α, and (**E**) IFN-γ at 5 months post injury were quantified using MILLIPLEX assay. Values presented as mean ± S.E.M. n = 6 (sham), 8 (moderate), and 5 (severe). Data analyzed by one-way ANOVA. * $p < 0.05$.

3.9. SCI, Heart, and Liver Innervation

To assess how SCI could potentially change innervation of both the heart and the liver, the percent of tyrosine hydrolase (TH) stain was measured in each tissue (Figure 10A,C). Between the sham and severe injury models for the heart, no significant difference in positive TH percentage was found (Figure 10B). Likewise, there was no significant difference in positive TH percentage in the liver (Figure 10D).

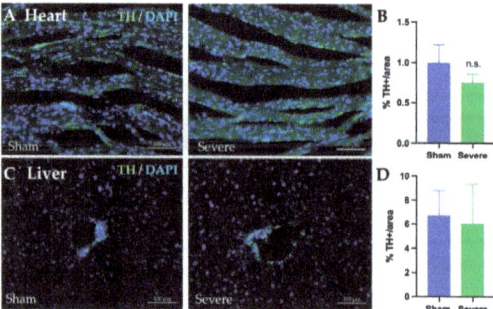

Figure 10. TH staining in the LV and liver. Heart (LVAW, **A**) and liver (**C**) 10 µm sections stained for tyrosine hydroxylase (TH) (green) and DAPI (blue) in both sham and sever SCI models. Heart

sections from both sham and severe SCI were analyzed for % area of positive TH stain (**B**). No significant differences in % positive was seen. Liver sections from both sham and severe SCI were also analyzed for % area of positive TH stain (**D**). Again, no significant differences in % positive was seen. Values presented as mean ± S.E.M. n = 6 (sham) and 5 (severe). Data analyzed by Student's T-test comparing the means of 2 groups. * $p < 0.05$. Scale bars = 100 µm.

4. Discussion

The main findings of this study are that chronic SCI at T8 level: (1) increases the liver echogenicity, which is associated with increased liver fibrosis; (2) reduces the LVID and increases the FS that are found to be associated with increased cardiac fibrosis and LV thickness indicating severe hypertrophy; (3) induces the sustained loss of motor functions; and (4) leads to the reduction in body weight, lean and fat percentage. Importantly, these perturbations in cardiometabolic functions vary significantly depending upon the severity of the injury and play a key role in determining the long-term health outcome following SCI.

4.1. SCI Severity and Hepatic Dysfunctions

The liver plays an essential role in metabolic function and SCI is associated with liver abnormalities in humans and rodents [37,39]. We observed a non-significant increase in liver echogenicity at 12 and 20 weeks after severe injury. Several factors may lead to changes in liver echogenicity including liver steatosis [68]. Changes in the hepatic echogenicity may be induced by the infiltration of pro-inflammatory cytokines and chemokines in the liver due to the trauma [40]. Interestingly, these changes in echogenicity were associated with an increase in fibrotic tissues in relation to the injury severity. In humans, ultrasound imaging is not routinely performed to assess liver dysfunction in people with chronic SCI [37]. Our data suggest that changes in echogenicity obtained from ultrasound imaging after chronic SCI, even if not significant, are correlated with significant increase in histological fibrotic changes of the liver. Therefore, because of the risks associated with a liver biopsy to assess for hepatic diseases, noninvasive examination of liver echogenicity following SCI may be of high interest to monitor the development of hepatic dysfunction in humans. This could be performed in addition to testing for serum markers such as alanine aminotransferase and aspartate transaminase (AST) [67].

Several studies have reported that SCI patients developed metabolic dysfunctions such as insulin resistance and impaired glucose tolerance [20,21,69,70]. Using IPGTT to assess glucose tolerance, our results revealed no differences between the groups at any time points up to 20 weeks after SCI. These results are consistent with a prior study reporting that glucose intolerance was not observed in SCI male mice at 56 or 84 days after T10 SCI transection [71]. However, the same study described an elevated fasting blood glucose in these mice. Another group reported that moderate T8 contusion in female rats led to no significant change in glucose levels at 23-days post SCI [67]. Importantly, female rats with a complete T3 transection showed a significant enhancement in glucose handling at 16 weeks post SCI, with lower serum insulin concentrations [72]. Our data do not show a change in insulin level at 18 weeks post SCI. However, these measurements of insulin levels were not performed on fasted animals. Future work is needed to better characterize the complex insulin/glucose relationship in mice models of SCI. Altogether, this suggests that the injury severity (contusion vs. transection), the level of the injury (high or low thoracic), and the timing post-SCI are important factors impacting metabolic functions [69]. Indeed, both the hepatic infiltration of fatty acids and/or inflammation following SCI and the disruption of the hepatic nervous system may impact hepatic functions. Our data suggest that severe T8 contusion does not alter hepatic TH innervation. However, it is of high interest to better understand how the level and severity of the injury may play a key role in directly or indirectly modulating the hepatic nervous system and the hepatic functions.

4.2. SCI Severity and Cardiac Functions

The development of cardiovascular dysfunction following SCI is one of the leading causes of death among SCI patients [73]. Cardiovascular dysfunction after SCI is dependent on the level and the degree of the injury [74]. Disruption of the cardiovascular nervous control by SCI leads to autonomic dysreflexia especially if the injury level is at T6 or above [46]. However, a T8 contusion model does not disrupt the cardiovascular sympathetic control, suggesting that the cardiac changes we have observed are due to other factors. Our data suggest no significant changes in TH innervation in the LV after chronic SCI. One could speculate that the reduction in survival observed in severe SCI (only 55% at 5-month post SCI) is the result of these cardiovascular complications. We could not confirm this hypothesis as we were not able collect the tissue from the animals found dead. Our results indicated that, during systole, both the LVID;s and volume were reduced in severe SCI at 16 weeks, and significantly at 20 weeks PI. This was correlated histologically with the increase in the left ventricle thickness. It is known that SCI individuals have smaller LV volumes and mass [75]. In rat models of SCI, West et al. reported a reduction in LV dimensions at 6 weeks post T3 SCI [76] and cardiac atrophy, reduced myocardium contractility, and increased fibrosis [77].

Our data showed an increase in the ejection fraction (EF) at 20 weeks PI in the severely injured group compared to the sham and moderate group. In humans, an EF >75% is a sign of hypertrophy cardiomyopathy. However, previous studies reported no differences in EF between SCI and able-bodied individuals despite LV volumes reduction [75]. In our data, EF is 58.1% in sham, 62.3% in moderate, and 70.4% in severe SCI. These severely injured mice also developed LV thickness and hypertrophy shown by histological analysis. While echocardiography scanning showed no significant differences in other cardiac parameters such as LV mass, SV, CO, HR, and LVPW, and LVAW thickness (Table 2), histological analysis revealed a significant change in LVPW, and LVAW thickness induced by severe SCI. Squair et al. observed a reduction in LVID;s, LVID;d, Volume;s and Volume;d [51]. They also reported a non-significant increase in EF in T3 severe contusion model in rat. However, we must acknowledge the limitation of this type of echo measurements and that short axis view analyses can infer volumetric measurements, and impact the EF calculated [78]. EF is calculated using the LV chamber volume during end systole (Volume;s) and end diastole (Volume;d) with this equation [EF = (Volume;d−Volume;s)/ Volume;d × 100]. Our hypothesis is that because of the LV hypertrophy in the severe SCI group, as measured by histology, the left ventricle contains a smaller amount of blood (reduced Volume;d). In this situation, with a Volume;s not decreasing proportionally, an increase in EF would be measured (as in our data). Because of this and the increase in perivascular fibrosis in the heart, we believe the severe SCI group present cardiac dysfunctions. Future experiments using blood pressure measurement, telemetric devices, or echocardiography using doppler analysis and B-mode/long-axis measurement will allow for the confirmation of these observations.

Another critical aspect of cardiac remodeling is the increase in collagen, often synonymous with fibrosis, in the LV tissue of both SCI groups, with more accumulation in the severity SCI. Outside of a SCI, myocardial fibrosis can be triggered by several factors including mechanical forces, inflammation [79], neurohormonal such as aldosterone [80,81], and others reviewed extensively here [82,83]. LV fibrosis can impair cardiac contractility function, reduce LV chamber size, lead to hypertrophic cardiomyopathy [84,85], LV dysfunction and heart failure [86]. One can speculate that even in moderate SCI, mice may develop hypertrophic cardiomyopathy at later chronic timepoints. The molecular mechanisms underlining these cardiac changes are not well understood. However, chronic inflammation is associated with metabolic syndrome phenotypes, which are causes of cardiovascular diseases. Therefore, sustained inflammatory cytokine activity after SCI may be a trigger for cardiac tissue damage and dysfunction. The direct impact of inflammation on cardiac alterations remains to be determined. Reduction of the systemic inflammation could be a potential target to reduce cardiac complications associated with chronic SCI.

LV thickening may be caused by several mechanisms, including increase in hypertension, diabetes, and aortic valve stenosis. We could not measure the potential changes in blood pressure over time and we did not observe changes in glucose levels. However, we observed significant increase in fibrosis in liver and LV. Therefore, it is possible that fibrosis occurs in other parts of heart, including on the aortic valve, leading to stenosis at chronic time points, and LV hypertrophy. Another possibility is the direct role of systemic inflammation on cardiac functions. Indeed, chronic low-grade inflammation leads to cardiomyopathies, including cardiomyocytes hypertrophy and dysfunctions [87–89]. Future work is necessary to understand the mechanism of LV thickening in this chronic T8 severe contusion model in mice, including the changes in cardiomyocytes size and numbers [51].

While we do not observe differences in TH staining in the heart and liver, we have to acknowledge that the T8 contusion model used here can impact innervation in other organs [45,46]. Therefore, any change in blood regulation in these organs induced by the dysregulation of the nervous system may overtime directly impact heart functions and induce hypertrophy and fibrosis through change in blood pressure. Additionally, more work is needed to understand how mid-thoracic SCI could precisely alter heart functions, despite the non-significant change in TH. Indeed, neural remodeling in the autonomic nervous system, and the balance between the sympathetic and parasympathetic systems, may be altered and induce further changes in cardiac functions and regulation. Interestingly, the autonomic nervous system is involved in detecting and modulating inflammation [90]. Therefore, change in the sympathetic tone can not only modulate heart function but also directly alter inflammation. Whether inflammation alters the sympathetic first after SCI of the reversed needs to be determined.

4.3. SCI Severity and Body Composition

Due to the severe trauma induced by SCI which increases the metabolic demand, significant changes in the body weight and body fat may occur [70]. In humans, reports have indicated that people with SCI exhibit a significant increase in body mass index (BMI) [91]. These changes may increase the body fat and reduce lean mass [7,24,92]. Our results showed a reduction in body weight and body fat and lean percentage in both SCI severity models, compared to the sham control group. Severely injured mice lost more body fat and lean mass than moderately injured mice. This prolonged reduction in body weight including fat mass was also reported in rats after 16 weeks of T3 SCI [72]. In this study, the authors related this reduction to possible permanent changes in gastrointestinal transit and absorption and not due to hypophagia. Interestingly, thoracic SCI at level T10 in rats maintained on a low-fat diet did not gain weight compared to SCI rats maintained on high fat diet after 12 weeks post injury, indicating that diet also plays an important role in changes in body composition [93]. Our results showed a reduction in fat and lean percentages compared to sham. This reduction in fat is correlated with the overall reduction in the level of triglycerides in the liver and plasma levels in severe SCI, although it is not significant. Previous work reported some pathological changes to lipid species early on following injury [39,94]. However, our data suggest that when examined 5 months after SCI, the lipid levels appear to be normal with a moderate SCI, and slightly reduced after a severe SCI. Potential increases or decreases within the lipid profile of SCI patients have been shown to be dependent upon numerous factors such as the level and severity of injury, age/sex, and time after injury [38,95,96]. Damage to the liver, notably fibrosis, does remain at this chronic timepoint, suggesting that the liver may be more prone to inflammation or differential response after high fat diet feeding. The lack of fat gain in rodent and the reduction in lipid (hepatic and circulating) is intriguing. Different types of diet, lower food intake, and changes in metabolism may explain the slower fat accumulation following SCI in mice. In this study, we did not monitor dietary intake, which would be recommended for future work. It will also be interesting to challenge this new metabolic state by shocking the system via a large uptake in fat. It would be interesting to see if the mice gain weight (and fat) at all at more chronic time points as aged mice do.

4.4. SCI Severity, Motor Function, and Injury Size

Regarding behavioral assessments, BMS testing indicated that, for both SCI severity models, mice did not fully recover their locomotor function at 20 weeks after SCI. Moderate SCI mice recovered better than severely injured mice. Functional recovery in mice is severity-dependent and is not complete in a moderate or severe contusion model of SCI, with animals reaching the maximum of the recovery several weeks after injury. Four months old mice injured at T8-10 (75 kdyn) contusion did not recover fully after 6 weeks post injury [97,98]. Our results assessed recovery at chronic time point (up to 5 months post-SCI) and demonstrate that functional recovery is severity dependent and that injured mice do not further recover over a long period of time.

Our results showed a significant increase in the spinal cord lesion size with the model of injury severity. It has been previously shown that there is a positive relationship between lesion severity and functional outcomes where increase in lesion size may lead to decreased outcomes [99]. Interestingly, liver dysfunction and inflammation at the time of SCI increases the spinal cord lesion size and worsens motor recovery [67]. The changes induced by SCI are affecting several organs and are severity dependent. This is apparent in individuals living with SCI because they are more prone to infections and cardiometabolic disorder [100]. Chronic exposure to increased levels of circulating inflammatory cytokines lead to liver dysfunction and metabolic disease [94]. We observed a significant increase in IL-1β and a trend for upregulation of IL-6 plasma concentrations in the severe group compared to the sham groups. Previous finding showed that IL-1β gene expression was upregulated in the hepatic tissue for at least 21 days post-injury [39]. Furthermore, IL-6 has been implicated in regulations of metabolic function induction of the hepatic acute phase proteins [101]. Hepatic IL-6 expression is increased in animal models of nonalcoholic fatty liver disease (NAFLD), which results in insulin resistance in mice [102]. Considering the role of the liver as a key organ in regulating metabolism, modulating the inflammatory response may reduce liver dysfunction, which in turn may reduce the onset of the severity of cardiometabolic dysfunctions.

5. Conclusions

In conclusion, our data suggest that mice with thoracic T8 injury develop numerous hepatic and cardiometabolic alterations over time. Further work will determine if changes in innervation in several organs after SCI, including inflammatory organs such as the spleen and the gastro-intestinal tract, can directly or indirectly influence these health issues. Importantly, it will be of high interest to determine if targeting inflammation will reduce these metabolic outcomes, as well as reduce the morbidity and mortality of people living with SCI.

Author Contributions: A.B.G. and C.G.G. conceived and designed the research; A.B.G. conducted the in vivo experiments and histology with assistance from C.J. A.S. conducted the experiments and analyses relating to the injury size and cytokine analysis. C.J. and A.J.D. conducted all analyses of TH staining, triglyceride, cholesterol, and insulin. A.J.R. and J.M.R. assisted in experimentation of triglyceride, cholesterol, and insulin levels. A.B.G., A.S., C.G.G., C.J. and A.J.D. wrote the manuscript. All authors have read and agreed to the published version of the manuscript.

Funding: This research was funded by Mission Connect, a program of TIRR Foundation, grant number 019-110.

Institutional Review Board Statement: The study was conducted and approved by the Institutional Animal Care Committee at Texas A&M University (IACUC 2018-0048). All the experiments reported here were reviewed and approved by the and were consistent with the NIH guidelines for animal care and use.

Informed Consent Statement: Not applicable.

Data Availability Statement: The data presented in this study are available on request from the corresponding author.

Acknowledgments: The authors would like to thank Graphit Science & Art for preparing the illustrations used in Figure 1, and Carl Tong at Texas A&M for the help with the ultrasound imaging. This work was supported by the Neuroscience and Experimental Therapeutics Bevahior Core at Texas A&M Health Science Center.

Conflicts of Interest: The authors declare no conflict of interest.

References

1. SCI Facts and Figures. *J. Spinal Cord Med.* **2017**, *40*, 872–873. [CrossRef] [PubMed]
2. Alizadeh, A.; Dyck, S.M.; Karimi-Abdolrezaee, S. Traumatic Spinal Cord Injury: An Overview of Pathophysiology, Models and Acute Injury Mechanisms. *Front. Neurol.* **2019**, *10*, 282. [CrossRef]
3. Ahuja, C.S.; Wilson, J.R.; Nori, S.; Kotter, M.R.N.; Druschel, C.; Curt, A.; Fehlings, M.G. Traumatic spinal cord injury. *Nat. Rev. Dis. Primers* **2017**, *3*, 17018. [CrossRef] [PubMed]
4. Sun, X.; Jones, Z.B.; Chen, X.M.; Zhou, L.; So, K.F.; Ren, Y. Multiple organ dysfunction and systemic inflammation after spinal cord injury: A complex relationship. *J. Neuroinflamm.* **2016**, *13*, 260. [CrossRef]
5. Smith, D.L., Jr.; Yarar-Fisher, C. Contributors to Metabolic Disease Risk Following Spinal Cord Injury. *Curr. Phys. Med. Rehabil. Rep.* **2016**, *4*, 190–199. [CrossRef] [PubMed]
6. Gill, S.; Sumrell, R.M.; Sima, A.; Cifu, D.X.; Gorgey, A.S. Waist circumference cutoff identifying risks of obesity, metabolic syndrome, and cardiovascular disease in men with spinal cord injury. *PLoS ONE* **2020**, *15*, e0236752. [CrossRef]
7. Gorgey, A.S.; Gater, D.R., Jr. Prevalence of Obesity After Spinal Cord Injury. *Top. Spinal Cord Inj. Rehabil.* **2007**, *12*, 1–7. [CrossRef]
8. Nash, M.S.; Mendez, A.J. A guideline-driven assessment of need for cardiovascular disease risk intervention in persons with chronic paraplegia. *Arch. Phys. Med. Rehabil.* **2007**, *88*, 751–757. [CrossRef]
9. Nash, M.S.; Gater, D.R., Jr. Cardiometabolic Disease and Dysfunction Following Spinal Cord Injury: Origins and Guideline-Based Countermeasures. *Phys. Med. Rehabil. Clin. N. Am.* **2020**, *31*, 415–436. [CrossRef]
10. Cornier, M.A.; Dabelea, D.; Hernandez, T.L.; Lindstrom, R.C.; Steig, A.J.; Stob, N.R.; Van Pelt, R.E.; Wang, H.; Eckel, R.H. The metabolic syndrome. *Endocr. Rev.* **2008**, *29*, 777–822. [CrossRef]
11. Eckel, R.H.; Grundy, S.M.; Zimmet, P.Z. The metabolic syndrome. *Lancet* **2005**, *365*, 1415–1428. [CrossRef]
12. Grundy, S.M.; Hansen, B.; Smith, S.C., Jr.; Cleeman, J.I.; Kahn, R.A.; American Heart, A.; National Heart, L.; Blood, I.; American Diabetes, A. Clinical management of metabolic syndrome: Report of the American Heart Association/National Heart, Lung, and Blood Institute/American Diabetes Association conference on scientific issues related to management. *Arterioscler. Thromb. Vasc. Biol.* **2004**, *24*, e19–e24. [CrossRef] [PubMed]
13. Buchholz, A.C.; Pencharz, P.B. Energy expenditure in chronic spinal cord injury. *Curr. Opin. Clin. Nutr. Metab. Care* **2004**, *7*, 635–639. [CrossRef]
14. Gurka, M.J.; Filipp, S.L.; DeBoer, M.D. Geographical variation in the prevalence of obesity, metabolic syndrome, and diabetes among US adults. *Nutr. Diabetes* **2018**, *8*, 14. [CrossRef] [PubMed]
15. Stein, C.J.; Colditz, G.A. The epidemic of obesity. *J. Clin. Endocrinol. Metab.* **2004**, *89*, 2522–2525. [CrossRef]
16. Gater, D.R., Jr.; Farkas, G.J.; Berg, A.S.; Castillo, C. Prevalence of metabolic syndrome in veterans with spinal cord injury. *J. Spinal Cord Med.* **2019**, *42*, 86–93. [CrossRef]
17. Shulman, G.I. Ectopic fat in insulin resistance, dyslipidemia, and cardiometabolic disease. *N. Engl. J. Med.* **2014**, *371*, 2237–2238. [CrossRef]
18. Bao, F.; Omana, V.; Brown, A.; Weaver, L.C. The systemic inflammatory response after spinal cord injury in the rat is decreased by alpha4beta1 integrin blockade. *J. Neurotrauma* **2012**, *29*, 1626–1637. [CrossRef]
19. Gorgey, A.S.; Wells, K.M.; Austin, T.L. Adiposity and spinal cord injury. *World J. Orthop.* **2015**, *6*, 567–576. [CrossRef]
20. Bauman, W.A.; Spungen, A.M. Metabolic changes in persons after spinal cord injury. *Phys. Med. Rehabil. Clin. N. Am.* **2000**, *11*, 109–140. [CrossRef]
21. Bauman, W.A.; Spungen, A.M. Carbohydrate and lipid metabolism in chronic spinal cord injury. *J. Spinal Cord Med.* **2001**, *24*, 266–277. [CrossRef] [PubMed]
22. Spungen, A.M.; Adkins, R.H.; Stewart, C.A.; Wang, J.; Pierson, R.N., Jr.; Waters, R.L.; Bauman, W.A. Factors influencing body composition in persons with spinal cord injury: A cross-sectional study. *J. Appl. Physiol. (1985)* **2003**, *95*, 2398–2407. [CrossRef] [PubMed]
23. Shojaei, M.H.; Alavinia, S.M.; Craven, B.C. Management of obesity after spinal cord injury: A systematic review. *J. Spinal Cord Med.* **2017**, *40*, 783–794. [CrossRef] [PubMed]
24. Gater, D.R., Jr. Obesity after spinal cord injury. *Phys. Med. Rehabil. Clin. N. Am.* **2007**, *18*, 333–351. [CrossRef]
25. Castro, M.J.; Apple, D.F., Jr.; Rogers, S.; Dudley, G.A. Influence of complete spinal cord injury on skeletal muscle mechanics within the first 6 months of injury. *Eur. J. Appl. Physiol.* **2000**, *81*, 128–131. [CrossRef]
26. Shah, P.K.; Stevens, J.E.; Gregory, C.M.; Pathare, N.C.; Jayaraman, A.; Bickel, S.C.; Bowden, M.; Behrman, A.L.; Walter, G.A.; Dudley, G.A.; et al. Lower-extremity muscle cross-sectional area after incomplete spinal cord injury. *Arch. Phys. Med. Rehabil.* **2006**, *87*, 772–778. [CrossRef] [PubMed]

27. Lee, M.Y.; Myers, J.; Hayes, A.; Madan, S.; Froelicher, V.F.; Perkash, I.; Kiratli, B.J. C-reactive protein, metabolic syndrome, and insulin resistance in individuals with spinal cord injury. *J. Spinal Cord Med.* **2005**, *28*, 20–25. [CrossRef]
28. Cragg, J.J.; Noonan, V.K.; Krassioukov, A.; Borisoff, J. Cardiovascular disease and spinal cord injury: Results from a national population health survey. *Neurology* **2013**, *81*, 723–728. [CrossRef]
29. Van der Scheer, J.W.; Totosy de Zepetnek, J.O.; Blauwet, C.; Brooke-Wavell, K.; Graham-Paulson, T.; Leonard, A.N.; Webborn, N.; Goosey-Tolfrey, V.L. Assessment of body composition in spinal cord injury: A scoping review. *PLoS ONE* **2021**, *16*, e0251142. [CrossRef]
30. Neto, F.R.; Lopes, G.H. Body composition modifications in people with chronic spinal cord injury after supervised physical activity. *J. Spinal Cord Med.* **2011**, *34*, 586–593. [CrossRef]
31. Felleiter, P.; Krebs, J.; Haeberli, Y.; Schmid, W.; Tesini, S.; Perret, C. Post-traumatic changes in energy expenditure and body composition in patients with acute spinal cord injury. *J. Rehabil. Med.* **2017**, *49*, 579–584. [CrossRef] [PubMed]
32. Cardus, D.; McTaggart, W.G. Body composition in spinal cord injury. *Arch. Phys. Med. Rehabil.* **1985**, *66*, 257–259. [CrossRef]
33. Kocina, P. Body composition of spinal cord injured adults. *Sports Med.* **1997**, *23*, 48–60. [CrossRef] [PubMed]
34. Bechmann, L.P.; Hannivoort, R.A.; Gerken, G.; Hotamisligil, G.S.; Trauner, M.; Canbay, A. The interaction of hepatic lipid and glucose metabolism in liver diseases. *J. Hepatol.* **2012**, *56*, 952–964. [CrossRef]
35. Rui, L. Energy metabolism in the liver. *Compr. Physiol.* **2014**, *4*, 177–197. [CrossRef]
36. Kitade, H.; Chen, G.; Ni, Y.; Ota, T. Nonalcoholic Fatty Liver Disease and Insulin Resistance: New Insights and Potential New Treatments. *Nutrients* **2017**, *9*, 387. [CrossRef]
37. Sipski, M.L.; Estores, I.M.; Alexander, C.J.; Guo, X.; Chandralapaty, S.K. Lack of justification for routine abdominal ultrasonography in patients with chronic spinal cord injury. *J. Rehabil. Res. Dev.* **2004**, *41*, 101–108. [CrossRef]
38. Rankin, K.C.; O'Brien, L.C.; Segal, L.; Khan, M.R.; Gorgey, A.S. Liver Adiposity and Metabolic Profile in Individuals with Chronic Spinal Cord Injury. *Biomed. Res. Int.* **2017**, *2017*, 1364818. [CrossRef]
39. Sauerbeck, A.D.; Laws, J.L.; Bandaru, V.V.; Popovich, P.G.; Haughey, N.J.; McTigue, D.M. Spinal cord injury causes chronic liver pathology in rats. *J. Neurotrauma* **2015**, *32*, 159–169. [CrossRef]
40. Campbell, S.J.; Zahid, I.; Losey, P.; Law, S.; Jiang, Y.; Bilgen, M.; van Rooijen, N.; Morsali, D.; Davis, A.E.; Anthony, D.C. Liver Kupffer cells control the magnitude of the inflammatory response in the injured brain and spinal cord. *Neuropharmacology* **2008**, *55*, 780–787. [CrossRef]
41. Hundt, H.; Fleming, J.C.; Phillips, J.T.; Lawendy, A.; Gurr, K.R.; Bailey, S.I.; Sanders, D.; Bihari, R.; Gray, D.; Parry, N.; et al. Assessment of hepatic inflammation after spinal cord injury using intravital microscopy. *Injury* **2011**, *42*, 691–696. [CrossRef] [PubMed]
42. Garshick, E.; Kelley, A.; Cohen, S.A.; Garrison, A.; Tun, C.G.; Gagnon, D.; Brown, R. A prospective assessment of mortality in chronic spinal cord injury. *Spinal Cord* **2005**, *43*, 408–416. [CrossRef]
43. Claydon, V.E.; Krassioukov, A.V. Orthostatic hypotension and autonomic pathways after spinal cord injury. *J. Neurotrauma* **2006**, *23*, 1713–1725. [CrossRef] [PubMed]
44. Ravensbergen, H.J.; de Groot, S.; Post, M.W.; Slootman, H.J.; van der Woude, L.H.; Claydon, V.E. Cardiovascular function after spinal cord injury: Prevalence and progression of dysfunction during inpatient rehabilitation and 5 years following discharge. *Neurorehabil. Neural. Repair.* **2014**, *28*, 219–229. [CrossRef] [PubMed]
45. Michael, F.M.; Patel, S.P.; Rabchevsky, A.G. Intraspinal Plasticity Associated With the Development of Autonomic Dysreflexia After Complete Spinal Cord Injury. *Front. Cell. Neurosci.* **2019**, *13*, 505. [CrossRef]
46. Hou, S.; Rabchevsky, A.G. Autonomic consequences of spinal cord injury. *Compr. Physiol.* **2014**, *4*, 1419–1453. [CrossRef]
47. West, C.R.; Mills, P.; Krassioukov, A.V. Influence of the neurological level of spinal cord injury on cardiovascular outcomes in humans: A meta-analysis. *Spinal Cord* **2012**, *50*, 484–492. [CrossRef]
48. West, C.R.; Poormasjedi-Meibod, M.S.; Manouchehri, N.; Williams, A.M.; Erskine, E.L.; Webster, M.; Fisk, S.; Morrison, C.; Short, K.; So, K.; et al. A porcine model for studying the cardiovascular consequences of high-thoracic spinal cord injury. *J. Physiol.* **2020**, *598*, 929–942. [CrossRef]
49. Lujan, H.L.; Janbaih, H.; DiCarlo, S.E. Dynamic interaction between the heart and its sympathetic innervation following T5 spinal cord transection. *J. Appl. Physiol. (1985)* **2012**, *113*, 1332–1341. [CrossRef]
50. Lujan, H.L.; Janbaih, H.; DiCarlo, S.E. Structural remodeling of the heart and its premotor cardioinhibitory vagal neurons following T(5) spinal cord transection. *J. Appl. Physiol. (1985)* **2014**, *116*, 1148–1155. [CrossRef]
51. Squair, J.W.; Liu, J.; Tetzlaff, W.; Krassioukov, A.V.; West, C.R. Spinal cord injury-induced cardiomyocyte atrophy and impaired cardiac function are severity dependent. *Exp. Physiol.* **2018**, *103*, 179–189. [CrossRef] [PubMed]
52. Squair, J.W.; West, C.R.; Popok, D.; Assinck, P.; Liu, J.; Tetzlaff, W.; Krassioukov, A.V. High Thoracic Contusion Model for the Investigation of Cardiovascular Function after Spinal Cord Injury. *J. Neurotrauma* **2017**, *34*, 671–684. [CrossRef] [PubMed]
53. Bhalala, O.G.; Pan, L.; North, H.; McGuire, T.; Kessler, J.A. Generation of Mouse Spinal Cord Injury. *Bio Protoc.* **2013**, *3*, e886. [CrossRef] [PubMed]
54. Gruner, J.A. A monitored contusion model of spinal cord injury in the rat. *J. Neurotrauma* **1992**, *9*, 123–126, discussion 126–128. [CrossRef]
55. Lee, J.K.; Geoffroy, C.G.; Chan, A.F.; Tolentino, K.E.; Crawford, M.J.; Leal, M.A.; Kang, B.; Zheng, B. Assessing spinal axon regeneration and sprouting in Nogo-, MAG-, and OMgp-deficient mice. *Neuron* **2010**, *66*, 663–670. [CrossRef]

56. Basso, D.M.; Fisher, L.C.; Anderson, A.J.; Jakeman, L.B.; McTigue, D.M.; Popovich, P.G. Basso Mouse Scale for locomotion detects differences in recovery after spinal cord injury in five common mouse strains. *J. Neurotrauma* **2006**, *23*, 635–659. [CrossRef]
57. Nixon, J.P.; Zhang, M.; Wang, C.; Kuskowski, M.A.; Novak, C.M.; Levine, J.A.; Billington, C.J.; Kotz, C.M. Evaluation of a quantitative magnetic resonance imaging system for whole body composition analysis in rodents. *Obesity* **2010**, *18*, 1652–1659. [CrossRef]
58. Pandit, H.; Tinney, J.P.; Li, Y.; Cui, G.; Li, S.; Keller, B.B.; Martin, R.C.G., 2nd. Utilizing Contrast-Enhanced Ultrasound Imaging for Evaluating Fatty Liver Disease Progression in Pre-clinical Mouse Models. *Ultrasound Med. Biol.* **2019**, *45*, 549–557. [CrossRef]
59. Ghnenis, A.B.; Burns, D.T.; Osimanjiang, W.; He, G.; Bushman, J.S. A Long-Term Pilot Study on Sex and Spinal Cord Injury Shows Sexual Dimorphism in Functional Recovery and Cardio-Metabolic Responses. *Sci. Rep.* **2020**, *10*, 2762. [CrossRef]
60. Zhao, Q.; Yan, T.; Li, L.; Chopp, M.; Venkat, P.; Qian, Y.; Li, R.; Wu, R.; Li, W.; Lu, M.; et al. Immune Response Mediates Cardiac Dysfunction after Traumatic Brain Injury. *J. Neurotrauma* **2019**, *36*, 619–629. [CrossRef]
61. Wu, C.; Yan, F.; Li, M.; Tu, Y.; Guo, Z.; Chen, Y.; Wu, Y.; Li, Q.; Yu, C.; Fu, Y.; et al. Whole-Mount Kidney Clearing and Visualization Reveal Renal Sympathetic Hyperinnervation in Heart Failure Mice. *Front. Physiol.* **2021**, *12*, 696286. [CrossRef] [PubMed]
62. Liu, J.; Rigel, D.F. Echocardiographic examination in rats and mice. *Methods Mol. Biol.* **2009**, *573*, 139–155. [CrossRef] [PubMed]
63. Tong, C.W.; Stelzer, J.E.; Greaser, M.L.; Powers, P.A.; Moss, R.L. Acceleration of crossbridge kinetics by protein kinase A phosphorylation of cardiac myosin binding protein C modulates cardiac function. *Circ. Res.* **2008**, *103*, 974–982. [CrossRef] [PubMed]
64. Chakraborty, A.; Barajas, S.; Lammoglia, G.M.; Reyna, A.J.; Morley, T.S.; Johnson, J.A.; Scherer, P.E.; Rutkowski, J.M. Vascular Endothelial Growth Factor-D (VEGF-D) Overexpression and Lymphatic Expansion in Murine Adipose Tissue Improves Metabolism in Obesity. *Am. J. Pathol.* **2019**, *189*, 924–939. [CrossRef] [PubMed]
65. Wang, D.; Patel, V.V.; Ricciotti, E.; Zhou, R.; Levin, M.D.; Gao, E.; Yu, Z.; Ferrari, V.A.; Lu, M.M.; Xu, J.; et al. Cardiomyocyte cyclooxygenase-2 influences cardiac rhythm and function. *Proc. Natl. Acad. Sci. USA* **2009**, *106*, 7548–7552. [CrossRef]
66. Jackson, S.J.; Andrews, N.; Ball, D.; Bellantuono, I.; Gray, J.; Hachoumi, L.; Holmes, A.; Latcham, J.; Petrie, A.; Potter, P.; et al. Does age matter? The impact of rodent age on study outcomes. *Lab. Anim.* **2017**, *51*, 160–169. [CrossRef]
67. Goodus, M.T.; Carson, K.E.; Sauerbeck, A.D.; Dey, P.; Alfredo, A.N.; Popovich, P.G.; Bruno, R.S.; McTigue, D.M. Liver inflammation at the time of spinal cord injury enhances intraspinal pathology, liver injury, metabolic syndrome and locomotor deficits. *Exp. Neurol.* **2021**, *342*, 113725. [CrossRef]
68. Mathiesen, U.L.; Franzen, L.E.; Aselius, H.; Resjo, M.; Jacobsson, L.; Foberg, U.; Fryden, A.; Bodemar, G. Increased liver echogenicity at ultrasound examination reflects degree of steatosis but not of fibrosis in asymptomatic patients with mild/moderate abnormalities of liver transaminases. *Dig. Liver. Dis.* **2002**, *34*, 516–522. [CrossRef]
69. Raymond, J.; Harmer, A.R.; Temesi, J.; van Kemenade, C. Glucose tolerance and physical activity level in people with spinal cord injury. *Spinal Cord* **2010**, *48*, 591–596. [CrossRef]
70. Gorgey, A.S.; Dolbow, D.R.; Dolbow, J.D.; Khalil, R.K.; Castillo, C.; Gater, D.R. Effects of spinal cord injury on body composition and metabolic profile—Part I. *J. Spinal Cord Med.* **2014**, *37*, 693–702. [CrossRef]
71. Graham, Z.A.; Liu, X.H.; Harlow, L.; Pan, J.; Azulai, D.; Tawfeek, H.A.; Wnek, R.D.; Mattingly, A.J.; Bauman, W.A.; Yarrow, J.F.; et al. Effects of a High-Fat Diet on Tissue Mass, Bone, and Glucose Tolerance after Chronic Complete Spinal Cord Transection in Male Mice. *Neurotrauma Rep.* **2020**, *1*, 17–31. [CrossRef] [PubMed]
72. Primeaux, S.D.; Tong, M.; Holmes, G.M. Effects of chronic spinal cord injury on body weight and body composition in rats fed a standard chow diet. *Am. J. Physiol. Regul. Integr. Comp. Physiol.* **2007**, *293*, R1102–R1109. [CrossRef]
73. Squair, J.W.; West, C.R.; Krassioukov, A.V. Neuroprotection, Plasticity Manipulation, and Regenerative Strategies to Improve Cardiovascular Function following Spinal Cord Injury. *J. Neurotrauma* **2015**, *32*, 609–621. [CrossRef] [PubMed]
74. Hagen, E.M.; Rekand, T.; Gronning, M.; Faerestrand, S. Cardiovascular complications of spinal cord injury. *Tidsskr. Nor. Laegeforen* **2012**, *132*, 1115–1120. [CrossRef] [PubMed]
75. Williams, A.M.; Gee, C.M.; Voss, C.; West, C.R. Cardiac consequences of spinal cord injury: Systematic review and meta-analysis. *Heart* **2019**, *105*, 217–225. [CrossRef] [PubMed]
76. West, C.R.; Squair, J.W.; McCracken, L.; Currie, K.D.; Somvanshi, R.; Yuen, V.; Phillips, A.A.; Kumar, U.; McNeill, J.H.; Krassioukov, A.V. Cardiac Consequences of Autonomic Dysreflexia in Spinal Cord Injury. *Hypertension* **2016**, *68*, 1281–1289. [CrossRef] [PubMed]
77. West, C.R.; Crawford, M.A.; Poormasjedi-Meibod, M.S.; Currie, K.D.; Fallavollita, A.; Yuen, V.; McNeill, J.H.; Krassioukov, A.V. Passive hind-limb cycling improves cardiac function and reduces cardiovascular disease risk in experimental spinal cord injury. *J. Physiol.* **2014**, *592*, 1771–1783. [CrossRef]
78. Lindsey, M.L.; Kassiri, Z.; Virag, J.A.I.; de Castro Bras, L.E.; Scherrer-Crosbie, M. Guidelines for measuring cardiac physiology in mice. *Am. J. Physiol. Heart Circ. Physiol.* **2018**, *314*, H733–H752. [CrossRef]
79. Kai, H.; Kuwahara, F.; Tokuda, K.; Imaizumi, T. Diastolic dysfunction in hypertensive hearts: Roles of perivascular inflammation and reactive myocardial fibrosis. *Hypertens Res.* **2005**, *28*, 483–490. [CrossRef]
80. Lijnen, P.; Petrov, V. Induction of cardiac fibrosis by aldosterone. *J. Mol. Cell. Cardiol.* **2000**, *32*, 865–879. [CrossRef]
81. Essick, E.E.; Sam, F. Cardiac hypertrophy and fibrosis in the metabolic syndrome: A role for aldosterone and the mineralocorticoid receptor. *Int. J. Hypertens* **2011**, *2011*, 346985. [CrossRef]

82. Kong, P.; Christia, P.; Frangogiannis, N.G. The pathogenesis of cardiac fibrosis. *Cell. Mol. Life Sci.* **2014**, *71*, 549–574. [CrossRef] [PubMed]
83. Diez, J. Mechanisms of cardiac fibrosis in hypertension. *J. Clin. Hypertens (Greenwich)* **2007**, *9*, 546–550. [CrossRef] [PubMed]
84. Ho, C.Y.; Lopez, B.; Coelho-Filho, O.R.; Lakdawala, N.K.; Cirino, A.L.; Jarolim, P.; Kwong, R.; Gonzalez, A.; Colan, S.D.; Seidman, J.G.; et al. Myocardial fibrosis as an early manifestation of hypertrophic cardiomyopathy. *N. Engl. J. Med.* **2010**, *363*, 552–563. [CrossRef]
85. Naser, J.A.; Anupraiwan, O.; Adigun, R.O.; Maleszewski, J.J.; Pislaru, S.V.; Pellikka, P.A.; Pislaru, C. Myocardial Stiffness by Cardiac Elastography in Hypertrophic Cardiomyopathy: Relationship With Myocardial Fibrosis and Clinical Outcomes. *JACC Cardiovasc. Imaging* **2021**, *14*, 2051–2053. [CrossRef] [PubMed]
86. Basso, C.; Thiene, G.; Corrado, D.; Buja, G.; Melacini, P.; Nava, A. Hypertrophic cardiomyopathy and sudden death in the young: Pathologic evidence of myocardial ischemia. *Hum. Pathol.* **2000**, *31*, 988–998. [CrossRef] [PubMed]
87. Frieler, R.A.; Mortensen, R.M. Immune cell and other noncardiomyocyte regulation of cardiac hypertrophy and remodeling. *Circulation* **2015**, *131*, 1019–1030. [CrossRef] [PubMed]
88. Mann, D.L. Innate immunity and the failing heart: The cytokine hypothesis revisited. *Circ. Res.* **2015**, *116*, 1254–1268. [CrossRef] [PubMed]
89. Wenzl, F.A.; Ambrosini, S.; Mohammed, S.A.; Kraler, S.; Luscher, T.F.; Costantino, S.; Paneni, F. Inflammation in Metabolic Cardiomyopathy. *Front. Cardiovasc. Med.* **2021**, *8*, 742178. [CrossRef]
90. Koopman, F.A.; van Maanen, M.A.; Vervoordeldonk, M.J.; Tak, P.P. Balancing the autonomic nervous system to reduce inflammation in rheumatoid arthritis. *J. Intern. Med.* **2017**, *282*, 64–75. [CrossRef]
91. Crane, D.A.; Little, J.W.; Burns, S.P. Weight gain following spinal cord injury: A pilot study. *J. Spinal Cord Med.* **2011**, *34*, 227–232. [CrossRef]
92. Castro, M.J.; Apple, D.F., Jr.; Hillegass, E.A.; Dudley, G.A. Influence of complete spinal cord injury on skeletal muscle cross-sectional area within the first 6 months of injury. *Eur. J. Appl. Physiol. Occup. Physiol.* **1999**, *80*, 373–378. [CrossRef] [PubMed]
93. Harris, K.K.; Himel, A.R.; Duncan, B.C.; Grill, R.J.; Grayson, B.E. Energy balance following diets of varying fat content: Metabolic dysregulation in a rodent model of spinal cord contusion. *Physiol. Rep.* **2019**, *7*, e14207. [CrossRef] [PubMed]
94. Goodus, M.T.; McTigue, D.M. Hepatic dysfunction after spinal cord injury: A vicious cycle of central and peripheral pathology? *Exp. Neurol.* **2020**, *325*, 113160. [CrossRef] [PubMed]
95. Laclaustra, M.; Van Den Berg, E.L.; Hurtado-Roca, Y.; Castellote, J.M. Serum lipid profile in subjects with traumatic spinal cord injury. *PLoS ONE* **2015**, *10*, e0115522. [CrossRef] [PubMed]
96. Raguindin, P.F.; Frankl, G.; Itodo, O.A.; Bertolo, A.; Zeh, R.M.; Capossela, S.; Minder, B.; Stoyanov, J.; Stucki, G.; Franco, O.H.; et al. The neurological level of spinal cord injury and cardiovascular risk factors: A systematic review and meta-analysis. *Spinal Cord* **2021**, *59*, 1135–1145. [CrossRef] [PubMed]
97. McFarlane, K.; Otto, T.E.; Bailey, W.M.; Veldhorst, A.K.; Donahue, R.R.; Taylor, B.K.; Gensel, J.C. Effect of Sex on Motor Function, Lesion Size, and Neuropathic Pain after Contusion Spinal Cord Injury in Mice. *J. Neurotrauma* **2020**, *37*, 1983–1990. [CrossRef]
98. Kakuta, Y.; Adachi, A.; Yokohama, M.; Horii, T.; Mieda, T.; Iizuka, Y.; Takagishi, K.; Chikuda, H.; Iizuka, H.; Nakamura, K. Spontaneous functional full recovery from motor and sensory deficits in adult mice after mild spinal cord injury. *Heliyon* **2019**, *5*, e01847. [CrossRef]
99. Fouad, K.; Hurd, C.; Magnuson, D.S. Functional testing in animal models of spinal cord injury: Not as straight forward as one would think. *Front. Integr. Neurosci.* **2013**, *7*, 85. [CrossRef]
100. Phillips, A.A.; Krassioukov, A.V. Contemporary Cardiovascular Concerns after Spinal Cord Injury: Mechanisms, Maladaptations, and Management. *J. Neurotrauma* **2015**, *32*, 1927–1942. [CrossRef]
101. Rose-John, S. Interleukin-6 Family Cytokines. *Cold Spring Harb. Perspect. Biol.* **2018**, *10*, a028415. [CrossRef] [PubMed]
102. Wieckowska, A.; Papouchado, B.G.; Li, Z.; Lopez, R.; Zein, N.N.; Feldstein, A.E. Increased hepatic and circulating interleukin-6 levels in human nonalcoholic steatohepatitis. *Am. J. Gastroenterol.* **2008**, *103*, 1372–1379. [CrossRef] [PubMed]

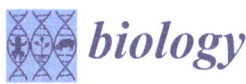

Article

Effects of Chronic High-Frequency rTMS Protocol on Respiratory Neuroplasticity Following C2 Spinal Cord Hemisection in Rats

Pauline Michel-Flutot [1], Isley Jesus [1], Valentin Vanhee [1], Camille H. Bourcier [1,2], Laila Emam [2], Abderrahim Ouguerroudj [1], Kun-Ze Lee [3], Lyandysha V. Zholudeva [4], Michael A. Lane [5], Arnaud Mansart [2], Marcel Bonay [1] and Stéphane Vinit [1,*]

[1] Université Paris-Saclay, UVSQ, Inserm, END-ICAP, 78000 Versailles, France; pauline.michel78280@yahoo.fr (P.M.-F.); isleyj@yahoo.com.br (I.J.); valentin.vanhee.pro@gmail.com (V.V.); camille.bourcier@uvsq.fr (C.H.B.); ouguerroudj.a@gmail.com (A.O.); marcel.bonay@bch.aphp.fr (M.B.)
[2] Université Paris-Saclay, UVSQ, Inserm, Infection et Inflammation (2I), 78000 Versailles, France; laila.emam@uvsq.fr (L.E.); arnaud.mansart@uvsq.fr (A.M.)
[3] Department of Biological Sciences, National Sun Yat-sen University, Kaohsiung 80424, Taiwan; kzlee@mail.nsysu.edu.tw
[4] Gladstone Institutes, San Francisco, CA 94158, USA; lvzholudeva@gmail.com
[5] Marion Murray Spinal Cord Research Center, Department of Neurobiology and Anatomy, Drexel University College of Medicine, Philadelphia, PA 19129, USA; mlane.neuro@gmail.com
* Correspondence: stephane.vinit@uvsq.fr; Tel.: +33-170-429-427

Simple Summary: High spinal cord injuries (SCIs) are known to lead to permanent diaphragmatic paralysis, and to induce deleterious post-traumatic inflammatory processes following cervical spinal cord injury. We used a noninvasive therapeutic tool (repetitive transcranial magnetic stimulation (rTMS)), to harness plasticity in spared descending respiratory circuit and reduce the inflammatory processes. Briefly, the results obtained in this present study suggest that chronic high-frequency rTMS can ameliorate respiratory dysfunction and elicit neuronal plasticity with a reduction in deleterious post-traumatic inflammatory processes in the cervical spinal cord post-SCI. Thus, this therapeutic tool could be adopted and/or combined with other therapeutic interventions in order to further enhance beneficial outcomes.

Abstract: High spinal cord injuries (SCIs) lead to permanent diaphragmatic paralysis. The search for therapeutics to induce functional motor recovery is essential. One promising noninvasive therapeutic tool that could harness plasticity in a spared descending respiratory circuit is repetitive transcranial magnetic stimulation (rTMS). Here, we tested the effect of chronic high-frequency (10 Hz) rTMS above the cortical areas in C2 hemisected rats when applied for 7 days, 1 month, or 2 months. An increase in intact hemidiaphragm electromyogram (EMG) activity and excitability (diaphragm motor evoked potentials) was observed after 1 month of rTMS application. Interestingly, despite no real functional effects of rTMS treatment on the injured hemidiaphragm activity during eupnea, 2 months of rTMS treatment strengthened the existing crossed phrenic pathways, allowing the injured hemidiaphragm to increase its activity during the respiratory challenge (i.e., asphyxia). This effect could be explained by a strengthening of respiratory descending fibers in the ventrolateral funiculi (an increase in GAP-43 positive fibers), sustained by a reduction in inflammation in the C1–C3 spinal cord (reduction in CD68 and Iba1 labeling), and acceleration of intracellular plasticity processes in phrenic motoneurons after chronic rTMS treatment. These results suggest that chronic high-frequency rTMS can ameliorate respiratory dysfunction and elicit neuronal plasticity with a reduction in deleterious post-traumatic inflammatory processes in the cervical spinal cord post-SCI. Thus, this therapeutic tool could be adopted and/or combined with other therapeutic interventions in order to further enhance beneficial outcomes.

Citation: Michel-Flutot, P.; Jesus, I.; Vanhee, V.; Bourcier, C.H.; Emam, L.; Ouguerroudj, A.; Lee, K.-Z.; Zholudeva, L.V.; Lane, M.A.; Mansart, A.; et al. Effects of Chronic High-Frequency rTMS Protocol on Respiratory Neuroplasticity Following C2 Spinal Cord Hemisection in Rats. *Biology* 2022, 11, 473. https://doi.org/10.3390/biology11030473

Academic Editors: Cédric G. Geoffroy and Warren Alilain

Received: 14 February 2022
Accepted: 16 March 2022
Published: 19 March 2022

Publisher's Note: MDPI stays neutral with regard to jurisdictional claims in published maps and institutional affiliations.

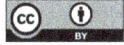

Copyright: © 2022 by the authors. Licensee MDPI, Basel, Switzerland. This article is an open access article distributed under the terms and conditions of the Creative Commons Attribution (CC BY) license (https://creativecommons.org/licenses/by/4.0/).

Keywords: spinal cord injury; repetitive transcranial magnetic stimulation; phrenic motor network; neuroplasticity; motoneuron excitability; diaphragm muscle

1. Introduction

High spinal cord injuries (SCIs) induce long-lasting neuromotor deficits, such as respiratory insufficiency [1]. Patients living with such injuries often rely on ventilatory assistance to survive, although some can be weaned off with time, exemplifying spontaneous plasticity. The rodent C2 hemisection (C2HS) model is one of the most common preclinical models to study respiratory system neuroplasticity and neuroinflammation. A C2HS disrupts descending input to ipsilateral phrenic motoneurons that innervate the diaphragm, the main inspiratory muscle, thus resulting in diaphragm hemiplegia [2–10]. The contralateral side remains intact, allowing the animal to survive.

Limited spontaneous recovery of the injured hemidiaphragm activity is observed in this model of SCI, characterized by a partial reactivation of phrenic motor networks and diaphragm activities. This reactivation is sustained by normally silent respiratory pathways crossing the spinal midline at the C3–C6 spinal cord levels, called the crossed phrenic phenomenon (CPP) [11–14]. However, this marginal spontaneous plasticity is too weak to contribute to significant ventilatory recovery following C2HS [15]. Strengthening the CPP and providing new intraspinal connections to the denervated motoneurons is a potential target for developing novel therapeutic tools in order to further improve respiratory function following high SCI.

A noninvasive approach to stimulate neural activity is transcranial magnetic stimulation (TMS), which involves applying a high output magnetic field above the neuronal areas. In fact, TMS applied as a single pulse or in a repetitive way (rTMS) is a noninvasive and painless method already used in the clinic to diagnose and treat many disorders [16–20], as well as a potential therapeutic tool in preclinical models of cognitive impairment [21,22]. This technique operates through its neuromodulatory effects on neuronal circuitry [23,24]. The potential of rTMS to improve outcomes following incomplete SCI has gained recognition in the past few years but has mainly been applied to enhance locomotor recovery [25–27] and sensorimotor restoration [27–29] in preclinical models of SCI.

We recently demonstrated that a single train of TMS delivered above the animals' motor threshold can induce a long-lasting increase in phrenic system excitability, as measured with diaphragm motor evoked potentials (MEPdia) [30]. While this study was focused on determining stimulation parameters in naïve, anesthetized rats, it demonstrated that MEPdia can be used as a reliable and reproducible technique for assessing phrenic system excitability during TMS [31–34]. While there is interest in the therapeutic potential of rTMS following SCI among researchers, little is known about the cellular and molecular mechanisms that sustain the neuromodulatory effects of acute or chronic rTMS. A few in vivo and in vitro studies have been conducted to elucidate potential cellular mechanisms [35–38], including excitatory neurotransmission via N-methyl-D-aspartic acid (NMDA) and α-amino-3-hydroxy-5-méthylisoxazol-4-propionate (AMPA) (GluR1 subunit) receptor pathways [37,39,40], and inhibitory neurotransmission via γ-aminobutyric acid (GABA) system [41,42]. For example, rTMS protocols can modulate the expression of neuronal activity markers such as c-fos. Low-frequency repetitive magnetic stimulation (rMS) has been shown to increase nuclear, neuronal c-fos expression in rat organotypic cortex brain slices [43], whereas rTMS theta-burst stimulation resulted in decreased neuronal c-fos expression [38]. In addition, repetitive magnetic stimulation (rMS) protocol on SH-SY5Y neuroblastoma cells induced an increase in cAMP and phospho-CREB expression [44]. In vivo, protocols using high-frequency repetitive trans-spinal magnetic stimulation (rTSMS) also resulted in reduced expression of markers for apoptosis and neuronal death, while the expression of markers of axonal growth and neuronal proliferation were upregulated. These results were accompanied by reduced axonal demyelination [45]. A deeper understanding of rTMS-regulated molecular signaling pathways following SCI could, therefore, help to harness the potential beneficial effects of rTMS as a therapeutic intervention.

The putative effects of rTMS on neuroinflammation are also of great interest. A few studies have used rMS on glial cells, but its effects are diverse and depend on the stimulation parameters used and the model studied [46]. Chronic low-frequency rTMS used on naive rats did not induce observable changes in astrocyte and microglial density, supporting the safety of this protocol regarding glial cell homeostasis in the normal/control condition [47]. However, conflicting results have been observed in in vivo studies. For instance, chronic high-frequency rTMS increased astrocytic and microglial density in a preclinical model of ischemia in gerbils (hippocampus) [48], whereas a decrease in cellular density in a preclinical model of T9 dorsal SCI (compression) [49]. In addition, some studies also showed a beneficial neuroinflammatory effect, observed through the decreased release of TNFα (proinflammatory cytokine) in substantia nigra in a model of Parkinson's disease [50,51].

To our knowledge, there have been no studies investigating the potential therapeutic effects of high-frequency rTMS on impaired respiratory function following cervical SCI, specifically at the phrenic circuit level. The present study aimed to test the hypothesis that chronic 10 Hz rTMS can improve respiratory function after SCI. Here, we test this hypothesis using cellular, molecular, and electrophysiological outcome measures to assess the potential therapeutic benefits of rTMS in a preclinical model of C2HS in adult, Sprague Dawley rats.

2. Materials and Methods

2.1. Ethics Statement

Adult Sprague Dawley male rats (Janvier, France; n = 41, 350–450 g) were used for this study. Experiments were approved by the Ethics Committee of the University of Versailles Saint-Quentin-en-Yvelines and complied with the French and European laws (EU Directive 2010/63/EU) regarding animal experimentation (Apafis #2017111516297308_v3).

Animals were dually housed in ventilated cages in a state-of-the-art animal care facility (2CARE animal facility, accreditation A78-322-3, France) on a 12 h light–dark cycle, with access to food and water ad libitum.

2.2. Chronic C2 Hemisection

2.2.1. Intrapleural CTB Injection and Surgery

Prior to anesthesia, animals were premedicated subcutaneously with buprenorphine (Buprécare, 0.03 mg/kg), trimethoprim, and sulfadoxine (Borgal 24%, 30 mg/kg), medetomidine (Médétor, 0.1 mg/kg) and carprofen (Rimadyl, 5 mg/kg). 10 min after the injections, animals were anesthetized with isoflurane (5% in 100% O_2) in a closed chamber. Rats were then intubated and ventilated with a rodent ventilator (model 683; Harvard Apparatus, South Natick, MA, USA), and anesthesia was maintained throughout the surgical procedure with isoflurane (2.5% in 100% O_2). For phrenic motoneuron retrograde labeling, intrapleural injections of cholera toxin B fragment were performed bilaterally in all animals (15 µL/side) using a custom needle (6 mm, 23 gauge, semi-blunt to avoid puncturing of the lung) and a 50 µL Hamilton syringe as described previously [52]. After skin and muscles were retracted, laminectomy and durotomy were performed at the C2 level. The spinal cord was then sectioned unilaterally (left side) with microscissors. To ensure the section of potentially remaining fibers, a microscalpel was used immediately after microscissors, as described previously [7].

2.2.2. Brainstem Neuronal Retrograde Labeling with Hydroxystilbamidine

For respiratory brainstem neuronal retrograde labeling, a sterilized piece of cotton was impregnated with 2 µL of 7% hydroxystilbamidine (Fluorogold) and left into the injury site for 20 min. Then, the lesion site was flushed with sterilized saline, and muscles and skin were then sutured closed. To reverse medetomidine-induced anesthesia, atipamezole (Revertor, 0.5 mg/kg) was intramuscularly injected. Isoflurane anesthesia was then turned off, and the endotracheal tube was removed when animals showed signs of wakefulness. All animals were kept 7 days postsurgery in their cage to recover before rTMS or Sham rTMS protocol was applied.

2.3. Repetitive TMS (rTMS) Protocol

rTMS protocol was performed using the magnetic stimulator MAGPRO R30 (Magventure, Farum, Denmark) connected to a figure-of-eight coil (Cool-B65), delivering a unique biphasic pulse with the intensity of the stimulus expressed as a percentage of a maximum output of the stimulator (% MO). The protocol (9 trains of 100 biphasic pulses, separated by 30 s intervals between trains delivered at 50% MO, 900 stimulations per protocol) was applied in awake restrained animals at −6 mm caudal to Bregma. This protocol induced a long-lasting increase in phrenic excitability in anesthetized, intact rats [30]. Control animals received a Sham rTMS protocol (e.g., no stimulation but the same time spent in the custom-designed restraining device, Figure 1). This rTMS protocol was applied 7 days postinjury for either 7 days (once a day), 1 month, or 2 months (once a day, 5 days per week) (Figure 1).

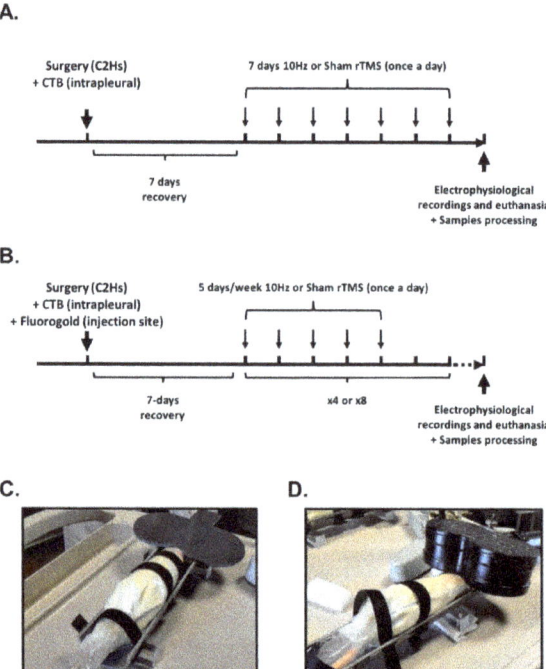

Figure 1. Protocols for 10 Hz or Sham rTMS following C2 spinal cord hemisection: (**A**) rTMS protocols for 7-day-treated groups; (**B**) rTMS protocols for 1-month- and 2-month-treated groups; (**C**) image of rat receiving Sham rTMS protocol; (**D**) image of rat receiving 10 Hz rTMS protocol.

2.4. Electrophysiological Recordings
2.4.1. Animal Preparation

Animals were randomly divided into 6 groups: 7-day Sham rTMS ($n = 8$); 7-day 10 Hz rTMS ($n = 9$); 1-month Sham rTMS ($n = 6$); 1-month 10 Hz rTMS ($n = 6$); 2-month Sham rTMS (*n* = 6); 2-month 10 Hz rTMS (*n* = 6). Electrophysiological recordings of diaphragm activity and excitability were used to functionally evaluate the effects of rTMS treatment on the phrenic motor circuit after completion of sham or 10 Hz rTMS. Briefly, anesthesia was induced using isoflurane (5% in 21% O_2 balanced) in an anesthesia chamber and maintained through a nose cone (2.5% in 100% air balanced). Animals were tracheotomized and pump-ventilated (Rodent Ventilator, model 683; Harvard Apparatus, South Natick, MA, USA). The ventilation rate (frequency > 72 breaths per minute, tidal volume: 2.5 mL) was adjusted to reduce the end-tidal CO_2 value below the animals' central apneic threshold throughout the experiment to avoid recording spontaneous diaphragm contractions. During the recordings, animals were placed on a heating pad to maintain a constant body temperature (37.5 ± 0.5 °C), and their rectal temperature was continuously monitored throughout the experiment. Arterial pressure was measured through a catheter inserted into the right femoral artery. Arterial and tracheal pressures were monitored continuously with transducers connected to a bridge amplifier (AD Instruments, Dunedin, New Zealand). The depth of anesthesia was confirmed by the absence of response to toe pinch. A laparotomy was performed, and the liver was gently moved dorsally to access the diaphragm. Gauze soaked with warm phosphate-buffered saline was placed on the liver to prevent dehydration. Both sides (ipsilateral and contralateral to the spinal cord lesion) of the diaphragm were implanted with two custom-made hooked bipolar electrodes into each mid-costal part of the diaphragm and left in place for the duration of the experiment for the measurement of (1) spontaneous diaphragm EMG during spontaneous poïkilocapnic normoxic or transient mild asphyxia breathing (by occlusion of the animal's nose for 15 s after disconnection of a tracheal tube from the ventilator) and (2) diaphragm MEP when $PETCO_2$ was below the apneic threshold.

2.4.2. Diaphragmatic EMG Recordings

EMGs were amplified (Model 1800; gain, 100; A-M Systems, Everett, WA, USA) and band pass-filtered (100 Hz to 10 kHz). The signals were digitized with an 8-channel Powerlab data acquisition device (Acquisition rate: 4 k/s; AD Instruments, Dunedin, New Zealand), connected to a computer, and analyzed using LabChart 7 Pro software (AD Instruments, Dunedin, New Zealand). The bilateral diaphragmatic EMGs were integrated (50 ms decay).

2.4.3. Diaphragmatic MEP Recordings

Next, the head of the animal was placed on a nonmagnetic, custom-made stereotaxic apparatus, which allowed its positioning from the center of the figure-of-eight coil to −6 mm from Bregma, at an angle of 0°, as previously described [30,31]. MEPdia induced by a single pulse of TMS was recorded (summation of 5 to 10 TMS pulses between 2 heartbeats, max 10 trials at 90% MO). These electromyographic signals were amplified (gain, 1 k; A-M Systems, Everett, WA, USA) and band pass-filtered (100 Hz to 10 kHz). The signals were then digitized with an 8-channel Powerlab data acquisition device (Acquisition rate: 100 k/s; AD Instruments, Dunedin, New Zealand) connected to a computer and analyzed using LabChart 8 Pro software (AD Instruments, Dunedin, New Zealand).

2.5. Tissue Processing

At the end of the experiment, animals were euthanized by intracardiac injection of pentobarbital (EXAGON, Axience), intracardially perfused with heparinized 0.9% NaCl (10 mL), followed by Antigenfix solution (DIAPATH). After perfusion, the C1–C6 spinal cord and brainstem were carefully dissected and stored at 4 °C in fixative for 24 h. After postfixation, tissues were cryoprotected for 48 h in 30% sucrose (in 0.9% NaCl), and stored at −80 °C. Frozen longitudinal (C1–C3 spinal cord) and transverse (C3–C6 spinal cord and brainstem) free-floating sections (30 µm) were cut using a Thermo Fisher cryostat. C1–C3, C3–C6, and brainstem sections were stored in a cryoprotectant solution (Sucrose 30%, ethylene glycol 30%, and PVP40 1% in PBS 1×) at −22 °C. Every fifth section from

C1–C3 was used for lesion reconstruction to examine the extent of C2 injury using cresyl violet histochemistry.

2.6. Histological Reconstruction of the Extent of C2 Injury

Longitudinal sections from the C1–C3 cord were used to assess the dorsoventral and mediolateral extent of injury in all animals. Brightfield microscopy was used to examine the cresyl violet-stained sections and recorded on a stereotaxic transverse plane of the C2 spinal cord. Each injury was then digitized and analyzed with ImageJ software (NIH). The extent of the injury on the injured side was calculated using a reference to a complete hemisection (which is 100% of the hemicord) and reported as a percentage (Figure 2), as described in our previous publication [7].

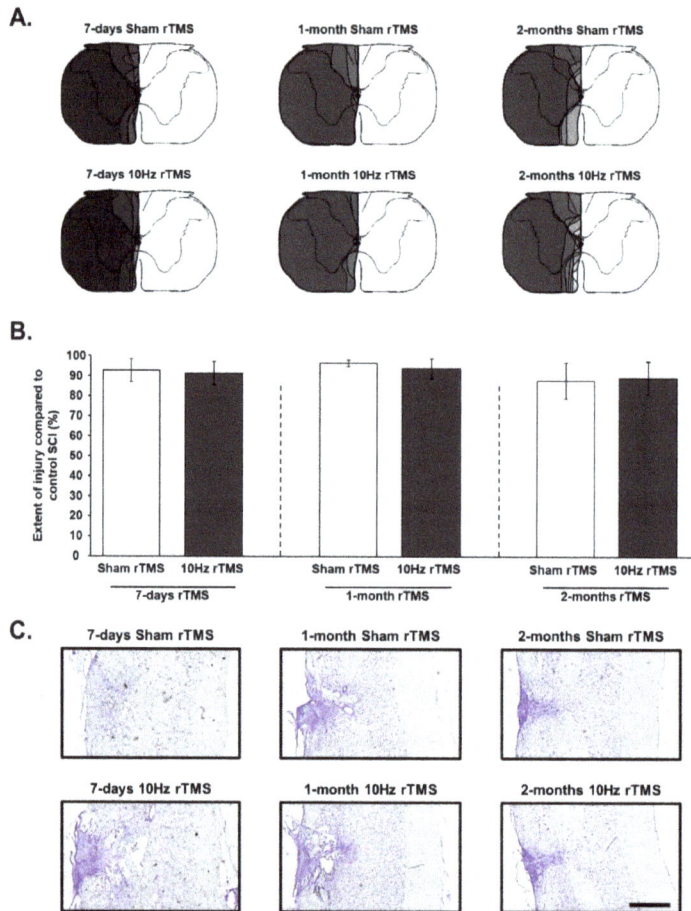

Figure 2. Extent of injury following a C2 spinal cord hemisection: (**A**) representative schematic diagrams of the extent of injury in each animal at 15 days postinjury (P.I.) for 7-day Sham and 10 Hz rTMS groups, 36 days P.I. for 1-month Sham and 10 Hz rTMS groups, and 64 days P.I. for 2-month Sham and 10 Hz rTMS groups; (**B**) extent of injury quantification in percentage compared with control spinal cord injury (SCI) 100%. The quantification has been made only in the ventral part where the phrenic motoneurons are located. There is no difference between the different groups (One Way ANOVA, $p = 0.235$); (**C**) representative image for each group stained in cresyl violet. Scale Bar: 1 mm.

2.7. Immunofluorescence

For immunofluorescence experiments, free-floating transverse sections of the C3–C6 spinal cord and brainstem were washed and placed in blocking solution (NDS 5% in PBS 1×) for 30 min and then incubated with the corresponding antibody in blocking solution (NDS 5%) overnight on an orbital shaker at 4 °C. After several PBS washes, sections were incubated in the corresponding secondary antibody for 2 h at room temperature, then washed again with PBS. The following primary antibodies were used: cholera toxin, B-subunit (CTB, Calbiochem, Saint-Quentin-Fallavier, France, 1/1000, goat polyclonal), CREB (Sigma, Saint-Quentin-Fallavier, France, 1/2000, rabbit polyclonal), GAP-43 (Sigma, Saint-Quentin-Fallavier, France, 1/2000, mouse monoclonal), nitric oxide synthase II (iNOS, Millipore-Merck, Guyancourt, France, 1/3000, rabbit polyclonal), CD68 (Millipore-Merck, Guyancourt, France, 1/300, mouse monoclonal), Iba1 (Abcam, Paris, France, 1/400, goat polyclonal), phospho-c-Jun (Ser63) II (Cell Signaling, Saint-Cyr-L'Ecole, France, 1/200, rabbit polyclonal), and GFAP (Millipore-Merck, Guyancourt, France, 1/4000, rabbit polyclonal). The secondary antibodies were linked to the fluorochromes Alexa Fluor 488, 594 (Molecular Probes, Illkirch, France, 1/2000) or 647 (Invitrogen, Illkirch, France, 1/2000). Biotinylated wisteria floribunda lectin (WFA, Vector laboratories, Les Ulis, France, 1/2000) with Alexa Fluor 488 Avidin (Molecular Probes, Illkirch, France, 1/1000) were used to labeled chondroitin sulfate proteoglycans (CSPGs). Images of the different sections were captured with a Hamamatsu ORCA-R^2 camera mounted on an Olympus IX83 P2ZF microscope or a 3dhistech panoramic slide scanner. Images were analyzed using ImageJ 1.53n software (NIH, USA).

2.8. Data Processing and Statistical Analyses

The amplitude (normalized to the corresponding sham group in arbitrary units, AU) of at least 5 double-integrated diaphragm EMG inspiratory bursts during normoxia and mild asphyxia was calculated for each animal from the injured and the intact sides with LabChart 7 Pro software (AD Instruments). Diaphragm MEP traces for each side (at least 5 MEPdia) were averaged and superimposed using LabChart Pro software (AD Instruments). The baseline-to-peak amplitude of the first wave of each superimposed MEPdia was calculated.

One-way ANOVA was performed between different groups for the extent of injury evaluation. Comparisons between intact and injured sides for diaphragmatic EMG and MEP and between eupnea and asphyxia for diaphragmatic EMG were performed by Student's paired t-test. Two-way ANOVA (Fisher LSD Method for multiple comparisons) was used to compare MEPdia throughout the experiment and between different rTMS protocols. Student's t-tests were used to compare values of the same side (intact or injured) between the different protocols (between 7-day, 1-month, and 2-month Sham rTMS or between 7-day, 1-month, and 2-month 10 Hz rTMS) and to compare Sham and 10 Hz rTMS group values for the same time point (at 7 days, 1 month, and 2 months). Paired t-tests were used to compare data from intact and injured sides of the same animal.

All data are presented as mean ± SD, and statistics were considered significant when $p < 0.05$. SigmaPlot 12.5 software was used for all analyses.

3. Results

3.1. rTMS-Induced Effects on Diaphragm Activity during Eupnea

Diaphragm activity was assessed by recording EMGdia amplitude for both intact and injured sides (Figure 3A). A reduction in EMGdia amplitude was observed 15 days postinjury (P.I.) for the injured side (7-day Sham rTMS = 0.06 ± 0.08 μV.s.s), compared with intact side (0.54 ± 0.20 μV.s.s, $p < 0.001$). This reduced diaphragm activity persisted for the injured side in Sham rTMS-treated animals at 36 days P.I. (0.00 ± 0.00 μV.s.s) and 64 days P.I. (0.03 ± 0.04 μV.s.s) ($p > 0.05$). The 10 Hz rTMS protocol did not induce a significant change in EMGdia amplitude on the side of the injury at any experimental time point (7 days: 0.01 ± 0.02 μV.s.s; 1-month rTMS: 0.01 ± 0.03 μV.s.s; 2-month rTMS: 0.03 ± 0.03 μV.s.s). For the intact side, no differences in diaphragm activity were observed between Sham rTMS group (0.54 ± 0.20 µV.s.s) and 10 Hz rTMS group (0.51 ± 0.21 µV.s.s) following 7 days of stimulation ($p = 0.772$). However, following 1 month of rTMS, 10 Hz treated animals (0.63 ± 0.15 µV.s.s) presented a significantly higher EMGdia amplitude, compared with Sham-treated animals (0.45 ± 0.10 µV.s.s, $p = 0.011$). After 2 months of rTMS, this difference between Sham-treated animals (0.67 ± 0.14 µV.s.s) and 10 Hz treated animals (0.64 ± 0.12 µV.s.s) disappeared ($p = 0.656$) due to an increase in EMGdia amplitude between 1 month (0.45 ± 0.10 µV.s.s) and 2 months (0.67 ± 0.14 µV.s.s) in the Sham group ($p = 0.039$) (Figure 3B).

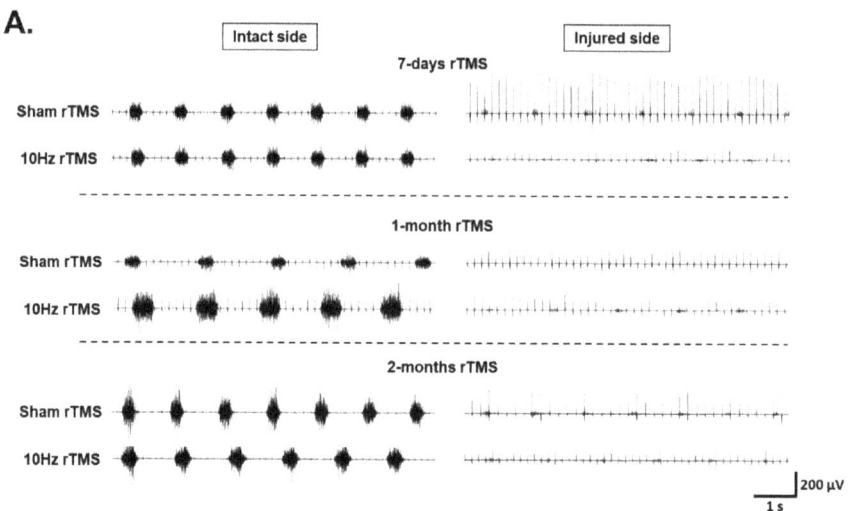

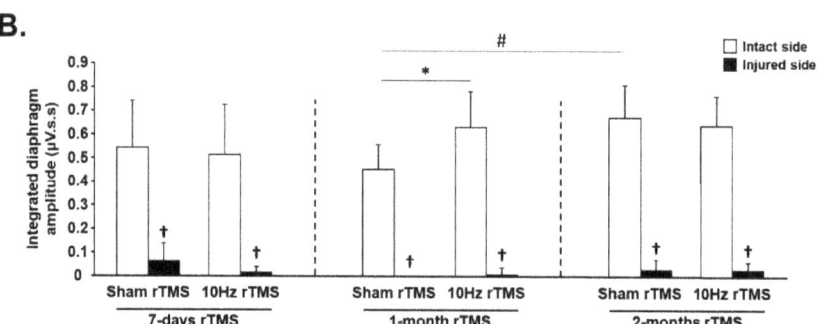

Figure 3. Diaphragm activity in C2 hemisected rats following chronic Sham and 10 Hz rTMS: (A) representative traces of raw diaphragm EMG of C2 hemisected rats, following 7-day, 1-month, or 2-month Sham or 10 Hz rTMS treatment; (B) integrated diaphragm amplitude for intact and injured sides of Sham or 10 Hz rTMS treated C2 hemisected animals following 7 days, 1 month, or 2 months of treatment. † $p < 0.001$, compared with intact side; * $p = 0.011$, intact side of Sham rTMS group vs. intact side of 10 Hz rTMS group following 1-month treatment. # $p = 0.039$, intact side of Sham rTMS group following 1-month treatment vs. corresponding group following 2 months of treatment.

3.2. rTMS-Induced Effects on Diaphragm Muscle Response to Respiratory Challenge

In addition to analyzing diaphragm activity during eupneic breathing, muscle activity was also analyzed during respiratory challenges (i.e., mild asphyxia). When challenged with mild asphyxia, there was no significant change in EMGdia amplitude, compared with eupneic breathing on the intact side at 7 days in Sham-treated animals, and 7-day and 1-month 10 Hz rTMS groups (Figure 4A,B,D, respectively). EMGdia on the intact side, however, significantly decreased with mild asphyxia challenge, compared to eupneic breathing, in 1- and 2-month Sham-treated groups, as well as the 2-month 10 Hz rTMS group (Figure 4C,E,F, respectively). In contrast, EMGdia on the injured side significantly increased with 10 Hz rTMS 2 months poststimulation (Figure 4F). No other statistically significant differences were observed.

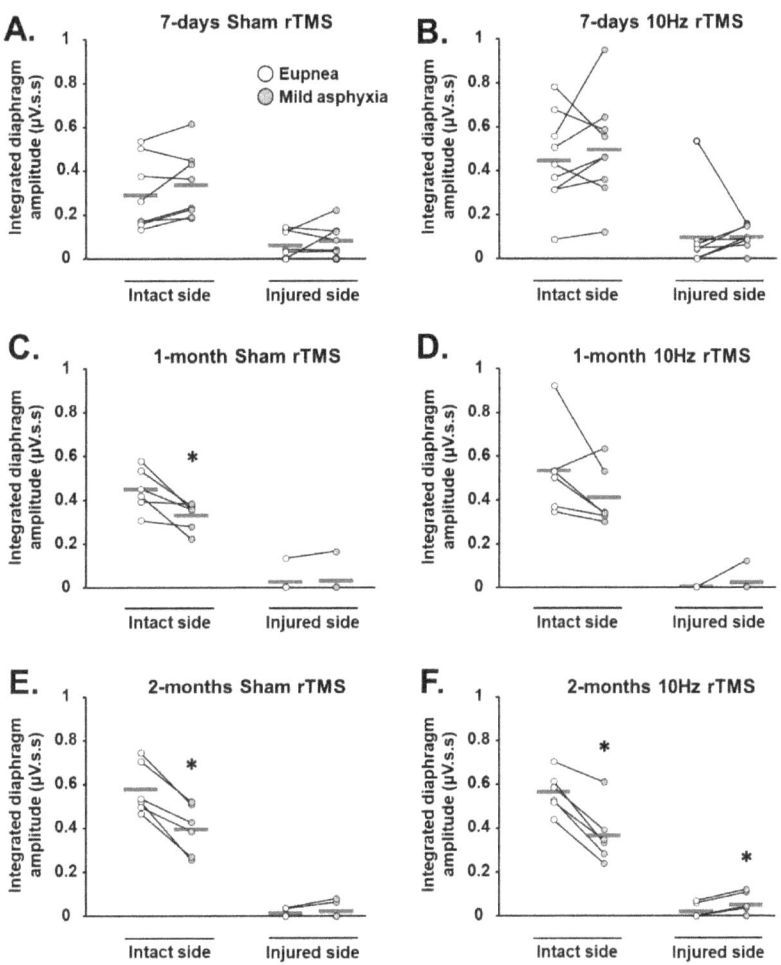

Figure 4. Diaphragm activity in C2 hemisected rats following chronic Sham and 10 Hz rTMS during respiratory challenge: integrated diaphragm amplitude for (**A**) 7-day Sham, (**B**) 7-day 10 Hz rTMS, (**C**) 1-month Sham, (**D**) 1-month 10 Hz rTMS, (**E**) 2-month Sham, and (**F**) 2-month 10 Hz rTMS groups in eupnea and during mild asphyxia. * $p < 0.05$ mild asphyxia, compared with eupnea (paired *t*-test). The red short line represent the mean value.

3.3. rTMS-Induced Effects on Phrenic System Excitability

MEPdia amplitudes were measured in response to a single pulse of TMS to evaluate phrenic excitability following rTMS protocols (Figure 5A). Significant differences in response were seen only between Sham-treated animals on the intact side from 1 to 2 months postinjury (MEPdia increased), and between intact and injured sides of Sham-treated animals at 1 month, with the injured side being significantly greater (Figure 5B). No other statistically significant differences were observed.

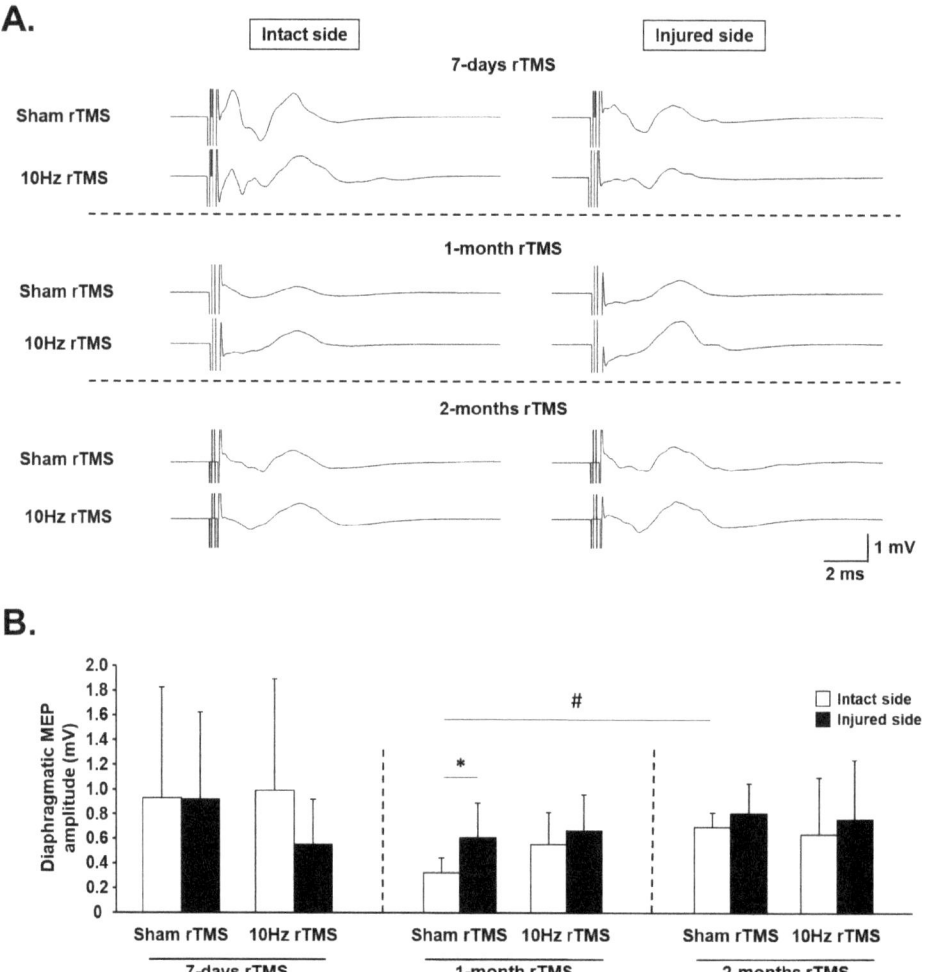

Figure 5. Diaphragm excitability in C2 hemisected rats following chronic Sham and 10 Hz rTMS: (**A**) representative traces of raw diaphragm MEP of C2 hemisected rats, following 7 days, 1 month, or 2 months of Sham or 10 Hz rTMS treatment; (**B**) MEP amplitude for intact and injured sides of Sham- or 10 Hz rTMS-treated C2 hemisected animals following 7 days, 1 month, or 2 months of treatment. * $p = 0.028$, intact side vs. injured side of Sham rTMS group following 1-month treatment. # $p < 0.001$, intact side of Sham rTMS group following 1-month treatment vs. corresponding group following 2 months of treatment.

3.4. rTMS-Induced Effects on Plasticity Markers in C3–C6 Spinal Cord

The expression of plasticity markers CREB and GAP-43 was evaluated at the C3–C6 spinal cord, the anatomical location of the phrenic motoneuron nucleus (Figure 6A). The percentage of cholera toxin beta (CTB, Figure 6A)-labeled phrenic motoneurons expressing CREB (Figure S1A) was significantly reduced for the intact side after 1 month of Sham or 10 Hz rTMS. In contrast, a reduction in CREB expression was seen on the injured side only in those animals treated with 10 Hz rTMS for 1 month (Figure 6B).

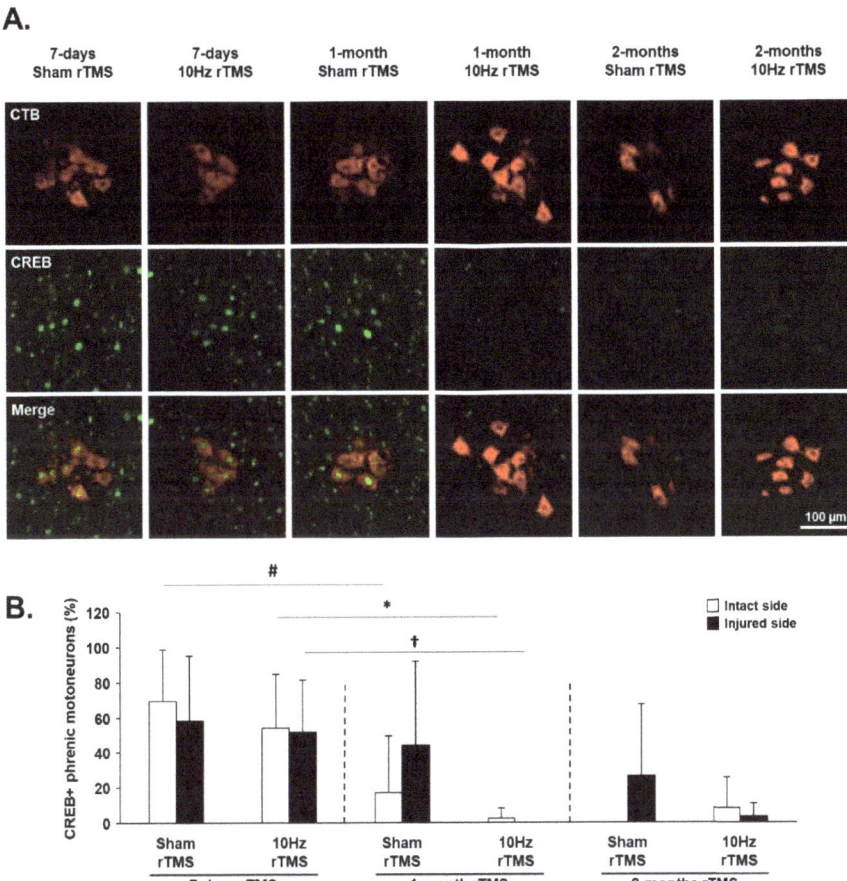

Figure 6. CREB expression in phrenic motoneurons following C2 hemisection: (**A**) representative images showing expression of CREB in denervated phrenic motoneurons labeled with CTB in C2 hemisected rats, following 7 days, 1 month or 2 months of Sham or 10 Hz rTMS treatment; (**B**) quantification of the percentage of CREB expressing phrenic motoneurons for intact and injured sides of Sham- or 10 Hz rTMS-treated C2 hemisected animals following 7 days, 1 month, or 2 months of treatment. There is no difference between the intact and the injured sides for the different groups (paired *t*-test for intact vs. injured side, $p > 0.05$); # 7-day Sham rTMS intact side, compared with 1-month Sham rTMS intact side, $p = 0.012$. * 7-day 10 Hz rTMS intact side, compared with 1-month 10 Hz rTMS intact side, $p = 0.007$. † 7-day 10 Hz rTMS injured side, compared with 1-month 10 Hz rTMS injured side, $p = 0.004$.

GAP-43 is normally synthesized in axonal growth cones; therefore, changes in GAP-43 immunofluorescence were evaluated in the phrenic motoneuron area in the C3–C6 spinal cord (Figure S1B and Figure 7A). The area labeled by antibodies against GAP-43 increased on the side of the injury 1 month after 10 Hz rTMS. No other significant differences were observed at any experimental time point on the intact or injured side (Figure 7B). Although there was significantly less GAP-43 labeling on the injured side, compared with the intact side in the ventrolateral funiculi of the spinal cord, no significant differences were seen between Sham- or 10 Hz treated animals across any of the time points exampled (Figure S2).

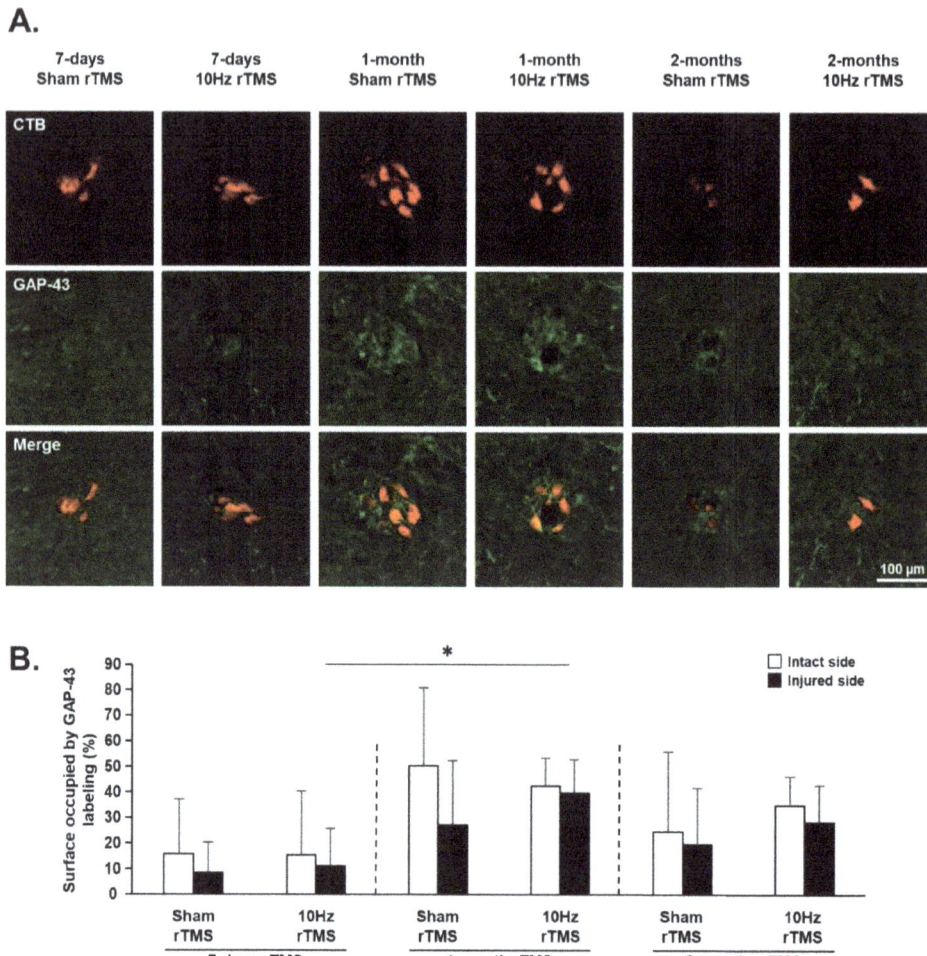

Figure 7. GAP-43 expression approximate to phrenic motoneurons following C2 hemisection: (**A**) representative images showing the surface occupied by GAP-43 labeling around denervated phrenic motoneurons labeled with CTB in C2 hemisected rats, following 7 days, 1 month, or 2 months of Sham or 10 Hz rTMS treatment; (**B**) quantification of the area occupied by GAP-43 labeling approximate to phrenic motoneurons on the intact and injured sides of Sham or 10 Hz rTMS-treated C2 hemisected animals following 7 days, 1 month, or 2 months of treatment. There is no difference between the intact and the injured sides for the different groups (paired t-test for intact vs. injured side, $p > 0.05$; * 7-day 10 Hz rTMS compared with 1-month 10 Hz rTMS for the injured side (Student's t-test, $p = 0.017$).

There was no difference in the expression of iNOS, which produces the reactive oxygen species nitric oxide, in phrenic motoneurons despite their denervation in any of the groups (Figure S3). There was also no difference in p-c-Jun and CREB expression in Fluorogold positive identified rostral ventral respiratory group (rVRG) neurons on the side of the injury when compared between 1 and 2 months of Sham or 10 Hz rTMS treatment (Figures S4 and S5, respectively), nor were there differences in CSPG expression in the rVRG (Figure S6).

3.5. rTMS-Induced Effects on Neuroinflammation

Immunohistochemistry against Iba1 (microglia) and CD68 (macrophages) was used to evaluate neuroinflammation in the injured C1–C3 spinal cord following 1 month and 2 months of rTMS treatment (Figure S7A). For the injured side, the area occupied by Iba1 labeling was reduced in 1-month 10 Hz rTMS-treated animals ($10.72 \pm 5.73\%$), compared with 1-month Sham rTMS-treated animals ($23.74 \pm 8.45\%$; $p < 0.05$) between -345 μm and $+345$ μm from lesion epicenter, as well as between -690 μm and -345 μm from lesion epicenter (1-month 10 Hz rTMS: $13.72 \pm 9.42\%$ vs. 1-month Sham rTMS: $24.46 \pm 6.31\%$; $p < 0.05$) (Figure S7B). No difference in CD68 labeling on the side of the injury was observed between groups (Figure S7D). For the intact side, there was no difference in Iba1 labeling between groups (Figure S7C). However, the area occupied by CD68 positive cells was reduced in the 2-month 10 Hz rTMS group ($0.02 \pm 0.03\%$), compared with 2-month Sham rTMS ($0.33 \pm 0.39\%$; $p < 0.05$) between -345 μm and $+345$ μm from lesion epicenter (Figure S7E).

Immunohistochemistry against GFAP (astrocytes) and WFA (CSPGs) was used to evaluate any rTMS-induced changes in the astroglial border of the lesion (Figure S8A). No difference in GFAP immunofluorescence was detected on either the injured or the intact sides (Figure S8B,C). WFA labeling was reduced in 2-month 10 Hz rTMS ($9.04 \pm 3.42\%$), compared with 1-month 10 Hz rTMS-treated animals ($17.14 \pm 9.54\%$; $p < 0.05$) on the side of the injury (Figure S8D). No differences were observed in WFA immunofluorescence on the intact side (Figure S8E).

4. Discussion

The present study is the first to investigate the therapeutic effects of chronic rTMS for enhancing respiratory function following cervical spinal cord injury (SCI) in a preclinical model. Our previous study already demonstrated that a single acute delivery of 10 Hz rTMS in anesthetized rats induced an increase in phrenic network excitability [30]. This 10 Hz magnetic stimulation is recognized for its long-term potentiation (LTP)-like effect [42,52]. We, therefore, hypothesized that chronic delivery of this protocol would induce beneficial effects on respiratory recovery after cervical SCI.

Contrary to our expectations, the analysis of EMGdia recordings showed the application of chronic 10 Hz rTMS had no effect on diaphragm activity on the side of the injury during eupnea, regardless of the duration of treatment. Conversely, an increase in diaphragm activity on the intact side after 1 month of treatment in injured animals was observed. Nontreated animals reached an EMGdia amplitude similar to those of treated animals at 9 weeks postinjury. These results might suggest that chronic 10 Hz rTMS strengthens spared descending respiratory pathways, reflecting a recovery plateau. Indeed, between 4 and 8 weeks post-C2 hemisection, a plateau in diaphragm activity has been observed when treated with intermittent hypoxia [53]. A similar observation was also found when a chronic protocol of intermittent hypoxia was applied following C2 hemisection in rats on diaphragm activity, with no difference between treated animals and normoxic animals after 3 weeks of treatment (spontaneous recovery reaches a ceiling/plateau by that time postinjury) [54]. Additionally, consistent with MEPdia results, the intact hemidiaphragm could better compensate for the paralyzed hemidiaphragm. Indeed, animals treated with 10 Hz rTMS did not differ significantly in MEP amplitude over time in either intact or injured hemidiaphragm. In contrast, Sham-treated animals had a reduced amplitude for the intact side, compared with the injured side following 1 month of treatment, and similar to those of rTMS-treated rats after 2 months of treatment. These results suggest that excitability of spared phrenic motoneurons is reduced in Sham-treated animals, whereas rTMS treatment maintained basal excitability in these motoneurons. Moreover, at 2 months post-rTMS treatment, an increased response to asphyxia was observed on the injured side, whereas no response was observed in Sham-treated animals. This reflects a strengthening of the existing CPP, which is consistent with evidence for spontaneous CPP 3 months post-C2 hemisection but not seen at 7 days postinjury [5].

The reduction in CREB expression in phrenic motoneurons occurred earlier postinjury in treated animals, suggesting that CREB signaling may contribute to treatment-driven plasticity. Moreover, the reduction in CD68 positive cells on the intact side of the C1–C3 spinal cord could reflect the anti-inflammatory effect of rTMS treatment, which may also contribute to neuroplasticity. Consistent with this finding, others have shown a reduction in GFAP and Iba1 labeling, which correlated with increased neuronal plasticity after rTSMS treatment [45,55]. Although these effects correlate with neuroplastic processes, no change in CREB or p-c-Jun expression was observed in respiratory brainstem neurons (putative ventral respiratory column) on the side of the injury, despite these molecules being involved in synaptic plasticity and axonal regeneration [56].

The present study also demonstrated no significant change in GAP-43 expression within white matter regions with treatment. This raises the question as to whether neuroplasticity is being mediated by spinal networks, which many recruit spinal interneurons within the phrenic network. This would be consistent with injured mice [57] and rats [58,59] displaying increased connectivity of spinal interneurons after cervical spinal cord injury. Furthermore, stimulating activity within spinal networks has also been shown to increase spinal interneuron activity and plasticity [60]. Based on these prior results, it is likely that stimulation with rTMS may also drive a degree of plasticity within these same phrenic interneuronal networks. This could also explain why phrenic motor activity on the side of injury was increased during asphyxia 2 months after chronic rTMS. Indeed, this observation could be an indication of strengthening of the CPP involving both spared descending pathways and interneuronal connectivity.

In this study, we chose to specifically stimulate at the cortical level to target neuronal networks connected to brainstem respiratory centers. Previous studies using repetitive magnetic stimulation employed a thoracic model of SCI, applying magnetic stimulation at the side of injury. Studies in mice demonstrated that 10 Hz acute or chronic rTSMS improved locomotor function after thoracic injury [45,61], but a lower frequency (0.2 Hz) of rTSMS in rats did not [40]. However, when combining stimulation with growth factor delivery and activity-based therapy, improved functional effects were observed [40].

More invasive spinal stimulation approaches, such as intraspinal and epidural stimulation, have also been used to elicit spinal neural plasticity [62–65]. High-frequency epidural stimulation was used at the level of the phrenic motor nucleus (C4 segment) in C1-transected animals to induce short-term facilitation of the phrenic motor circuit [64]. This has been demonstrated within the denervated phrenic motor pool after C2HS in rats with increased growth factor expression (e.g., VEGF and BDNF) [66].

5. Conclusions

Even though epidural stimulation is a promising technique, it is surgically invasive, and accordingly, less invasive approaches than that used in the present study may be more readily applied in the clinic. Despite some promise with TMS, the results from the present study may reflect the fact that 10 Hz rTMS alone may be insufficient to stimulate significant functional diaphragmatic recovery. Combining the rTMS protocol employed in the present study with other therapeutic interventions (e.g., activity-based therapy [40,67]) may be more efficacious.

Supplementary Materials: The following are available online at https://www.mdpi.com/article/10.3390/biology11030473/s1, Figure S1: Representative C3–C6 spinal cord sections labeled for CTB and CREB or GAP-43, Figure S2: GAP-43 expression in C3–C6 ventrolateral funiculi following C2 hemisection, Figure S3: iNOS expression in phrenic motoneurons following C2 hemisection, Figure S4: p-c-Jun expression in injured rVRG neurons, Figure S5: CREB expression in injured rVRG neurons, Figure S6: CSPG expression in in the area around injured rVRG neurons, Figure S7: Iba1 and CD68 expression in the C1–C3 spinal cord following C2 hemisection, Figure S8: GFAP and WFA expression in the C1–C3 spinal cord following C2 hemisection.

Author Contributions: P.M.-F.: Conceptualization, experimental design, investigation, project administration, formal analysis, visualization, writing—original draft preparation. I.J.: investigation. V.V.: investigation. C.H.B.: investigation. L.E.: investigation. A.O.: investigation. K.-Z.L.: writing—review and editing. L.V.Z.: writing—review and editing. M.A.L.: writing—review and editing. A.M.: investigation, writing—review and editing. M.B.: writing—review and editing. S.V.: conceptualization, experimental design, investigation, supervision, project administration, funding acquisition, writing—review and editing. All authors have read and agreed to the published version of the manuscript.

Funding: This research was funded by the Chancellerie des Universités de Paris (Legs Poix) (SV, MB), the Fondation de France (SV), the Fondation Médisite (SV), INSERM (MB, SV, AM), Université de Versailles Saint-Quentin-en-Yvelines (SV, AM), the National Institutes of Health, NINDS, R01 NS104291 (MAL) and F32 NS119348 (LVZ), the Lisa Dean Moseley Foundation (MAL), and Ministry of Science and Technology 109-2636-B-110-001 (KZL). The supporters had no role in study design, data collection, and analysis, decision to publish, or preparation of the manuscript.

Institutional Review Board Statement: The study was conducted according to the guidelines of the Declaration of Helsinki, and approved by the Ethics Committee of the University of Versailles Saint-Quentin-en-Yvelines (Comité d'éthique n°047) and complied with the French and European laws (EU Directive 2010/63/EU) regarding animal experimentation (Apafis #2017111516297308_v3).

Informed Consent Statement: Not applicable.

Data Availability Statement: The data presented in this study are available on request from the corresponding author.

Acknowledgments: This study has benefited from the facilities of CYMAGES and histology (UFR SVS, UVSQ, Université Paris-Saclay, 78180 Montigny-le-Bretonneux, France).

Conflicts of Interest: The authors declare no conflict of interest.

References

1. Winslow, C.; Rozovsky, J. Effect of spinal cord injury on the respiratory system. *Am. J. Phys. Med. Rehabil.* **2003**, *82*, 803–814. [CrossRef] [PubMed]
2. Golder, F.J.; Reier, P.J.; Bolser, D.C. Altered respiratory motor drive after spinal cord injury: Supraspinal and bilateral effects of a unilateral lesion. *J. Neurosci.* **2001**, *21*, 8680–8689. [CrossRef]
3. Lane, M.A.; Lee, K.-Z.; Fuller, D.D.; Reier, P.J. Spinal circuitry and respiratory recovery following spinal cord injury. *Respir. Physiol. Neurobiol.* **2009**, *169*, 123–132. [CrossRef] [PubMed]
4. Vinit, S.; Gauthier, P.; Stamegna, J.C.; Kastner, A. High cervical lateral spinal cord injury results in long-term ipsilateral hemidiaphragm paralysis. *J. Neurotrauma* **2006**, *23*, 1137–1146. [CrossRef] [PubMed]
5. Vinit, S.; Kastner, A. Descending bulbospinal pathways and recovery of respiratory motor function following spinal cord injury. *Respir. Physiol. Neurobiol.* **2009**, *169*, 115–122. [CrossRef] [PubMed]
6. Alilain, W.J.; Horn, K.P.; Hu, H.; Dick, T.E.; Silver, J. Functional regeneration of respiratory pathways after spinal cord injury. *Nature* **2011**, *475*, 196–200. [CrossRef]
7. Keomani, E.; Deramaudt, T.B.; Petitjean, M.; Bonay, M.; Lofaso, F.; Vinit, S. A murine model of cervical spinal cord injury to study post-lesional respiratory neuroplasticity. *J. Vis. Exp.* **2014**, *87*, e51235. [CrossRef]
8. Porter, W.T. The Path of the Respiratory Impulse from the Bulb to the Phrenic Nuclei. *J. Physiol.* **1895**, *17*, 455–485. [CrossRef]
9. Nantwi, K.D.; El-Bohy, A.A.; Schrimsher, G.W.; Reier, P.J.; Goshgarian, H.G. Spontaneous Functional Recovery in a Paralyzed Hemidiaphragm Following Upper Cervical Spinal Cord Injury in Adult Rats. *Neurorehabil. Neural Repair* **1999**, *13*, 225–234. [CrossRef]
10. Lee, K.Z.; Huang, Y.J.; Tsai, I.L. Respiratory motor outputs following unilateral midcervical spinal cord injury in the adult rat. *J. Appl. Physiol.* **2014**, *116*, 395–405. [CrossRef]
11. Goshgarian, H.G. Invited Review: The crossed phrenic phenomenon: A model for plasticity in the respiratory pathways following spinal cord injury. *J. Appl. Physiol.* **2003**, *94*, 795–810. [CrossRef] [PubMed]
12. Ghali, M.G.Z. The crossed phrenic phenomenon. *Neural Regen. Res.* **2017**, *12*, 845–864. [CrossRef]
13. Goshgarian, H.G. The crossed phrenic phenomenon and recovery of function following spinal cord injury. *Respir. Physiol. Neurobiol.* **2009**, *169*, 85–93. [CrossRef] [PubMed]
14. Fuller, D.D.; Golder, F.J.; Olson, E.B., Jr.; Mitchell, G.S. Recovery of phrenic activity and ventilation after cervical spinal hemisection in rats. *J. Appl. Physiol.* **2006**, *100*, 800–806. [CrossRef]
15. Dougherty, B.J.; Lee, K.Z.; Lane, M.A.; Reier, P.J.; Fuller, D.D. Contribution of the spontaneous crossed-phrenic phenomenon to inspiratory tidal volume in spontaneously breathing rats. *J. Appl. Physiol.* **2012**, *112*, 96–105. [CrossRef] [PubMed]

16. Martin, D.M.; McClintock, S.M.; Forster, J.J.; Lo, T.Y.; Loo, C.K. Cognitive enhancing effects of rTMS administered to the prefrontal cortex in patients with depression: A systematic review and meta-analysis of individual task effects. *Depress. Anxiety* 2017, *34*, 1029–1039. [CrossRef]
17. Jassova, K.; Albrecht, J.; Ceresnakova, S.; Papezova, H.; Anders, M. Repetitive transcranial magnetic stimulation significantly influences the eating behavior in depressive patients. *Neuropsychiatr. Dis. Treat.* 2019, *15*, 2579–2586. [CrossRef]
18. McClintock, S.M.; Reti, I.M.; Carpenter, L.L.; McDonald, W.M.; Dubin, M.; Taylor, S.F.; Cook, I.A.; O'Reardon, J.; Husain, M.M.; Wall, C.; et al. Consensus Recommendations for the Clinical Application of Repetitive Transcranial Magnetic Stimulation (rTMS) in the Treatment of Depression. *J. Clin. Psychiatry* 2018, *79*, 3651. [CrossRef]
19. Yan, T.; Xie, Q.; Zheng, Z.; Zou, K.; Wang, L. Different frequency repetitive transcranial magnetic stimulation (rTMS) for posttraumatic stress disorder (PTSD): A systematic review and meta-analysis. *J. Psychiatr. Res.* 2017, *89*, 125–135. [CrossRef]
20. Kozel, F.A. Clinical Repetitive Transcranial Magnetic Stimulation for Posttraumatic Stress Disorder, Generalized Anxiety Disorder, and Bipolar Disorder. *Psychiatr. Clin. N. Am.* 2018, *41*, 433–446. [CrossRef]
21. Ma, Q.; Geng, Y.; Wang, H.L.; Han, B.; Wang, Y.Y.; Li, X.L.; Wang, L.; Wang, M.W. High Frequency Repetitive Transcranial Magnetic Stimulation Alleviates Cognitive Impairment and Modulates Hippocampal Synaptic Structural Plasticity in Aged Mice. *Front. Aging Neurosci.* 2019, *11*, 235. [CrossRef] [PubMed]
22. Wang, H.; Geng, Y.; Han, B.; Qiang, J.; Li, X.; Sun, M.; Wang, Q.; Wang, M. Repetitive transcranial magnetic stimulation applications normalized prefrontal dysfunctions and cognitive-related metabolic profiling in aged mice. *PLoS ONE* 2013, *8*, e81482. [CrossRef]
23. Kobayashi, M.; Pascual-Leone, A. Transcranial magnetic stimulation in neurology. *Lancet Neurol.* 2003, *2*, 145–156. [CrossRef]
24. Ziemann, U.; Paulus, W.; Nitsche, M.A.; Pascual-Leone, A.; Byblow, W.D.; Berardelli, A.; Siebner, H.R.; Classen, J.; Cohen, L.G.; Rothwell, J.C. Consensus: Motor cortex plasticity protocols. *Brain Stimul.* 2008, *1*, 164–182. [CrossRef]
25. Poirrier, A.L.; Nyssen, Y.; Scholtes, F.; Multon, S.; Rinkin, C.; Weber, G.; Bouhy, D.; Brook, G.; Franzen, R.; Schoenen, J. Repetitive Transcranial Magnetic Stimulation Improves Open Field Locomotor Recovery after Low but Not High Thoracic Spinal Cord Compression-Injury in Adult Rats. *J. Neurosci. Res.* 2004, *75*, 253–261. [CrossRef] [PubMed]
26. Marufa, S.A.; Hsieh, T.H.; Liou, J.C.; Chen, H.Y.; Peng, C.W. Neuromodulatory effects of repetitive transcranial magnetic stimulation on neural plasticity and motor functions in rats with an incomplete spinal cord injury: A preliminary study. *PLoS ONE* 2021, *16*, e0252965. [CrossRef]
27. Krishnan, V.S.; Shin, S.S.; Belegu, V.; Celnik, P.; Reimers, M.; Smith, K.R.; Pelled, G. Multimodal Evaluation of TMS—Induced Somatosensory Plasticity and Behavioral Recovery in Rats with Contusion Spinal Cord Injury. *Front. Neurosci.* 2019, *13*, 387. [CrossRef] [PubMed]
28. Ellaway, P.H.; Vásquez, N.; Craggs, M. Induction of central nervous system plasticity by repetitive transcranial magnetic stimulation to promote sensorimotor recovery in incomplete spinal cord injury. *Front. Integr. Neurosci.* 2014, *8*, 42. [CrossRef]
29. Petrosyan, H.A.; Alessi, V.; Sisto, S.A.; Kaufman, M.; Arvanian, V.L. Transcranial magnetic stimulation (TMS) responses elicited in hindlimb muscles as an assessment of synaptic plasticity in spino-muscular circuitry after chronic spinal cord injury. *Neurosci. Lett.* 2017, *642*, 37–42. [CrossRef]
30. Michel-Flutot, P.; Zholudeva, L.V.; Randelman, M.L.; Deramaudt, T.B.; Mansart, A.; Alvarez, J.-C.; Lee, K.-Z.; Petitjean, M.; Bonay, M.; Lane, M.A.; et al. High frequency repetitive Transcranial Magnetic Stimulation promotes long lasting phrenic motoneuron excitability via GABAergic networks. *Respir. Physiol. Neurobiol.* 2021, *292*, 103704. [CrossRef]
31. Vinit, S.; Keomani, E.; Deramaudt, T.B.; Spruance, V.M.; Bezdudnaya, T.; Lane, M.A.; Bonay, M.; Petitjean, M. Interdisciplinary approaches of transcranial magnetic stimulation applied to a respiratory neuronal circuitry model. *PLoS ONE* 2014, *9*, e113251. [CrossRef]
32. Vinit, S.; Keomani, E.; Deramaudt, T.B.; Bonay, M.; Petitjean, M. Reorganization of Respiratory Descending Pathways following Cervical Spinal Partial Section Investigated by Transcranial Magnetic Stimulation in the Rat. *PLoS ONE* 2016, *11*, e0148180. [CrossRef] [PubMed]
33. Lee, K.Z.; Liou, L.M.; Vinit, S.; Ren, M.Y. Rostral-Caudal Effect of Cervical Magnetic Stimulation on the Diaphragm Motor Evoked Potential after Cervical Spinal Cord Contusion in the Rat. *J. Neurotrauma* 2022. [CrossRef] [PubMed]
34. Lee, K.Z.; Liou, L.M.; Vinit, S. Diaphragm Motor-Evoked Potential Induced by Cervical Magnetic Stimulation following Cervical Spinal Cord Contusion in the Rat. *J. Neurotrauma* 2021, *38*, 2122–2140. [CrossRef] [PubMed]
35. Gersner, R.; Kravetz, E.; Feil, J.; Pell, G.; Zangen, A. Long-term effects of repetitive transcranial magnetic stimulation on markers for neuroplasticity: Differential outcomes in anesthetized and awake animals. *J. Neurosci. Off. J. Soc. Neurosci.* 2011, *31*, 7521–7526. [CrossRef] [PubMed]
36. Benali, A.; Trippe, J.; Weiler, E.; Mix, A.; Petrasch-Parwez, E.; Girzalsky, W.; Eysel, U.T.; Erdmann, R.; Funke, K. Theta-burst transcranial magnetic stimulation alters cortical inhibition. *J. Neurosci.* 2011, *31*, 1193–1203. [CrossRef]
37. Vlachos, A.; Muller-Dahlhaus, F.; Rosskopp, J.; Lenz, M.; Ziemann, U.; Deller, T. Repetitive magnetic stimulation induces functional and structural plasticity of excitatory postsynapses in mouse organotypic hippocampal slice cultures. *J. Neurosci.* 2012, *32*, 17514–17523. [CrossRef]
38. Volz, L.J.; Benali, A.; Mix, A.; Neubacher, U.; Funke, K. Dose-dependence of changes in cortical protein expression induced with repeated transcranial magnetic theta-burst stimulation in the rat. *Brain Stimul.* 2013, *6*, 598–606. [CrossRef]
39. Hunanyan, A.S.; Petrosyan, H.A.; Alessi, V.; Arvanian, V.L. Repetitive spinal electromagnetic stimulation opens a window of synaptic plasticity in damaged spinal cord: Role of NMDA receptors. *J. Neurophysiol.* 2012, *107*, 3027–3039. [CrossRef]

40. Petrosyan, H.A.; Alessi, V.; Hunanyan, A.S.; Sisto, S.A.; Arvanian, V.L. Spinal electro-magnetic stimulation combined with transgene delivery of neurotrophin NT-3 and exercise: Novel combination therapy for spinal contusion injury. *J. Neurophysiol.* **2015**, *114*, 2923–2940. [CrossRef]
41. Trippe, J.; Mix, A.; Aydin-Abidin, S.; Funke, K.; Benali, A. theta burst and conventional low-frequency rTMS differentially affect GABAergic neurotransmission in the rat cortex. *Exp. Brain Res.* **2009**, *199*, 411–421. [CrossRef]
42. Lenz, M.; Galanis, C.; Muller-Dahlhaus, F.; Opitz, A.; Wierenga, C.J.; Szabo, G.; Ziemann, U.; Deller, T.; Funke, K.; Vlachos, A. Repetitive magnetic stimulation induces plasticity of inhibitory synapses. *Nat. Commun.* **2016**, *7*, 10020. [CrossRef]
43. Hausmann, A.; Marksteiner, J.; Hinterhuber, H.; Humpel, C. Magnetic stimulation induces neuronal c-fos via tetrodotoxin-sensitive sodium channels in organotypic cortex brain slices of the rat. *Neurosci. Lett.* **2001**, *310*, 105–108. [CrossRef]
44. Hellmann, J.; Jüttner, R.; Roth, C.; Bajbouj, M.; Kirste, I.; Heuser, I.; Gertz, K.; Endres, M.; Kronenberg, G. Repetitive magnetic stimulation of human-derived neuron-like cells activates cAMP-CREB pathway. *Eur. Arch. Psychiatry Clin. Neurosci.* **2012**, *262*, 87–91. [CrossRef]
45. Chalfouh, C.; Guillou, C.; Hardouin, J.; Delarue, Q.; Li, X.; Duclos, C.; Schapman, D.; Marie, J.P.; Cosette, P.; Guérout, N. The Regenerative Effect of Trans-spinal Magnetic Stimulation After Spinal Cord Injury: Mechanisms and Pathways Underlying the Effect. *Neurotherapeutics* **2020**, *17*, 2069–2088. [CrossRef] [PubMed]
46. Cullen, C.L.; Young, K.M. How Does Transcranial Magnetic Stimulation Influence Glial Cells in the Central Nervous System? *Front. Neural Circuits* **2016**, *10*, 26. [CrossRef] [PubMed]
47. Liebetanz, D.; Fauser, S.; Michaelis, T.; Czéh, B.; Watanabe, T.; Paulus, W.; Frahm, J.; Fuchs, E. Safety aspects of chronic low-frequency transcranial magnetic stimulation based on localized proton magnetic resonance spectroscopy and histology of the rat brain. *J. Psychiatr. Res.* **2003**, *37*, 277–286. [CrossRef]
48. Rauš, S.; Selaković, V.; Manojlović-Stojanoski, M.; Radenović, L.; Prolić, Z.; Janać, B. Response of hippocampal neurons and glial cells to alternating magnetic field in gerbils submitted to global cerebral ischemia. *Neurotox. Res.* **2013**, *23*, 79–91. [CrossRef]
49. Kim, J.Y.; Choi, G.S.; Cho, Y.W.; Cho, H.; Hwang, S.J.; Ahn, S.H. Attenuation of spinal cord injury-induced astroglial and microglial activation by repetitive transcranial magnetic stimulation in rats. *J. Korean Med. Sci.* **2013**, *28*, 295–299. [CrossRef]
50. Yang, X.; Song, L.; Liu, Z. The effect of repetitive transcranial magnetic stimulation on a model rat of Parkinson's disease. *Neuroreport* **2010**, *21*, 268–272. [CrossRef]
51. Aftanas, L.I.; Gevorgyan, M.M.; Zhanaeva, S.Y.; Dzemidovich, S.S.; Kulikova, K.I.; Al'perina, E.L.; Danilenko, K.V.; Idova, G.V. Therapeutic Effects of Repetitive Transcranial Magnetic Stimulation (rTMS) on Neuroinflammation and Neuroplasticity in Patients with Parkinson's Disease: A Placebo-Controlled Study. *Bull. Exp. Biol. Med.* **2018**, *165*, 195–199. [CrossRef] [PubMed]
52. Lenz, M.; Platschek, S.; Priesemann, V.; Becker, D.; Willems, L.M.; Ziemann, U.; Deller, T.; Muller-Dahlhaus, F.; Jedlicka, P.; Vlachos, A. Repetitive magnetic stimulation induces plasticity of excitatory postsynapses on proximal dendrites of cultured mouse CA1 pyramidal neurons. *Brain Struct. Funct.* **2015**, *220*, 3323–3337. [CrossRef] [PubMed]
53. Doperalski, N.J.; Fuller, D.D. Long-term facilitation of ipsilateral but not contralateral phrenic output after cervical spinal cord hemisection. *Exp. Neurol.* **2006**, *200*, 74–81. [CrossRef] [PubMed]
54. Navarrete-Opazo, A.; Vinit, S.; Dougherty, B.J.; Mitchell, G.S. Daily acute intermittent hypoxia elicits functional recovery of diaphragm and inspiratory intercostal muscle activity after acute cervical spinal injury. *Exp. Neurol.* **2015**, *266*, 1–10. [CrossRef] [PubMed]
55. Robac, A.; Neveu, P.; Hugede, A.; Garrido, E.; Nicol, L.; Delarue, Q.; Guérout, N. Repetitive Trans Spinal Magnetic Stimulation Improves Functional Recovery and Tissue Repair in Contusive and Penetrating Spinal Cord Injury Models in Rats. *Biomedicines* **2021**, *9*, 1827. [CrossRef] [PubMed]
56. Mahar, M.; Cavalli, V. Intrinsic mechanisms of neuronal axon regeneration. *Nat. Rev. Neurosci.* **2018**, *19*, 323–337. [CrossRef] [PubMed]
57. Zholudeva, L.V.; Karliner, J.S.; Dougherty, K.J.; Lane, M.A. Anatomical Recruitment of Spinal V2a Interneurons into Phrenic Motor Circuitry after High Cervical Spinal Cord Injury. *J. Neurotrauma* **2017**, *34*, 3058–3065. [CrossRef]
58. Lane, M.A.; Lee, K.Z.; Salazar, K.; O'Steen, B.E.; Bloom, D.C.; Fuller, D.D.; Reier, P.J. Respiratory function following bilateral mid-cervical contusion injury in the adult rat. *Exp. Neurol.* **2012**, *235*, 197–210. [CrossRef]
59. Satkunendrarajah, K.; Karadimas, S.K.; Laliberte, A.M.; Montandon, G.; Fehlings, M.G. Cervical excitatory neurons sustain breathing after spinal cord injury. *Nature* **2018**, *562*, 419–422. [CrossRef]
60. Streeter, K.A.; Sunshine, M.D.; Patel, S.R.; Gonzalez-Rothi, E.J.; Reier, P.J.; Baekey, D.M.; Fuller, D.D. Mid-cervical interneuron networks following high cervical spinal cord injury. *Respir. Physiol. Neurobiol.* **2020**, *271*, 103305. [CrossRef]
61. Leydeker, M.; Delva, S.; Tserlyuk, I.; Yau, J.; Wagdy, M.; Hawash, A.; Bendaoud, S.; Mohamed, S.; Wieraszko, A.; Ahmed, Z. The effects of 15 Hz trans-spinal magnetic stimulation on locomotor control in mice with chronic contusive spinal cord injury. *Electromagn. Biol. Med.* **2013**, *32*, 155–164. [CrossRef] [PubMed]
62. Edgerton, V.R.; Harkema, S. Epidural stimulation of the spinal cord in spinal cord injury: Current status and future challenges. *Expert Rev. Neurother.* **2011**, *11*, 1351–1353. [CrossRef] [PubMed]
63. Bonizzato, M.; James, N.D.; Pidpruzhnykova, G.; Pavlova, N.; Shkorbatova, P.; Baud, L.; Martinez-Gonzalez, C.; Squair, J.W.; DiGiovanna, J.; Barraud, Q.; et al. Multi-pronged neuromodulation intervention engages the residual motor circuitry to facilitate walking in a rat model of spinal cord injury. *Nat. Commun.* **2021**, *12*, 1925. [CrossRef]

64. Bezdudnaya, T.; Lane, M.A.; Marchenko, V. Paced breathing and phrenic nerve responses evoked by epidural stimulation following complete high cervical spinal cord injury in rats. *J. Appl. Physiol.* **2018**, *125*, 687–696. [CrossRef] [PubMed]
65. Mercier, L.M.; Gonzalez-Rothi, E.J.; Streeter, K.A.; Posgai, S.S.; Poirier, A.S.; Fuller, D.D.; Reier, P.J.; Baekey, D.M. Intraspinal microstimulation and diaphragm activation after cervical spinal cord injury. *J. Neurophysiol.* **2017**, *117*, 767–776. [CrossRef] [PubMed]
66. Dale, E.A.; Sunshine, M.D.; Kelly, M.N.; Mitchell, G.S.; Fuller, D.D.; Reier, P.J. Chronic, closed-loop, cervical epidural stimulation elicits plasticity in diaphragm motor output and upregulates spinal neurotrophic factor gene expression. *FASEB J.* **2019**, *33*, 843.10. [CrossRef]
67. Jesus, I.; Michel-Flutot, P.; Deramaudt, T.B.; Paucard, A.; Vanhee, V.; Vinit, S.; Bonay, M. Effects of aerobic exercise training on muscle plasticity in a mouse model of cervical spinal cord injury. *Sci. Rep.* **2021**, *11*, 112. [CrossRef] [PubMed]

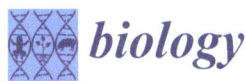

Article

Diaphragmatic Activity and Respiratory Function Following C3 or C6 Unilateral Spinal Cord Contusion in Mice

Afaf Bajjig [1], Pauline Michel-Flutot [2], Tiffany Migevent [1], Florence Cayetanot [1], Laurence Bodineau [1], Stéphane Vinit [2,†] and Isabelle Vivodtzev [1,*,†]

[1] Inserm, UMR_S1158 Neurophysiologie Respiratoire Expérimentale et Clinique, Sorbonne Université, 75013 Paris, France; afaf.bajjig@sorbonne-universite.fr (A.B.); tiffanymigevent77@gmail.com (T.M.); florence.cayetanot@sorbonne-universite.fr (F.C.); laurence.bodineau@sorbonne-universite.fr (L.B.)
[2] Inserm, END-ICAP, Université Paris-Saclay, UVSQ, 78000 Versailles, France; pauline.michel-flutot@uvsq.fr (P.M.-F.); stephane.vinit@uvsq.fr (S.V.)
* Correspondence: isabelle.vivodtzev@sorbonne-universite.fr
† These authors contributed equally to this work.

Simple Summary: Tetraplegia is one of the most devastating conditions that an individual can sustain and affects more than 2.5 million people worldwide. Tetraplegia not only affects mobility but also impacts spontaneous breathing such that survivors can be rendered ventilator dependent and have increased mortality. Although no treatment can restore respiratory function after tetraplegia, there is a need for more exploratory studies defining therapeutic approaches to ameliorate respiratory decline in tetraplegia. Here, we studied two models of tetraplegia mimicking human forms of injury, using spinal cord contusion in mice, either above the third cervical metameric segment (C3 model) or below the sixth cervical metameric segment (C6 model) innervation of the phrenic nerves. These nerves are responsible for contraction of the diaphragm, the main inspiratory muscle. Using measurements of spontaneous breathing and muscle activity of the diaphragm, we found reduced diaphragmatic activity in both models, but only the C3 model led to reduced spontaneous breathing similar to what is seen in humans with tetraplegia. Moreover, we found a decline in basal contractility of the diaphragm in the C3 model only. We conclude that the C3 model is an appropriate model to explore interventions aimed at restoring breathing following tetraplegia.

Abstract: The majority of spinal cord injuries (SCIs) are cervical (cSCI), leading to a marked reduction in respiratory capacity. We aimed to investigate the effect of hemicontusion models of cSCI on both diaphragm activity and respiratory function to serve as preclinical models of cervical SCI. Since phrenic motoneuron pools are located at the C3–C5 spinal level, we investigated two models of preclinical cSCI mimicking human forms of injury, namely, one above (C3 hemicontusion—C3HC) and one below phrenic motoneuron pools (C6HC) in wild-type swiss OF-1 mice, and we compared their effects on respiratory function using whole-body plethysmography and on diaphragm activity using electromyography (EMG). At 7 days post-surgery, both C3HC and C6HC damaged spinal cord integrity above the lesion level, suggesting that C6HC potentially alters C5 motoneurons. Although both models led to decreased diaphragmatic EMG activity in the injured hemidiaphragm compared to the intact one (−46% and −26% in C3HC and C6HC, respectively, both $p = 0.02$), only C3HC led to a significant reduction in tidal volume and minute ventilation compared to sham surgery (−25% and −20% vs. baseline). Moreover, changes in EMG amplitude between respiratory bursts were observed post-C3HC, reflecting a change in phrenic motoneuronal excitability. Hence, C3HC and C6HC models induced alteration in respiratory function proportionally to injury level, and the C3HC model is a more appropriate model for interventional studies aiming to restore respiratory function in cSCI.

Keywords: spinal cord injury; contusion model; respiratory function; diaphragmatic activity; phrenic motoneurons

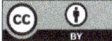

1. Introduction

Spinal cord injury (SCI) prevalence is estimated at 500,000 individuals worldwide each year [1]. Most cases of SCI happen at the cervical level [2,3], leading not only to locomotor impairment but also marked respiratory dysfunction. Indeed, cervical SCI at or above the level of phrenic motor neurons (C3 to C5) interrupts descending medullary spinal respiratory pathways and causes complete or partial diaphragm paralysis. As a result, forced vital capacity and total lung capacity are proportionally reduced with an increasing level and severity of injury [4], and only mechanical ventilation can ensure sufficient breathing in patients with the highest level of injury (C4 or above) [5]. Notably, almost all tetraplegic patients use mechanical ventilation (MV) acutely after injury, and many remain dependent on it. Moreover, even when patients are weaned from diurnal MV, most of them (60%) are still dependent on nocturnal ventilation support due to sleep-disordered breathing [6]. Furthermore, efficient diaphragmatic activity is needed to ensure coughing and sneezing abilities, both crucial for airway clearance in order to prevent respiratory infections [7]. Hence, respiratory dysfunction after SCI not only compromises comfort and life quality but also increases morbidity and mortality rates in patients living with such high injuries [8].

Currently, there is no efficient treatment that can be used to fully restore respiratory function in cervical SCI. Implanted phrenic stimulation (diaphragm pacing) allows some patients to be weaned from MV [9], but this procedure is invasive and only possible when phrenic nerve conduction is preserved, therefore allowing less than 10% of patients with SCI above C4 to be treated with diaphragm pacing [10]. Similarly, the restoration of diaphragm innervation by using the nerve transfer approach is limited by the need for the donor and their axons to have previously been innervated by the respiratory centers [11,12], making this approach complicated and limiting. Nevertheless, a growing number of interventional studies using pharmacological strategies, such as the modulation of noradrenergic, serotonergic or dopaminergic neurotransmission, or neuromechanical devices, such as electrical stimulation, robotic assistance or even the brain–computer interface, are suggesting that respiratory neuroplasticity may be enhanced to improve spontaneous ventilation after SCI [13,14]. Moreover, few non-invasive therapeutics such as intermittent hypoxia protocols demonstrated their ability to induce substantial respiratory recovery in rodent preclinical models [15–19] of cervical injury as well as in human patients [20–22]. There is a need for more exploratory studies searching for a pharmacological agent, intervention or combinatorial approaches to further ameliorate the respiratory outcome following cervical SCI.

One of the most challenging aspects of medical research is ensuring that benefits found based on animal data can be translated to humans. Therefore, current and developing studies need representative preclinical models of cSCI to allow a better understanding of respiratory physiopathology after SCI and to unravel the benefit of therapeutic approaches. Currently, most studies investigating respiratory physiopathology, the neuroplasticity of medullary spinal axonal regeneration and phrenic motoneurons nuclei reinnervation following high SCI use the C2 hemisection in rat [22–25] and mouse [26–28] models. These studies have unraveled fundamental concepts of respiratory physiopathology after SCI [23,27] and provided bases for putative therapeutics to cure SCI [15,24,29]. However, section models are not ideal for investigating SCI pathophysiology because transections are scarce in clinical settings [24,29–31]. Contusion models may be more appropriate since they lead to spared motoneurons and not death of all neurons. Moreover, respiratory recovery after C2 injuries can be linked to cross-phrenic phenomena typical of C2 injury [32], whose existence is still debated in humans [33]. Hence, it may be relevant to use injury occurring at the phrenic motoneurons innervation level (C3–C5 in rodents) in a manner similar to that in previous publications [15,34–40]. Furthermore, despite recent progress in the generation of transgenic rats, there is currently almost no alternative to mice for studying the roles of specific genes after SCI. Indeed, when hypotheses are confirmed, further projects would need to explore and confirm the effect on genetically engineered lines. Hence, mouse models of cervical hemicontusion would be helpful to study the recovery of respiratory function after SCI with interventions.

To date, very few studies have sought to characterize the respiratory physiopathology in the mouse model of cervical hemicontusion. Of note, Charles Nicaise and colleagues previously reported diaphragm deficits and phrenic motor neuron degeneration following C4/C5 SCI in mice [41,42]. These were pioneering studies showing the diaphragmatic impact of cervical hemicontusion in mice. However, since phrenic nuclei are located in the C3–C5 region in mice [42–44], it is likely that some phrenic motoneurons at the C3 level survive after C4/5 injury. On the contrary, although complete T8 contusion decreases tidal volume and minute ventilation in rats [42], it is not known whether respiration dysfunction occurs after mid-cervical SCI without direct damage to the phrenic motoneuron (MN). Lastly, respiratory function has been measured following bilateral mid-cervical contusion injury at the C3/C4 level, but only in rats [39]. Therefore, it would be interesting to assess the effect of unilateral phrenic MN denervation after C3 hemicontusion as compared to intercostal and abdominal denervation after C6 hemicontusion in a mouse model of SCI.

Furthermore, pulmonary volume has not been characterized after hemicervical contusion in mice. However, it is a direct, accurate and precise reflection of respiratory function and may be an interesting tool to investigate, especially given that it can be evaluated non-invasively at different time points and provide the functional effect of putative therapeutic strategies to restore impaired breathing. In the present study, we aimed to develop and investigate the effect of C3 and C6 hemicontusion models on both diaphragm activity and respiratory function to serve as preclinical models of cervical SCI in interventional studies with the aim of restoring respiratory function in SCI.

2. Materials and Methods
2.1. Animals and Experimental Design

Adult WT Swiss OF-1 (Charles River, France) male mice of 20–30 g (10–12 weeks old) were housed in ventilated cages with controlled humidity, light and temperature. Animals were first housed in cages in groups of 5 before surgery and then in cages in groups of 2 after surgery. Only two animals needed to be separated due to showing aggressive behavior toward other males. *Ad libitum* food and water were provided in an enriched cage environment. All experiments reported in this manuscript conformed to the policies laid out by the Guide for the Care and Use of Laboratory Animals in the EU Directive 2010/63/EU for animal experiments. These experiments were approved by the Ethics Committee Charles Darwin CEEACD/N°5 (Project authorization APAFIS No. 2020070317412138 v3).

Thirty-five animals were included in this study and were divided into 3 groups: (1) laminectomy ($n = 5$) or no surgery for one control mouse (sham/control, $n = 6$); (2) unilateral SCI at the C3 level (C3HC, $n = 12$); and (3) unilateral SCI at the C6 level (C6HC, $n = 17$). Two mice did not survive C3 hemicontusion and died during surgery, and one responded by self-mutilation on the 5th day and was excluded from the study. For all animals, terminal procedures were performed at J + 7 days post-lesion. From the 32 animals, 26 animals received plethysmography before and after surgery ($n = 7$ C3HC, $n = 13$ C6HC and $n = 6$ sham/control), and among these, 9 also received diaphragmatic electromyogram (EMG, $n = 4$ C3HC, $n = 4$ C6HC and $n = 1$ control) before being used for histologic analyses. In addition, 6 received EMG only ($n = 2$ C3HC and $n = 4$ C6HC) before being used for histologic analyses.

2.2. Unilateral Cervical Spinal Cord Contusion

Animals were placed in a closed chamber for anesthesia induction with isoflurane (4%) maintained throughout the procedure with a facial mask (1.5–2.5% isoflurane). As previously described in a study using a mouse model of cervical contusion targeting C4 and C5 levels [41], the dorsal skin and underlying muscles above the second cervical up to the first thoracic vertebrae were retracted. A dorsal laminectomy was performed to expose the spinal cord. A precision Impactor Device (RWD life science; 68,099 II) with a 1.5 mm tip impactor was used to perform the hemicontusion. The impactor parameters had a mean depth of 2.29 ± 0.41 mm, a speed of 2.41 ± 0.29 m/s and a dwell time of 0.50 ± 0.01 s (mean ± SEM) for the two injury types (not different for C3 and C6 epicenters). After contusion, sutures were used to close the wounds and skin. The isoflurane vaporizer was turned off, and the mice received subcutaneous injections of analgesia (buprenorphine, 0.1 mg/kg: QN02AE01, CEVA). After surgery, the animals were placed on a heated pad to recover. The animals were then placed in a cage containing water and a recovery diet gel, both in a small Petri dish, and then solid food was provided in the cage. Food and water were also provided on the top grid of the cage. Analgesia was maintained for at least 3 days following injury.

2.3. Breathing Recording Using Plethysmography

Before and 7 days after spinal cord contusion, respiratory variables were measured (tidal volume—V_T, breathing frequency—B_f, minute ventilation—V_E, inspiratory time—Ti and expiratory time—Te). One-hour plethysmography recordings were obtained for each mouse. The animals were placed in 400 mL chambers, breathing spontaneously and not constrained. Plethysmography does not require anesthesia and is a non-invasive procedure. The air in the chambers was constantly renewed by a pump at a flow rate of 0.5 L/min. The plethysmography chamber was hermetic, sealed and composed of 2 sections: a 150 mL reference chamber and a 250 mL chamber wherein the animal was placed. Before baseline measurements, the animals were placed in ventilated and enriched cages in the animal facility for one week for acclimatization. Subsequently, three-day plethysmography acclimation was conducted to familiarize the animals with the plethysmography chambers (Emka, France). This phase limited stress and resulted in calm animals, thereby allowing successful recordings with plethysmography software (Emka IOX software, Paris, France) on the 4th and 5th days of the week. The success rate (Sr) was obtained from the ratio of validated cycles (i.e., signals matching respiratory cycles) and the number of detected cycles for each 20 s period. Sr = 100% indicates that all detected respiratory cycles were validated by the software. We considered only measurements of respiratory function with Sr > 60. Mean Sr was similar between groups (76 ± 4, 75 ± 6 and 78 ± 10 in C3HC, C6HC and sham groups, respectively). Baseline recordings were performed for two consecutive days to check for data reproducibility. Post-surgery measurement was performed on day 7 to rule out any putative effect of analgesia.

2.4. Electrophysiological Recording of the Diaphragm

Electromyogram (EMG) was performed on 7 days post-injury. Anesthesia was induced using intraperitoneal injection of ketamine (QN01AX03, Virbac, Nice, France) (100 mg/kg) and xylazine (QN05CM92, Bayer, Leverkusen, Germany) (10 mg/kg). The animals were placed supine on a heating pad to maintain physiologic and constant body temperature (37.5 ± 1 °C). A laparotomy was performed to expose the diaphragm. Electromyogram (EMG) of the crural portion of the diaphragm ipsilateral and contralateral to the spinal cord lesion was obtained via handmade bipolar surface silver electrodes placed on the muscles during spontaneous poïkilocapnic normoxic breathing. EMG was amplified (Model 1800; gain, 100; A-M Systems, Everett, WA, USA) and bandpass filtered (100 Hz–10 kHz). Signals were digitized with Powerlab data acquisition hardware/software (Acquisition rate: 4 k/s; AD Instruments, Dunedin, New Zealand) connected to a computer and analyzed using LabChart 7 Pro software (AD Instruments, Dunedin, New Zealand). EMG was integrated (50 ms decay). After the experiment, the animals were euthanized with exsanguination, followed by intracardiac perfusion of saline and 4% paraformaldehyde (4 °C) for tissue fixation and subsequent harvesting.

2.5. Tissue Processing

After fixation, the C1-C8 segment of the spinal cord was dissected and immediately placed in cold 4% paraformaldehyde (P6148 Sigma-Aldrich, Darmstadt, Germany) for 48 h and then cryoprotected in 30% sucrose (in 0.9% NaCl, S9888, Sigma-Aldrich, Darmstadt, Germany) for 48 h and stored at −80 °C. Frozen transversal (C1–C5 or C4–C8 spinal cord) free-floating sections (30 µm) were obtained using a Thermo Fisher CryoStar NX70 cryostat. Spinal cord sections were stored in a cryoprotectant solution (sucrose 30% (pharma grade, 141621, AppliChem, Darmstadt, Germany), ethylene glycol 30% (BP230-4, Fisher Scientific, Illkirch, France) and polyvinylpyrrolidone 40 (PVP40-100G; Sigma-Aldrich 1% in phosphate-buffered saline (PBS) 1X) (BP665-1; Fisher Scientific, Illkirch, France) at −22 °C. Every fifth section from C1–C5 or C4–C8 was used for lesion evaluation to examine the extent of injury using cresyl violet histochemistry: 10 min in cresyl violet solution (0.001% cresyl violet acetate (C5042-10G, Sigma-Aldrich, Darmstadt, Germany) and 0.125% glacial acetic acid (A/0400/PB15, Fisher Scientific, Illkirch, France) in distilled water), 1 min in 70% ethanol, 1 min in 95% ethanol, 2 × 1 min in 100% ethanol (E/0600DF/17, Fisher Scientific, Illkirch, France) and 2 min in xylene (X/0100/PB17, Fischer Scientific, Illkirch, France). Then, they were coverslipped using Eukitt® mounting medium, and slide microphotographs were taken with a slide scanner (Aperio AT2, Leica, France).

2.6. Immunohistofluorescence

Immunohistodetection of markers of interest was performed on spinal cord samples from C3HC and C6HC for qualitative assessments. Free-floating transverse sections of the C1–C5 or C4–C8 spinal cord stored in cryoprotectant solution were washed 3 times in PBS 1X and placed in blocking solution (normal donkey serum (NDS) 5% and 0.2% Triton 100X in PBS 1X) for 30 min and then incubated with primary antibodies using ionized calcium-binding adaptor protein-1 (Iba1) (Abcam ab5076, 1/400, goat polyclonal) and glial fibrillary acidic protein (GFAP (Millipore-Merck AB5804, 1/4000, rabbit polyclonal) in blocking solution overnight in an orbital shaker at 4 °C. After 3 PBS 1X washes, sections were incubated in the corresponding secondary antibodies Alexa Fluor 488 Donkey anti-rabbit (Molecular Probes A21206, 1/2000, ThermoFisher, Rockford, IL, USA) and Alexa Fluor 647 Donkey anti-goat (Molecular Probes A21447, 1/2000, ThermoFisher, Rockford, IL, USA) for 2 h at room temperature, and they were then washed again 3 times with PBS 1X. Sections were then incubated with NeuroTrace™ 530/615 (N21482, Invitrogen, Waltham, MA, USA), a neuronal marker (Nissl stain), for 10 min and then washed again 3 times with PBS 1X. Images of the different sections were captured with a Hamamatsu ORCA-R^2 camera mounted on an Olympus IX83 P2ZF scanning microscope.

2.7. Data Processing and Statistical Analyses

EMG analyses. The amplitude of at least 10 double-integrated diaphragmatic EMG inspiratory bursts during normoxia was calculated for each animal from the injured and the intact sides using LabChart 7 Pro software (AD Instruments). For inter-inspiratory burst basal signal analysis during normoxia, the amplitude of a minimum of 5 basal diaphragmatic EMG signals was calculated using LabChart 7.

Statistical analyses. Data are presented as mean ± standard deviation (SD) or median (interquartiles), and differences were considered significant at $p < 0.05$. GraphPad Prism software 9.3.1 was used for all statistical analyses. Normality of the data was checked with the Shapiro–Wilk test. Within-group comparisons (weight loss, EMG activity and respiratory variables) were performed using paired t-test or Wilcoxon's test (for non-parametric data and for groups with $n < 7$ animals), and between-group comparisons were performed using 2-way analysis of variance (diaphragmatic EMG and interburst) with the type of lesion and side (injured vs. intact) as factors. Between-group comparisons for changes in weight, V_T, B_f and V_E after 7 days were performed using 2-way repeated measures analysis of variance (ANOVA) with post hoc Bonferroni. The relationship between changes in V_T (post/pre ratio) and in hemidiaphragmatic activity (injured/intact EMG ratio) was assessed using simple regression analysis and Pearson coefficient correlation.

3. Results

3.1. Physiologic Effect of Cervical Contusion

Body weight loss was observed in both groups (after C3HC and C6HC), with no difference between groups in weight change at 7 days post-lesion (Table 1) being noted. After slight, daily decreases, body weight stabilized after the fifth day post-lesion in both groups. After C3HC, complete ipsilateral forelimb paralysis was observed, whereas partial paralysis was observed after C6HC.

Table 1. Respiratory variables following C3 or C6 hemicontusion.

Variables		Sham	C3HC	C6HC
Weight (g)	day of surgery	38 (9)	41 ± 5	37 ± 3
	day 1	-	38 ± 3	35 ± 2
	day 2	-	36 ± 4	34 ± 2
	day 5	-	33 ± 3	33 ± 3
	day 7	39 (12)	34 ± 3	34 ± 3
V_T (µL/g)	pre	14.7 (5.2)	14.3 ± 3.6	14.9 ± 2.6
	7 d post	17.5 (5.7)	10.1 [#ab] ± 2.1	14.2 ± 2.5
V_T (mL)	pre	0.56 (0.11)	0.59 ± 0.2	0.56 ± 0.1
	7 d post	0.62 (0.20)	0.36 * ± 0.1	0.48 * ± 0.1
B_f (rpm)	pre	226 (117)	233 ± 25	250 ± 59
	7 d post	264 (165)	273 * ± 36	248 ± 54
V_E (mL/min)	pre	146 (85)	139 ± 52	144 ± 52
	7 d post	160 (151)	98 [#a] ± 24	122 ± 44
Ti (ms)	pre	107 (55)	111 ± 12	98 ± 21
	7 d post	98 * (58)	96 ± 14	90 ± 18
Te (ms)	pre	168 (82)	179 ± 26	171 ± 47
	7 d post	155 (90)	150 * ± 38	179 ± 47

Definitions of abbreviations: V_T, tidal volume; B_f, breathing frequency; V_E, minute ventilation; Ti, inspiratory time; Te, expiratory time. * within-group comparison: $p < 0.05$. # between-group comparison $p < 0.05$. [a] post hoc comparison with sham: $p < 0.01$; [b] post hoc comparison with C6HC: $p < 0.001$.

3.2. Histological Analysis of C3 and C6 Hemicontusions

Histological analyses are shown in Figures 1 and 2. Seven days after hemicontusion, the spinal cord transverse sections stained with cresyl violet (Nissl body labeling) displayed tissue damage at the site of injury following C3HC or C6HC (Figures 1A,B and 2). GFAP-positive cells (astrocytes), Iba1-positive cells (microglia and macrophages) and NeuroTrace labeling (neurons) showed the anatomical cell composition of the site of injury in both models (Figure 1C,D). Note the absence of GFAP labeling at the site of injury, as well as the blurred NeuroTrace labeling and ameboid Iba1-positive cells at the site of injury. In addition, as shown in Figure 2, the extent of the lesion reached 600 µm rostral and caudal to the lesion epicenter for both C3HC and C6HC.

3.3. Respiratory Function Following C3 or C6 Hemicontusion

Plethysmography measurements are presented in Figure 3 and Table 1. There was a significant reduction in V_T at 7 days post-surgery after C3HC when corrected for weight loss (post vs. pre: 10.1 ± 2.1 vs. 14.3 ± 3.6 µL/g, −25%) compared to C6HC (14.2 ± 2.50 vs. 14.9 ± 2.6 µL/g, −5%) and sham (17.9 ± 4.6 vs. 14.9 ± 2.6 µL/g, +15%) (RM ANOVA, $p = 0.01$, Figure 3). There was also an increase in B_f in the C3HC group 7 days after surgery (273 ± 36 vs. 233 ± 25, $p = 0.04$), but differences were not observed in the two other groups. Lastly, changes in V_E were significantly different between the groups: 7 days after surgery, V_E was lower in C3HC than in sham but not C6HC (post vs. pre: 98 ± 22 vs. 139 ± 49 mL/min, −20%, $p = 0.02$) (Figure 3 and Table 1).

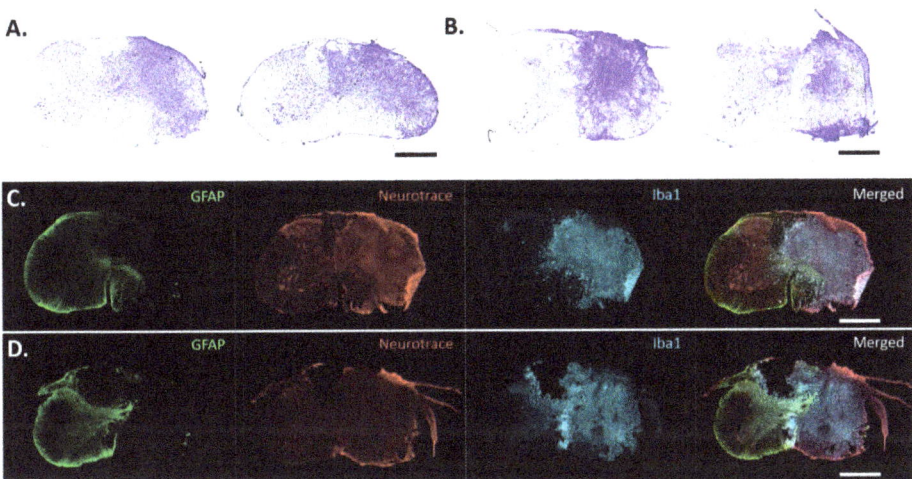

Figure 1. Examples of extent of injury to C3 and C6 spinal segments in mice 7 days post-contusion. Representative examples of cresyl violet staining at the injured site 7 days post-contusion for C3- ($n = 6$) (**A**) and C6- ($n = 6$) (**B**) injured groups. Representative images showing immunolabeling of glial fibrillary acidic protein (GFAP) (glial cells, in green), NeuroTrace (neurons in red) and ionized calcium-binding adaptor protein-1 (Iba1) (microglia, aqua) for C3-contused group (**C**) and C6-contused group (**D**). Note that half of the spinal cord is completely injured by the contusion for both groups, and no neurons remained in the scar. Scale bar: 500 µm.

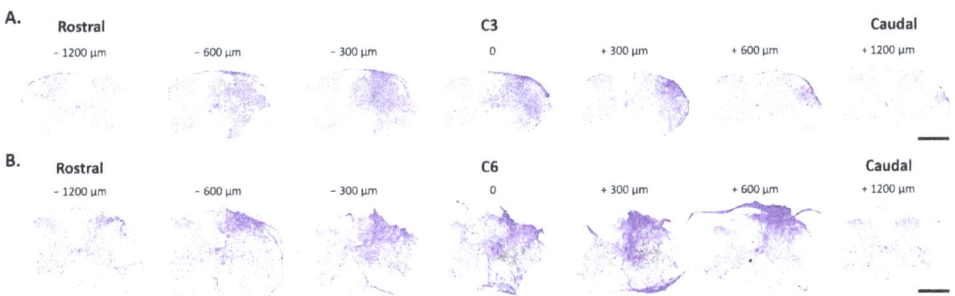

Figure 2. Representative rostro-caudal extent of contusion injury in C3- (A) and C6- (B) contused groups, where 0 represents the epicenter of the injury. Each picture is separated by 300 µm width. Note that the injury extends more than 2000 µm from the epicenter. Scale bar: 500 µm.

3.4. Diaphragmatic Activity Following C3 or C6 Hemicontusion

Diaphragm activity is shown in Figure 4. Seven days post-lesion, the activity in the ipsilateral (injured) hemidiaphragm showed a greater reduction than that in the contralateral (intact) hemidiaphragm after both C3HC (0.78 ± 0.43 vs. 1.62 ± 0.68 A.U. normalized to control, -46% $p = 0.02$) and C6HC (0.88 ± 0.42 vs. 1.21 ± 0.53 A.U. normalized to sham, $-p = 0.02$). The reduction in the injured hemidiaphragm compared to the intact one after C3HC tended to be significantly more pronounced than after C6HC (-46% vs. -27%, 2 ways RM ANOVA, $p = 0.07$) and was associated with increased activity of the intact hemidiaphragm (Figure 4C). In addition, the EMG amplitude recordings of two inspiratory interbursts on the injured side of the C3 mice was increased at 7 days post-injury compared to the intact side and to the C6 recordings (Figure 4D; injured side: 18 ± 15 vs. intact side:

3 ± 4 mV in C3HC compared to injured side: 4 ± 5 vs. intact side: 4 ± 3 mV in C6HC; two-way ANOVA; $p = 0.01$). Lastly, we found a significant correlation between changes in tidal volume (hemicontusion group vs. intact group) and changes in diaphragm activity (ipsilateral hemidiaphragm vs. contralateral hemidiaphragm) ($r = 0.72$, $p = 0.01$, Figure 5).

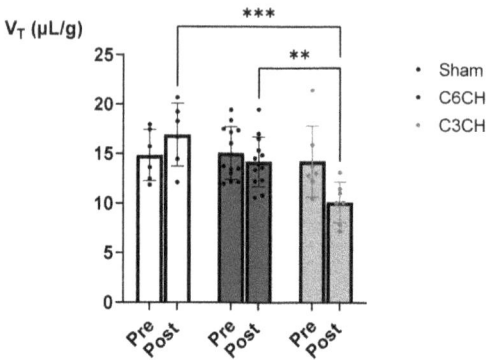

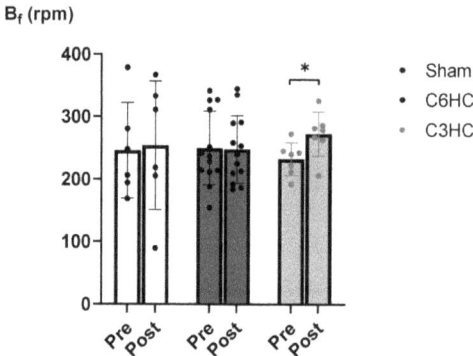

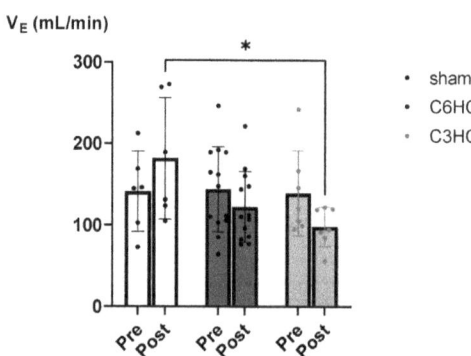

Figure 3. Respiratory pattern following C3 and C6 hemicontusions (HCs). Mean $\pm$ SD of tidal volume (V_T), breathing frequency (B_f) and minute ventilation (V_E) before and 7 days after sham surgery, C6HC or C3HC. *** $p < 0.001$, ** $p < 0.01$, * $p < 0.05$. Bonferroni post hoc analysis: V_T at 7 days post-C3HC was significantly lower than in sham and C6CH groups, and VE at 7 days post-C3HC was significantly lower than in sham.

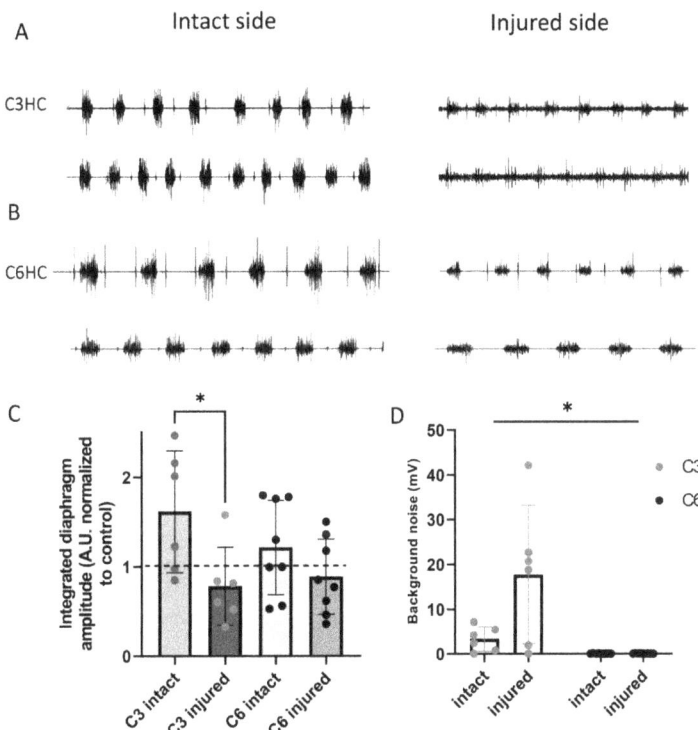

Figure 4. Diaphragm activity following C3 and C6 hemicontusions (HCs). Representative examples of diaphragmatic EMG in two mice 7 days after C3 hemicontusion (**A**) or C6 hemicontusion (**B**) and mean +/− SD in each group of animals (**C**). Amplitude recordings of 2 inspiratory interbursts and of the ECGs in injured and intact sides after C3 and C6 hemicontusions (**D**) * $p < 0.05$.

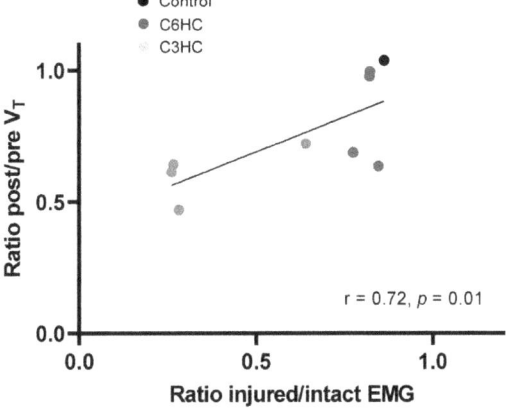

Figure 5. Relationship between changes in respiratory function and diaphragmatic activity. Simple linear relationship between diaphragmatic EMG activity of the injured side and that of the intact side (injured-to-intact ratio) and changes in tidal volume (ratio of post/pre values) 7 days post-lesion in animals after performing both plethysmography and EMG recordings (Pearson correlation coefficient).

4. Discussion

The present study compared for the first time two distinct models of cervical spinal cord injury differentially impacting the phrenic MN pool, and it demonstrates their respective effects on diaphragmatic activity and respiratory function in adult mice. Although the mice tolerated and survived after surgery similarly in both models, C3 hemicontusion had a more deleterious impact on both diaphragmatic activity and respiratory function, which were closely correlated. Moreover, we found a significant increase in interburst diaphragmatic activity in the C3HC model, suggesting impaired contractility. These rodent C3HC and C6HC injury models induce alterations in respiratory function proportionally to the level of injury, suggesting that the C3HC model is more appropriate for interventional studies aiming to restore respiratory function in cSCI.

Mid-cervical contusion models in mice were developed ten years ago by Nicaise and collaborators [41,42] but have been poorly studied since then due to the small animal size and challenging surgery procedures. Unilateral models allow for better survival of animals following surgery and reduce mortality rates. In the present study, we were interested in comparing two models of mid-cervical hemicontusion, which differ in terms of their impact on phrenic MNs. Indeed, the C3HC model may, in theory, lead to ipsilateral denervation below C3 and, hence, to the removal of the whole pool of phrenic MNs, reducing diaphragmatic activity, while C6HC would allow for preservation of the phrenic MN pool but may still impact the extra-diaphragmatic muscles involved in respiration. Our qualitative assessment of NeuroTrace on the lesion site 7 days after C3HC and C6HC (Figure 1C,D) showed unilateral destruction of neuron cell bodies and white matter in all animals, suggesting that neuronal conduction below the lesion site may be compromised in these animals. Moreover, GFAP and Iba1 staining was also limited to the border of the lesion site, suggesting that the injured tissue at 7 days post-HC was scar fibrotic tissue without any visible cystic cavities, as opposed to what has previously been observed in section or contusion in rat models [45–47]. Indeed, a recent study from our group reported increased expressions of Iba1 and GFAP after C2 hemisection in rats, suggesting that, similar to hemisection, hemicontusions may also induce recruitment and activation of microglia, macrophages and astrocytes 7 days post-HC around the lesion site [48].

Furthermore, as shown in Figure 2, both contusion types extended rostro-caudally. As a result, it is likely that not only does C6HC impact extra-diaphragmatic respiratory muscles via denervation of the conduction below the site of the lesion (intercostal denervation, for example), but it may also partly damage phrenic conduction at the C5 MN pool. Similar extension of the lesion (up to 600 μm) has recently been reported in mice after C5 hemicontusion [49], although other authors showed that double hemicontusion at C4 and C5 impacted their respective spinal segments [41,42]. Differences between studies may derive from technical aspects of the impactor device. We used a new pneumatic and electric system controlling for depth, velocity and dwell time of the impact. Nevertheless, despite a slight impact on the C5 spinal segment, C6HC caused considerably less damage to respiratory function than did C3HC.

A primary finding of the present study is the reduction in tidal volume after C3HC compared to the sham lesion and to C6HC. Our results corroborate previous findings in rats. Choi et al. previously reported a reduction in V_T and V_E after C4/5 double hemicontusion in rats even when considering weight reduction after SCI [37]. Moreover, Warren et al. previously showed that spinal cord contusion at the C3 level leads to decreased V_T under "normal" breathing conditions at an acute stage, which is similar to the results of our study (7 days post-surgery), but also at chronic stages up to 3 weeks post-trauma [25]. Recently, Chiu et al. confirmed that mid-cervical contusion causes a significant reduction in V_T that remains at the chronic injury stage [50]. However, to the best of our knowledge our study shows for the first time the effect of mid-cervical contusion in a mouse model of C3 injury. Furthermore, since reduced ventilation was not found after C6HC, i.e., when phrenic MNs are less damaged (C5 spinal level), the present study strongly suggests that damaged phrenic MNs are responsible for the reduction in V_T volume during resting breathing in mice after hemicontusion. Moreover, B_f increased after C3HC. This may be explained by an attempt to compensate for the reduced V_T to maintain V_E, as demonstrated in other studies. Indeed, a similar change in the respiratory pattern (lower V_T and increased B_f) has been reported in rats after C4/5 [37,38]. In our study, this increase was not sufficient to restore normal ventilation, which was still 20% lower than baseline values (Figure 3). Of note, C3HC led to a significant reduction in tidal volume compared to C6HC. This result suggests that the C3HC model has a more deleterious effect on respiratory function and would, therefore, be a better model to study the effect of SCI on ventilatory recovery with interventions.

In parallel with reduced respiratory function, C3HC was also associated with altered diaphragmatic activity. Indeed, we found a greater deficit in diaphragmatic EMG with a higher injury level, suggesting that less spontaneous recovery occurs after injury. This may be due to the fact that C3HC induced deafferentation of all the phrenic MNs on the injury side, leading to greater loss of phrenic MN drive and less diaphragmatic contraction on the injured side. Similarly, C3/C4 contusion in the rat induced permanent hemidiaphragm paralysis without inducing phrenic MN neuronal loss [51]. Moreover, a previous study reported permanent diaphragm deficit after C4/5 hemicontusion in mice and showed that it may last up to 6 weeks post-injury [41]. In addition, these results are similar to those obtained in rat models of C2 hemisection [24,52], suggesting that the C3HC model has effects comparable to those of the complete unilateral denervation of phrenic MN pools, allowing for investigation of respiratory function recovery without the potential interference of the crossed phrenic phenomenon [23,27]. In fact, diaphragm activity and pulmonary volume were closely related (Figure 5), such that the reduction in V_T after C3HC was proportional to the reduced activity of the injured hemidiaphragm. In other words, V_T measurement could be a good functional marker of reduced diaphragmatic activity 7 days post-injury in these mice.

Lastly, the increased background noise observed between bursts after C3HC may reflect a change in phrenic motoneuronal excitability that was not observed after C6HC. This phenomenon has been previously reported and attributed to phrenic MN desynchronization or even spastic activity on the injured side following cervical C2 hemisection in mice [26]. Indeed, C3HC interrupts inhibitory projections from the Bötzinger complex of expiratory neurons [53], which could increase MN excitability, leading to spontaneous diaphragmatic EMG firing during the expiratory phase. In the present study, the massive injury induced by the contusion at C3 could have led to a larger inflammatory response than that of the cervical C2 hemisection, leading to persistent interburst activity compared to the hemisected animals. In fact, this interburst activity disappeared 7 d post-hemisection in mice [26]. Longer C3 post-contusion time is needed to confirm this phenomenon and to better describe the pathophysiological mechanisms.

5. Conclusions

The present study describes for the first time the comparative impact of C3 and C6 hemicontusions on both diaphragmatic activity and respiratory function. Our results suggest that the C3HC model has a more deleterious impact on spontaneous ventilation than the C6HC model, possibly due to greater damage to phrenic MN pools and diaphragmatic activity. Further studies are needed to confirm the motoneuronal loss and better explain the alteration in diaphragmatic activity; however, C3HC seems to be an appropriate model for interventional studies aiming to restore respiratory function in cSCI. Such models are critical to investigate respiratory neuroplasticity induced by pharmacological and/or interventional therapeutics, such as changes in neuronal networks, motoneuron excitability and synaptic connectivity. From the clinical perspective, this model will help in the identification of new treatment modalities to enable the restoration of respiratory function in cervical SCI.

Author Contributions: Conceptualization, I.V. and S.V.; methodology, I.V. and S.V.; software, A.B., T.M. and P.M.-F.; validation, F.C., L.B., S.V. and I.V.; formal analysis, A.B., T.M., P.M.-F., I.V. and S.V.; investigation, A.B., T.M., P.M.-F., I.V. and S.V.; resources, A.B., T.M., P.M.-F., I.V. and S.V.; data curation, A.B., T.M., P.M.-F. and I.V. writing—original draft preparation, A.B. and I.V.; writing—review and editing, P.M.-F., F.C., L.B., S.V. and I.V.; visualization, P.M.-F. and S.V.; supervision, I.V.; project administration, I.V.; funding acquisition, I.V. and S.V. All authors have read and agreed to the published version of the manuscript.

Funding: This research was funded by *"La Fondation du Souffle"* (I.V.); Inserm (I.V., F.C. and L.B.), Sorbonne university (I.V., F.C. and L.B.), Chancellerie des Universités de Paris (Legs Poix) (S.V.), the Fondation de France (S.V.), the Fondation Médisite (S.V.) and Université de Versailles Saint-Quentin-en-Yvelines (S.V.).

Institutional Review Board Statement: Ethics Committee Charles Darwin CEEACD/N°5 (Project authorization APAFIS No. 2020070317412138 v3).

Informed Consent Statement: Not applicable.

Data Availability Statement: Data supporting reported results are available on request from the corresponding author.

Acknowledgments: The authors are grateful to *La Fondation du Souffle*, Inserm, Sorbonne University, Chancellerie des Universités de Paris, Fondation Médisite and Université de Versailles Saint-Quentin-en-Yvelines and to J. Andrew Taylor for editorial input.

Conflicts of Interest: The authors declare no conflict of interest.

References

1. OMS. Spinal Cord Injury. Available online: http://www.who.int/mediacentre/factsheets/fs384/en/ (accessed on 19 November 2013).
2. Van den Berg, M.E.; Castellote, J.M.; Mahillo-Fernandez, I.; de Pedro-Cuesta, J. Incidence of spinal cord injury worldwide: A systematic review. *Neuroepidemiology* **2010**, *34*, 184–192; discussion 192. [CrossRef] [PubMed]
3. Jackson, A.B.; Dijkers, M.; DeVivo, M.J.; Poczatek, R.B. A demographic profile of new traumatic spinal cord injuries: Change and stability over 30 years. *Arch. Phys. Med. Rehabil.* **2004**, *85*, 1740–1748. [CrossRef] [PubMed]
4. Winslow, C.; Rozovsky, J. Effect of spinal cord injury on the respiratory system. *Am. J. Phys. Med. Rehabil.* **2003**, *82*, 803–814. [CrossRef] [PubMed]
5. Hou, Y.F.; Lv, Y.; Zhou, F.; Tian, Y.; Ji, H.Q.; Zhang, Z.S.; Guo, Y. Development and validation of a risk prediction model for tracheostomy in acute traumatic cervical spinal cord injury patients. *Eur. Spine J.* **2015**, *24*, 975–984. [CrossRef] [PubMed]
6. Sankari, A.; Bascom, A.; Oomman, S.; Badr, M.S. Sleep disordered breathing in chronic spinal cord injury. *J. Clin. Sleep Med.* **2014**, *10*, 65–72. [CrossRef]
7. Mantilla, C.B.; Sieck, G.C. Phrenic motor unit recruitment during ventilatory and non-ventilatory behaviors. *Respir. Physiol. Neurobiol.* **2011**, *179*, 57–63. [CrossRef]
8. DeVivo, M.J.; Black, K.J.; Stover, S.L. Causes of death during the first 12 years after spinal cord injury. *Arch. Phys. Med. Rehabil.* **1993**, *74*, 248–254. [CrossRef]
9. Le Pimpec-Barthes, F.; Legras, A.; Arame, A.; Pricopi, C.; Boucherie, J.C.; Badia, A.; Panzini, C.M. Diaphragm pacing: The state of the art. *J. Thorac. Dis.* **2016**, *8*, S376–S386. [CrossRef]
10. Assouad, J.; Masmoudi, H.; Gonzalez-Bermejo, J.; Morelot-Panzini, C.; Diop, M.; Grunenwald, D.; Similowski, T. Diaphragm pacing after bilateral implantation of intradiaphragmatic phrenic stimulation electrodes through a transmediastinal endoscopic minimally invasive approach: Pilot animal data. *Eur. J. Cardiothorac. Surg.* **2012**, *42*, 333–339. [CrossRef]
11. Senjaya, F.; Midha, R. Nerve transfer strategies for spinal cord injury. *World Neurosurg.* **2013**, *80*, e319–e326. [CrossRef]
12. Gauthier, P.; Baussart, B.; Stamegna, J.C.; Tadie, M.; Vinit, S. Diaphragm recovery by laryngeal innervation after bilateral phrenicotomy or complete C2 spinal section in rats. *Neurobiol. Dis.* **2006**, *24*, 53–66. [CrossRef] [PubMed]
13. Pizzolato, C.; Gunduz, M.A.; Palipana, D.; Wu, J.; Grant, G.; Hall, S.; Dennison, R.; Zafonte, R.D.; Lloyd, D.G.; Teng, Y.D. Non-invasive approaches to functional recovery after spinal cord injury: Therapeutic targets and multimodal device interventions. *Exp. Neurol.* **2021**, *339*, 113612. [CrossRef] [PubMed]
14. Bezdudnaya, T.; Lane, M.A.; Marchenko, V. Paced breathing and phrenic nerve responses evoked by epidural stimulation following complete high cervical spinal cord injury in rats. *J. Appl. Physiol.* **2018**, *125*, 687–696. [CrossRef] [PubMed]
15. Gonzalez-Rothi, E.J.; Lee, K.Z. Intermittent hypoxia and respiratory recovery in pre-clinical rodent models of incomplete cervical spinal cord injury. *Exp. Neurol.* **2021**, *342*, 113751. [CrossRef] [PubMed]
16. Navarrete-Opazo, A.; Mitchell, G.S. Therapeutic potential of intermittent hypoxia: A matter of dose. *Am. J. Physiol.-Regul. Integr. Comp. Physiol.* **2014**, *307*, R1181–R1197. [CrossRef]
17. Lin, M.T.; Vinit, S.; Lee, K.Z. Functional role of carbon dioxide on intermittent hypoxia induced respiratory response following mid-cervical contusion in the rat. *Exp. Neurol.* **2021**, *339*, 113610. [CrossRef]

18. Randelman, M.; Zholudeva, L.V.; Vinit, S.; Lane, M.A. Respiratory Training and Plasticity after Cervical Spinal Cord Injury. *Front. Cell. Neurosci.* **2021**, *15*, 700821. [CrossRef]
19. Vinit, S.; Lovett-Barr, M.R.; Mitchell, G.S. Intermittent hypoxia induces functional recovery following cervical spinal injury. *Respir. Physiol. Neurobiol.* **2009**, *169*, 210–217. [CrossRef]
20. Tester, N.J.; Fuller, D.D.; Fromm, J.S.; Spiess, M.R.; Behrman, A.L.; Mateika, J.H. Long-term facilitation of ventilation in humans with chronic spinal cord injury. *Am. J. Respir. Crit. Care Med.* **2014**, *189*, 57–65. [CrossRef]
21. Sandhu, M.S.; Rymer, W.Z. Brief exposure to systemic hypoxia enhances plasticity of the central nervous system in spinal cord injured animals and man. *Curr. Opin. Neurol.* **2021**, *34*, 819–824. [CrossRef]
22. Sutor, T.; Cavka, K.; Vose, A.K.; Welch, J.F.; Davenport, P.; Fuller, D.D.; Mitchell, G.S.; Fox, E.J. Single-session effects of acute intermittent hypoxia on breathing function after human spinal cord injury. *Exp. Neurol.* **2021**, *342*, 113735. [CrossRef] [PubMed]
23. Goshgarian, H.G. Invited Review: The crossed phrenic phenomenon: A model for plasticity in the respiratory pathways following spinal cord injury. *J. Appl. Physiol.* **2003**, *94*, 795–810. [CrossRef] [PubMed]
24. Vinit, S.; Gauthier, P.; Stamegna, J.-C.; Kastner, A. High Cervical Lateral Spinal Cord Injury Results in Long-Term Ipsilateral Hemidiaphragm Paralysis. *J. Neurotrauma* **2006**, *23*, 1137–1146. [CrossRef] [PubMed]
25. Warren, P.M.; Campanaro, C.; Jacono, F.J.; Alilain, W.J. Mid-cervical spinal cord contusion causes robust deficits in respiratory parameters and pattern variability. *Exp. Neurol.* **2018**, *306*, 122–131. [CrossRef] [PubMed]
26. Michel-Flutot, P.; Mansart, A.; Deramaudt, B.T.; Jesus, I.; Lee, K.; Bonay, M.; Vinit, S. Permanent diaphragmatic deficits and spontaneous respiratory plasticity in a mouse model of incomplete cervical spinal cord injury. *Respir. Physiol. Neurobiol.* **2021**, *284*, 103568. [CrossRef] [PubMed]
27. Minor, K.H.; Akison, L.K.; Goshgarian, H.G.; Seeds, N.W. Spinal cord injury-induced plasticity in the mouse—The crossed phrenic phenomenon. *Exp. Neurol.* **2006**, *200*, 486–495. [CrossRef] [PubMed]
28. Mantilla, C.B.; Greising, S.M.; Stowe, J.M.; Zhan, W.-Z.; Sieck, G.C. TrkB kinase activity is critical for recovery of respiratory function after cervical spinal cord hemisection. *Exp. Neurol.* **2014**, *261*, 190–195. [CrossRef]
29. Vinit, S.; Kastner, A. Descending bulbospinal pathways and recovery of respiratory motor function following spinal cord injury. *Respir. Physiol. Neurobiol.* **2009**, *169*, 115–122. [CrossRef]
30. Cheriyan, T.; Ryan, D.J.; Weinreb, J.H.; Cheriyan, J.; Paul, J.C.; Lafage, V.; Kirsch, T.; Errico, T.J. Spinal cord injury models: A review. *Spinal Cord* **2014**, *52*, 588–595. [CrossRef]
31. Alilain, W.J.; Horn, K.P.; Hu, H.; Dick, T.E.; Silver, J. Functional regeneration of respiratory pathways after spinal cord injury. *Nature* **2011**, *475*, 196–200. [CrossRef]
32. Goshgarian, H.G. The crossed phrenic phenomenon and recovery of function following spinal cord injury. *Respir. Physiol. Neurobiol.* **2009**, *169*, 85–93. [CrossRef] [PubMed]
33. Ghali, M.G.Z. The crossed phrenic phenomenon. *Neural Regen. Res.* **2017**, *12*, 845–864. [CrossRef] [PubMed]
34. Zholudeva, L.V.; Iyer, N.; Qiang, L.; Spruance, V.M.; Randelman, M.L.; White, N.W.; Bezdudnaya, T.; Fischer, I.; Sakiyama-Elbert, S.E.; Lane, M.A. Transplantation of Neural Progenitors and V2a Interneurons after Spinal Cord Injury. *J. Neurotrauma* **2018**, *35*, 2883–2903. [CrossRef] [PubMed]
35. Lee, K.Z.; Liou, L.M.; Vinit, S. Diaphragm Motor-Evoked Potential Induced by Cervical Magnetic Stimulation following Cervical Spinal Cord Contusion in the Rat. *J. Neurotrauma* **2021**, *38*, 2122–2140. [CrossRef] [PubMed]
36. Khurram, O.U.; Fogarty, M.J.; Rana, S.; Vang, P.; Sieck, G.C.; Mantilla, C.B. Diaphragm muscle function following midcervical contusion injury in rats. *J. Appl. Physiol.* **2019**, *126*, 221–230. [CrossRef]
37. Choi, H.; Liao, W.L.; Newton, K.M.; Onario, R.C.; King, A.M.; Desilets, F.C.; Woodard, E.J.; Eichler, M.E.; Frontera, W.R.; Sabharwal, S.; et al. Respiratory abnormalities resulting from midcervical spinal cord injury and their reversal by serotonin 1A agonists in conscious rats. *J. Neurosci.* **2005**, *25*, 4550–4559. [CrossRef]
38. Golder, F.J.; Fuller, D.D.; Lovett-Barr, M.R.; Vinit, S.; Resnick, D.K.; Mitchell, G.S. Breathing patterns after mid-cervical spinal contusion in rats. *Exp. Neurol.* **2011**, *231*, 97–103. [CrossRef]
39. Lane, M.A.; Lee, K.Z.; Salazar, K.; O'Steen, B.E.; Bloom, D.C.; Fuller, D.D.; Reier, P.J. Respiratory function following bilateral mid-cervical contusion injury in the adult rat. *Exp. Neurol.* **2012**, *235*, 197–210. [CrossRef]
40. Wen, M.H.; Lee, K.Z. Diaphragm and Intercostal Muscle Activity after Mid-Cervical Spinal Cord Contusion in the Rat. *J. Neurotrauma* **2018**, *35*, 533–547. [CrossRef]
41. Nicaise, C. Degeneration of Phrenic Motor Neurons Induces Long-Term Diaphragm Deficits following Mid-Cervical Spinal Contusion in Mice. *J. Neurotrauma* **2012**, *29*, 2748–2760. [CrossRef]
42. Nicaise, C.; Hala, T.J.; Frank, D.M.; Parker, J.L.; Authelet, M.; Leroy, K.; Brion, J.-P.; Wright, M.C.; Lepore, A.C. Phrenic motor neuron degeneration compromises phrenic axonal circuitry and diaphragm activity in a unilateral cervical contusion model of spinal cord injury. *Exp. Neurol.* **2012**, *235*, 539–552. [CrossRef] [PubMed]
43. Vandeweerd, J.-M.; Hontoir, F.; De Knoop, A.; De Swert, K.; Nicaise, C. Retrograde Neuroanatomical Tracing of Phrenic Motor Neurons in Mice. *J. Vis. Exp.* **2018**, *132*, e56758. [CrossRef] [PubMed]
44. Qiu, K.; Lane, M.A.; Lee, K.Z.; Reier, P.J.; Fuller, D.D. The phrenic motor nucleus in the adult mouse. *Exp. Neurol.* **2010**, *226*, 254–258. [CrossRef] [PubMed]

45. Robac, A.; Neveu, P.; Hugede, A.; Garrido, E.; Nicol, L.; Delarue, Q.; Guérout, N. Repetitive Trans Spinal Magnetic Stimulation Improves Functional Recovery and Tissue Repair in Contusive and Penetrating Spinal Cord Injury Models in Rats. *Biomedicines* **2021**, *9*, 1827. [CrossRef] [PubMed]
46. Xia, Y.; Zhao, T.; Li, J.; Li, L.; Hu, R.; Hu, S.; Feng, H.; Lin, J. Antisense vimentin cDNA combined with chondroitinase ABC reduces glial scar and cystic cavity formation following spinal cord injury in rats. *Biochem. Biophys. Res. Commun.* **2008**, *377*, 562–566. [CrossRef] [PubMed]
47. Von Boxberg, Y.; Salim, C.; Soares, S.; Baloui, H.; Alterio, J.; Ravaille-Veron, M.; Nothias, F. Spinal cord injury-induced up-regulation of AHNAK, expressed in cells delineating cystic cavities, and associated with neoangiogenesis. *Eur. J. Neurosci.* **2006**, *24*, 1031–1041. [CrossRef] [PubMed]
48. Michel-Flutot, P.; Jesus, I.; Vanhee, V.; Bourcier, C.H.; Emam, L.; Ouguerroudj, A.; Lee, K.Z.; Zholudeva, L.V.; Lane, M.A.; Mansart, A.; et al. Effects of Chronic High-Frequency rTMS Protocol on Respiratory Neuroplasticity Following C2 Spinal Cord Hemisection in Rats. *Biology* **2022**, *11*, 473. [CrossRef]
49. Huang, Z.; Huang, Z.; Kong, G.; Lin, J.; Liu, J.; Yang, Z.; Li, R.; Wu, X.; Alaeiilkhchi, N.; Jiang, H.; et al. Anatomical and behavioral outcomes following a graded hemi-contusive cervical spinal cord injury model in mice. *Behav. Brain Res.* **2022**, *419*, 113698. [CrossRef]
50. Chiu, T.-T.; Lee, K.-Z. Impact of cervical spinal cord injury on the relationship between the metabolism and ventilation in rats. *J. Appl. Physiol.* **2021**, *131*, 1799–1814. [CrossRef]
51. Baussart, B.; Stamegna, J.C.; Polentes, J.; Tadié, M.; Gauthier, P. A new model of upper cervical spinal contusion inducing a persistent unilateral diaphragmatic deficit in the adult rat. *Neurobiol. Dis.* **2006**, *22*, 562–574. [CrossRef]
52. Goshgarian, H.G. The role of cervical afferent nerve fiber inhibition of the crossed phrenic phenomenon. *Exp. Neurol.* **1981**, *72*, 211–225. [CrossRef]
53. Tian, G.F.; Peever, J.H.; Duffin, J. Bötzinger-complex expiratory neurons monosynaptically inhibit phrenic motoneurons in the decerebrate rat. *Exp. Brain Res.* **1998**, *122*, 149–156. [CrossRef] [PubMed]

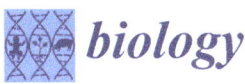

Review

Role of Descending Serotonergic Fibers in the Development of Pathophysiology after Spinal Cord Injury (SCI): Contribution to Chronic Pain, Spasticity, and Autonomic Dysreflexia

Gizelle N. K. Fauss, Kelsey E. Hudson and James W. Grau *

Department of Psychological and Brain Sciences, Texas A&M University, College Station, TX 77843, USA; gizellefauss@gmail.com (G.N.K.F.); kelsey3hudson@tamu.edu (K.E.H.)
* Correspondence: j-grau@tamu.edu; Tel.: +1-979-845-2584

Simple Summary: Fiber pathways that descend from the brain to the spinal cord drive motor behavior and modulate incoming sensory signals and the capacity to change (plasticity). A subset of these fibers release the neurotransmitter serotonin (5-HT), which can affect spinal cord function in alternative ways depending upon the region innervated and the receptor type engaged. The present paper examines the dampening (inhibitory) effect of serotonin and how a disruption in this process contributes to pathophysiology after spinal cord injury (SCI). After briefly reviewing the underlying anatomy and receptor types, we discuss how damage to serotonergic fibers can enable a state of over-excitation that interferes with adaptive learning and contributes to the development of pain, spasticity, and the dysregulation of autonomic function (autonomic dysreflexia). Recent work has shown that these effects arise, in part, because there is a shift in how the neurotransmitter gamma-aminobutyric acid (GABA) affects neural transmission within the spinal cord, a modification that lessens its inhibitory effect. Clinical implications of these results are discussed.

Citation: Fauss, G.N.K.; Hudson, K.E.; Grau, J.W. Role of Descending Serotonergic Fibers in the Development of Pathophysiology after Spinal Cord Injury (SCI): Contribution to Chronic Pain, Spasticity, and Autonomic Dysreflexia. *Biology* **2022**, *11*, 234. https://doi.org/10.3390/biology11020234

Academic Editors: Cédric G. Geoffroy and Warren Alilain

Received: 31 December 2021
Accepted: 29 January 2022
Published: 1 February 2022

Publisher's Note: MDPI stays neutral with regard to jurisdictional claims in published maps and institutional affiliations.

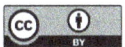

Copyright: © 2022 by the authors. Licensee MDPI, Basel, Switzerland. This article is an open access article distributed under the terms and conditions of the Creative Commons Attribution (CC BY) license (https://creativecommons.org/licenses/by/4.0/).

Abstract: As the nervous system develops, nerve fibers from the brain form descending tracts that regulate the execution of motor behavior within the spinal cord, incoming sensory signals, and capacity to change (plasticity). How these fibers affect function depends upon the transmitter released, the receptor system engaged, and the pattern of neural innervation. The current review focuses upon the neurotransmitter serotonin (5-HT) and its capacity to dampen (inhibit) neural excitation. A brief review of key anatomical details, receptor types, and pharmacology is provided. The paper then considers how damage to descending serotonergic fibers contributes to pathophysiology after spinal cord injury (SCI). The loss of serotonergic fibers removes an inhibitory brake that enables plasticity and neural excitation. In this state, noxious stimulation can induce a form of over-excitation that sensitizes pain (nociceptive) circuits, a modification that can contribute to the development of chronic pain. Over time, the loss of serotonergic fibers allows prolonged motor drive (spasticity) to develop and removes a regulatory brake on autonomic function, which enables bouts of unregulated sympathetic activity (autonomic dysreflexia). Recent research has shown that the loss of descending serotonergic activity is accompanied by a shift in how the neurotransmitter GABA affects neural activity, reducing its inhibitory effect. Treatments that target the loss of inhibition could have therapeutic benefit.

Keywords: spinal cord injury; monoamines; serotonin; GABA; neuromodulation; pain; autonomic dysreflexia; spasticity; ionic plasticity

1. Introduction

In early development, neural excitability within the spinal cord is enabled, a process that fosters the emergence of neural circuits coupled by coherent patterns of activity [1]. Over time, operational modules form that help to organize motor behavior and regulate the transmission of sensory signals to the brain. As a stable network emerges, inhibitory processes develop that limit excitability and plastic potential. Part of this transformation is tied to a local alteration, attributed to a strengthening of the inhibitory potential of the neurotransmitter gamma-aminobutyric acid (GABA) [1]. Paralleling this change, serotonergic fibers from the brain innervate the spinal cord. These projections can have a neuromodulatory effect that can either facilitate or inhibit neural function depending upon the region/cellular systems innervated and the receptor systems engaged.

Damage to descending serotonergic fibers can impair motor performance and remove a homeostatic brake on neural activity that can fuel pathology after spinal cord injury (SCI). How serotonin (5-HT) modulates motor behavior (e.g., locomotion, respiration) and regeneration has been amply reviewed elsewhere [2–9]. Likewise, its role in regulating incoming pain (nociceptive) signals has been well covered [10–12]. The current review focuses on a different aspect of serotonergic function, how damage to these fiber pathways contributes to pathophysiology after SCI.

We begin with a brief review of the underlying anatomy, the receptor types engaged, how these affect neural functions, and the pharmacological tools used to study serotonergic systems. We then describe how a complete SCI (spinal cord transection) enables neural activity within the caudal tissue, a state that fosters plasticity. Attenuating inhibition, this places the spinal cord in a vulnerable state wherein strong noxious stimulation can sensitize neurons within the dorsal horn, a modification that interferes with adaptive learning, promotes cell loss when the spinal cord is bruised (contused), and can drive the development of chronic pain. The loss of serotonergic fibers has also been linked to the sustained motor activity (spasticity) and the dysregulation of autonomic function. The latter can allow nociceptive signals to trigger bouts of unregulated sympathetic activity (autonomic dysreflexia).

New work suggests that the loss of serotonergic activity enables over-excitation within the spinal cord because it transforms the action of GABA, recapitulating an earlier developmental state wherein its capacity to inhibit neural excitation is reduced. We discuss the neurobiological mechanisms that mediate these alterations and how treatments designed to quiet neural activity after SCI can bring therapeutic benefit.

2. Serotonin Function in the Uninjured Nervous System
2.1. Overview of Descending Pathways and Their Function

Traditionally, serotonergic systems within the rat brain were categorized into groups (B1–B9) by location, with B1 being the most caudal [13]. For the purposes of this review, we will focus on the medullary groups (B1–B3) of serotonergic fibers that descend into the spinal cord [14,15]. For further details on anatomy, see [16–18]. Groups B1 through B3 occupy regions of the raphe pallidus nucleus (B1), raphe obscurus nucleus (B2), and raphe magnus nucleus (B3). Serotonergic fibers project through the white matter of the spinal cord and terminate in three main regions: the dorsal horn, ventral horn, and intermediate zone (Figure 1). Fibers that terminate in the dorsal horn, a region that modulates nociception and sensory function, are mainly sourced from the raphe magnus nucleus and the adjacent reticular formation (the rostral ventrolateral medulla, group B3) [14,15,19]. These fibers travel through the dorsolateral fasciculus (DLF) and terminate primarily in laminae I and II of the dorsal horn. Motoneurons in the ventral horn (primary lamina IX) receive input from descending serotonergic fibers from the raphe obscurus and raphe pallidus (groups B1 and B2) [14]. In the thoracic cord, sympathetic neurons receive descending serotonergic inputs that are sourced from the ventrolateral medulla (group B3) [14].

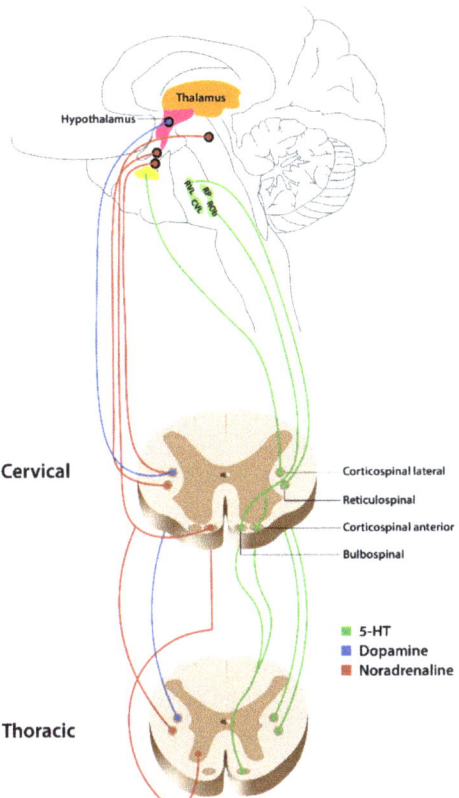

Figure 1. Serotonin (5-HT), noradrenaline, and dopamine projections to the spinal cord.

2.1.1. Regulation of Sensory Processes and Pain

The prominent sources of serotonergic efferents for nociception are the rostral ventral medulla (RVM) and the raphe magnus nucleus [14,15,20]. Within the dorsal horn, serotonergic fibers are most dense in the superficial laminae of the dorsal horn (laminae I and II) but the deeper laminae (IV–VI) also display serotonergic terminals [21,22]. Traditionally, modulation of nociception within the dorsal horn has been considered mainly inhibitory [23,24]. However, more recent data examining the effect of engaging alternative classes of 5-HT receptors suggest bidirectional modulation of nociception [16]. From this new perspective, it is not expected that engaging neurons within the raphe magnus or the rostral ventral medulla will necessarily induce antinociception. The outcome observed varies across stimulus parameters and both hyperalgesia and analgesia can be elicited by RVM stimulation [25–29]. Similarly, Ren and colleagues found that engaging vagal afferents projecting to the RVM could trigger facilitation or inhibition of nociception [30,31]. More recent reports have found specific "ON-cells" and "OFF-cells" in the RVM and raphe magnus that drive the facilitation and inhibition of pain, respectively [32,33].

Whether 5-HT has an antinociceptive or pronociceptive effect depends in large measure upon the receptor type engage (Tables 1 and 2). $5\text{-HT}_{1A/B/D}$ and 5-HT_7 are primarily antinociceptive while 5-HT_2 and 5-HT_3 are pronociceptive [34]. It is important to note that this grouping is general and that there is evidence for both anti- and pro-nociception for several of these receptors.

Table 1. Distribution and function of alternative 5-HT receptors (SC = spinal cord; SCI = spinal cord injury; DRG = dorsal root ganglion).

Receptor		Receptor Type	Location in SC	Normal Function	Function after SCI
5-HT$_1$	1A	Gi/o	Primarily in laminae I and II [35]; Cell bodies in dorsal and ventral horns and intermediate zone [36–38]	Antinociception [39,40]; Pronociception [41,42]; Enhances motoneurons [43]; Micturition reflex facilitation [44–49]; Inhibits motor function [50,51]	Locomotor recovery [52–54]; Antinociception [39]
	1B		Intermediate zone [35,55]; Dorsal horn (laminae I and IV) [35,55,56]	Antinociception [40,57]	Mitigating spasms [58]; Inhibits mono- and polysynaptic reflexes [58,59]
	1D		Superficial dorsal horn [60,61]; γ motoneurons in ventral horn [62]	Antinociception [57]; Inhibits monosynaptic reflexes [63]	Inhibits bladder activity [64]; Inhibits mono- and polysynaptic reflexes [65]
	1E				
	1F		DRG [66]	Antinociception [67,68]	Mitigating Spasms [58]
5-HT$_2$	2A	Gαq	Laminae II and II of dorsal horn [69]; Ventral horn [70]	Antinociception [71,72]; Pronociception [40,73,74]; Protects adaptive learning [75]; Sexual behavior [76,77]; Micturition reflex facilitation [78,79]; Motor function [50,51,80–82]	Functional motor recovery [83,84]; Respiratory recovery [85]; Bladder recovery [79]
	2B		Dorsal horn [86]; DRG [86,87]; Motoneurons [88]	Pronociception [86,87,89]	Functional motor recovery [83]; Mitigates spasms [83,90]; Respiration [88]
	2C		Most parts of spinal gray (except lamina II) [91] and superficial dorsal horn [92]	Spinal reflexes [93]; Inhibit motor activity [94]; Micturition reflex inhibition [78,79,95,96]	Functional motor recovery [83,97]; Mitigates spasms [83,90]
5-HT$_3$	3A 3B 3C 3D 3E	Ligand-gated ion channel	In spinal gray matter [91,98]; Laminae VI through X in dorsal horn [91]; DRG [99]	Pronociception [40,100,101]; Antinociception [102,103]; Micturition facilitation [104]	Motor recovery [105]
5-HT$_4$		GαS	Ventral horn [106]	Pronociception [107]; Micturition reflex facilitation [45]	Locomotor recovery [54,108,109]
5-HT$_5$	5A 5B	Gi/o	Laminae I and II of dorsal horn [110] Not expressed in humans [113]	Antinociception [111,112]; Micturition function [110]	
5-HT$_6$		GαS	Superficial dorsal horn and lamina IX [114]; DRG [115]	Pronociception [116]	
5-HT$_7$		GαS	Superficial laminae [117]; Laminae VII and VIII [118]	Pronociception [119,120]; Antinociception [120,121]; Micturition reflex facilitation [122,123]; Motor function [51,81,82,124]	

Table 2. Common serotonergic agonists and antagonists.

Receptor		Agonists	Antagonists	Non-Selective Agonists	Non-Selective Antagonists
5-HT$_1$	1A	8-OH-DPAT (5-HT1A/7) [125]; Diprpyl-5-CT and Gepirone [126]	WAY-100635 [127]; BMY 7378, NAN-190, MDL 75005 EF; SDZ 216525 [126]; NAD-299 [49]		Propranolol [116]; Spiperone and Pindolol [126]
	1B	TFMPP and mCPP [128]; L-694247, RU 24969 [129], 5-CT, CP 93129 [126]	Quipazine [128], Methiothepin, SB-244289 and SB-216641 [126] BRL-15572 [126,130]; Ketanserin and Ritanserin [126]		
	1D	Gr-46611 [130]			
	1E				
	1F	Lasmiditan (COL-144; LY573144) [68]; LY344864 and LY334370 [126]			
5-HT$_2$	2A	DOI (5-HT$_{2A/2C}$) [131]; TCB-2 [71]; Quipazine [132]	Ketanserin; Ritanserin (5-HT$_{2A/2c}$) [133]; MDL 100907, SB 200646A, SB 206553 [126] RS-127445 [95]; SB 204741 [126] D-MC-5-H-dibenzo [130]; N-desmethylclozapine [71]; SB-242084 [96,126], RS-102221 [126]	DOM [134]; SB 200646 (5-HT$_{2B/2C}$) and SB 206553 (5-HT$_{2B/2C}$) [126]	Ketanserin [116]; Methysergide (5-HT$_{1/2}$) [135]
	2B	α-methey-5-HT [136]; SB 204741, Yohimbine [126]			
	2C	MK-212 [130]; WAY-161503 [71]; RO-600175 [96]			
5-HT$_3$	3A 3B 3C 3D 3E	SR-57227 [137]; 2-methyl-5-HT [134]; PBG [126]	Ondansetron (Zofran3), Alosetron [138], Granisetron, Tropisetron, MDL 72 222 [126]		Tropisetron [116]
5-HT$_4$			GR 113808 and SB204070 [126]		
5-HT$_5$	5A 5B				
5-HT$_6$		EMD-386088 [117]	SB-271046 [139]; SB-399885, SB-258585 [116]; Ro 04-6790 and Ro 63-0563 [126]		
5-H7$_1$		LP-211 [140]; E-57431, AS-19 [141]; E-55888 [142]	SB-269970 [119,143]; SB-656104 [140]; SB-258719 [141,142]; LP44 [123]		

Work suggests that 5-HT$_{1A}$ suppresses nociception by post-synaptically blocking dorsal horn neuronal activity [144–149]. There are also reports of 5-HT$_{1A}$ receptor involvement in pronociception [41,42]. 5-HT$_{1B/D}$ receptors, on the other hand, appear to only have an antinociceptive effect [40,57]. 5-HT$_7$ receptors have multiple effects in modulating nociception depending on the physiological condition of the organism and the location of the receptors. In healthy rats, 5-HT$_7$ receptor agonists exert a pronociceptive effect [121]. In neuropathic conditions however, 5-HT$_7$ receptor agonists have an antinociceptive effect at the level of the spinal cord and pronociceptive effects at the periphery [120,121]. When agonists are administered systemically, however, the antinociceptive effect predominates over the pronociceptive effect in the periphery [120].

Pronociception is primarily mediated by $5\text{-HT}_{2A/B}$ and 5-HT_3 receptors. Similar to 5-HT_{1A} receptors, there is evidence of both pronociception [40,73,74] and antinociception from 5-HT_{2A} receptors [71,72]. Unlike 5-HT_{2A} receptor, 5-HT_{2B} receptors appear to have only a pronociceptive effect [86,87,89]. While 5-HT_3 receptors have also been characterized as pronociceptive [40,100,101], there are reports of antinociceptive actions [102,103].

2.1.2. Regulation of Motor Behavior

It is well recognized that 5-HT also regulates locomotion and motor behavior [54,132,150–158]. For reviews, see [159,160]. For motor control, 5-HT pathways originate from the B1 and B2 regions of the medulla and project to the motoneurons and interneurons in laminae VII and VIII of the spinal cord [118,161–163]. The two main receptors that facilitate locomotion are 5-HT_{2A} [50,51,80–82] and 5-HT7 [51,81,82,124,164]. 5-HT_{1A} and 5-HT_{2C}, however, are associated with inhibition of locomotor activity [50,51,94]. Importantly, 5-HT is also heavily involved in the neuromodulation of central pattern generator (CPG) activity [2,108,154]. Indeed, after SCI, CPG activity can be re-elicited by targeting 5-HT [54,84,165–167].

2.1.3. Regulation of Autonomic Function

There are five major brain regions that modulate sympathetic function: the rostral ventromedial medulla, the rostral ventrolateral medulla (RVLM), the caudal raphe nucleus, the A5 region of the brainstem, and the periventricular nucleus of the hypothalamus [168–171]. Descending supraspinal vasomotor fibers that innervate sympathetic preganglionic neurons (SPNs) express numerous neurotransmitters including amino acids, catecholamines, and neuropeptides. Notably, serotonergic and noradrenergic inputs to SPNs are sourced from the caudal raphe nuclei and the A5 region of the RVLM, respectively [170]. These regions send projections to SPNs in the intermediolateral cell column throughout the T1-L2 segments of the spinal cord and regulate sympathetic outflow [172–174]. The RVLM is the primary source of input to supraspinal vasomotor pathways in the spinal cord that regulate cardiovascular function [175,176]. These fibers terminate in the dorsal and lateral funiculi in the spinal cord [177–179]. While sympathetic postganglionic fibers are driven by neurons from the T1-L2 region of the spinal cord innervate blood vessels throughout the body, the heart is innervated by SPNs innervated by neurons from the T1-T4 region of the spinal cord. Damage to this region can remove a regulatory brake on autonomic function, enabling the emergence of autonomic dysreflexia (AD) [18].

5-HT also affects parasympathetic function, an effect that is largely mediated by 5-HT_{1A} receptors. These signaling pathways have been implicated in parasympathetic control of respiration [180,181], heart rate [182–186], and micturition [44–49]. Other 5-HT receptors have been associated with micturition facilitation (5-HT_{2A}, 5-HT_3, 5-HT_4, 5-HT_7) [45,78,79,104,122], inhibition (5-HT_{2C}) [78,79,95,96], and general function (5-HT_5) [110].

2.2. Overview of How 5-HT Affects Neural Function within the Spinal Cord

The functional consequences of engaging alternative 5-HT receptors vary with the mechanism engaged and location within the spinal cord (Table 1). The 5-HT_1 and 5-HT_5 receptor families are negatively coupled to adenylyl cyclase through $G_{i/o}$-proteins. Their activation leads to decreased production of cyclic adenosine monophosphate (cAMP), which ultimately leads to an inhibitory effect on neuronal firing [17,126,138]. The $G_{i/o}$ receptor types are mainly found within the superficial dorsal horn of the spinal cord [35,55,56,60,61,110]. Other locations include the intermediate zone (5-HT_{1B}) [35,55], ventral horn (5-HT_{1D}) [62], and dorsal root ganglia (DRG) (5-HT_{1F}) [66].

The 5-HT_2 receptor family is positively coupled (via G_q proteins) to phospholipase C, which activates protein kinase C (PKC) and leads to increased accumulation of intracellular Ca^{2+}. This class of receptors has an excitatory influence on neuronal activity. 5-HT_2 receptors are primarily found within the spinal cord dorsal horn [69,86,91,92], with some expression in the ventral horn [69,70,88,91] and DRG (5-HT_{2B}) [86,87] as well.

5-HT$_4$, 5-HT$_6$, and 5-HT$_7$ receptors are positively coupled (via Gα_S proteins) to adenylyl cyclase, which, through protein kinase A, leads to an inactivation of K+ currents, exerting an excitatory effect on neuronal activity. The Gα_S receptor family is primarily distributed in the ventral horn of the spinal cord [106,114,118]. 5-HT$_6$ and 5-HT$_7$ can also be found in the dorsal horn [114,117] and 5-HT$_6$ can also be found in the DRG [115].

Lastly, 5-HT$_3$ receptors are exceptional to the 5-HT receptor family in that they are the only receptors that are ligand-gated and cation-permeable [17,187]. Upon activation, they enhance phospholipase C activity and facilitate neuronal excitability. 5-HT$_3$ can be found throughout the spinal gray matter [91,98] and the DRG [99].

3. Impact of SCI on 5-HT Function

3.1. Impact of Injury on 5-HT Levels

5-HT response to SCI has been extensively studied (for review, see [83]). While the specific time course varies with species and SCI model, destruction of 5-HT fibers can induce an upregulation of 5-HT receptor expression that may last up to 3 weeks [92,156,188–196], with some reporting an extended effect sustained for 6 weeks [197] to 8 weeks [36]. Levels usually return to normal within 60 days [189,193] or earlier [198]. Higher levels have been reported within a few hours of injury [156,196,199] and after 24 h [192]. The upregulation of 5-HT, or its major metabolite (5-HT$_{1AA}$), is associated with edema, increased vascular permeability, and decreased spinal cord blood flow [199,200].

After the initial increase, 5-HT levels decline [201,202]. Faden et al. examined 5-HT fiber immunoreactivity after a moderate to severe injury in rats [203]. After a severe injury, there was a near complete loss of 5-HT immunoreactivity within the lumbar spinal cord two weeks after injury, which was associated with severe spastic paraparesis (a decline in the capacity to move the hind legs accompanied by increased muscle tone and stiffness). In the moderately injured animals, they found a complete loss of staining in the dorsal horn and reduced staining in the ventral horn. In line with this less severe decrease of immunoreactivity, the rats showed moderate, spastic paraparesis. They concluded that loss of 5-HT fibers correlated with the severity of the SCI. Not surprisingly, motor scores were significantly correlated with changes in 5-HT staining in the ventral horn but not in the dorsal horn. This was attributed to the fact that the SCI significantly damaged the fibers in the dorsal region and that these fibers are linked to antinociception rather than motor function.

On the other hand, Saruhashi and colleagues reported that the recovery of serotonergic fibers correlates with gains in functional performance [204,205]. In a hemisection model [205], they found that 5-HT immunoreactive (5-HT+) fibers show increased expression in the ipsilateral cord after 4 weeks and that this predicts the time course and extent of locomotor recovery. The authors suggest the increased expression to be evidence of re-innervation. Similarly, in a later study [204], they found that an increase in 5-HT transporter terminal expression in the lumbosacral ventral horn also significantly correlates with locomotor recovery. Hashimoto, in 1991, found that 5-HT and norepinephrine (NE) are significantly correlated with neurologic score 14 days post-injury and thus suggest that they both participate in functional recovery [206]. Due to the disparate activity of 5-HT within the cord at different phases of injury, it is possible that 5-HT neurons have distinct roles in the progression of neural damage in the immediate phases of injury and in the recovery of function in the chronic phase of injury.

3.2. Acute Effects of Impaired Serotonergic Activity

3.2.1. Descending Serotonergic Fibers Can Quell Nociceptive Sensitization

Damage to descending serotonergic fiber tracts will reduce 5-HT release independent of variation in presynaptic transmitter levels. The acute effect of damage to descending pathways on neural function within the lumbosacral spinal cord has been studied using a full thoracic transection, providing evidence that 5-HT release maintains a brake on neural activity within the dorsal horn that counters the development of over-excitation.

Work in this area was fueled by studies examining the effect of driving nociceptive input to the lumbosacral spinal cord after brain function was disrupted (e.g., by decerebration) or communication with the brain was blocked (by means of a rostral thoracic transection). Under these conditions, electrical stimulation of the sciatic nerve at an intensity that engages myelinated (delta) and unmyelinated (c) nociceptive fibers can induce a state of over-excitation within the lumbosacral dorsal horn [207]. Peripheral application of a chemical irritant (e.g., formalin) has a similar effect [208]. This phenomenon is often studied using the irritant capsaicin, which engages nociceptive fibers that express the transient receptor vanilloid 1 (TRPV1) receptor [209]. Treatment with capsaicin induces a lasting increase in neural excitability within the dorsal horn [210–212], a form of central sensitization [211]. At a cellular level, central sensitization within the spinal cord is correlated with increased expression of the immediate early proto-oncogene c-fos and the phosphorylation of the protein extracellular-signal-regulated kinase (pERK) [213]. At a behavioral level, nociceptive sensitization can transform how animals respond to light touch, leading to a withdrawal response when mechanical receptors are stimulated using calibrated (von Frey) filaments [214]. This alteration is of particular interest because it parallels the development of pain to touch (allodynia), a feature of neuropathic pain.

Interest in nociceptive sensitization was fueled by the observation that exposure to noxious stimulation can have a lasting effect, suggesting it may contribute to the maintenance of chronic pain [215]. Further work revealed that this memory-like effect depended upon signal pathways implicated in brain-dependent learning and memory, such as the N-methyl-D-aspartate (NMDA) receptor (NMDAR), calcium/calmodulin-dependent protein kinase II (CaMKII), and the trafficking/activation (phosphorylation) of α-amino-3-hydroxy-5-methyl-4-isoxazolepropionic acid (AMPA) receptors [210]. The link to brain-dependent learning and memory was further supported by work demonstrating that nociceptive stimulation can induce a form of long-term potentiation (LTP) within the dorsal horn and that this effect too depends upon the NMDAR [215,216]. Interestingly, nociceptive stimulation induces long-term depression (LTD) rather than LTP if the spinal cord is intact [217], implying that descending fibers normally inhibit the development of LTP.

Additional work revealed that brain systems inhibit the development of LTP within the dorsal horn via serotonergic fibers that descend through the dorsolateral funiculus (DLF), which inhibit nociceptive activity by engaging 5-HT$_{1A}$ receptors [148,207,218–222]. This inhibitory effect has been related to the downregulation of adenylate cyclase and enhanced flow of K$^+$ out of the cell [223]. Engaging the 5-HT$_{1A}$ receptor can also counter the development of spinally mediated LTP by depressing voltage-dependent Ca^{2+} channel activity, which attenuates postsynaptic Ca^{2+} influx [148].

Recent work has shown that descending serotonergic systems also inhibit the development of spinally mediated nociceptive sensitization in response to treatment with capsaicin. Supporting this, Huang et al. (2016) showed that both behavioral (enhanced mechanical reactivity) and cellular indices of sensitization are amplified when communication to the brain is cut by means of a rostral thoracic (T2) transection [224]. Here too, the quieting effect was linked to serotonergic fibers that descend thru the DLF [127]. Supporting this, rostral cuts limited to the DLF fostered the development of nociceptive sensitization within the lumbosacral spinal cord. In animals that had undergone a complete transection, intrathecal (i.t.) application of 5-HT$_{1A}$ agonist (8-OH-DPAT) to the lumbosacral region countered the development of nociceptive sensitization. Conversely, i.t. application of a 5-HT$_{1A}$ antagonist (WAY-100635) in intact animals allowed nociceptive sensitization to develop. Taken together, the results suggest that descending 5-HT fibers normally quell the development of nociceptive sensitization, suggesting that this phenomenon may play a limited role in the maintenance of chronic pain in the absence of injury and/or inflammation. The corollary to this is that nociceptive sensitization is especially relevant to the emergence of chronic pain after SCI.

3.2.2. Only Uncontrollable Stimulation Induces Nociceptive Sensitization

Further work revealed that the development of nociceptive sensitization within the spinal cord is modulated by behavioral control [225]. Behavioral control was introduced by applying noxious stimulation to one hind leg (via electrodes implanted in the tibialis anterior muscle) whenever the limb was extended [226]. Under these conditions, animals soon learn to maintain the leg in a flexed position, which minimizes exposure to noxious stimulation, a form of learning known as instrumental conditioning [227]. Subsequent work revealed that this learning involved an intraspinal modification and the NMDAR [228,229].

To show that introducing behavioral control mattered, animals in a second group were experimentally coupled (yoked) to those with behavioral control (master) [226]. Each animal in the yoked condition received electrical stimulation (shock) at the same time, and for the same duration, as its master partner but independent of leg position. Yoked rats that received this uncontrollable stimulation did not exhibit an increase in flexion duration—they failed to learn. Furthermore, they failed to learn when subsequently tested with controllable stimulation applied to the opposite leg, implying that treatment with uncontrollable stimulation induces a kind of learning deficit. Subsequent work showed that exposure to just 6 min of intermittent electrical stimulation applied in an uncontrollable manner impairs learning for up to 48 h [230].

Further research suggested that uncontrollable stimulation interferes with learning because it induces a state of over-excitation within the spinal cord, a form of nociceptive sensitization that saturates NMDAR-mediated plasticity and thereby interferes with the capacity to modify selective behavioral responses. Supporting this hypothesis, exposure to uncontrollable, but not controllable, electrical stimulation enhances reactivity to mechanical stimulation [231,232]. Furthermore, treatments that induce central sensitization (e.g., application of the irritants formalin, carrageenan, capsaicin) impair adaptive learning [231–233]. This learning impairment has been linked to an upregulation of the pro-inflammatory cytokine tumor necrosis factor (TNF) and the trafficking of Ca^{2+} permeable AMPARs [234,235].

3.2.3. Uncontrollable Stimulation Increases Tissue Loss and Impairs Recovery after a Contusion Injury

Because over-excitation after SCI can foster cell death [236], exposure to noxious stimulation could increase tissue loss (secondary injury). This is clinically important because many injuries are accompanied by additional tissue damage (polytrauma) and invasive surgery is often needed to relieve pressure at the site of injury. To explore these issues, rats received a bruising (contusion injury) to the lower thoracic spinal cord using a surgical impactor. Nociceptive fibers were engaged the next day by exposing animals to intermittent electrical stimulation to the tail or the irritant capsaicin applied to one hind paw. Both treatments impaired long-term behavioral recovery [237,238]. Importantly, noxious electrical stimulation only impaired behavioral recovery if given in an uncontrollable manner [237]; stimulation had no effect when animals had behavioral control. Further analyses revealed that noxious stimulation increased the area of tissue loss at the site of injury and that this effect was related to increased expression of TNF [237,239]. Noxious stimulation also engages interleukin-1 beta (IL-1ß), IL 18, and signals related to cell death (caspase 1, 3, and 8) [238,239].

While it is not known whether 5-HT can counter the acute adverse effect nociceptive stimulation has on recovery, there is evidence that targeting spinal 5-HT soon after injury can improve cell survival and reduce neural damage. Bharne et al. found that giving spinally injured mice a 5-HT antagonist (ritanersin) and an alpha-melanocyte stimulating hormone resulted in reduced demyelination, necrosis and cyst formation, and improved locomotor recovery [240]. Administration of the SSRI fluoxetine after SCI had a 5-HT-dependent modulatory effect on matrix metalloproteinase-9 (MMP-9) activation that lessened hemorrhage and the breakdown of the blood-spinal cord barrier (BSCB) [241]. The drug also improved long-term locomotor recovery. In a later publication [242], they found that fluoxetine alleviates cell death (oligodendrocyte cell death) by inhibiting microglial activation after SCI.

3.2.4. Descending 5-HT Fibers Help Preserve the Capacity to Learn

Consistent with prior work, exposure to uncontrollable stimulation does not induce a spinally mediated learning impairment in the absence of injury [75]. In these experiments, rats were given uncontrollable intermittent electrical stimulation to the tail using a computer program that emulated the variable pattern produced by an animal that had behavioral control (master). As previously reported, Crown et al. showed that noxious stimulation induced a learning impairment in animals that had received a rostral (T2) transection [230]. However, when the same amount of stimulation was given prior to T2 transection, it had no effect on spinal function, implying that brain-dependent processes normally act to preserve the capacity for adaptive learning to enable selective modifications within the spinal network. Interestingly, inhibiting brain processes with the anesthetic pentobarbital had an effect analogous to spinal transection, allowing noxious stimulation to induce a learning impairment [243]. This observation is clinically important because it suggests that nociceptive signals during medical procedures under anesthesia may adversely affect spinal function.

Here too, brain systems counter the adverse effects of uncontrollable stimulation via serotonergic fibers that descend in the DLF to engage the 5-HT_{1A} receptor [75]. Supporting this, noxious stimulation induced a learning impairment in animals that had spinal injuries limited to the DLF. Replacing 5-HT via intrathecal (i.t.) application of a 5-HT_{1A} agonist (8-OH-DPAT) blocked the adverse effect uncontrollable stimulation has on learning in transected rats. Conversely, when uninjured rats were given a 5-HT_{1A} receptor antagonist (WAY 100635 i.t.) prior to spinal transection, uncontrollable stimulation induced a spinally mediated learning impairment [75]. The observation that engaging the 5-HT_{1A} receptor can have a protective effect is consistent with other work demonstrating that 8-OH-DPAT attenuates NMDA mediated overexcitation and cell death [244] and inhibits NMDA evoked intracellular signaling cascades in vitro [245].

Taken together, research suggests that engaging nociceptive fibers can induce a form of maladaptive plasticity after SCI that impairs long-term recovery [246,247]. These adverse effects are modulated by behavioral control and brain systems which exert a protective effect via descending serotonergic fibers [225].

3.2.5. Behavioral Control and Brain-Derived Neurotrophic Factor (BDNF) Counter the Adverse Effects of Noxious Stimulation

Work by Crown et al. revealed that introducing behavioral control does more than counter the immediate (acute) effects of nociceptive stimulation; it engages a lasting protective effect that blocks the development of a learning impairment when animals are subsequently exposed to uncontrollable stimulation [248]. It also counters the development of capsaicin-induced nociceptive sensitization [232]. In addition, after a learning impairment has been induced by exposure to uncontrollable stimulation, it can be reversed by training animals with controllable stimulation (in the presence of a drug that temporarily blocks the expression of the learning deficit) [248].

These protective/restorative effects have been related to an upregulation of BDNF [249,250]. Supporting this, the beneficial effect of training is blocked by i.t. application of an immunoglobulin (IgG) for the tropomyosin receptor kinase B (TrkB) receptor (TrkB-IgG) that sequesters BDNF. Conversely, i.t. application of BDNF can substitute for behavioral training to prevent the induction and expression of the learning deficit [250]. Application of BDNF to the lumbosacral region also counters behavioral and cellular signs of capsaicin-induced nociceptive sensitization [251]. Likewise, exercise and locomotor training increase the expression of BDNF [252,253] which attenuate behavioral signs of chronic pain and spasticity after injury [254,255].

The results reviewed above suggest that BDNF has a restorative effect after SCI. These findings stand in contrast to other work that suggests BDNF contributes to the development of nociceptive sensitization in uninjured animals [256–259], an effect that has been related to inflammation and the activation of microglia [260]. The implication is that BDNF can have a bidirectional effect on neural excitability and plasticity. This may help maintain the balance between excitatory and inhibitory transmission, providing a kind of autoregulatory homeostasis [261–263]. This suggests that the effect of BDNF on spinal cord function depends upon factors related to neuronal injury and the overall state of neural excitation [264,265]. After injury, when the effect of nociceptive stimulation on neuronal excitation is amplified, BDNF has a quieting effect; in the absence of injury, activity-dependent BDNF release may promote nociceptive sensitization. It is not currently known whether this transformation of BDNF function is tied to factors related to the cellular context in which it acts (e.g., cellular signals tied to the general level of neural excitation (e.g., intracellular Ca^{2+} concentration)), or the presence/absence of descending fibers (and cellular signals engaged by these pathways). It has been suggested [266] that the switch in BDNF function is related to the expression of phospholipase C (PLC), an effector of 5-HT receptor activation; when PLC is present, BDNF promotes neural excitation, whereas in its absence BDNF has a quieting effect. Supporting this, Garraway et al. showed that BDNF promotes neural excitability in the presence of PLC [267]. The hypothesis also predicts that treatments that engage PLC should promote the development of over-excitation and impair adaptive learning in spinally transected animals. As predicted, treatment with an agonist dihydroxyphenylglcine (DHPG) for the metabotropic glutamate receptor 1 (mGluR1), which engages PLC, induces a learning impairment [268].

Taken together, the results suggest that uncontrollable and controllable stimulation have opposing effects on spinal cord plasticity; the former disables the capacity to learn whereas the latter has an enabling effect. Because these effects involve the modulation of plasticity (the plasticity of plasticity), they have been characterized as forms of meta-plasticity [127,269]. The same could be suggested for descending serotonergic fibers that modulate plastic potential within the dorsal horn [148].

3.3. Long-Term Effects of Impaired Serotonergic Activity

3.3.1. Damage to Serotonergic Pathways Promotes the Development of Neuropathic Pain

Further work has detailed the long-term consequences of damage to 5-HT fibers, which can dysregulate nociceptive transmission and foster the development of neuropathic pain. Work in SCI models of neuropathic pain has shown that serotonergic fibers respond differentially to injury depending on the location. Bruce et al., in 2002, examined serotonergic structural changes after a clip-compression injury (T12) in rats and found that tactile allodynia and hyperalgesia are associated with a reduction in serotonergic fibers caudal to the injury [270]. These findings are supported by other work that linked below-level allodynia to the loss of descending 5-HT fibers after SCI [271]. However, Bruce et al. also found an increase in immunoreactivity for serotonergic fibers rostral to the injury, raising the question of whether the development of pain is due to the increase in faciliatory fibers or the loss of inhibition. Continuing the work of Bruce et al., Oatway and collaborators have found that 5-HT$_3$ receptors (5-HT$_3$R), known for being pronociceptive in pain transmission, facilitate at-level mechanical allodynia after a thoracic SCI [272]. They attribute this effect to the increase in 5-HT fibers immediately rostral to their T13 compression injury. Furthermore, Chen et al. found that a sustained delivery of a 5-HT$_3$ receptor antagonist, given intravenously over multiple days, reduces at- and below-level mechanical allodynia in rats with thoracic SCI [273].

Outside of SCI, injury to the peripheral nervous system (PNS) can lead to similar adverse effects within the dorsal horn. Sprouting of descending serotonergic fibers in the dorsal horn that modulate nociceptive transmission has been found in models of afferent nerve injury [35,274] and traumatic brain injury (TBI) [275].

3.3.2. Damage to Serotonergic Pathways Fosters Spasticity

Spasticity after SCI is a product of overactive, unregulated motor neurons within the spinal cord that create muscle spasms. Weeks after disconnection from supraspinal input, spinal motoneurons compensate for the loss of 5-HT by transitioning into an excitable state, easily responsive to excitatory transmitters such as glutamate [276–279]. This leads to the activation of 5-HT receptors that facilitate sustained firing of voltage-gated persistent Ca^{2+} and Na^+ currents (also called persistent inward currents, PICs) and cause muscle contractions [280]. PICs and spasms are easily triggered by innocuous stimuli such as touch or muscle stretching [281]. Murray et al. [58,90,97] showed that this effect is due to the activity of $5\text{-}HT_2$ receptors. Supporting this, they found that tail spasms in rats after chronic transection injury are associated with constitutively active $5\text{-}HT_2$ receptors. Furthermore, administration of a $5\text{-}HT_2$ inverse agonist SB206553 (cyproheptadine) decreased the magnitude of the PICs and reduced the spasms in the rats. In the follow-up studies, they found that $5\text{-}HT_{2B}$ and $5\text{-}HT_{2C}$ receptors are responsible for the facilitation of motoneuron PICs [90]. Interestingly, they also demonstrated that $5\text{-}HT_{1B/1F}$ agonists can restore serotonergic inhibition of sensory transmission without affecting motoneuron function [58]. The authors showed that the pharmacologic control of $5\text{-}HT_2$ PICs is clinically relevant by administering the inverse agonist to spinally injured humans with evoked leg muscle spasms [97]. The drug significantly decreased muscle spasms. A subsequent study replicated the prior observation that cyproheptadine decreases CaPICs and showed that a serotonin reuptake inhibitor increased spastic muscle activity, further supporting the hyperactivity of 5-HT receptors [282]. The authors stress caution in choosing the dose of the drugs to preserve residual function of the motoneurons. When given at a high dose, cyproheptadine dramatically reduced weight support in rats with a staggered hemisection [97]. In addition, low doses of cyproheptadine have been shown to improve locomotor function in human SCI patients [283].

3.3.3. Damage to Serotonergic Pathways Fosters Autonomic Function

Sympathetic dysfunction, in the form of blood pressure and cardiac impairment, is a prevalent comorbidity in SCI patients with high thoracic injuries. It often takes the form of a condition known as autonomic dysreflexia (AD), characterized by acute bouts of hypertension and bradycardia induced by innocuous or nociceptive stimuli below the injury (such as bladder or colorectal distension). It is well known that descending monoaminergic fibers are involved in spinal sympathetic regulation; spinal $5\text{-}HT_{1A/2A}$ receptors regulate blood pressure [284–287], activation of descending 5-HT axons produce elevations in arterial pressure [288], and adrenal receptors are involved in cardiac dysfunction induced by AD [289]. AD often occurs as a result of the loss of descending sympathetic fibers above the T6 region [18]. Loss of high thoracic supraspinal input can lead to the development of unmodulated sympathetic reflexes and decreased vasomotor tone that results in significant unregulated changes in blood pressure and heart rate that can be life threatening. Additionally, AD is associated with maladaptive fiber sprouting [290,291] and anatomic reorganization [292–296].

Loss of serotonergic fibers can foster the development of AD. In a rat model of severe SCI, it was found that a decline in 5-HT+ fibers located in the intermediolateral cell column of the spinal cord was associated with the severity of AD [297]. Intrathecal administration of a $5\text{-}HT_{2A}$ agonist restored resting mean arterial pressure (MAP) and blocked the colon distension-induced AD while a $5\text{-}HT_{2A}$ antagonist (ketanserin) had no effect on hypertension [297]. The serotonergic fibers were further characterized in a study in 2013 that examined axon regeneration using biotinylated dextran amine (BDA) injected into the rostral ventrolateral medulla to anterogradely trace the vasomotor pathways [179]. The authors observed localized labeling within the DLF throughout the cervical and thoracic spinal segments and, surprisingly, within the ventral white matter. A T4 hemisection that disrupted DLF fibers did not abolish the labeling or result in hemodynamic dysfunction. Only a complete bilateral transection injury that disrupted all supraspinal vasomotor pathways promoted the development of AD. In a subsequent study, the authors attempted to restore basal cardiovascular functions by injecting either brainstem-derived neural stem cells or spinal cord-derived neural stem cells into the T4 transection site [298]. While they found that both grafts mitigated AD, only the brainstem-derived cells displayed axonal growth and functional innervation. Additionally, graft-derived catecholaminergic and serotonergic neurons extended from the injury site and formed synaptic connections with the surrounding host tissue, suggesting that the regeneration of these fibers contributed to the cardiovascular functional recovery. Significant re-innervation was also observed when 5-HT+ neuron-enriched embryonic raphe nucleus-derived neural stem cells were grafted into the lesion site of T4 transected rats [299]. Functional innervation of serotonergic circuits regulating autonomic activity was associated with restored MAP and the alleviation of naturally occurring as well as artificially induced AD. These effects were mediated by the activity of the 5-HT$_{2A}$ receptor, evidenced by the reversal of the grafting treatment with the 5-HT$_{2A}$ antagonist, ketanserin. Lastly, in a study examining the effects of 5-HT$_{2A}$ receptors and dopamine receptors in a rat model of AD, it was found that only 5-HT$_{2A}$ receptor blockade restored hemodynamic parameters [300].

Recent studies have shown that AD after SCI is associated with cardiac dysfunction, in the form of unregulated heart rate and reduced contractility. A study in 2020 compared cardiovascular outcomes after a T2 transection or C6 transection in rats [301]. It was found that hemodynamic function and cardiac outcomes were different after 12 weeks based on the location of injury. The authors reported that C6-injured rats display hypertension and bradycardia while the T2 transected rats exhibit tachycardia. Relative to T2 transected rats, the C6 transected rats had reduced sympathetic tonus support to maintain arterial blood pressure. These results shine a light on the variability of AD symptoms found in human patients that differ in injury location and severity. In a study specifically examining cardiac function as a response to AD, spinally transected rats (T3) were given repeated episodes of AD 2 weeks after injury to allow for normal secondary injury mechanisms to occur. Repetitively induced AD resulted in significant cardiac dysfunction evidenced by reduced basal contractility and the desensitized β-adrenergic receptors. The desensitization of the β-adrenergic receptors was surprising because other studies find that AD increases sensitivity [289]. The desensitization could be attributed to the repeated induction of AD as well the increased circulating catecholamines that occur during episodes of AD [302,303]. A similar pattern of cardiac dysfunction was observed in human SCI patients with recurring episodes of AD. With the increased risk of heart disease in SCI patients [304,305], these results could indicate a link between AD and the development of heart disease.

Spinal sympathetic adrenergic receptors are also involved in immunosuppression after high thoracic injury. Lucin and colleagues found an association between hypothalamic–pituitary–adrenal (HPA) axis and sympathetic nervous system dysfunction and the reduction of antibody synthesis and elevated splenocyte apoptosis [306]. These effects were mediated by NE acting on β2-adrenergic receptors and could be reversed with pharmacological blockade. Pharmacological blockade of both glucocorticoids (GC) and β2-adrenergic receptors has similar restorative effects and diminishes SCI-induced splenic lymphopenia and lymphocyte Bim levels (a pro-apoptotic protein) [307]. While the effects of the immunosuppression could only be found in the T3 transection model, the effects could be mimicked in the T9 contusion model with the application of a β2-adrenergic agonist. A study in 2013 associated the immunosuppressive effects of high thoracic SCI with AD [308]. They found episodes of AD increased as a function of time post-SCI and that experimental activation of AD exacerbated the immunosuppression and splenic atrophy. These effects were also alleviated by pharmacological inhibition of NE and GC receptors.

3.3.4. SCI Facilitates Pulvinar Reorganization and Dysfunction

In this review, we have discussed how descending serotonergic circuits contribute to significant dysfunction after SCI. It is important to note however, that supraspinal circuits are also affected by SCI. Pulvinar dysfunction in the thalamus has been observed in patients with complete SCI [309]. The pulvinar nucleus is known to play an important role in contextual multi-sensory processing and gating [310–312]. Importantly, the excitability of pulvinar neurons is modulated by 5-HT [313]. Specifically, 5-HT was found to have a hyperpolarizing effect. After SCI, there is a reorganization of supraspinal circuits to compensate for the lack of proprioceptive feedback. A functional magnetic resonance imaging (fMRI) study found an increase in functional connectivity between the left pulvinar nucleus and regions of the left inferior frontal gyrus and left inferior parietal lobe in patients with complete SCI [309]. The authors suggest that the lack of afferents from lower motor centers could create an imbalance in sensory weighting, initiating a compensatory increase in cross-talk between multisensory association cortices through the pulvinar nucleus. Given this, the pulvinar could be a promising therapeutic target after SCI.

4. Descending Serotonergic Fibers Regulate the Inhibitory Effect of GABA

The findings reviewed above suggest that the loss of descending 5-HT fibers promotes the development of maladaptive plasticity by enabling a state of over-excitation that can fuel cell death and foster the development of spasticity, pain, and autonomic dysreflexia. This dampening effect has been traditionally linked to the direct consequences of engaging the 5-HT$_{1A}$ receptor, which has an inhibitory effect on neural activity (see Section 2.2). More recent work has revealed a secondary consequence of interrupting 5-HT function, related to an alteration in how the neurotransmitter GABA affects neural excitability, which may help to explain its broad effect on spinal function. This new perspective is motivated by two observations that challenge traditional views of how GABA affects neural activity.

4.1. Pretreatment with a GABA-A Antagonist Blocks the Development of Nociceptive Sensitization after SCI

The standard view of GABA function presumes it inhibits neural activity, an effect that is primarily mediated by the activation of the GABA-A receptor, an ionotropic receptor that regulates the flow of the anion Cl^- across the cellular membrane [314]. In the adult central nervous system (CNS), neurons maintain a low intracellular concentration of Cl^- [1]. As a consequence, engaging the GABA-A receptor allows the anion to flow into the cell, which has a hyperpolarizing (inhibitory) effect.

Within the uninjured adult spinal cord, GABAergic interneurons regulate neural excitation and plastic potential, exerting an inhibitory effect that modulates motor excitability and quiets nociceptive activity [315]. Neural inhibition also limits plasticity, which helps preserve neural circuits over time. Given this characterization, it is naturally anticipated that local application of a GABA-A antagonist (e.g., bicuculline) would remove a brake on neural activity to promote motor output, the transmission of sensory signals to the brain, and plasticity. As predicted, i.t. bicuculline has a pronociceptive effect that enhances behavioral reactivity to noxious and non-noxious stimuli, inducing a state akin to nociceptive sensitization [316–321]. Conversely, administration of a GABA-A agonist (e.g., muscimol), or implanting cells that express GABA, attenuates neural excitation and behavioral reactivity [322–324].

Contrary to the standard view are data demonstrating that blocking the GABA-A receptor can sometimes have an antinociceptive effect that counters the development of nociceptive sensitization. For example, in diabetic rats, pretreatment with bicuculline attenuates the enhanced mechanical reactivity (allodynia) elicited by peripheral treatment with the irritant formalin [325]. Likewise, in rats that have undergone a thoracic (T2) transection, bicuculline reduces the nociceptive sensitization elicited by noxious electrical stimulation, capsaicin, and inflammation [224]. Here, blocking GABA does not remove a brake on neural excitation; instead, the opposite is observed, which suggests that after SCI engaging the GABA-A receptor can have a paradoxical effect that drives, rather than inhibits, neural sensitization.

4.2. Alterations in Intracellular Cl⁻ Impact How GABA Affects Neural Activity

A second observation that led to a paradigm shift stemmed from the recognition that there is a developmental shift in how GABA affects neural activity [326,327]. This alteration is driven by changes in the intracellular concentration of Cl^-, which is controlled by two membrane bound proteins, the K^+-Cl^- cotransporter (KCC2) and the Na^+-K^+-Cl^- cotransporter (NKCC1) that regulate the outward and inward flow of Cl^-, respectively [326,328–330]. Because NKCC1 develops first, the inward flow of Cl^- is augmented early in development, which maintains a high intracellular concentration of the anion [331]. Under these conditions, engaging the GABA-A receptor allows Cl^- to flow out of the cell, which has a depolarizing (excitatory) effect [326,327]. Later in development, there is increased expression of KCC2, which lowers the intracellular concentration of Cl^-. Now, engaging the GABA-A receptor allows Cl^- to enter the cell, producing a hyperpolarization that inhibits neural activity.

What transformed the view of GABA function is the recognition that intracellular Cl^- concentration is dynamically regulated in the adult CNS, a phenomenon known as ionic plasticity [332,333]. Evidence suggests that this change is largely due to a downregulation of KCC2, which attenuates the hyperpolarizing effect of engaging the GABA-A receptor. Indeed, if KCC2 is sufficiently downregulated, engaging the GABA-A receptor can have a depolarizing effect that drives neural activity and plasticity. Evidence suggests that a downregulation of KCC2 can foster the development of hippocampal LTP and contributes to a number of disease states, including epilepsy, addiction, and diabetes [1,325,326,334–337]. Of particular import in the present context, SCI has been shown to downregulate KCC2 caudal to the injury, a transformation that removes a brake on neural activity and plasticity [328,338–340]. While this may benefit recovery by enabling the adaptive re-wiring of neural circuits [127], it also removes a governor on neural excitation, which enables nociceptive sensitization and the development of neuropathic pain [315,328]. The downregulation of KCC2 also contributes to the emergence of prolonged muscle activity (spasticity) after injury and the weakening of inhibitory processes essential to rhythmic locomotion [339,341]. In addition, a GABA-dependent over-excitation impairs the adaptive re-wiring of neural circuits and the capacity to learn [342,343].

The discovery that a downregulation of KCC2 contributes to pain and spasticity after SCI has fueled the exploration of a new class of treatments, designed to re-establish GABAergic inhibition by promoting KCC2 activity (e.g., CLP-290, a KCC2 activator) or by reducing the inward flow of Cl^- with a NKCC1 inhibitor (e.g., bumetanide) [328,340]. Evidence suggests that these treatments can promote the adaptive re-wiring of spinal circuits, foster behavioral recovery, and attenuate the development of spasticity and pain [224,339,343]. The realization that SCI brings a shift in how GABA affects neural activity also helps to explain the paradoxical effect of blocking the GABA-A receptor after injury—because injury leads to a high concentration of intracellular Cl^-, engaging the GABA-A receptor has a depolarizing effect. Under these conditions, pretreatment with the GABA-A antagonist would be expected to have an antinociceptive effect that counters the development of nociceptive sensitization [224].

4.3. Exercise and Training Re-Establish GABAergic Inhibition after Injury

We noted earlier that exercise and locomotor training can have a therapeutic influence after SCI, promoting motor behavior and attenuating the maintenance of chronic pain and spasticity [255,344]. New data have revealed that locomotor training has these effects, in part, because it helps to re-establish GABAergic inhibition by upregulating KCC2 [345]. Because GABAergic inhibition plays an essential role in the execution of rhythmic behavior [341], this fosters the recovery of stepping. In addition, it helps to explain why step training and exercise attenuate chronic pain and spasticity. The beneficial effect of locomotor training and exercise after SCI may be related to increased expression of BDNF, which upregulates KCC2 after injury [345]. Indeed, blocking BDNF counters the behavioral benefit of training and its effect on KCC2, suggesting that BDNF expression plays an essential role [344,346]. As noted earlier, BDNF also attenuates nociceptive sensitization after SCI and this effect too has been related to an upregulation of KCC2 [251].

We discussed above how BDNF can have opposing effects on nociceptive processing, countering the development of sensitization after SCI but generally promoting neural excitability in the absence of injury [256–258]. These alternative effects may be explained by its opposing action on KCC2. After SCI, BDNF upregulates the expression of KCC2, which would counter the maintenance of pain and spasticity [254,339]. In the absence of injury, BDNF downregulates KCC2 within the spinal cord, which would fuel nociceptive sensitization and the development of neuropathic pain [258,260,347,348]. The key question then becomes why does BDNF have opposite effects on KCC2 in injured and uninjured animals? One suggestion is that this is determined by the signal pathways engaged [266,332,333]. BDNF binds to the TrkB receptor, which can activate both Shc (src homology 2 domain containing transforming protein) and PLC. How these pathways affect KCC2 depends upon PLC: If PLC is absent, KCC2 is upregulated; if PLC is engaged, KCC2 is downregulated. In line with this hypothesis, PLC is downregulated within the spinal cord after injury and upregulated by locomotor training [255,345]. Alternatively, the effect of BDNF on KCC2 may be modulated by the intracellular concentration of Ca^{2+} leading to a downregulation when the concentration is high and an upregulation when Ca^{2+} levels are low [326]. Supporting this, neural injury does not transform how BDNF acts if the depolarizing shift is blocked with bumetanide [349].

4.4. The Shift in GABA Function Is Tied to the Loss of Descending 5-HT Fibers

Recent data has linked the downregulation of KCC2 after SCI to the loss of serotonergic fibers that descend through the DLF [127]. Supporting this, lesions limited to this region can flip how bicuculline affects the development of nociceptive sensitization. In sham operated rats, the drug has a pronociceptive effect. After bilateral lesions of the DLF at T2, KCC2 is downregulated and bicuculline has an antinociceptive effect [127]. Likewise, in uninjured animals, pretreatment with a 5-HT_{1A} antagonist (i.t.) reverses the action of bicuculline, causing it to have an antinociceptive effect that counters the development of capsaicin-induced nociceptive sensitization. Conversely, after a complete SCI (T2 transection) i.t. administration of a 5-HT_{1A} agonist (8-OH-DPAT) upregulates KCC2 and re-establishes the pronociceptive effect of bicuculline.

A key unanswered question concerns the impact of these manipulations on the affective/motivational consequences of nociceptive stimulation. Does the loss of descending serotonergic fibers, and the consequent switch in GABA function, alter the sensory signal relayed to the brain? To explore this issue, we examined the effect of bicuculline treatment on capsaicin-induced pain in a place conditioning task, wherein animals experience different treatments prior to being placed in distinctive environments (contexts) [127]. Rats received bilateral cuts of the DLF at T2 or a sham surgery. Over the next two days, the key groups were treated with capsaicin before they were placed in each context. On one day, animals received bicuculline (i.t.) prior to capsaicin treatment; on the other, they received the drug vehicle before capsaicin. Prior work has established that animals exhibit a conditioned aversion to the context where they experience greater pain [350]. In the present case, the focal question concerns the effect of bicuculline treatment on capsaicin-induced pain. If GABA inhibits pain, blocking GABA should enhance the painfulness of capsaicin, inducing a stronger aversion to that context. To establish whether this occurred, animals were given a preference test where they were free to enter either context. As expected, sham operated rats showed an aversion to the context where they had received bicuculline before capsaicin, implying that blocking GABA-A receptors within the spinal cord enhanced pain. However, bicuculline had the opposite effect in DLF-lesioned rats. These animals preferred the context where they had received bicuculline prior to capsaicin treatment, implying that the GABA-A antagonist had an antinociceptive effect. The results reinforce the claim that, after SCI, the engagement of the GABA-A receptor by GABA promotes nociceptive activity and pain.

Other research has shown that a disruption in descending serotonergic fibers contributes to the downregulation of KCC2 that drives spasticity and motor impairments [339,341]. Here, however, 5-HT appears to act via the 5-HT$_2$ receptor [351]. Pretreatment with a 5-HT$_2$ agonist ((4-bromo-3,6-dimethoxy benzocyclobuten-1-yl)methylamine hydrobromide (TCB-2)) upregulated KCC2 after SCI and attenuated mechanical and thermal hyperalgesia. TCB-2 did not, however, attenuate the development of neuropathic pain induced by peripheral nerve injury in SCI rats [352]. Interestingly, treatment with TCB-2 also counters the stress-induced downregulation of KCC2 within the ventral tegmental area, a modification that contributes to alcohol self-administration [335,353].

Serotonergic innervation may also help to explain the transformation in BDNF function, which Rivera et al. linked to the expression of PLC—an effector of engaging 5-HT receptors [266,332]. In adult animals, descending 5-HT fibers would drive PLC signaling, which would cause BDNF to downregulate KCC2 and foster nociceptive sensitization. Damage to descending 5-HT fibers would reduce PLC activity and transform the action of BDNF, causing it to upregulate KCC2.

While the above may help to explain the change in BDNF function, some key questions remain unanswered: (1) How does the development of descending fibers upregulate KCC2?; and (2) Why does damage to these pathways have the opposite effect? Regarding the first question, prior work has shown that the shift in GABA function coincides with the innervation of descending fibers [354,355]. Furthermore, transecting the spinal cord at an early age (before fibers reach the caudal spinal cord) blocks the upregulation of KCC2. Finally, prolonged treatment with a 5-HT$_2$ agonist (DOI) during the first postnatal week can substitute for the lost innervation in transected animals to re-establish GABAergic inhibition [351]. As to the second question, the reduction in KCC2 observed after SCI in adults could be tied to the inhibitory effect of descending fibers. In vitro, artificially driving neural activity leads to a downregulation of KCC2 [266,332]. Likewise, epileptic activity can drive KCC2 down. From this perspective, KCC2 is downregulated after SCI because damage to descending serotonergic fibers removes a source of tonic inhibition, resulting in a state of prolonged neural activity. Under these circumstances, removing a brake on neural activity is biologically efficient and could help neurons survive in the face of increased metabolic load [326,332]. Interestingly, the initiation of this process may depend upon BDNF; blocking BDNF before neural activity is increased, or the spinal cord is cut, counters the downregulation of KCC2 [266,339].

5. Role of Other Monoamines

Monoaminergic neuromodulation within the spinal cord includes not only serotonin, but NE and dopamine as well. While descending serotonergic fibers have been the main focus of this review, it is important to acknowledge the role of the other monoamines.

5.1. Noradrenergic Fiber Pathways

Noradrenergic projections to in the spinal cord (Figure 1) are primarily sourced from the C1 and C2 medullary nuclei, the A$_5$ and A$_6$ nuclei in the locus coeruleus, and the A$_7$ pontine region [17]. The intermediolateral cell column and the ventral horn are recipients of noradrenergic input from the A5 and A6 regions, respectively, while the dorsal horn receives input predominately from the A$_7$ region. There are three major classes of adrenoreceptors (Tables 3 and 4). The $\alpha_{1A/B/D}$ are characterized as excitatory through their positive coupling to G$_{q/11}$ proteins. The $\alpha_{2A/B/C}$ receptors are characterized as inhibitory via their inhibition of adenylyl cyclase through G$_{i/o}$ proteins and their suppression of Ca^{2+} currents. Lastly, β-adrenoreceptors (β$_{1/2/3/4}$) stimulate neuronal activity via Gs proteins.

Table 3. Distribution and function of alternative norepinephrine receptors (SC = spinal cord; SCI = spinal cord injury).

Receptor	Receptor Type		Location in SC	Normal Function	Function after SCI
α_1	α_{1A} α_{1B} α_{1C}	$G_{q/11}$	Dorsal horn, intermediate cell column, and ventral horn [17]; motoneurons [356]	Antinociception [17]; motor behavior, pronociception, autonomic processing [17]	Spontaneous motoneuron activity7; spasticity [357]; Sympathetic neurovascular function [358,359]; micturition [360,361]
α_2	α_{2A} α_{2B} α_{2C}	$G_{i/o}$	Superficial dorsal horn and deeper laminae, and lamina X [17]; motoneurons [356] Dorsal horn [17] Dorsal horn and DRG [17]; motoneurons [356]	Antinociception [17,362,363]; inhibits sympathetic outflow [17]	Locomotor recovery [364]; mediates bowel dysfunction [365]; reflex/muscle spasticity [366,367]; neurological recovery [368]
β	β_1 β_2 β_3 β_4	Gs		Cardiac function [369]	Micturition [370], locomotor recovery [371,372], cardiac function [369]

Table 4. Common noradrenergic agonists and antagonists.

Receptor		Agonists	Antagonists	Non-Selective Agonists	Non-Selective Antagonists
α_1	α_{1A} α_{1B} α_{1C}	Methoxamine (A61603) [357]	WB4010 [357], prozosin [357], BRL44408 [373], silodosin, naftopidil [374], tamsulosin [361]	REC15/2739 [357]; methoxamine [358], phenylephrine [358–360]	Terazosin [360,375]
α_2	α_{2A} α_{2B} α_{2C}	Clonidine, UK14303 [357,376], Guanfacine [377]	Atipamezole [373] ARC239 [373]	Dexmedetomidine [368,378], guanabenz, UK-14304 [376], tianidine [367]; medetomidine [379]	Yohimbine, RX821001(2) [357], rauwolscine, idazoxan [376], efaroxan [373]
β	β_1 β_2 β_3 β_4	Dobutamine [369] Formoterol [371,372] Vibegron [370]	ICI118551 [385] SR59230A [385]		Propranolol [380,381], carvedilol [382,383], nadolol [384]

Adrenoreceptors' involvement in spinal cord neuromodulation is extensive. Traditionally, in conditions of early SCI, NE's activities are known to be involved in hemorrhagic necrosis [386–389], blood pressure/blood flow [390–392], and motor function [387,393–395]. Nociception is regulated by α2-adrenergic receptors which inhibit activity of deep dorsal horn neurons [362,363], and in neuropathic pain models of SCI, catecholaminergic fibers have shown evidence of maladaptive plasticity and fiber sprouting after thoracic transection [396,397]. Lastly, spinal sympathetic β-adrenoreceptors have been shown to be involved in immunosuppression after high thoracic SCI [306,307], and these effects have also been linked to AD [308].

5.2. Dopaminergic Fiber Pathways

Descending dopaminergic projections (Figure 1) originate from the A11 region of the periventricular posterior hypothalamus [17]. These fibers can be detected in the intermediolateral cell column and the ventral horn, but they are primarily found in the dorsal horn and lamina X. Dopamine receptors are classified into two families, D_1-like and D_2-like (Tables 5 and 6). D_1-like receptors include D_1 and D_5 receptors and they have an excitatory action upon neural activation via G_q proteins through stimulation of adenylyl cyclase [17]. D_2-like receptors include D_2, D_3, and D_4 and they inhibit adenylyl cyclase through $G_{i/o}$ proteins and thus suppress neural activity.

Table 5. Distribution and function of alternative dopamine receptors (SC = spinal cord; SCI = spinal cord injury).

Receptor		Receptor Type	Location in SC	Normal Function	Function after SCI
D_1-like	D_1 D_5	G_q	Throughout the spinal cord [17]	Pronociception [17]	Micturition [398,399], cardiovascular function [400], pronociception [401]
D_2-like	D_2 D_3 D_4	$G_{i/o}$	Superficial laminae and lamina X [17] Dorsal horn [17] Dorsal horn (check this one) [17]	Antinociception, pronociception [17]	Micturition [398,399], cardiovascular function [400], antinociception [401]

Table 6. Common dopaminergic agonists and antagonists.

Receptor		Agonists	Antagonists	Non-Selective Agonists	Non-Selective Antagonists
D_1-like	D_1 D_5	SKF 38393 [398,399,402] [403]	SCH 23390 [398–400,402,403], SCH 39166 [401,404]	Aripiprazole [405], apomorphine [300,398,400,406], SKF 83959 [402]	
	D_2	Quinpirole [399,402,403,407], Ropinirole [408], sumanirole [409], B-HT 920, bromocriptine [410,411], LY 141865 [412]	Remoxipride [398,399], domperidone [400,413], metoclopramide [400], eticlopride [414], L-741,626 [402], (−)-sulpiride [403,410], haloperidol [411]		
D_2-like	D_3 D_4	Pramipexole [401,404], ropinirole [408]			

While research on the role of spinal cord dopamine is growing, there is relatively little known regarding its contribution to pathology after SCI [415–417]. There is evidence it is involved in pain modulation. Supporting this, systemic administration of D_2 receptor agonists elicit antinociception while D_1 receptor agonists elicit pronociception [17,403,410–413]. In an SCI model, targeting D_2 receptors has been shown to alleviate pain-related behaviors and even improved secondary injury by reducing inflammation and MMP-9 expression [407]. Lastly, dopaminergic agonists administered to the preganglionic neurons within the intermediolateral cell column have been shown to elicit hypotension and bradycardia [400,418–420].

Recent work has found that dopamine receptors play an active role in micturition after SCI. In a male rat thoracic (T10) transection model, it was found that spinal D1 receptors tonically suppress tonic external urethral sphincter (EUS) activity to enable voiding while the activation of D2 receptors facilitates voiding [399]. Work in a complete transection female rat model showed similar results where pharmacologic activation of D1 receptors after SCI inhibits urine storage and enhances voiding by differentially modulating (EUS) tonic and bursting patterns, respectively [398]. Additionally, they found that pharmacologic activation of D2 receptors with quinpirole improves voiding by enhancing EUS bursting.

6. Conclusions

6.1. Summary

We have described how damage to descending serotonergic fibers can contribute to pathophysiology after SCI. These effects include an amplification of nociceptive signaling that fosters the development of acute nociceptive sensitization, impairs adaptive learning and locomotor recovery, and promotes the development of neuropathic pain, spasticity, and autonomic dysreflexia. In many cases, these adverse effects appear tied to a loss of activity at 5-HT$_{1A}$ and 5-HT$_2$ receptors. New research has shown that the loss of serotonergic activity downregulates the co-transporter KCC2 caudal to injury, bringing a reduction in the inhibitory effect of GABA. It was suggested that this modification may provide a cellular context that fosters pathophysiology, to augment the adverse effects of nociceptive input, impair locomotor function, and drive spasticity. Treatments that bolster 5-HT function after injury may bring benefit by restoring GABAergic inhibition. Likewise, the pathophysiological consequences of damage to serotonergic fibers may be lessened by treatments that target ionic plasticity.

6.2. Limitations and Issues for Future Research

We described above how noxious stimulation can induce a state of over-excitation in the spinal cord and undermine recovery after injury [231,237]. We have also shown that pain input after injury engages pro-inflammatory cytokines and signals related to cell death [238]. More recently we discovered that nociceptive stimulation after SCI promotes hemorrhage at the site of injury [421]. Because blood borne contents are neurotoxic [422], the infiltration of blood would expand the area of tissue loss (secondary injury). Our review of serotonergic regulation of spinal systems has emphasized how these fiber tracts can quell over-excitation and thereby have a protective effect. Given these observations, we naturally hypothesized that noxious stimulation would lead to greater tissue loss and hemorrhage after a contusion injury if communication with the brain was cut. We found exactly the opposite—that disrupting communication with the brain by means of a surgical or pharmacological transection at T2 blocks nociception-induced hemorrhage in rats that had a lower thoracic contusion injury [423,424]. A T2 transection also blocked the activation of pro-inflammatory cytokines, and signals indicative of cell death, at the site of injury. Furthermore, a pharmacological transection at T2 blocked the adverse effect nociceptive stimulation has on long-term recovery [423]. Because a rostral transection is sufficient to downregulate KCC2 in the caudal tissue [224], these findings imply that the shift in GABA function does not, by itself, enable nociception-induced hemorrhage after injury [425]. The implication is that an additional, brain-dependent, process is engaged that plays an essential role in driving pain-induced tissue loss after injury. We have hypothesized that this adverse effect may be linked to a nociception-induced surge in blood pressure [426]. From this perspective, local alterations may enable nociceptive sensitization (setting the stage for chronic pain) and place the tissue in a vulnerable state (e.g., by weakening the blood spinal cord barrier). A surge in blood pressure/flow could then lead to hemorrhage, increasing inflammation and cell death at the site of injury.

A related issue that requires additional research concerns the dissociation of the time-course of injury-induced changes in KCC2 and the development of chronic pain/spasticity. Injury causes a reduction in KCC2 sufficient to transform the action of GABA within 24 h [224]. Yet, spasticity and enhanced pain generally do not develop until weeks later [239,339,427]. Again, the findings imply that a downregulation in KCC2 is not sufficient to produce these effects—that other processes and events play an essential role. Key processes may include the engagement of nociceptive fibers, hemodynamic dysregulation, and factors related to stress.

Additional research is also needed to explore the contribution of these processes to other pathophysiological features of SCI. One unknown concerns the contribution of ionic plasticity to autonomic dysreflexia. Likewise, while it is known that a downregulation of KCC2 contributes to a maladaptive consequence of morphine treatment (spinally mediated hyperalgesia) [333], it is not known whether this effect mediates the adverse effect acute morphine has on tissue sparing and long-term recovery [428,429]. Finally, it should be noted that our review has focused upon how serotonergic fibers and ionic plasticity affect lumbosacral function. A parallel line of work has explored the consequences of cervical injury on respiratory function, demonstrating a BDNF-dependent benefit of intermittent hypoxia [9,430]. Here too, descending serotonergic fibers play an essential modulatory role. However, in this model, ionic plasticity may contribute little to pathophysiology or recovery [431].

Author Contributions: Writing—original draft preparation, G.N.K.F. and K.E.H.; Writing—review and editing, G.N.K.F., J.W.G. and K.E.H.; Visualization, G.N.K.F. and J.W.G.; Supervision, J.W.G.; Project administration, J.W.G.; Funding acquisition, J.W.G. All authors have read and agreed to the published version of the manuscript.

Funding: This research was funded by the National Institute of Neurological Disorders and Stroke (NS104422), and the Office of the Assistant Secretary of Defense for Health Affairs, through the Spinal Cord Injury Research Program under award no. W81XWH-18-1-0807.

Institutional Review Board Statement: Not applicable.

Informed Consent Statement: Not applicable.

Data Availability Statement: Not applicable.

Acknowledgments: The authors would like to thank J.A. Reynolds for his help with the figure.

Conflicts of Interest: The authors declare no conflict of interest.

References

1. Ben-Ari, Y.; Khalilov, I.; Kahle, K.T.; Cherubini, E. The GABA Excitatory/Inhibitory Shift in Brain Maturation and Neurological Disorders. *Neuroscientist* **2012**, *18*, 467–486. [CrossRef] [PubMed]
2. Ghosh, M.; Pearse, D.D. The role of the serotonergic system in locomotor recovery after spinal cord injury. *Front. Neural Circuits* **2014**, *8*, 151. [CrossRef] [PubMed]
3. Hachoumi, L.; Sillar, K.T. Developmental stage-dependent switching in the neuromodulation of vertebrate locomotor central pattern generator networks. *Dev. Neurobiol.* **2020**, *80*, 42–57. [CrossRef] [PubMed]
4. Perrin, F.E.; Noristani, H.N. Serotonergic mechanisms in spinal cord injury. *Exp. Neurol.* **2019**, *318*, 174–191. [CrossRef]
5. Perrier, J.F.; Cotel, F. Serotonergic modulation of spinal motor control. *Curr. Opin. Neurobiol.* **2015**, *33*, 1–7. [CrossRef]
6. Slawinska, U.; Miazga, K.; Jordan, L.M. The role of serotonin in the control of locomotor movements and strategies for restoring locomotion after spinal cord injury. *Acta Neurobiol. Exp.* **2014**, *74*, 172–187.
7. Jordan, L.M.; Slawinska, U. Chapter 12—Modulation of rhythmic movement: Control of coordination. *Prog. Brain Res.* **2011**, *188*, 181–195. [CrossRef]
8. Cummings, K.J.; Hodges, M.R. The serotonergic system and the control of breathing during development. *Respir. Physiol. Neurobiol.* **2019**, *270*, 103255. [CrossRef]
9. Fields, D.P.; Mitchell, G.S. Spinal metaplasticity in respiratory motor control. *Front. Neural Circuits* **2015**, *9*, 2. [CrossRef]
10. Bannister, K.; Dickenson, A.H. What do monoamines do in pain modulation? *Curr. Opin. Supportive Palliat. Care* **2017**, *10*, 143–148. [CrossRef]
11. Bardoni, R. Serotonergic Modulation of Nociceptive Circuits in Spinal Cord Dorsal Horn. *Curr. Neuropharmacol.* **2019**, *17*, 1133–1145. [CrossRef]
12. Liu, Q.Q.; Yao, X.X.; Gao, S.H.; Li, R.; Li, B.J.; Yang, W.; Cui, R.J. Role of 5-HT receptors in neuropathic pain: Potential therapeutic implications. *Pharmacol. Res.* **2020**, *159*, 104949. [CrossRef]
13. Dahlstroem, A.; Fuxe, K. Evidence for the existence of monoamine-containing neurons in the central nervous system. I. Demonstration of monoamines in the cell bodies of brain stem neurons. *Acta Physiol. Scand.* **1964**, *62* (Suppl. S232), 231–255.
14. Törk, I. Anatomy of the serotonergic system. *Ann. N. Y. Acad. Sci.* **1990**, *600*, 9–34. [CrossRef]
15. Bowker, R.M.; Westlund, K.N.; Sullivan, M.C.; Coulter, J.D. Organization of descending serotonergic projections to the spinal cord. *Prog. Brain Res.* **1982**, *57*, 239–265. [CrossRef]
16. Benarroch, E.E. Descending monoaminergic pain modulation: Bidirectional control and clinical relevance. *Neurology* **2008**, *71*, 217–221. [CrossRef]
17. Millan, M.J. Descending control of pain. *Prog. Neurobiol.* **2002**, *66*, 355–474. [CrossRef]
18. Eldahan, K.C.; Rabchevsky, A.G. Autonomic dysreflexia after spinal cord injury: Systemic pathophysiology and methods of management. *Auton. Neurosci.* **2018**, *209*, 59–70. [CrossRef]
19. Bowker, R.M.; Westlund, K.N.; Coulter, J.D. Origins of serotonergic projections to the spinal cord in rat: An immunocytochemical-retrograde transport study. *Brain Res.* **1981**, *226*, 187–199. [CrossRef]
20. Bowker, R.M.; Westlund, K.N.; Sullivan, M.C.; Wilber, J.F.; Coulter, J.D. Descending serotonergic, peptidergic and cholinergic pathways from the raphe nuclei: A multiple transmitter complex. *Brain Res.* **1983**, *288*, 33–48. [CrossRef]

21. Basbaum, A.I.; Fields, H.L. Endogenous pain control systems: Brainstem spinal pathways and endorphin circuitry. *Annu. Rev. Neurosci.* **1984**, *7*, 309–338. [CrossRef]
22. Stewart, W.; Maxwell, D.J. Morphological evidence for selective modulation by serotonin of a subpopulation of dorsal horn cells which possess the neurokinin-1 receptor. *Eur. J. Neurosci.* **2000**, *12*, 4583–4588.
23. Millan, M.J. Endorphins and nociception: An overview. *Methods Find. Exp. Clin. Pharmacol.* **1982**, *4*, 445–462.
24. Fields, H.L.; Basbaum, A.I. Brainstem control of spinal pain-transmission neurons. *Annu. Rev. Physiol.* **1978**, *40*, 217–248. [CrossRef]
25. Zhuo, M.; Gebhart, G.F. Characterization of descending facilitation and inhibition of spinal nociceptive transmission from the nuclei reticularis gigantocellularis and gigantocellularis pars alpha in the rat. *J. Neurophysiol.* **1992**, *67*, 1599–1614. [CrossRef]
26. Zhuo, M.; Gebhart, G.F. Spinal serotonin receptors mediate descending facilitation of a nociceptive reflex from the nuclei reticularis gigantocellularis and gigantocellularis pars alpha in the rat. *Brain Res.* **1991**, *550*, 35–48. [CrossRef]
27. Zhuo, M.; Gebhart, G.F. Characterization of descending inhibition and facilitation from the nuclei reticularis gigantocellularis and gigantocellularis pars alpha in the rat. *Pain* **1990**, *42*, 337–350. [CrossRef]
28. Zhuo, M.; Gebhart, G.F. Biphasic modulation of spinal nociceptive transmission from the medullary raphe nuclei in the rat. *J. Neurophysiol.* **1997**, *78*, 746–758. [CrossRef] [PubMed]
29. Gebhart, G.F. Descending modulation of pain. *Neurosci. Biobehav. Rev.* **2004**, *27*, 729–737. [CrossRef] [PubMed]
30. Ren, K.; Randich, A.; Gebhart, G.F. Vagal afferent modulation of a nociceptive reflex in rats: Involvement of spinal opioid and monoamine receptors. *Brain Res.* **1988**, *446*, 285–294. [CrossRef]
31. Ren, K.; Randich, A.; Gebhart, G.F. Spinal serotonergic and kappa opioid receptors mediate facilitation of the tail flick reflex produced by vagal afferent stimulation. *Pain* **1991**, *45*, 321–329. [CrossRef]
32. Mason, P.; Gao, K.; Genzen, J.R. Serotonergic raphe magnus cell discharge reflects ongoing autonomic and respiratory activities. *J. Neurophysiol.* **2007**, *98*, 1919–1927. [CrossRef]
33. Heinricher, M.M.; Morgan, M.M.; Tortorici, V.; Fields, H.L. Disinhibition of off-cells and antinociception produced by an opioid action within the rostral ventromedial medulla. *Neuroscience* **1994**, *63*, 279–288. [CrossRef]
34. Ossipov, M.H.; Morimura, K.; Porreca, F. Descending pain modulation and chronification of pain. *Curr. Opin. Support. Palliat. Care* **2014**, *8*, 143–151. [CrossRef]
35. Marlier, L.; Teilhac, J.R.; Cerruti, C.; Privat, A. Autoradiographic mapping of 5-HT1, 5-HT1A, 5-HT1B and 5-HT2 receptors in the rat spinal cord. *Brain Res.* **1991**, *550*, 15–23. [CrossRef]
36. Otoshi, C.K.; Walwyn, W.M.; Tillakaratne, N.J.; Zhong, H.; Roy, R.R.; Edgerton, V.R. Distribution and localization of 5-HT(1A) receptors in the rat lumbar spinal cord after transection and deafferentation. *J. Neurotrauma* **2009**, *26*, 575–584. [CrossRef]
37. Kia, H.K.; Miquel, M.C.; Brisorgueil, M.J.; Daval, G.; Riad, M.; El Mestikawy, S.; Hamon, M.; Vergé, D. Immunocytochemical localization of serotonin1A receptors in the rat central nervous system. *J. Comp. Neurol.* **1996**, *365*, 289–305. [CrossRef]
38. Talley, E.M.; Bayliss, D.A. Postnatal development of 5-HT(1A) receptor expression in rat somatic motoneurons. *Dev. Brain Res.* **2000**, *122*, 1–10. [CrossRef]
39. Colpaert, F.C. 5-HT(1A) receptor activation: New molecular and neuroadaptive mechanisms of pain relief. *Curr. Opin. Investig. Drugs* **2006**, *7*, 40–47.
40. Kayser, V.; Elfassi, I.E.; Aubel, B.; Melfort, M.; Julius, D.; Gingrich, J.A.; Hamon, M.; Bourgoin, S. Mechanical, thermal and formalin-induced nociception is differentially altered in 5-HT1A$^{-/-}$, 5-HT1B$^{-/-}$, 5-HT2A$^{-/-}$, 5-HT3A$^{-/-}$ and 5-HTT$^{-/-}$ knock-out male mice. *Pain* **2007**, *130*, 235–248. [CrossRef]
41. Ali, Z.; Wu, G.; Kozlov, A.; Barasi, S. The actions of 5-HT1 agonists and antagonists on nociceptive processing in the rat spinal cord: Results from behavioural and electrophysiological studies. *Brain Res.* **1994**, *661*, 83–90. [CrossRef]
42. Alhaider, A.A.; Wilcox, G.L. Differential roles of 5-hydroxytryptamine1A and 5-hydroxytryptamine1B receptor subtypes in modulating spinal nociceptive transmission in mice. *J. Pharmacol. Exp. Ther.* **1993**, *265*, 378–385.
43. Perrier, J.F.; Cotel, F. Serotonin differentially modulates the intrinsic properties of spinal motoneurons from the adult turtle. *J. Physiol.* **2008**, *586*, 1233–1238. [CrossRef]
44. Lecci, A.; Giuliani, S.; Santicioli, P.; Maggi, C.A. Involvement of 5-hydroxytryptamine1A receptors in the modulation of micturition reflexes in the anesthetized rat. *J. Pharmacol. Exp. Ther.* **1992**, *262*, 181–189.
45. Ishizuka, O.; Gu, B.; Igawa, Y.; Nishizawa, O.; Pehrson, R.; Andersson, K.E. Role of supraspinal serotonin receptors for micturition in normal conscious rats. *Neurourol. Urodyn.* **2002**, *21*, 225–230. [CrossRef]
46. Testa, R.; Guarneri, L.; Poggesi, E.; Angelico, P.; Velasco, C.; Ibba, M.; Cilia, A.; Motta, G.; Riva, C.; Leonardi, A. Effect of several 5-hydroxytryptamine(1A) receptor ligands on the micturition reflex in rats: Comparison with WAY 100635. *J. Pharmacol. Exp. Ther.* **1999**, *290*, 1258–1269.
47. Conley, R.K.; Williams, T.J.; Ford, A.P.D.W.; Ramage, A.G. The role of α1-adrenoceptors and 5-HT1A receptors in the control of the micturition reflex in male anaesthetized rats. *Br. J. Pharmacol.* **2001**, *133*, 61–72. [CrossRef]
48. Kakizaki, H.; Yoshiyama, M.; Koyanagi, T.; De Groat, W.C. Effects of WAY100635, a selective 5-HT1A-receptor antagonist on the micturition-reflex pathway in the rat. *Am. J. Physiol. Regul. Integr. Comp. Physiol.* **2001**, *280*, R1407–R1413. [CrossRef]
49. Pehrson, R.; Ojteg, G.; Ishizuka, O.; Andersson, K.E. Effects of NAD-299, a new, highly selective 5-HT1A receptor antagonist, on bladder function in rats. *Naunyn-Schmiedeberg's Arch. Pharmacol.* **2002**, *366*, 528–536. [CrossRef] [PubMed]

50. Beato, M.; Nistri, A. Serotonin-induced inhibition of locomotor rhythm of the rat isolated spinal cord is mediated by the 5-HT1 receptor class. *Proc. Biol. Sci.* **1998**, *265*, 2073–2080. [CrossRef]
51. Dunbar, M.J.; Tran, M.A.; Whelan, P.J. Endogenous extracellular serotonin modulates the spinal locomotor network of the neonatal mouse. *J. Physiol.* **2010**, *588*, 139–156. [CrossRef] [PubMed]
52. Antri, M.; Mouffle, C.; Orsal, D.; Barthe, J.Y. 5-HT1A receptors are involved in short- and long-term processes responsible for 5-HT-induced locomotor function recovery in chronic spinal rat. *Eur. J. Neurosci.* **2003**, *18*, 1963–1972. [CrossRef] [PubMed]
53. Jackson, D.A.; White, S.R. Receptor subtypes mediating facilitation by serotonin of excitability of spinal motoneurons. *Neuropharmacology* **1990**, *29*, 787–797. [CrossRef]
54. Landry, E.S.; Lapointe, N.P.; Rouillard, C.; Levesque, D.; Hedlund, P.B.; Guertin, P.A. Contribution of spinal 5-HT1A and 5-HT7 receptors to locomotor-like movement induced by 8-OH-DPAT in spinal cord-transected mice. *Eur. J. Neurosci.* **2006**, *24*, 535–546. [CrossRef]
55. Thor, K.B.; Nickolaus, S.; Helke, C.J. Autoradiographic localization of 5-hydroxytryptamine1A, 5-hydroxytryptamine1B and 5-hydroxytryptamine1C/2 binding sites in the rat spinal cord. *Neuroscience* **1993**, *55*, 235–252. [CrossRef]
56. Laporte, A.M.; Doyen, C.; Nevo, I.T.; Chauveau, J.; Hauw, J.J.; Hamon, M. Autoradiographic mapping of serotonin 5-HT1A, 5-HT1D, 5-HT2A and 5-HT3 receptors in the aged human spinal cord. *J. Chem. Neuroanat.* **1996**, *11*, 67–75. [CrossRef]
57. Kayser, V.; Aubel, B.; Hamon, M.; Bourgoin, S. The antimigraine 5-HT 1B/1D receptor agonists, sumatriptan, zolmitriptan and dihydroergotamine, attenuate pain-related behaviour in a rat model of trigeminal neuropathic pain. *Br. J. Pharmacol.* **2002**, *137*, 1287–1297. [CrossRef]
58. Murray, K.C.; Stephens, M.J.; Rank, M.; D'Amico, J.; Gorassini, M.A.; Bennett, D.J. Polysynaptic excitatory postsynaptic potentials that trigger spasms after spinal cord injury in rats are inhibited by 5-HT1B and 5-HT1F receptors. *J. Neurophysiol.* **2011**, *106*, 925–943. [CrossRef]
59. Honda, M.; Tanabe, M.; Ono, H. Serotonergic depression of spinal monosynaptic transmission is mediated by 5-HT1B receptors. *Eur. J. Pharmacol.* **2003**, *482*, 155–161. [CrossRef]
60. Potrebic, S.; Ahn, A.H.; Skinner, K.; Fields, H.L.; Basbaum, A.I. Peptidergic nociceptors of both trigeminal and dorsal root ganglia express serotonin 1D receptors: Implications for the selective antimigraine action of triptans. *J. Neurosci.* **2003**, *23*, 10988–10997. [CrossRef]
61. Ahn, A.H.; Basbaum, A.I. Tissue injury regulates serotonin 1D receptor expression: Implications for the control of migraine and inflammatory pain. *J. Neurosci.* **2006**, *26*, 8332–8338. [CrossRef]
62. Enjin, A.; Leão, K.E.; Mikulovic, S.; Le Merre, P.; Tourtellotte, W.G.; Kullander, K. Sensorimotor function is modulated by the serotonin receptor 1d, a novel marker for gamma motor neurons. *Mol. Cell. Neurosci.* **2012**, *49*, 322–332. [CrossRef]
63. Honda, M.; Imaida, K.; Tanabe, M.; Ono, H. Endogenously released 5-hydroxytryptamine depresses the spinal monosynaptic reflex via 5-HT1D receptors. *Eur. J. Pharmacol.* **2004**, *503*, 55–61. [CrossRef]
64. Gu, B.; Olejar, K.J.; Reiter, J.P.; Thor, K.B.; Dolber, P.C. Inhibition of bladder activity by 5-hydroxytryptamine1 serotonin receptor agonists in cats with chronic spinal cord injury. *J. Pharmacol. Exp. Ther.* **2004**, *310*, 1266–1272. [CrossRef]
65. D'Amico, J.M.; Li, Y.; Bennett, D.J.; Gorassini, M.A. Reduction of spinal sensory transmission by facilitation of 5-HT1B/D receptors in noninjured and spinal cord-injured humans. *J. Neurophysiol.* **2013**, *109*, 1485–1493. [CrossRef]
66. Classey, J.D.; Bartsch, T.; Goadsby, P.J. Distribution of 5-HT(1B), 5-HT(1D) and 5-HT(1F) receptor expression in rat trigeminal and dorsal root ganglia neurons: Relevance to the selective anti-migraine effect of triptans. *Brain Res.* **2010**, *1361*, 76–85. [CrossRef]
67. Agosti, R.M. 5HT1F- and 5HT7-receptor agonists for the treatment of migraines. *CNS Neurol. Disord. Drug Targets* **2007**, *6*, 235–237. [CrossRef]
68. Ferrari, M.D.; Färkkilä, M.; Reuter, U.; Pilgrim, A.; Davis, C.; Krauss, M.; Diener, H.C. Acute treatment of migraine with the selective 5-HT1F receptor agonist lasmiditan–a randomised proof-of-concept trial. *Cephalalgia* **2010**, *30*, 1170–1178. [CrossRef]
69. Doly, S.; Madeira, A.; Fischer, J.; Brisorgueil, M.J.; Daval, G.; Bernard, R.; Vergé, D.; Conrath, M. The 5-HT2A receptor is widely distributed in the rat spinal cord and mainly localized at the plasma membrane of postsynaptic neurons. *J. Comp. Neurol.* **2004**, *472*, 496–511. [CrossRef]
70. Pompeiano, M.; Palacios, J.M.; Mengod, G. Distribution of the serotonin 5-HT2 receptor family mRNAs: Comparison between 5-HT2A and 5-HT2C receptors. *Brain Res. Mol. Brain Res.* **1994**, *23*, 163–178. [CrossRef]
71. Xie, D.J.; Uta, D.; Feng, P.Y.; Wakita, M.; Shin, M.C.; Furue, H.; Yoshimura, M. Identification of 5-HT receptor subtypes enhancing inhibitory transmission in the rat spinal dorsal horn in vitro. *Mol. Pain* **2012**, *8*, 58. [CrossRef] [PubMed]
72. Iwasaki, T.; Otsuguro, K.; Kobayashi, T.; Ohta, T.; Ito, S. Endogenously released 5-HT inhibits A and C fiber-evoked synaptic transmission in the rat spinal cord by the facilitation of GABA/glycine and 5-HT release via 5-HT(2A) and 5-HT(3) receptors. *Eur. J. Pharmacol.* **2013**, *702*, 149–157. [CrossRef] [PubMed]
73. Aira, Z.; Buesa, I.; Gallego, M.; García del Caño, G.; Mendiable, N.; Mingo, J.; Rada, D.; Bilbao, J.; Zimmermann, M.; Azkue, J.J. Time-dependent cross talk between spinal serotonin 5-HT2A receptor and mGluR1 subserves spinal hyperexcitability and neuropathic pain after nerve injury. *J. Neurosci.* **2012**, *32*, 13568–13581. [CrossRef] [PubMed]
74. Obata, H.; Saito, S.; Ishizaki, K.; Goto, F. Antinociception in rat by sarpogrelate, a selective 5-HT(2A) receptor antagonist, is peripheral. *Eur. J. Pharmacol.* **2000**, *404*, 95–102. [CrossRef]
75. Crown, E.D.; Grau, J.W. Evidence that descending serotonergic systems protect spinal cord plasticity against the disruptive effect of uncontrollable stimulation. *Exp. Neurol.* **2005**, *196*, 164–176. [CrossRef]

76. Watson, N.V.; Gorzalka, B.B. DOI-induced inhibition of copulatory behavior in male rats: Reversal by 5-HT2 antagonists. *Pharmacol. Biochem. Behav.* **1991**, *39*, 605–612. [CrossRef]
77. Rössler, A.S.; Bernabé, J.; Denys, P.; Alexandre, L.; Giuliano, F. Effect of the 5-HT receptor agonist DOI on female rat sexual behavior. *J. Sex. Med.* **2006**, *3*, 432–441. [CrossRef]
78. Mbaki, Y.; Gardiner, J.; McMurray, G.; Ramage, A.G. 5-HT 2A receptor activation of the external urethral sphincter and 5-HT 2C receptor inhibition of micturition: A study based on pharmacokinetics in the anaesthetized female rat. *Eur. J. Pharmacol.* **2012**, *682*, 142–152. [CrossRef]
79. Chen, J.; Gu, B.; Wu, G.; Tu, H.; Si, J.; Xu, Y.; Andersson, K.E. The effect of the 5-HT2A/2C receptor agonist DOI on micturition in rats with chronic spinal cord injury. *J. Urol.* **2013**, *189*, 1982–1988. [CrossRef]
80. Gordon, I.T.; Whelan, P.J. Monoaminergic control of cauda-equina-evoked locomotion in the neonatal mouse spinal cord. *J. Neurophysiol.* **2006**, *96*, 3122–3129. [CrossRef]
81. Liu, J.; Jordan, L.M. Stimulation of the parapyramidal region of the neonatal rat brain stem produces locomotor-like activity involving spinal 5-HT7 and 5-HT2A receptors. *J. Neurophysiol.* **2005**, *94*, 1392–1404. [CrossRef]
82. Pearlstein, E.; Ben Mabrouk, F.; Pflieger, J.F.; Vinay, L. Serotonin refines the locomotor-related alternations in the in vitro neonatal rat spinal cord. *Eur. J. Neurosci.* **2005**, *21*, 1338–1346. [CrossRef]
83. Nardone, R.; Holler, Y.; Thomschewski, A.; Holler, P.; Lochner, P.; Golaszewski, S.; Brigo, F.; Trinka, E. Serotonergic transmission after spinal cord injury. *J. Neural Transm.* **2015**, *122*, 279–295. [CrossRef]
84. Antri, M.; Orsal, D.; Barthe, J.Y. Locomotor recovery in the chronic spinal rat: Effects of long-term treatment with a 5-HT2 agonist. *Eur. J. Neurosci.* **2002**, *16*, 467–476. [CrossRef]
85. Zhou, S.Y.; Basura, G.J.; Goshgarian, H.G. Serotonin(2) receptors mediate respiratory recovery after cervical spinal cord hemisection in adult rats. *J. Appl. Physiol.* **2001**, *91*, 2665–2673. [CrossRef]
86. Pineda-Farias, J.B.; Velázquez-Lagunas, I.; Barragán-Iglesias, P.; Cervantes-Durán, C.; Granados-Soto, V. 5-HT(2B) Receptor Antagonists Reduce Nerve Injury-Induced Tactile Allodynia and Expression of 5-HT(2B) Receptors. *Drug Dev. Res.* **2015**, *76*, 31–39. [CrossRef]
87. Lin, S.Y.; Chang, W.J.; Lin, C.S.; Huang, C.Y.; Wang, H.F.; Sun, W.H. Serotonin receptor 5-HT2B mediates serotonin-induced mechanical hyperalgesia. *J. Neurosci.* **2011**, *31*, 1410–1418. [CrossRef]
88. MacFarlane, P.M.; Vinit, S.; Mitchell, G.S. Serotonin 2A and 2B receptor-induced phrenic motor facilitation: Differential requirement for spinal NADPH oxidase activity. *Neuroscience* **2011**, *178*, 45–55. [CrossRef]
89. Cervantes-Durán, C.; Vidal-Cantú, G.C.; Barragán-Iglesias, P.; Pineda-Farias, J.B.; Bravo-Hernández, M.; Murbartián, J.; Granados-Soto, V. Role of peripheral and spinal 5-HT2B receptors in formalin-induced nociception. *Pharmacol. Biochem. Behav.* **2012**, *102*, 30–35. [CrossRef]
90. Murray, K.C.; Stephens, M.J.; Ballou, E.W.; Heckman, C.J.; Bennett, D.J. Motoneuron excitability and muscle spasms are regulated by 5-HT2B and 5-HT2C receptor activity. *J. Neurophysiol.* **2011**, *105*, 731–748. [CrossRef]
91. Fonseca, M.I.; Ni, Y.G.; Dunning, D.D.; Miledi, R. Distribution of serotonin 2A, 2C and 3 receptor mRNA in spinal cord and medulla oblongata. *Mol. Brain Res.* **2001**, *89*, 11–19. [CrossRef]
92. Ren, L.Q.; Wienecke, J.; Chen, M.; Møller, M.; Hultborn, H.; Zhang, M. The time course of serotonin 2C receptor expression after spinal transection of rats: An immunohistochemical study. *Neuroscience* **2013**, *236*, 31–46. [CrossRef]
93. Machacek, D.W.; Garraway, S.M.; Shay, B.L.; Hochman, S. Serotonin 5-HT(2) receptor activation induces a long-lasting amplification of spinal reflex actions in the rat. *J. Physiol.* **2001**, *537*, 201–207. [CrossRef]
94. Halberstadt, A.L.; van der Heijden, I.; Ruderman, M.A.; Risbrough, V.B.; Gingrich, J.A.; Geyer, M.A.; Powell, S.B. 5-HT(2A) and 5-HT(2C) receptors exert opposing effects on locomotor activity in mice. *Neuropsychopharmacology* **2009**, *34*, 1958–1967. [CrossRef]
95. Mbaki, Y.; Ramage, A.G. Investigation of the role of 5-HT2 receptor subtypes in the control of the bladder and the urethra in the anaesthetized female rat. *Br. J. Pharmacol.* **2008**, *155*, 343–356. [CrossRef]
96. Conlon, K.; Miner, W.; McCleary, S.; McMurray, G. Identification of 5-HT(2C) mediated mechanisms involved in urethral sphincter reflexes in a guinea-pig model of urethral function. *BJU Int.* **2012**, *110*, E113–E117. [CrossRef]
97. Murray, K.C.; Nakae, A.; Stephens, M.J.; Rank, M.; D'Amico, J.; Harvey, P.J.; Li, X.; Harris, R.L.; Ballou, E.W.; Anelli, R.; et al. Recovery of motoneuron and locomotor function after spinal cord injury depends on constitutive activity in 5-HT2C receptors. *Nat. Med.* **2010**, *16*, 694–700. [CrossRef]
98. Morales, M.; Battenberg, E.; Bloom, F.E. Distribution of neurons expressing immunoreactivity for the 5HT3 receptor subtype in the rat brain and spinal cord. *J. Comp. Neurol.* **1998**, *402*, 385–401. [CrossRef]
99. Morales, M.; McCollum, N.; Kirkness, E.F. 5-HT(3)-receptor subunits A and B are co-expressed in neurons of the dorsal root ganglion. *J. Comp. Neurol.* **2001**, *438*, 163–172. [CrossRef]
100. Smith, M.I.; Banner, S.E.; Sanger, G.J. 5-HT4 receptor antagonism potentiates inhibition of intestinal allodynia by 5-HT3 receptor antagonism in conscious rats. *Neurosci. Lett.* **1999**, *271*, 61–64. [CrossRef]
101. Doak, G.J.; Sawynok, J. Formalin-induced nociceptive behavior and edema: Involvement of multiple peripheral 5-hydroxytryptamine receptor subtypes. *Neuroscience* **1997**, *80*, 939–949. [CrossRef]
102. Alhaider, A.A.; Lei, S.Z.; Wilcox, G.L. Spinal 5-HT3 receptor-mediated antinociception: Possible release of GABA. *J. Neurosci.* **1991**, *11*, 1881–1888. [CrossRef] [PubMed]

103. Khasabov, S.G.; Lopez-Garcia, J.A.; Asghar, A.U.; King, A.E. Modulation of afferent-evoked neurotransmission by 5-HT3 receptors in young rat dorsal horn neurones in vitro: A putative mechanism of 5-HT3 induced anti-nociception. *Br. J. Pharmacol.* **1999**, *127*, 843–852. [CrossRef] [PubMed]
104. Espey, M.J.; Du, H.J.; Downie, J.W. Serotonergic modulation of spinal ascending activity and sacral reflex activity evoked by pelvic nerve stimulation in cats. *Brain Res.* **1998**, *798*, 101–108. [CrossRef]
105. Guertin, P.A.; Steuer, I. Ionotropic 5-HT3 receptor agonist-induced motor responses in the hindlimbs of paraplegic mice. *J. Neurophysiol.* **2005**, *94*, 3397–3405. [CrossRef] [PubMed]
106. Suwa, B.; Bock, N.; Preusse, S.; Rothenberger, A.; Manzke, T. Distribution of serotonin 4(a) receptors in the juvenile rat brain and spinal cord. *J. Chem. Neuroanat.* **2014**, *55*, 67–77. [CrossRef]
107. Godínez-Chaparro, B.; López-Santillán, F.J.; Orduña, P.; Granados-Soto, V. Secondary mechanical allodynia and hyperalgesia depend on descending facilitation mediated by spinal 5-HT$_4$, 5-HT$_6$ and 5-HT$_7$ receptors. *Neuroscience* **2012**, *222*, 379–391. [CrossRef]
108. Sławińska, U.; Miazga, K.; Cabaj, A.M.; Leszczyńska, A.N.; Majczyński, H.; Nagy, J.I.; Jordan, L.M. Grafting of fetal brainstem 5-HT neurons into the sublesional spinal cord of paraplegic rats restores coordinated hindlimb locomotion. *Exp. Neurol.* **2013**, *247*, 572–581. [CrossRef]
109. Sławińska, U.; Miazga, K.; Jordan, L.M. 5-HT$_2$ and 5-HT$_7$ receptor agonists facilitate plantar stepping in chronic spinal rats through actions on different populations of spinal neurons. *Front. Neural Circuits* **2014**, *8*, 95. [CrossRef]
110. Doly, S.; Fischer, J.; Brisorgueil, M.J.; Vergé, D.; Conrath, M. 5-HT5A receptor localization in the rat spinal cord suggests a role in nociception and control of pelvic floor musculature. *J. Comp. Neurol.* **2004**, *476*, 316–329. [CrossRef]
111. Cervantes-Durán, C.; Rocha-González, H.I.; Granados-Soto, V. Peripheral and spinal 5-HT receptors participate in the pronociceptive and antinociceptive effects of fluoxetine in rats. *Neuroscience* **2013**, *252*, 396–409. [CrossRef]
112. Muñoz-Islas, E.; Vidal-Cantú, G.C.; Bravo-Hernández, M.; Cervantes-Durán, C.; Quiñonez-Bastidas, G.N.; Pineda-Farias, J.B.; Barragán-Iglesias, P.; Granados-Soto, V. Spinal 5-HT$_5$A receptors mediate 5-HT-induced antinociception in several pain models in rats. *Pharmacol. Biochem. Behav.* **2014**, *120*, 25–32. [CrossRef]
113. Grailhe, R.; Grabtree, G.W.; Hen, R. Human 5-HT(5) receptors: The 5-HT(5A) receptor is functional but the 5-HT(5B) receptor was lost during mammalian evolution. *Eur. J. Pharmacol.* **2001**, *418*, 157–167. [CrossRef]
114. Gérard, C.; Martres, M.P.; Lefèvre, K.; Miquel, M.C.; Vergé, D.; Lanfumey, L.; Doucet, E.; Hamon, M.; el Mestikawy, S. Immunolocalization of serotonin 5-HT6 receptor-like material in the rat central nervous system. *Brain Res.* **1997**, *746*, 207–219. [CrossRef]
115. Gérard, C.; el Mestikawy, S.; Lebrand, C.; Adrien, J.; Ruat, M.; Traiffort, E.; Hamon, M.; Martres, M.P. Quantitative RT-PCR distribution of serotonin 5-HT6 receptor mRNA in the central nervous system of control or 5,7-dihydroxytryptamine-treated rats. *Synapse* **1996**, *23*, 164–173. [CrossRef]
116. Castañeda-Corral, G.; Rocha-González, H.I.; Araiza-Saldaña, C.I.; Ambriz-Tututi, M.; Vidal-Cantú, G.C.; Granados-Soto, V. Role of peripheral and spinal 5-HT6 receptors according to the rat formalin test. *Neuroscience* **2009**, *162*, 444–452. [CrossRef]
117. Doly, S.; Fischer, J.; Brisorgueil, M.J.; Vergé, D.; Conrath, M. Pre- and postsynaptic localization of the 5-HT7 receptor in rat dorsal spinal cord: Immunocytochemical evidence. *J. Comp. Neurol.* **2005**, *490*, 256–269. [CrossRef]
118. Noga, B.R.; Johnson, D.M.; Riesgo, M.I.; Pinzon, A. Locomotor-activated neurons of the cat. I. Serotonergic innervation and co-localization of 5-HT7, 5-HT2A, and 5-HT1A receptors in the thoraco-lumbar spinal cord. *J. Neurophysiol.* **2009**, *102*, 1560–1576. [CrossRef]
119. Yesilyurt, O.; Seyrek, M.; Tasdemir, S.; Kahraman, S.; Deveci, M.S.; Karakus, E.; Halici, Z.; Dogrul, A. The critical role of spinal 5-HT7 receptors in opioid and non-opioid type stress-induced analgesia. *Eur. J. Pharmacol.* **2015**, *762*, 402–410. [CrossRef]
120. Brenchat, A.; Zamanillo, D.; Hamon, M.; Romero, L.; Vela, J.M. Role of peripheral versus spinal 5-HT(7) receptors in the modulation of pain undersensitizing conditions. *Eur. J. Pain* **2012**, *16*, 72–81. [CrossRef]
121. Viguier, F.; Michot, B.; Hamon, M.; Bourgoin, S. Multiple roles of serotonin in pain control mechanisms–implications of 5-HT$_7$ and other 5-HT receptor types. *Eur. J. Pharmacol.* **2013**, *716*, 8–16. [CrossRef]
122. Read, K.E.; Sanger, G.J.; Ramage, A.G. Evidence for the involvement of central 5-HT7 receptors in the micturition reflex in anaesthetized female rats. *Br. J. Pharmacol.* **2003**, *140*, 53–60. [CrossRef]
123. Gang, W.; Hongjian, T.; Jasheng, C.; Jiemin, S.; Zhong, C.; Yuemin, X.; Baojun, G.; Andersson, K.E. The effect of the 5-HT7 serotonin receptor agonist, LP44, on micturition in rats with chronic spinal cord injury. *Neurourol. Urodyn.* **2014**, *33*, 1165–1170. [CrossRef] [PubMed]
124. Liu, J.; Akay, T.; Hedlund, P.B.; Pearson, K.G.; Jordan, L.M. Spinal 5-HT7 receptors are critical for alternating activity during locomotion: In vitro neonatal and in vivo adult studies using 5-HT7 receptor knockout mice. *J. Neurophysiol.* **2009**, *102*, 337–348. [CrossRef] [PubMed]
125. Meuser, T.; Pietruck, C.; Gabriel, A.; Xie, G.X.; Lim, K.J.; Pierce Palmer, P. 5-HT7 receptors are involved in mediating 5-HT-induced activation of rat primary afferent neurons. *Life Sci.* **2002**, *71*, 2279–2289. [CrossRef]
126. Barnes, N.M.; Sharp, T. A review of central 5-HT receptors and their function. *Neuropharmacology* **1999**, *38*, 1083–1152. [CrossRef]
127. Huang, Y.J.; Grau, J.W. Ionic plasticity and pain: The loss of descending serotonergic fibers after spinal cord injury transforms how GABA affects pain. *Exp. Neurol.* **2018**, *306*, 105–116. [CrossRef] [PubMed]
128. Brown, L.; Amedro, J.; Williams, G.; Smith, D. A pharmacological analysis of the rat spinal cord serotonin (5-HT) autoreceptor. *Eur. J. Pharmacol.* **1988**, *145*, 163–171. [CrossRef]

129. Eide, P.K.; Joly, N.M.; Hole, K. The role of spinal cord 5-HT1A and 5-HT1B receptors in the modulation of a spinal nociceptive reflex. *Brain Res.* **1990**, *536*, 195–200. [CrossRef]
130. Jeong, C.Y.; Choi, J.I.; Yoon, M.H. Roles of serotonin receptor subtypes for the antinociception of 5-HT in the spinal cord of rats. *Eur. J. Pharmacol.* **2004**, *502*, 205–211. [CrossRef] [PubMed]
131. Kjørsvik, A.; Tjølsen, A.; Hole, K. Activation of spinal serotonin(2A/2C) receptors augments nociceptive responses in the rat. *Brain Res.* **2001**, *910*, 179–181. [CrossRef]
132. Landry, E.S.; Guertin, P.A. Differential effects of 5-HT1 and 5-HT2 receptor agonists on hindlimb movements in paraplegic mice. *Prog. Neuro-Psychopharmacol. Biol. Psychiatry* **2004**, *28*, 1053–1060. [CrossRef]
133. Rahman, W.; Bannister, K.; Bee, L.A.; Dickenson, A.H. A pronociceptive role for the 5-HT2 receptor on spinal nociceptive transmission: An in vivo electrophysiological study in the rat. *Brain Res.* **2011**, *1382*, 29–36. [CrossRef]
134. Fone, K.C.; Robinson, A.J.; Marsden, C.A. Characterization of the 5-HT receptor subtypes involved in the motor behaviours produced by intrathecal administration of 5-HT agonists in rats. *Br. J. Pharmacol.* **1991**, *103*, 1547–1555. [CrossRef]
135. Espey, M.J.; Downie, J.W.; Fine, A. Effect of 5-HT receptor and adrenoceptor antagonists on micturition in conscious cats. *Eur. J. Pharmacol.* **1992**, *221*, 167–170. [CrossRef]
136. Holohean, A.M.; Hackman, J.C. Mechanisms intrinsic to 5-HT2B receptor-induced potentiation of NMDA receptor responses in frog motoneurones. *Br. J. Pharmacol.* **2004**, *143*, 351–360. [CrossRef]
137. Guo, W.; Miyoshi, K.; Dubner, R.; Gu, M.; Li, M.; Liu, J.; Yang, J.; Zou, S.; Ren, K.; Noguchi, K.; et al. Spinal 5-HT3 receptors mediate descending facilitation and contribute to behavioral hypersensitivity via a reciprocal neuron-glial signaling cascade. *Mol. Pain* **2014**, *10*, 35. [CrossRef]
138. Nichols, D.E.; Nichols, C.D. Serotonin receptors. *Chem. Rev.* **2008**, *108*, 1614–1641. [CrossRef]
139. Finn, D.P.; Fone, K.C.; Beckett, S.R.; Baxter, J.A.; Ansell, L.; Marsden, C.A.; Chapman, V. The effects of pharmacological blockade of the 5-HT(6) receptor on formalin-evoked nociceptive behaviour, locomotor activity and hypothalamo-pituitary-adrenal axis activity in rats. *Eur. J. Pharmacol.* **2007**, *569*, 59–63. [CrossRef]
140. Martínez-García, E.; Leopoldo, M.; Lacivita, E.; Terrón, J.A. Increase of capsaicin-induced trigeminal Fos-like immunoreactivity by 5-HT(7) receptors. *Headache* **2011**, *51*, 1511–1519. [CrossRef]
141. Brenchat, A.; Nadal, X.; Romero, L.; Ovalle, S.; Muro, A.; Sánchez-Arroyos, R.; Portillo-Salido, E.; Pujol, M.; Montero, A.; Codony, X.; et al. Pharmacological activation of 5-HT7 receptors reduces nerve injury-induced mechanical and thermal hypersensitivity. *Pain* **2010**, *149*, 483–494. [CrossRef] [PubMed]
142. Brenchat, A.; Ejarque, M.; Zamanillo, D.; Vela, J.M.; Romero, L. Potentiation of morphine analgesia by adjuvant activation of 5-HT7 receptors. *J. Pharmacol. Sci.* **2011**, *116*, 388–391. [CrossRef] [PubMed]
143. Amaya-Castellanos, E.; Pineda-Farias, J.B.; Castañeda-Corral, G.; Vidal-Cantú, G.C.; Murbartián, J.; Rocha-González, H.I.; Granados-Soto, V. Blockade of 5-HT7 receptors reduces tactile allodynia in the rat. *Pharmacol. Biochem. Behav.* **2011**, *99*, 591–597. [CrossRef] [PubMed]
144. Cervo, L.; Rossi, C.; Tatarczynska, E.; Samanin, R. Role of 5-HT1A receptors in the antinociceptive action of 8-hydroxy-2-(di-n-propylamino)tetralin in the rat. *Eur. J. Pharmacol.* **1994**, *263*, 187–191. [CrossRef]
145. Bardin, L.; Tarayre, J.P.; Koek, W.; Colpaert, F.C. In the formalin model of tonic nociceptive pain, 8-OH-DPAT produces 5-HT1A receptor-mediated, behaviorally specific analgesia. *Eur. J. Pharmacol.* **2001**, *421*, 109–114. [CrossRef]
146. El-Yassir, N.; Fleetwood-Walker, S.M.; Mitchell, R. Heterogeneous effects of serotonin in the dorsal horn of rat: The involvement of 5-HT1 receptor subtypes. *Brain Res.* **1988**, *456*, 147–158. [CrossRef]
147. Garraway, S.M.; Hochman, S. Pharmacological characterization of serotonin receptor subtypes modulating primary afferent input to deep dorsal horn neurons in the neonatal rat. *Br. J. Pharmacol.* **2001**, *132*, 1789–1798. [CrossRef]
148. Garraway, S.M.; Hochman, S. Serotonin increases the incidence of primary afferent-evoked long-term depression in rat deep dorsal horn neurons. *J. Neurophysiol.* **2001**, *85*, 1864–1872. [CrossRef]
149. Gjerstad, J.; Tjølsen, A.; Hole, K. The effect of 5-HT1A receptor stimulation on nociceptive dorsal horn neurones in rats. *Eur. J. Pharmacol.* **1996**, *318*, 315–321. [CrossRef]
150. Barbeau, H.; Rossignol, S. The effects of serotonergic drugs on the locomotor pattern and on cutaneous reflexes of the adult chronic spinal cat. *Brain Res.* **1990**, *514*, 55–67. [CrossRef]
151. Barbeau, H.; Rossignol, S. Initiation and modulation of the locomotor pattern in the adult chronic spinal cat by noradrenergic, serotonergic and dopaminergic drugs. *Brain Res.* **1991**, *546*, 250–260. [CrossRef]
152. Cazalets, J.R.; Sqalli-Houssaini, Y.; Clarac, F. Activation of the central pattern generators for locomotion by serotonin and excitatory amino acids in neonatal rat. *J. Physiol.* **1992**, *455*, 187–204. [CrossRef]
153. Cowley, K.C.; Schmidt, B.J. A comparison of motor patterns induced by N-methyl-D-aspartate, acetylcholine and serotonin in the in vitro neonatal rat spinal cord. *Neurosci. Lett.* **1994**, *171*, 147–150. [CrossRef]
154. Feraboli-Lohnherr, D.; Barthe, J.Y.; Orsal, D. Serotonin-induced activation of the network for locomotion in adult spinal rats. *J. Neurosci. Res.* **1999**, *55*, 87–98. [CrossRef]
155. Kiehn, O.; Kjaerulff, O. Spatiotemporal characteristics of 5-HT and dopamine-induced rhythmic hindlimb activity in the in vitro neonatal rat. *J. Neurophysiol.* **1996**, *75*, 1472–1482. [CrossRef]

156. Ung, R.V.; Landry, E.S.; Rouleau, P.; Lapointe, N.P.; Rouillard, C.; Guertin, P.A. Role of spinal 5-HT2 receptor subtypes in quipazine-induced hindlimb movements after a low-thoracic spinal cord transection. *Eur. J. Neurosci.* **2008**, *28*, 2231–2242. [CrossRef]
157. Madriaga, M.A.; McPhee, L.C.; Chersa, T.; Christie, K.J.; Whelan, P.J. Modulation of locomotor activity by multiple 5-HT and dopaminergic receptor subtypes in the neonatal mouse spinal cord. *J. Neurophysiol.* **2004**, *92*, 1566–1576. [CrossRef]
158. Nishimaru, H.; Takizawa, H.; Kudo, N. 5-Hydroxytryptamine-induced locomotor rhythm in the neonatal mouse spinal cord in vitro. *Neurosci. Lett.* **2000**, *280*, 187–190. [CrossRef]
159. Slawinska, U.; Jordan, L.M. Serotonergic influences on locomotor circuits. *Curr. Opin. Physiol.* **2019**, *8*, 7. [CrossRef]
160. Miles, G.B.; Sillar, K.T. Neuromodulation of Vertebrate Locomotor Control Networks. *Physiology* **2011**, *26*, 393–411. [CrossRef]
161. Alvarez, F.J.; Pearson, J.C.; Harrington, D.; Dewey, D.; Torbeck, L.; Fyffe, R.E. Distribution of 5-hydroxytryptamine-immunoreactive boutons on alpha-motoneurons in the lumbar spinal cord of adult cats. *J. Comp. Neurol.* **1998**, *393*, 69–83. [CrossRef]
162. Hammar, I.; Bannatyne, B.A.; Maxwell, D.J.; Edgley, S.A.; Jankowska, E. The actions of monoamines and distribution of noradrenergic and serotoninergic contacts on different subpopulations of commissural interneurons in the cat spinal cord. *Eur. J. Neurosci.* **2004**, *19*, 1305–1316. [CrossRef]
163. Ballion, B.; Branchereau, P.; Chapron, J.; Viala, D. Ontogeny of descending serotonergic innervation and evidence for intraspinal 5-HT neurons in the mouse spinal cord. *Dev. Brain Res.* **2002**, *137*, 81–88. [CrossRef]
164. Cabaj, A.M.; Majczynski, H.; Couto, E.; Gardiner, P.F.; Stecina, K.; Slawinska, U.; Jordan, L.M. Serotonin controls initiation of locomotion and afferent modulation of coordination via 5-HT7 receptors in adult rats. *J. Physiol.* **2017**, *595*, 301–320. [CrossRef]
165. Schmidt, B.J.; Jordan, L.M. The role of serotonin in reflex modulation and locomotor rhythm production in the mammalian spinal cord. *Brain Res. Bull.* **2000**, *53*, 689–710. [CrossRef]
166. Courtine, G.; Gerasimenko, Y.; van den Brand, R.; Yew, A.; Musienko, P.; Zhong, H.; Song, B.; Ao, Y.; Ichiyama, R.M.; Lavrov, I.; et al. Transformation of nonfunctional spinal circuits into functional states after the loss of brain input. *Nat. Neurosci.* **2009**, *12*, 1333–1342. [CrossRef]
167. Fouad, K.; Rank, M.M.; Vavrek, R.; Murray, K.C.; Sanelli, L.; Bennett, D.J. Locomotion after spinal cord injury depends on constitutive activity in serotonin receptors. *J. Neurophysiol.* **2010**, *104*, 2975–2984. [CrossRef]
168. Calaresu, F.R.; Yardley, C.P. Medullary basal sympathetic tone. *Annu. Rev. Physiol.* **1988**, *50*, 511–524. [CrossRef] [PubMed]
169. Chalmers, J.; Arnolda, L.; Llewellyn-Smith, I.; Minson, J.; Pilowsky, P.; Suzuki, S. Central neurons and neurotransmitters in the control of blood pressure. *Clin. Exp. Pharmacol. Physiol.* **1994**, *21*, 819–829. [CrossRef] [PubMed]
170. Jansen, A.S.; Nguyen, X.V.; Karpitskiy, V.; Mettenleiter, T.C.; Loewy, A.D. Central command neurons of the sympathetic nervous system: Basis of the fight-or-flight response. *Science* **1995**, *270*, 644–646. [CrossRef] [PubMed]
171. Llewellyn-Smith, I.J. Anatomy of synaptic circuits controlling the activity of sympathetic preganglionic neurons. *J. Chem. Neuroanat.* **2009**, *38*, 231–239. [CrossRef]
172. Pyner, S.; Coote, J.H. Evidence that sympathetic preganglionic neurones are arranged in target-specific columns in the thoracic spinal cord of the rat. *J. Comp. Neurol.* **1994**, *342*, 15–22. [CrossRef]
173. Tang, F.R.; Tan, C.K.; Ling, E.A. A light-microscopic study of the intermediolateral nucleus following injection of CB-HRP and fluorogold into the superior cervical ganglion of the rat. *J. Auton. Nerv. Syst.* **1995**, *50*, 333–338. [CrossRef]
174. Zagon, A.; Smith, A.D. Monosynaptic projections from the rostral ventrolateral medulla oblongata to identified sympathetic preganglionic neurons. *Neuroscience* **1993**, *54*, 729–743. [CrossRef]
175. Granata, A.R.; Ruggiero, D.A. Evidence of disynaptic projections from the rostral ventrolateral medulla to the thoracic spinal cord. *Brain Res.* **1998**, *781*, 329–334. [CrossRef]
176. Guyenet, P.G.; Haselton, J.R.; Sun, M.K. Sympathoexcitatory neurons of the rostroventrolateral medulla and the origin of the sympathetic vasomotor tone. *Prog. Brain Res.* **1989**, *81*, 105–116. [CrossRef]
177. Furlan, J.C.; Fehlings, M.G.; Shannon, P.; Norenberg, M.D.; Krassioukov, A.V. Descending vasomotor pathways in humans: Correlation between axonal preservation and cardiovascular dysfunction after spinal cord injury. *J. Neurotrauma* **2003**, *20*, 1351–1363. [CrossRef]
178. Kerr, F.W.; Alexander, S. Descending Autonomic Pathways in the Spinal Cord. *Arch. Neurol.* **1964**, *10*, 249–261. [CrossRef]
179. Hou, S.; Lu, P.; Blesch, A. Characterization of supraspinal vasomotor pathways and autonomic dysreflexia after spinal cord injury in F344 rats. *Auton. Neurosci.* **2013**, *176*, 54–63. [CrossRef]
180. Bootle, D.J.; Adcock, J.J.; Ramage, A.G. Involvement of central 5-HT1A receptors in the reflex activation of pulmonary vagal motoneurones by inhaled capsaicin in anaesthetized cats. *Br. J. Pharmacol.* **1996**, *117*, 724–728. [CrossRef]
181. Bootle, D.J.; Adcock, J.J.; Ramage, A.G. The role of central 5-HT receptors in the bronchoconstriction evoked by inhaled capsaicin in anaesthetised guinea-pigs. *Neuropharmacology* **1998**, *37*, 243–250. [CrossRef]
182. Bogle, R.G.; Pires, J.G.; Ramage, A.G. Evidence that central 5-HT1A-receptors play a role in the von Bezold-Jarisch reflex in the rat. *Br. J. Pharmacol.* **1990**, *100*, 757–760. [CrossRef] [PubMed]
183. Futuro-Neto, H.A.; Pires, J.G.; Gilbey, M.P.; Ramage, A.G. Evidence for the ability of central 5-HT1A receptors to modulate the vagal bradycardia induced by stimulating the upper airways of anesthetized rabbits with smoke. *Brain Res.* **1993**, *629*, 349–354. [CrossRef]

184. Dando, S.B.; Skinner, M.R.; Jordan, D.; Ramage, A.G. Modulation of the vagal bradycardia evoked by stimulation of upper airway receptors by central 5-HT1 receptors in anaesthetized rabbits. *Br. J. Pharmacol.* **1998**, *125*, 409–417. [CrossRef]
185. Skinner, M.R.; Ramage, A.G.; Jordan, D. Modulation of reflexly evoked vagal bradycardias by central 5-HT1A receptors in anaesthetized rabbits. *Br. J. Pharmacol.* **2002**, *137*, 861–873. [CrossRef]
186. Wang, Y.; Ramage, A.G. The role of central 5-HT(1A) receptors in the control of B-fibre cardiac and bronchoconstrictor vagal preganglionic neurones in anaesthetized cats. *J. Physiol.* **2001**, *536*, 753–767. [CrossRef]
187. Zhang, M. Normal Distribution and Plasticity of Serotonin Receptors after Spinal Cord Injury and Their Impacts on Motor Outputs. In *Recovery of Motor Function Following Spinal Cord Injury*; IntechOpen: Rijeka, Croatia, 2016. [CrossRef]
188. Laporte, A.M.; Fattaccini, C.M.; Lombard, M.C.; Chauveau, J.; Hamon, M. Effects of dorsal rhizotomy and selective lesion of serotonergic and noradrenergic systems on 5-HT1A, 5-HT1B, and 5-HT3 receptors in the rat spinal cord. *J. Neural. Transm. Gen. Sect.* **1995**, *100*, 207–223. [CrossRef]
189. Giroux, N.; Rossignol, S.; Reader, T.A. Autoradiographic study of alpha1- and alpha2-noradrenergic and serotonin1A receptors in the spinal cord of normal and chronically transected cats. *J. Comp. Neurol.* **1999**, *406*, 402–414. [CrossRef]
190. Lee, J.K.; Johnson, C.S.; Wrathall, J.R. Up-regulation of 5-HT2 receptors is involved in the increased H-reflex amplitude after contusive spinal cord injury. *Exp. Neurol.* **2007**, *203*, 502–511. [CrossRef]
191. Fuller, D.D.; Baker-Herman, T.L.; Golder, F.J.; Doperalski, N.J.; Watters, J.J.; Mitchell, G.S. Cervical spinal cord injury upregulates ventral spinal 5-HT2A receptors. *J. Neurotrauma* **2005**, *22*, 203–213. [CrossRef]
192. Kong, X.Y.; Wienecke, J.; Chen, M.; Hultborn, H.; Zhang, M. The time course of serotonin 2A receptor expression after spinal transection of rats: An immunohistochemical study. *Neuroscience* **2011**, *177*, 114–126. [CrossRef]
193. Kong, X.Y.; Wienecke, J.; Hultborn, H.; Zhang, M. Robust upregulation of serotonin 2A receptors after chronic spinal transection of rats: An immunohistochemical study. *Brain Res.* **2010**, *1320*, 60–68. [CrossRef]
194. Kao, T.; Shumsky, J.S.; Jacob-Vadakot, S.; Himes, B.T.; Murray, M.; Moxon, K.A. Role of the 5-HT2C receptor in improving weight-supported stepping in adult rats spinalized as neonates. *Brain Res.* **2006**, *1112*, 159–168. [CrossRef]
195. Hayashi, Y.; Jacob-Vadakot, S.; Dugan, E.A.; McBride, S.; Olexa, R.; Simansky, K.; Murray, M.; Shumsky, J.S. 5-HT precursor loading, but not 5-HT receptor agonists, increases motor function after spinal cord contusion in adult rats. *Exp. Neurol.* **2010**, *221*, 68–78. [CrossRef]
196. Salzman, S.K.; Hirofuji, E.; Llados-Eckman, C.; MacEwen, G.D.; Beckman, A.L. Monoaminergic responses to spinal trauma. Participation of serotonin in posttraumatic progression of neural damage. *J. Neurosurg.* **1987**, *66*, 431–439. [CrossRef]
197. Navarrett, S.; Collier, L.; Cardozo, C.; Dracheva, S. Alterations of serotonin 2C and 2A receptors in response to T10 spinal cord transection in rats. *Neurosci. Lett.* **2012**, *506*, 74–78. [CrossRef]
198. Cornide-Petronio, M.E.; Fernández-López, B.; Barreiro-Iglesias, A.; Rodicio, M.C. Traumatic injury induces changes in the expression of the serotonin 1A receptor in the spinal cord of lampreys. *Neuropharmacology* **2014**, *77*, 369–378. [CrossRef]
199. Sharma, H.S.; Olsson, Y.; Dey, P.K. Early accumulation of serotonin in rat spinal cord subjected to traumatic injury. Relation to edema and blood flow changes. *Neuroscience* **1990**, *36*, 725–730. [CrossRef]
200. Siegal, T. Participation of Serotonergic Mechanisms in the Pathophysiology of Experimental Neoplastic Spinal Cord Compression. *Neurology* **1991**, *41*, 574–580. [CrossRef]
201. Shapiro, S.; McBride, W.; Sartorius, C.; Chernet, E.; Sanders, S.; Hall, P. Quantification of Changes in Serotonin Uptake with Spinal Cord Injury. *Neurosurgery* **1990**, *26*, 424–428. [CrossRef]
202. Oliveras, J.L.; Bourgoin, S.; Hery, F.; Besson, J.M.; Hamon, M. The topographical distribution of serotoninergic terminals in the spinal cord of the cat: Biochemical mapping by the combined use of microdissection and microassay procedures. *Brain Res.* **1977**, *138*, 393–406. [CrossRef]
203. Faden, A.I.; Gannon, A.; Basbaum, A.I. Use of Serotonin Immunocytochemistry as a Marker of Injury Severity After Experimental Spinal Trauma in Rats. *Brain Res.* **1988**, *450*, 94–100. [CrossRef]
204. Saruhashi, Y.; Matsusue, Y.; Fujimiya, M. The recovery of 5-HT transporter and 5-HT immunoreactivity in injured rat spinal cord. *Arch. Orthop. Trauma Surg.* **2009**, *129*, 1279–1285. [CrossRef] [PubMed]
205. Saruhashi, Y.; Young, W.; Perkins, R. The recovery of 5-HT immunoreactivity in lumbosacral spinal cord and locomotor function after thoracic hemisection. *Exp. Neurol.* **1996**, *139*, 203–213. [CrossRef]
206. Hashimoto, T.; Fukuda, N. Contribution of serotonin neurons to the functional recovery after spinal cord injury in rats. *Brain Res.* **1991**, *539*, 263–270. [CrossRef]
207. Gjerstad, J.; Tjolsen, A.; Hole, K. Induction of long-term potentiation of single wide dynamic range neurones in the dorsal horn is inhibited by descending pathways. *Pain* **2001**, *91*, 263–268. [CrossRef]
208. Le Bars, D.; Gozariu, M.; Cadden, S.W. Animal models of nociception. *Pharmacol. Rev.* **2001**, *53*, 597–652.
209. Willis, W.D. Mechanisms of central sensitization of nociceptive dorsal horn neurons. In *Spinal Cord Plasticity*; Springer: Boston, MA, USA, 2001; pp. 127–161.
210. Ji, R.R.; Kohno, T.; Moore, K.A.; Woolf, C.J. Central sensitization and LTP: Do pain and memory share similar mechanisms? *Trends Neurosci.* **2003**, *26*, 696–705. [CrossRef]
211. Latremoliere, A.; Woolf, C.J. Central Sensitization: A Generator of Pain Hypersensitivity by Central Neural Plasticity. *J. Pain* **2009**, *10*, 895–926. [CrossRef]
212. Sandkühler, J. Models and mechanisms of hyperalgesia and allodynia. *Physiol. Rev.* **2009**, *89*, 707–758. [CrossRef]

213. Gao, Y.J.; Ji, R.R. c-Fos and pERK, which is a better marker for neuronal activation and central sensitization after noxious stimulation and tissue injury? *Open Pain J.* **2009**, *2*, 11–17. [CrossRef]
214. Woolf, C.J. Central sensitization: Implications for the diagnosis and treatment of pain. *Pain* **2011**, *152*, S2–S15. [CrossRef]
215. Sandkuhler, J. Learning and memory in pain pathways. *Pain* **2000**, *88*, 113–118. [CrossRef]
216. Sandkühler, J.; Liu, X. Induction of long-term potentiation at spinal synapses by noxious stimulation or nerve injury. *Eur. J. Neurosci.* **1998**, *10*, 2476–2480. [CrossRef]
217. Liu, X.G.; Morton, C.R.; Azkue, J.J.; Zimmermann, M.; Sandkuhler, J. Long-term depression of C-fibre-evoked spinal field potentials by stimulation of primary afferent A delta-fibres in the adult rat. *Eur. J. Neurosci.* **1998**, *10*, 3069–3075. [CrossRef]
218. Hains, B.C.; Fullwood, S.D.; Eaton, M.J.; Hulsebosch, C.E. Subdural engraftment of serotonergic neurons following spinal hemisection restores spinal serotonin, downregulates serotonin transporter, and increases BDNF tissue content in rat. *Brain Res.* **2001**, *913*, 35–46. [CrossRef]
219. Hains, B.C.; Johnson, K.M.; McAdoo, D.J.; Eaton, M.J.; Hulsebosch, C.E. Engraftment of serotonergic precursors enhances locomotor function and attenuates chronic central pain behavior following spinal hemisection injury in the rat. *Exp. Neurol.* **2001**, *171*, 361–378. [CrossRef]
220. Hains, B.C.; Yucra, J.A.; Eaton, M.J.; Hulsebosch, C.E. Intralesion transplantation of serotonergic precursors enhances locomotor recovery but has no effect on development of chronic central pain following hemisection injury in rats. *Neurosci. Lett.* **2002**, *324*, 222–226. [CrossRef]
221. Bardin, L.; Schmidt, J.; Alloui, A.; Eschalier, A. Effect of intrathecal administration of serotonin in chronic pain models in rats. *Eur. J. Pharmacol.* **2000**, *409*, 37–43. [CrossRef]
222. Hains, B.C.; Yucra, J.A.; Hulsebosch, C.E. Reduction of pathological and behavioral deficits following spinal cord contusion injury with the selective cyclooxygenase-2 inhibitor NS-398. *J. Neurotrauma* **2001**, *18*, 409–423. [CrossRef]
223. Grau, J.W.; Huie, J.R.; Lee, K.C.; Hoy, K.C.; Huang, Y.J.; Turtle, J.D.; Strain, M.M.; Baumbauer, K.M.; Miranda, R.M.; Hook, M.A.; et al. Metaplasticity and behavior: How training and inflammation affect plastic potential within the spinal cord and recovery after injury. *Front. Neural Circuits* **2014**, *8*, 23. [CrossRef]
224. Huang, Y.J.; Lee, K.H.; Murphy, L.; Garraway, S.M.; Grau, J.W. Acute spinal cord injury (SCI) transforms how GABA affects nociceptive sensitization. *Exp. Neurol.* **2016**, *285*, 82–95. [CrossRef]
225. Grau, J.W.; Huie, J.R.; Garraway, S.M.; Hook, M.A.; Crown, E.D.; Baumbauer, K.M.; Lee, K.H.; Hoy, K.C.; Ferguson, A.R. Impact of behavioral control on the processing of nociceptive stimulation. *Front. Physiol.* **2012**, *3*, 21. [CrossRef]
226. Grau, J.W.; Barstow, D.G.; Joynes, R.L. Instrumental learning within the spinal cord: I. Behavioral properties. *Behav. Neurosci.* **1998**, *112*, 1366–1386. [CrossRef]
227. Grau, J.W.; Baine, R.E.; Bean, P.A.; Davis, J.A.; Fauss, G.N.; Henwood, M.K.; Hudson, K.E.; Johnston, D.T.; Tarbet, M.M.; Strain, M.M. Learning to promote recovery after spinal cord injury. *Exp. Neurol.* **2020**, *330*, 113334. [CrossRef]
228. Joynes, R.L.; Ferguson, A.R.; Crown, E.D.; Patton, B.C.; Grau, J.W. Instrumental learning within the spinal cord: V. Evidence the behavioral deficit observed after noncontingent nociceptive stimulation reflects an intraspinal modification. *Behav. Brain Res.* **2003**, *141*, 159–170. [CrossRef]
229. Joynes, R.L.; Grau, J.W. Instrumental learning within the spinal cord: III. Prior exposure to noncontingent shock induces a behavioral deficit that is blocked by an opioid antagonist. *Neurobiol. Learn. Mem.* **2004**, *82*, 35–51. [CrossRef]
230. Crown, E.D.; Ferguson, A.R.; Joynes, R.L.; Grau, J.W. Instrumental learning within the spinal cord: IV. Induction and retention of the behavioral deficit observed after noncontingent shock. *Behav. Neurosci.* **2002**, *116*, 1032–1051. [CrossRef]
231. Ferguson, A.R.; Crown, E.D.; Grau, J.W. Nociceptive plasticity inhibits adaptive learning in the spinal cord. *Neuroscience* **2006**, *141*, 421–431. [CrossRef]
232. Hook, M.A.; Huie, J.R.; Grau, J.W. Peripheral inflammation undermines the plasticity of the isolated spinal cord. *Behav. Neurosci.* **2008**, *122*, 233–249. [CrossRef]
233. Ferguson, A.R.; Huie, J.R.; Crown, E.D.; Grau, J.W. Central nociceptive sensitization vs. spinal cord training: Opposing forms of plasticity that dictate function after complete spinal cord injury. *Front. Physiol.* **2012**, *3*, 14. [CrossRef] [PubMed]
234. Huie, J.R.; Stuck, E.D.; Lee, K.H.; Irvine, K.A.; Beattie, M.S.; Bresnahan, J.C.; Grau, J.W.; Ferguson, A.R. AMPA Receptor Phosphorylation and Synaptic Colocalization on Motor Neurons Drive Maladaptive Plasticity below Complete Spinal Cord Injury. *eNeuro* **2015**, *2*, 16. [CrossRef] [PubMed]
235. Huie, J.R.; Baumbauer, K.M.; Lee, K.H.; Bresnahan, J.C.; Beattie, M.S.; Ferguson, A.R.; Grau, J.W. Glial Tumor Necrosis Factor Alpha (TNF alpha) Generates Metaplastic Inhibition of Spinal Learning. *PLoS ONE* **2012**, *7*, e39751. [CrossRef] [PubMed]
236. Beattie, M.S.; Hermann, G.E.; Rogers, R.C.; Bresnahan, J.C. Cell death in models of spinal cord injury. In *Spinal Cord Trauma: Regeneration, Neural Repair and Functional Recovery*; McKerracher, L., Doucet, G., Rossignol, S., Eds.; Progress in Brain Research; Elsevier: Amsterdam, The Netherlands, 2002; Volume 137, pp. 37–47.
237. Grau, J.W.; Washburn, S.N.; Hook, M.A.; Ferguson, A.R.; Crown, E.D.; Garcia, G.; Bolding, K.A.; Miranda, R.C. Uncontrollable stimulation undermines recovery after spinal cord injury. *J. Neurotrauma* **2004**, *21*, 1795–1817. [CrossRef]
238. Turtle, J.D.; Strain, M.M.; Reynolds, J.A.; Huang, Y.J.; Lee, K.H.; Henwood, M.K.; Garraway, S.M.; Grau, J.W. Pain Input After Spinal Cord Injury (SCI) Undermines Long-Term Recovery and Engages Signal Pathways That Promote Cell Death. *Front. Syst. Neurosci.* **2018**, *12*, 14. [CrossRef]

239. Garraway, S.M.; Woller, S.A.; Huie, J.R.; Hartman, J.J.; Hook, M.A.; Miranda, R.C.; Huang, Y.J.; Ferguson, A.R.; Grau, J.W. Peripheral noxious stimulation reduces withdrawal threshold to mechanical stimuli after spinal cord injury: Role of tumor necrosis factor alpha and apoptosis. *Pain* **2014**, *155*, 2344–2359. [CrossRef]
240. Bharne, A.P.; Upadhya, M.A.; Kokare, D.M.; Subhedar, N.K. Effect of alpha-melanocyte stimulating hormone on locomotor recovery following spinal cord injury in mice: Role of serotonergic system. *Neuropeptides* **2011**, *45*, 25–31. [CrossRef]
241. Lee, J.Y.; Kim, H.S.; Choi, H.Y.; Oh, T.H.; Ju, B.G.; Yune, T.Y. Valproic acid attenuates blood-spinal cord barrier disruption by inhibiting matrix metalloprotease-9 activity and improves functional recovery after spinal cord injury. *J. Neurochem.* **2012**, *121*, 818–829. [CrossRef]
242. Lee, J.Y.; Kang, S.R.; Yune, T.Y. Fluoxetine prevents oligodendrocyte cell death by inhibiting microglia activation after spinal cord injury. *J. Neurotrauma* **2015**, *32*, 633–644. [CrossRef]
243. Washburn, S.N.; Patton, B.C.; Ferguson, A.R.; Hudson, K.L.; Grau, J.W. Exposure to intermittent nociceptive stimulation under pentobarbital anesthesia disrupts spinal cord function in rats. *Psychopharmacology* **2007**, *192*, 243–252. [CrossRef]
244. Madhavan, L.; Freed, W.J.; Anantharam, V.; Kanthasamy, A.G. 5-hydroxytryptamine 1A receptor activation protects against N-methyl-D-aspartate-induced apoptotic cell death in striatal and mesencephalic cultures. *J. Pharmacol. Exp. Ther.* **2003**, *304*, 913–923. [CrossRef]
245. Maura, G.; Marcoli, M.; Pepicelli, O.; Rosu, C.; Viola, C.; Raiteri, M. Serotonin inhibition of the NMDA receptor/nitric oxide/cyclic GMP pathway in human neocortex slices: Involvement of 5-HT(2C) and 5-HT(1A) receptors. *Br. J. Pharmacol.* **2000**, *130*, 1853–1858. [CrossRef]
246. Ferguson, A.R.; Huie, J.R.; Crown, E.D.; Baumbauer, K.M.; Hook, M.A.; Garraway, S.M.; Lee, K.H.; Hoy, K.C.; Grau, J.W. Maladaptive spinal plasticity opposes spinal learning and recovery in spinal cord injury. *Front. Physiol.* **2012**, *3*, 17. [CrossRef]
247. Grau, J.W.; Huang, Y.J.; Turtle, J.D.; Strain, M.M.; Miranda, R.C.; Garraway, S.M.; Hook, M.A. When Pain Hurts: Nociceptive Stimulation Induces a State of Maladaptive Plasticity and Impairs Recovery after Spinal Cord Injury. *J. Neurotrauma* **2017**, *34*, 1873–1890. [CrossRef]
248. Crown, E.D.; Grau, J.W. Preserving and restoring behavioral potential within the spinal cord using an instrumental training paradigm. *J. Neurophysiol.* **2001**, *86*, 845–855. [CrossRef]
249. Gomez-Pinilla, F.; Huie, J.R.; Ying, Z.; Ferguson, A.R.; Crown, E.D.; Baumbauer, K.M.; Edgerton, V.R.; Grau, J.W. BDNF and learning: Evidence that instrumental training promotes learning within the spinal cord by up-regulating BDNF expression. *Neuroscience* **2007**, *148*, 893–906. [CrossRef]
250. Huie, J.R.; Garraway, S.M.; Baumbauer, K.M.; Hoy, K.C.; Beas, B.S.; Montgomery, K.S.; Bizon, J.L.; Grau, J.W. Brain-derived neurotrophic factor promotes adaptive plasticity within the spinal cord and mediates the beneficial effects of controllable stimulation. *Neuroscience* **2012**, *200*, 74–90. [CrossRef]
251. Huang, Y.J.; Lee, K.H.; Grau, J.W. Complete spinal cord injury (SCI) transforms how brain derived neurotrophic factor (BDNF) affects nociceptive sensitization. *Exp. Neurol.* **2017**, *288*, 38–50. [CrossRef]
252. Weishaupt, N.; Blesch, A.; Fouad, K. BDNF: The career of a multifaceted neurotrophin in spinal cord injury. *Exp. Neurol.* **2012**, *238*, 254–264. [CrossRef]
253. Ying, Z.; Roy, R.R.; Edgerton, V.R.; Gomez-Pinilla, F. Exercise restores levels of neurotrophins and synaptic plasticity following spinal cord injury. *Exp. Neurol.* **2005**, *193*, 411–419. [CrossRef]
254. Boyce, V.S.; Mendell, L.M. Neurotrophins and spinal circuit function. *Front. Neural Circuits* **2014**, *8*, 59. [CrossRef]
255. Tashiro, S.; Shinozaki, M.; Mukaino, M.; Renault-Mihara, F.; Toyama, Y.; Liu, M.G.; Nakamura, M.; Okano, H. BDNF Induced by Treadmill Training Contributes to the Suppression of Spasticity and Allodynia After Spinal Cord Injury via Upregulation of KCC2. *Neurorehabil. Neural Repair* **2015**, *29*, 677–689. [CrossRef]
256. Merighi, A.; Bardoni, R.; Salio, C.; Lossi, L.; Ferrini, F.; Prandini, M.; Zonta, M.; Gustincich, S.; Carmignoto, G. Presynaptic functional trkB receptors mediate the release of excitatory neurotransmitters from primary afferent terminals in lamina II (substantia gelatinosa) of postnatal rat spinal cord. *Dev. Neurobiol.* **2008**, *68*, 457–475. [CrossRef]
257. Pezet, S.; Cunningham, J.; Patel, J.; Grist, J.; Gavazzi, I.; Lever, I.J.; Malcangio, M. BDNF modulates sensory neuron synaptic activity by a facilitation of GABA transmission in the dorsal horn. *Mol. Cell. Neurosci.* **2002**, *21*, 51–62. [CrossRef]
258. Smith, P.A. BDNF: No gain without pain? *Neuroscience* **2014**, *283*, 107–123. [CrossRef]
259. Zhou, L.-J.; Zhong, Y.; Ren, W.-J.; Li, Y.-Y.; Zhang, T.; Liu, X.-G. BDNF induces late-phase LTP of C-fiber evoked field potentials in rat spinal dorsal horn. *Exp. Neurol.* **2008**, *212*, 507–514. [CrossRef] [PubMed]
260. Coull, J.A.M.; Beggs, S.; Boudreau, D.; Boivin, D.; Tsuda, M.; Inoue, K.; Gravel, C.; Salter, M.W.; De Koninck, Y. BDNF from microglia causes the shift in neuronal anion gradient underlying neuropathic pain. *Nature* **2005**, *438*, 1017–1021. [CrossRef] [PubMed]
261. Cunha, C.; Brambilla, R.; Thomas, K.L. A simple role for BDNF in learning and memory? *Front. Mol. Neurosci.* **2010**, *3*, 1. [CrossRef] [PubMed]
262. Turrigiano, G.G. The Self-Tuning Neuron: Synaptic Scaling of Excitatory Synapses. *Cell* **2008**, *135*, 422–435. [CrossRef]
263. Rutherford, L.C.; Nelson, S.B.; Turrigiano, G.G. BDNF has opposite effects on the quantal amplitude of pyramidal neuron and interneuron excitatory synapses. *Neuron* **1998**, *21*, 521–530. [CrossRef]
264. Desai, N.S.; Rutherford, L.C.; Turrigiano, G.G. BDNF regulates the intrinsic excitability of cortical neurons. *Learn Mem.* **1999**, *6*, 284–291. [CrossRef]

265. Schinder, A.F.; Berninger, B.; Poo, M. Postsynaptic target specificity of neurotrophin-induced presynaptic potentiation. *Neuron* 2000, *25*, 151–163. [CrossRef]
266. Rivera, C.; Voipio, J.; Thomas-Crusells, J.; Li, H.; Emri, Z.; Sipila, S.; Payne, J.A.; Minichiello, L.; Saarma, M.; Kaila, K. Mechanism of activity-dependent downregulation of the neuron-specific K-Cl cotransporter KCC2. *J. Neurosci.* 2004, *24*, 4683–4691. [CrossRef]
267. Garraway, S.M.; Petruska, J.C.; Mendell, L.M. BDNF sensitizes the response of lamina II neurons to high threshold primary afferent inputs. *Eur. J. Neurosci.* 2003, *18*, 2467–2476. [CrossRef]
268. Ferguson, A.R.; Bolding, K.A.; Huie, J.R.; Hook, M.A.; Santillano, D.R.; Miranda, R.C.; Grau, J.W. Group I metabotropic glutamate receptors control metaplasticity of spinal cord learning through a protein kinase C-dependent mechanism. *J. Neurosci.* 2008, *28*, 11939–11949. [CrossRef]
269. Abraham, W.C. Metaplasticity: Tuning synapses and networks for plasticity. *Nat. Rev. Neurosci.* 2008, *9*, 387. [CrossRef]
270. Bruce, J.C.; Oatway, M.A.; Weaver, L.C. Chronic pain after clip-compression injury of the rat spinal cord. *Exp. Neurol.* 2002, *178*, 33–48. [CrossRef]
271. Hains, B.C.; Everhart, A.W.; Fullwood, S.D.; Hulsebosch, C.E. Changes in serotonin, serotonin transporter expression and serotonin denervation supersensitivity: Involvement in chronic central pain after spinal hemisection in the rat. *Exp. Neurol.* 2002, *175*, 347–362. [CrossRef]
272. Oatway, M.A.; Chen, Y.; Weaver, L.C. The 5-HT3 receptor facilitates at-level mechanical allodynia following spinal cord injury. *Pain* 2004, *110*, 259–268. [CrossRef]
273. Chen, Y.; Oatway, M.A.; Weaver, L.C. Blockade of the 5-HT3 receptor for days causes sustained relief from mechanical allodynia following spinal cord injury. *J. Neurosci. Res.* 2009, *87*, 418–424. [CrossRef]
274. Wang, Y.X.; Bowersox, S.S.; Pettus, M.; Gao, D. Antinociceptive properties of fenfluramine, a serotonin reuptake inhibitor, in a rat model of neuropathy. *J. Pharmacol. Exp. Ther.* 1999, *291*, 1008–1016. [PubMed]
275. Irvine, K.A.; Sahbaie, P.; Ferguson, A.R.; Clark, J.D. Enhanced descending pain facilitation in acute traumatic brain injury. *Exp. Neurol.* 2019, *320*, 112976. [CrossRef] [PubMed]
276. Hultborn, H.; Denton, M.E.; Wienecke, J.; Nielsen, J.B. Variable amplification of synaptic input to cat spinal motoneurones by dendritic persistent inward current. *J. Physiol.* 2003, *552*, 945–952. [CrossRef] [PubMed]
277. Jacobs, B.L.; Martín-Cora, F.J.; Fornal, C.A. Activity of medullary serotonergic neurons in freely moving animals. *Brain Res. Rev.* 2002, *40*, 45–52. [CrossRef]
278. Perrier, J.F.; Delgado-Lezama, R. Synaptic release of serotonin induced by stimulation of the raphe nucleus promotes plateau potentials in spinal motoneurons of the adult turtle. *J. Neurosci.* 2005, *25*, 7993–7999. [CrossRef]
279. Hounsgaard, J.; Hultborn, H.; Jespersen, B.; Kiehn, O. Bistability of alpha-motoneurones in the decerebrate cat and in the acute spinal cat after intravenous 5-hydroxytryptophan. *J. Physiol.* 1988, *405*, 345–367. [CrossRef]
280. Li, Y.R.; Gorassini, M.A.; Bennett, D.J. Role of persistent sodium and calcium currents in motoneuron firing and spasticity in chronic spinal rats. *J. Neurophysiol.* 2004, *91*, 767–783. [CrossRef]
281. Bennett, D.J.; Sanelli, L.; Cooke, C.L.; Harvey, P.J.; Gorassini, M.A. Spastic long-lasting reflexes in the awake rat after sacral spinal cord injury. *J. Neurophysiol.* 2004, *91*, 2247–2258. [CrossRef]
282. D'Amico, J.M.; Murray, K.C.; Li, Y.; Chan, K.M.; Finlay, M.G.; Bennett, D.J.; Gorassini, M.A. Constitutively active 5-HT2/α1 receptors facilitate muscle spasms after human spinal cord injury. *J. Neurophysiol.* 2013, *109*, 1473–1484. [CrossRef]
283. Wainberg, M.; Barbeau, H.; Gauthier, S. The effects of cyproheptadine on locomotion and on spasticity in patients with spinal cord injuries. *J. Neurol. Neurosurg. Psychiatry* 1990, *53*, 754–763. [CrossRef]
284. Ramage, A.G. Central cardiovascular regulation and 5-hydroxytryptamine receptors. *Brain Res. Bull.* 2001, *56*, 425–439. [CrossRef]
285. Ramage, A.G.; Villalon, C.M. 5-hydroxytryptamine and cardiovascular regulation. *Trends Pharmacol. Sci.* 2008, *29*, 472–481. [CrossRef]
286. Coote, J.H. Bulbospinal serotonergic pathways in the control of blood pressure. *J. Cardiovasc. Pharmacol.* 1990, *15* (Suppl. S7), S35–S41. [CrossRef]
287. Lewis, D.I.; Coote, J.H. The influence of 5-hydroxytryptamine agonists and antagonists on identified sympathetic preganglionic neurones in the rat, in vivo. *Br. J. Pharmacol.* 1990, *99*, 667–672. [CrossRef]
288. Chalmers, J.P.; Pilowsky, P.M.; Minson, J.B.; Kapoor, V.; Mills, E.; West, M.J. Central serotonergic mechanisms in hypertension. *Am. J. Hypertens.* 1988, *1*, 79–83. [CrossRef]
289. Brock, J.A.; Yeoh, M.; McLachlan, E.M. Enhanced neurally evoked responses and inhibition of norepinephrine reuptake in rat mesenteric arteries after spinal transection. *Am. J. Physiol. Heart Circ. Physiol.* 2006, *290*, H398–H405. [CrossRef]
290. Hou, S.; Duale, H.; Rabchevsky, A.G. Intraspinal sprouting of unmyelinated pelvic afferents after complete spinal cord injury is correlated with autonomic dysreflexia induced by visceral pain. *Neuroscience* 2009, *159*, 369–379. [CrossRef]
291. Cameron, A.A.; Smith, G.M.; Randall, D.C.; Brown, D.R.; Rabchevsky, A.G. Genetic manipulation of intraspinal plasticity after spinal cord injury alters the severity of autonomic dysreflexia. *J. Neurosci.* 2006, *26*, 2923–2932. [CrossRef]
292. Weaver, L.C.; Verghese, P.; Bruce, J.C.; Fehlings, M.G.; Krenz, N.R.; Marsh, D.R. Autonomic dysreflexia and primary afferent sprouting after clip-compression injury of the rat spinal cord. *J. Neurotrauma* 2001, *18*, 1107–1119. [CrossRef]
293. Llewellyn-Smith, I.J.; Weaver, L.C. Changes in synaptic inputs to sympathetic preganglionic neurons after spinal cord injury. *J. Comp. Neurol.* 2001, *435*, 226–240. [CrossRef]

294. Krassioukov, A.V.; Johns, D.G.; Schramm, L.P. Sensitivity of sympathetically correlated spinal interneurons, renal sympathetic nerve activity, and arterial pressure to somatic and visceral stimuli after chronic spinal injury. *J. Neurotrauma* **2002**, *19*, 1521–1529. [CrossRef] [PubMed]
295. Rabchevsky, A.G. Segmental organization of spinal reflexes mediating autonomic dysreflexia after spinal cord injury. *Prog. Brain Res.* **2006**, *152*, 265–274. [CrossRef] [PubMed]
296. Michael, F.M.; Patel, S.P.; Rabchevsky, A.G. Intraspinal Plasticity Associated With the Development of Autonomic Dysreflexia After Complete Spinal Cord Injury. *Front. Cell. Neurosci.* **2019**, *13*, 10. [CrossRef] [PubMed]
297. Cormier, C.M.; Mukhida, K.; Walker, G.; Marsh, D.R. Development of autonomic dysreflexia after spinal cord injury is associated with a lack of serotonergic axons in the intermediolateral cell column. *J. Neurotrauma* **2010**, *27*, 1805–1818. [CrossRef]
298. Hou, S.; Tom, V.J.; Graham, L.; Lu, P.; Blesch, A. Partial restoration of cardiovascular function by embryonic neural stem cell grafts after complete spinal cord transection. *J. Neurosci.* **2013**, *33*, 17138–17149. [CrossRef]
299. Hou, S.P.; Saltos, T.M.; Mironets, E.; Trueblood, C.T.; Connors, T.M.; Tom, V.J. Grafting Embryonic Raphe Neurons Reestablishes Serotonergic Regulation of Sympathetic Activity to Improve Cardiovascular Function after Spinal Cord Injury. *J. Neurosci.* **2020**, *40*, 1248–1264. [CrossRef]
300. Trueblood, C.T.; Iredia, I.W.; Collyer, E.S.; Tom, V.J.; Hou, S. Development of Cardiovascular Dysfunction in a Rat Spinal Cord Crush Model and Responses to Serotonergic Interventions. *J. Neurotrauma* **2019**, *36*, 1478–1486. [CrossRef]
301. Lujan, H.L.; DiCarlo, S.E. Direct comparison of cervical and high thoracic spinal cord injury reveals distinct autonomic and cardiovascular consequences. *J. Appl. Physiol.* **2020**, *128*, 554–564. [CrossRef]
302. Mathias, C.J.; Christensen, N.J.; Corbett, J.L.; Frankel, H.L.; Spalding, J.M. Plasma catecholamines during paroxysmal neurogenic hypertension in quadriplegic man. *Circ. Res.* **1976**, *39*, 204–208. [CrossRef]
303. Leman, S.; Bernet, F.; Sequeira, H. Autonomic dysreflexia increases plasma adrenaline level in the chronic spinal cord-injured rat. *Neurosci. Lett.* **2000**, *286*, 159–162. [CrossRef]
304. Garshick, E.; Kelley, A.; Cohen, S.A.; Garrison, A.; Tun, C.G.; Gagnon, D.; Brown, R. A prospective assessment of mortality in chronic spinal cord injury. *Spinal Cord* **2005**, *43*, 408–416. [CrossRef]
305. Wu, J.C.; Chen, Y.C.; Liu, L.; Chen, T.J.; Huang, W.C.; Cheng, H.; Tung-Ping, S. Increased risk of stroke after spinal cord injury: A nationwide 4-year follow-up cohort study. *Neurology* **2012**, *78*, 1051–1057. [CrossRef]
306. Lucin, K.M.; Sanders, V.M.; Jones, T.B.; Malarkey, W.B.; Popovich, P.G. Impaired antibody synthesis after spinal cord injury is level dependent and is due to sympathetic nervous system dysregulation. *Exp. Neurol.* **2007**, *207*, 75–84. [CrossRef]
307. Lucin, K.M.; Sanders, V.M.; Popovich, P.G. Stress hormones collaborate to induce lymphocyte apoptosis after high level spinal cord injury. *J. Neurochem.* **2009**, *110*, 1409–1421. [CrossRef]
308. Zhang, Y.; Guan, Z.; Reader, B.; Shawler, T.; Mandrekar-Colucci, S.; Huang, K.; Weil, Z.; Bratasz, A.; Wells, J.; Powell, N.D.; et al. Autonomic Dysreflexia Causes Chronic Immune Suppression after Spinal Cord Injury. *J. Neurosci.* **2013**, *33*, 12970–12981. [CrossRef]
309. Karunakaran, K.D.; Yuan, R.; He, J.; Zhao, J.; Cui, J.L.; Zang, Y.F.; Zhang, Z.; Alvarez, T.L.; Biswal, B.B. Resting-State Functional Connectivity of the Thalamus in Complete Spinal Cord Injury. *Neurorehabil. Neural Repair* **2020**, *34*, 122–133. [CrossRef]
310. Chou, X.L.; Fang, Q.; Yan, L.; Zhong, W.; Peng, B.; Li, H.; Wei, J.; Tao, H.W.; Zhang, L.I. Contextual and cross-modality modulation of auditory cortical processing through pulvinar mediated suppression. *eLife* **2020**, *9*, e54157. [CrossRef]
311. Fang, Q.; Chou, X.L.; Peng, B.; Zhong, W.; Zhang, L.I.; Tao, H.W. A Differential Circuit via Retino-Colliculo-Pulvinar Pathway Enhances Feature Selectivity in Visual Cortex through Surround Suppression. *Neuron* **2020**, *105*, 355–369.e6. [CrossRef]
312. Ibrahim, L.A.; Mesik, L.; Ji, X.Y.; Fang, Q.; Li, H.F.; Li, Y.T.; Zingg, B.; Zhang, L.I.; Tao, H.W. Cross-Modality Sharpening of Visual Cortical Processing through Layer-1-Mediated Inhibition and Disinhibition. *Neuron* **2016**, *89*, 1031–1045. [CrossRef]
313. Monckton, J.E.; McCormick, D.A. Neuromodulatory role of serotonin in the ferret thalamus. *J. Neurophysiol.* **2002**, *87*, 2124–2136. [CrossRef]
314. Goodman, L.S.; Gillman, A.; Brunton Laurence, L.; Lazo John, S.; Parker Keith, L. *Goodman & Gilman's: The Pharmacological Basis of Therapeutics*; McGraw-Hill Education: New York, NY, USA, 2006.
315. Lu, Y.; Zheng, J.; Xiong, L.; Zimmermann, M.; Yang, J. Spinal cord injury-induced attenuation of GABAergic inhibition in spinal dorsal horn circuits is associated with down-regulation of the chloride transporter KCC2 in rat. *J. Physiol.* **2008**, *586*, 5701–5715. [CrossRef]
316. Baba, H.; Ji, R.R.; Kohno, T.; Moore, K.A.; Ataka, T.; Wakai, A.; Okamoto, M.; Woolf, C.J. Removal of GABAergic inhibition facilitates polysynaptic A fiber-mediated excitatory transmission to the superficial spinal dorsal horn. *Mol. Cell. Neurosci.* **2003**, *24*, 818–830. [CrossRef]
317. Dougherty, K.J.; Hochman, S. Spinal cord injury causes plasticity in a subpopulation of lamina I GABAergic interneurons. *J. Neurophysiol.* **2008**, *100*, 212–223. [CrossRef]
318. Roberts, L.A.; Beyer, C.; Komisaruk, B.R. Nociceptive responses to altered GABAergic activity at the spinal cord. *Life Sci.* **1986**, *39*, 1667–1674. [CrossRef]
319. Sivilotti, L.; Woolf, C.J. The contribution of GABAA and glycine receptors to central sensitization: Disinhibition and touch-evoked allodynia in the spinal cord. *J. Neurophysiol.* **1994**, *72*, 169–179. [CrossRef]
320. Zhang, Z.; Hefferan, M.P.; Loomis, C.W. Topical bicuculline to the rat spinal cord induces highly localized allodynia that is mediated by spinal prostaglandins. *Pain* **2001**, *92*, 351–361. [CrossRef]

321. Sorkin, L.S.; Puig, S.; Jones, D.L. Spinal bicuculline produces hypersensitivity of dorsal horn neurons: Effects of excitatory amino acid antagonists. *Pain* **1998**, *77*, 181–190. [CrossRef]
322. Hwang, J.H.; Yaksh, T.L. The effect of spinal GABA receptor agonists on tactile allodynia in a surgically-induced neuropathic pain model in the rat. *Pain* **1997**, *70*, 15–22. [CrossRef]
323. Kaneko, M.; Hammond, D.L. Role of spinal gamma-aminobutyric acidA receptors in formalin-induced nociception in the rat. *J. Pharmacol. Exp. Ther.* **1997**, *282*, 928–938.
324. Jergova, S.; Hentall, I.D.; Gajavelli, S.; Varghese, M.S.; Sagen, J. Intraspinal transplantation of GABAergic neural progenitors attenuates neuropathic pain in rats: A pharmacologic and neurophysiological evaluation. *Exp. Neurol.* **2012**, *234*, 39–49. [CrossRef]
325. Jolivalt, C.G.; Lee, C.A.; Ramos, K.M.; Calcutt, N.A. Allodynia and hyperalgesia in diabetic rats are mediated by GABA and depletion of spinal potassium-chloride co-transporters. *Pain* **2008**, *140*, 48–57. [CrossRef] [PubMed]
326. Kaila, K.; Price, T.J.; Payne, J.A.; Puskarjov, M.; Voipio, J. Cation-chloride cotransporters in neuronal development, plasticity and disease. *Nat. Rev. Neurosci.* **2014**, *15*, 637–654. [CrossRef] [PubMed]
327. Fiumelli, H.; Woodin, M.A. Role of activity-dependent regulation of neuronal chloride homeostasis in development. *Curr. Opin. Neurobiol.* **2007**, *17*, 81–86. [CrossRef] [PubMed]
328. Cramer, S.W.; Baggott, C.; Cain, J.; Tilghman, J.; Allcock, B.; Miranpuri, G.; Rajpal, S.; Sun, D.; Resnick, D. The role of cation-dependent chloride transporters in neuropathic pain following spinal cord injury. *Mol. Pain* **2008**, *4*, 36. [CrossRef]
329. Medina, I.; Friedel, P.; Rivera, C.; Kahle, K.T.; Kourdougli, N.; Uvarov, P.; Pellegrino, C. Current view on the functional regulation of the neuronal K^+–Cl^- cotransporter KCC2. *Front. Cell. Neurosci.* **2014**, *8*, 18. [CrossRef]
330. Kahle, K.T.; Deeb, T.Z.; Puskarjov, M.; Silayeva, L.; Liang, B.; Kaila, K.; Moss, S.J. Modulation of neuronal activity by phosphorylation of the K–Cl cotransporter KCC2. *Trends Neurosci.* **2013**, *36*, 726–737. [CrossRef]
331. Ben-Ari, Y. Excitatory actions of GABA during development: The nature of the nurture. *Nat. Rev. Neurosci.* **2002**, *3*, 728–739. [CrossRef]
332. Rivera, C.; Voipio, J.; Kaila, K. Two developmental switches in GABAergic signalling: The K^+–Cl^- cotransporter KCC2 and carbonic anhydrase CAVII. *J. Physiol.* **2005**, *562*, 27–36. [CrossRef]
333. Ferrini, F.; De Koninck, Y. Microglia control neuronal network excitability via BDNF signalling. *Neural Plast.* **2013**, *2013*, 429815. [CrossRef]
334. Ostroumov, A.; Thomas, A.M.; Kimmey, B.A.; Karsch, J.S.; Doyon, W.M.; Dani, J.A. Stress Increases Ethanol Self-Administration via a Shift toward Excitatory GABA Signaling in the Ventral Tegmental Area. *Neuron* **2016**, *92*, 493–504. [CrossRef]
335. Ostroumov, A.; Dani, J.A. Convergent Neuronal Plasticity and Metaplasticity Mechanisms of Stress, Nicotine, and Alcohol. *Annu. Rev. Pharmacol. Toxicol.* **2018**, *58*, 547–566. [CrossRef]
336. Wang, W.; Gong, N.; Xu, T.L. Downregulation of KCC2 following LTP-contributes to EPSP-spike potentiation in rat hippocampus. *Biochem. Biophys. Res. Commun.* **2006**, *343*, 1209–1215. [CrossRef]
337. Ostroumov, A.; Dani, J.A. Inhibitory Plasticity of Mesocorticolimbic Circuits in Addiction and Mental Illness. *Trends Neurosci.* **2018**, *41*, 898–910. [CrossRef]
338. Drew, G.M.; Siddall, P.J.; Duggan, A.W. Mechanical allodynia following contusion injury of the rat spinal cord is associated with loss of GABAergic inhibition in the dorsal horn. *Pain* **2004**, *109*, 379–388. [CrossRef]
339. Boulenguez, P.; Liabeuf, S.; Bos, R.; Bras, H.; Jean-Xavier, C.; Brocard, C.; Stil, A.; Darbon, P.; Cattaert, D.; Delpire, E.; et al. Down-regulation of the potassium-chloride cotransporter KCC2 contributes to spasticity after spinal cord injury. *Nat. Med.* **2010**, *16*, 302–307. [CrossRef]
340. Hasbargen, T.; Ahmed, M.M.; Miranpuri, G.; Li, L.; Kahle, K.T.; Resnick, D.; Sun, D. Role of NKCC1 and KCC2 in the development of chronic neuropathic pain following spinal cord injury. *Ann. N. Y. Acad. Sci.* **2010**, *1198*, 168–172. [CrossRef]
341. Gackière, F.; Vinay, L. Serotonergic modulation of post-synaptic inhibition and locomotor alternating pattern in the spinal cord. *Front. Neural Circuits* **2014**, *8*, 102. [CrossRef]
342. Ferguson, A.R.; Washburn, S.N.; Crown, E.D.; Grau, J.W. GABA(A) receptor activation is involved in noncontingent shock inhibition of instrumental conditioning in spinal rats. *Behav. Neurosci.* **2003**, *117*, 799–812. [CrossRef]
343. Chen, B.; Li, Y.; Yu, B.; Zhang, Z.; Brommer, B.; Williams, P.R.; Liu, Y.; Hegarty, S.V.; Zhou, S.; Zhu, J.; et al. Reactivation of Dormant Relay Pathways in Injured Spinal Cord by KCC2 Manipulations. *Cell* **2018**, *174*, 1599. [CrossRef]
344. Beverungen, H.; Klaszky, S.C.; Klaszky, M.; Cote, M.P. Rehabilitation Decreases Spasticity by Restoring Chloride Homeostasis through the Brain-Derived Neurotrophic Factor-KCC2 Pathway after Spinal Cord Injury. *J. Neurotrauma* **2020**, *37*, 846–859. [CrossRef]
345. Cote, M.P.; Gandhi, S.; Zambrotta, M.; Houle, J.D. Exercise Modulates Chloride Homeostasis after Spinal Cord Injury. *J. Neurosci.* **2014**, *34*, 8976–8987. [CrossRef] [PubMed]
346. Lee-Hotta, S.; Uchiyama, Y.; Kametaka, S. Role of the BDNF-TrkB pathway in KCC2 regulation and rehabilitation following neuronal injury: A mini review. *Neurochem. Int.* **2019**, *128*, 32–38. [CrossRef] [PubMed]
347. Zhang, W.; Liu, L.Y.; Xu, T.L. Reduced potassium-chloride co-transporter expression in spinal cord dorsal horn neurons contributes to inflammatory pain hypersensitivity in rats. *Neuroscience* **2008**, *152*, 502–510. [CrossRef] [PubMed]
348. Beggs, S.; Salter, M.W. Microglia-neuronal signalling in neuropathic pain hypersensitivity 2.0. *Curr. Opin. Neurobiol.* **2010**, *20*, 474–480. [CrossRef]

349. Shulga, A.; Thomas-Crusells, J.; Sigl, T.; Blaesse, A.; Mestres, P.; Meyer, M.; Yan, Q.; Kaila, K.; Saarma, M.; Rivera, C.; et al. Posttraumatic GABA(A)-mediated $[Ca^{2+}](i)$ increase is essential for the induction of brain-derived neurotrophic factor-dependent survival of mature central neurons. *J. Neurosci.* **2008**, *28*, 6996–7005. [CrossRef]
350. King, T.; Vera-Portocarrero, L.; Gutierrez, T.; Vanderah, T.W.; Dussor, G.; Lai, J.; Fields, H.L.; Porreca, F. Unmasking the tonic-aversive state in neuropathic pain. *Nat. Neurosci.* **2009**, *12*, 1364–1366. [CrossRef]
351. Bos, R.; Sadlaoud, K.; Boulenguez, P.; Buttigieg, D.; Liabeuf, S.; Brocard, C.; Haase, G.; Bras, H.; Vinay, L. Activation of 5-HT2A receptors upregulates the function of the neuronal K–Cl cotransporter KCC2. *Proc. Natl. Acad. Sci. USA* **2013**, *110*, 348–353. [CrossRef]
352. Sánchez-Brualla, I.; Boulenguez, P.; Brocard, C.; Liabeuf, S.; Viallat-Lieutaud, A.; Navarro, X.; Udina, E.; Brocard, F. Activation of 5-HT(2A) Receptors Restores KCC2 Function and Reduces Neuropathic Pain after Spinal Cord Injury. *Neuroscience* **2018**, *387*, 48–57. [CrossRef]
353. Kimmey, B.A.; Ostroumov, A.; Dani, J.A. 5-HT$_{2A}$ receptor activation normalizes stress-induced dysregulation of GABAergic signaling in the ventral tegmental area. *Proc. Natl. Acad. Sci. USA* **2019**, *116*, 27028–27034. [CrossRef]
354. Jean-Xavier, C.; Sharples, S.A.; Mayr, K.A.; Lognon, A.P.; Whelan, P.J. Retracing your footsteps: Developmental insights to spinal network plasticity following injury. *J. Neurophysiol.* **2018**, *119*, 521–536. [CrossRef]
355. Jean-Xavier, C.; Pflieger, J.F.; Liabeuf, S.; Vinay, L. Inhibitory postsynaptic potentials in lumbar motoneurons remain depolarizing after neonatal spinal cord transection in the rat. *J. Neurophysiol.* **2006**, *96*, 2274–2281. [CrossRef]
356. Rekling, J.C.; Funk, G.D.; Bayliss, D.A.; Dong, X.W.; Feldman, J.L. Synaptic control of motoneuronal excitability. *Physiol. Rev.* **2000**, *80*, 767–852. [CrossRef]
357. Rank, M.M.; Murray, K.C.; Stephens, M.J.; D'Amico, J.; Gorassini, M.A.; Bennett, D.J. Adrenergic receptors modulate motoneuron excitability, sensory synaptic transmission and muscle spasms after chronic spinal cord injury. *J. Neurophysiol.* **2011**, *105*, 410–422. [CrossRef]
358. Al Dera, H.; Brock, J.A. Changes in sympathetic neurovascular function following spinal cord injury. *Auton. Neurosci.* **2018**, *209*, 25–36. [CrossRef]
359. Streijger, F.; So, K.; Manouchehri, N.; Gheorghe, A.; Okon, E.B.; Chan, R.M.; Ng, B.; Shortt, K.; Sekhon, M.S.; Griesdale, D.E.; et al. A Direct Comparison between Norepinephrine and Phenylephrine for Augmenting Spinal Cord Perfusion in a Porcine Model of Spinal Cord Injury. *J. Neurotrauma* **2018**, *35*, 1345–1357. [CrossRef]
360. Miyazato, M.; Oshiro, T.; Chancellor, M.B.; de Groat, W.C.; Yoshimura, N.; Saito, S. An alpha1-adrenoceptor blocker terazosin improves urine storage function in the spinal cord in spinal cord injured rats. *Life Sci.* **2013**, *92*, 125–130. [CrossRef]
361. Mitsui, T.; Shumsky, J.S.; Lepore, A.C.; Murray, M.; Fischer, I. Transplantation of neuronal and glial restricted precursors into contused spinal cord improves bladder and motor functions, decreases thermal hypersensitivity, and modifies intraspinal circuitry. *J. Neurosci.* **2005**, *25*, 9624–9636. [CrossRef]
362. Pertovaara, A. Noradrenergic pain modulation. *Prog. Neurobiol.* **2006**, *80*, 53–83. [CrossRef]
363. Pertovaara, A.; Kauppila, T.; Jyväsjärvi, E.; Kalso, E. Involvement of supraspinal and spinal segmental alpha-2-adrenergic mechanisms in the medetomidine-induced antinociception. *Neuroscience* **1991**, *44*, 705–714. [CrossRef]
364. Kwaśniewska, A.; Miazga, K.; Majczyński, H.; Jordan, L.M.; Zawadzka, M.; Sławińska, U. Noradrenergic Components of Locomotor Recovery Induced by Intraspinal Grafting of the Embryonic Brainstem in Adult Paraplegic Rats. *Int. J. Mol. Sci.* **2020**, *21*, 5520. [CrossRef]
365. Xu, P.; Guo, S.; Xie, Y.; Liu, Z.; Liu, C.; Zhang, X.; Yang, D.; Gong, H.; Chen, Y.; Du, L.; et al. Effects of highly selective sympathectomy on neurogenic bowel dysfunction in spinal cord injury rats. *Sci. Rep.* **2021**, *11*, 15892. [CrossRef]
366. Li, Y.; Harvey, P.J.; Li, X.; Bennett, D.J. Spastic long-lasting reflexes of the chronic spinal rat studied in vitro. *J. Neurophysiol.* **2004**, *91*, 2236–2246. [CrossRef]
367. Corleto, J.A.; Bravo-Hernández, M.; Kamizato, K.; Kakinohana, O.; Santucci, C.; Navarro, M.R.; Platoshyn, O.; Cizkova, D.; Lukacova, N.; Taylor, J.; et al. Thoracic 9 Spinal Transection-Induced Model of Muscle Spasticity in the Rat: A Systematic Electrophysiological and Histopathological Characterization. *PLoS ONE* **2015**, *10*, e0144642. [CrossRef]
368. Gao, J.; Sun, Z.; Xiao, Z.; Du, Q.; Niu, X.; Wang, G.; Chang, Y.W.; Sun, Y.; Sun, W.; Lin, A.; et al. Dexmedetomidine modulates neuroinflammation and improves outcome via alpha2-adrenergic receptor signaling after rat spinal cord injury. *Br. J. Anaesth.* **2019**, *123*, 827–838. [CrossRef]
369. DeVeau, K.M.; Harman, K.A.; Squair, J.W.; Krassioukov, A.V.; Magnuson, D.S.K.; West, C.R. A comparison of passive hindlimb cycling and active upper-limb exercise provides new insights into systolic dysfunction after spinal cord injury. *Am. J. Physiol. Heart Circ. Physiol.* **2017**, *313*, H861–H870. [CrossRef]
370. Shimizu, N.; Gotoh, D.; Nishimoto, M.; Hashimoto, M.; Saito, T.; Fujita, K.; Hirayama, A.; Yoshimura, N.; Uemura, H. Efficacy of vibegron, a novel β3-adrenoreceptor agonist, for lower urinary tract dysfunction in mice with spinal cord injury. *Int. J. Urol.* **2021**, *28*, 1068–1072. [CrossRef]
371. Scholpa, N.E.; Simmons, E.C.; Tilley, D.G.; Schnellmann, R.G. β(2)-adrenergic receptor-mediated mitochondrial biogenesis improves skeletal muscle recovery following spinal cord injury. *Exp. Neurol.* **2019**, *322*, 113064. [CrossRef]
372. Scholpa, N.E.; Williams, H.; Wang, W.; Corum, D.; Narang, A.; Tomlinson, S.; Sullivan, P.G.; Rabchevsky, A.G.; Schnellmann, R.G. Pharmacological Stimulation of Mitochondrial Biogenesis Using the Food and Drug Administration-Approved β(2)-

Adrenoreceptor Agonist Formoterol for the Treatment of Spinal Cord Injury. *J. Neurotrauma* **2019**, *36*, 962–972. [CrossRef] [PubMed]
373. Fuchigami, T.; Kakinohana, O.; Hefferan, M.P.; Lukacova, N.; Marsala, S.; Platoshyn, O.; Sugahara, K.; Yaksh, T.L.; Marsala, M. Potent suppression of stretch reflex activity after systemic or spinal delivery of tizanidine in rats with spinal ischemia-induced chronic spastic paraplegia. *Neuroscience* **2011**, *194*, 160–169. [CrossRef] [PubMed]
374. Ishida, H.; Yamauchi, H.; Ito, H.; Akino, H.; Yokoyama, O. α1D-Adrenoceptor blockade increases voiding efficiency by improving external urethral sphincter activity in rats with spinal cord injury. *Am. J. Physiol. Regul. Integr. Comp. Physiol.* **2016**, *311*, R971–R978. [CrossRef] [PubMed]
375. Rivas, D.A.; Chancellor, M.B.; Huang, B.; Salzman, S.K. Autonomic dysreflexia in a rat model spinal cord injury and the effect of pharmacologic agents. *Neurourol. Urodyn.* **1995**, *14*, 141–152. [CrossRef]
376. Morrison, S.F.; Ge, Y.Z. Adrenergic modulation of a spinal sympathetic reflex in the rat. *J. Pharmacol. Exp. Ther.* **1995**, *273*, 380–385.
377. Yaksh, T.L.; Pogrel, J.W.; Lee, Y.W.; Chaplan, S.R. Reversal of nerve ligation-induced allodynia by spinal alpha-2 adrenoceptor agonists. *J. Pharmacol. Exp. Ther.* **1995**, *272*, 207–214.
378. Rong, H.; Zhao, Z.; Feng, J.; Lei, Y.; Wu, H.; Sun, R.; Zhang, Z.; Hou, B.; Zhang, W.; Sun, Y.; et al. The effects of dexmedetomidine pretreatment on the pro- and anti-inflammation systems after spinal cord injury in rats. *Brain Behav. Immun.* **2017**, *64*, 195–207. [CrossRef]
379. Molina, C.; Herrero, J.F. The influence of the time course of inflammation and spinalization on the antinociceptive activity of the alpha2-adrenoceptor agonist medetomidine. *Eur. J. Pharmacol.* **2006**, *532*, 50–60. [CrossRef]
380. Sakitani, N.; Iwasawa, H.; Nomura, M.; Miura, Y.; Kuroki, H.; Ozawa, J.; Moriyama, H. Mechanical Stress by Spasticity Accelerates Fracture Healing After Spinal Cord Injury. *Calcif. Tissue Int.* **2017**, *101*, 384–395. [CrossRef]
381. Lemmens, S.; Nelissen, S.; Dooley, D.; Geurts, N.; Peters, E.M.J.; Hendrix, S. Stress Pathway Modulation Is Detrimental or Ineffective for Functional Recovery after Spinal Cord Injury in Mice. *J. Neurotrauma* **2020**, *37*, 564–571. [CrossRef]
382. Karatas, Y.; Cengiz, S.L.; Esen, H.; Toker, A.; Savas, C. Effect of Carvedilol on Secondary Damage in Experimental Spinal Cord Injury in Rats. *Turk. Neurosurg.* **2015**, *25*, 930–935. [CrossRef]
383. Liu, D.; Huang, Y.; Li, B.; Jia, C.; Liang, F.; Fu, Q. Carvedilol promotes neurological function, reduces bone loss and attenuates cell damage after acute spinal cord injury in rats. *Clin. Exp. Pharmacol. Physiol.* **2015**, *42*, 202–212. [CrossRef]
384. Vega, J.L.; Ganea, D.; Jonakait, G.M. Acute down-regulation of antibody production following spinal cord injury: Role of systemic catecholamines. *J. Neuropathol. Exp. Neurol.* **2003**, *62*, 848–854. [CrossRef]
385. Zhang, X.; Hartung, J.E.; Bortsov, A.V.; Kim, S.; O'Buckley, S.C.; Kozlowski, J.; Nackley, A.G. Sustained stimulation of β(2)- and β(3)-adrenergic receptors leads to persistent functional pain and neuroinflammation. *Brain Behav. Immun.* **2018**, *73*, 520–532. [CrossRef]
386. Schoultz, T.W.; Deluca, D.C.; Reding, D.L. Norepinephrine Levels in the Traumatized Spinal Cord of Catecholamine-Depleted Cats. *Brain Res.* **1976**, *109*, 367–374. [CrossRef]
387. Osterholm, J.L.; Mathews, G.J. Altered norepinephrine metabolism, following experimental spinal cord injury. 2. Protection against traumatic spinal cord hemorrhagic necrosis by norepinephrine synthesis blockade with alpha methyl tyrosine. *J. Neurosurg.* **1972**, *36*, 395–401. [CrossRef]
388. Vise, W.M.; Yashon, D.; Hunt, W.E. Mechanisms of norepinephrine accumulation within sites of spinal cord injury. *J. Neurosurg.* **1974**, *40*, 76–82. [CrossRef]
389. Alderman, J.L.; Osterholm, J.L.; Damore, B.R.; Williams, H.D.; Irvin, J.D. The Influence of the Adrenal Gland Upon Actue Spinal Cord Injury. *Life Sci.* **1980**, *26*, 1627–1632. [CrossRef]
390. Crawford, R.A.; Griffiths, I.R.; McCulloch, J. The Effect of Norepinephrine on Spinal Cord Circulation and its Possible Implications in Pathogenesis of Acute Spinal Trauma. *J. Neurosurg.* **1977**, *47*, 567–576. [CrossRef]
391. Rawe, S.E.; Lee, W.A.; Perot, P.L., Jr. The histopathology of experimental spinal cord trauma. The effect of systemic blood pressure. *J. Neurosurg.* **1978**, *48*, 1002–1007. [CrossRef]
392. Rawe, S.E.; Roth, R.H.; Collins, W.F. Norepinephrine levels in experimental spinal cord trauma. Part 2: Histopathological study of hemorrhagic necrosis. *J. Neurosurg.* **1977**, *46*, 350–357. [CrossRef] [PubMed]
393. Kurihara, M. Role of monoamines in experimental spinal cord injury in rats. Relationship between Na^+–K^+-ATPase and lipid peroxidation. *J. Neurosurg.* **1985**, *62*, 743–749. [CrossRef] [PubMed]
394. Osterholm, J.L.; Mathews, G.J. A proposed biochemical mechanism for traumatic spinal cord hemorrhagic necrosis. Successful therapy for severe injuries by metabolic blockade. *Trans. Am. Neurol. Assoc.* **1971**, *96*, 187–191. [PubMed]
395. Osterholm, J.L. The pathophysiological response to spinal cord injury. The current status of related research. *J. Neurosurg.* **1974**, *40*, 5–33. [CrossRef]
396. Kalous, A.; Osborne, P.B.; Keast, J.R. Acute and chronic changes in dorsal horn innervation by primary afferents and descending supraspinal pathways after spinal cord injury. *J. Comp. Neurol.* **2007**, *504*, 238–253. [CrossRef]
397. Kalous, A.; Osborne, P.B.; Keast, J.R. Spinal cord compression injury in adult rats initiates changes in dorsal horn remodeling that may correlate with development of neuropathic pain. *J. Comp. Neurol.* **2009**, *513*, 668–684. [CrossRef]
398. Hou, S.; DeFinis, J.H.; Daugherty, S.L.; Tang, C.; Weinberger, J.; de Groat, W.C. Deciphering Spinal Endogenous Dopaminergic Mechanisms That Modulate Micturition Reflexes in Rats with Spinal Cord Injury. *eNeuro* **2021**, *8*, 1–20. [CrossRef]

399. Qiao, Y.; Brodnik, Z.D.; Zhao, S.; Trueblood, C.T.; Li, Z.; Tom, V.J.; España, R.A.; Hou, S. Spinal Dopaminergic Mechanisms Regulating the Micturition Reflex in Male Rats with Complete Spinal Cord Injury. *J. Neurotrauma* **2021**, *38*, 803–817. [CrossRef]
400. Lahlou, S. Enhanced hypotensive response to intravenous apomorphine in chronic spinalized, conscious rats: Role of spinal dopamine D(1) and D(2) receptors. *Neurosci. Lett.* **2003**, *349*, 115–119. [CrossRef]
401. Rodgers, H.M.; Patton, R.; Yow, J.; Zeczycki, T.N.; Kew, K.; Clemens, S.; Brewer, K.L. Morphine resistance in spinal cord injury-related neuropathic pain in rats is associated with alterations in dopamine and dopamine-related metabolomics. *J. Pain* **2021**, in press. [CrossRef]
402. Bao, Y.N.; Dai, W.L.; Fan, J.F.; Ma, B.; Li, S.S.; Zhao, W.L.; Yu, B.Y.; Liu, J.H. The dopamine D1-D2DR complex in the rat spinal cord promotes neuropathic pain by increasing neuronal excitability after chronic constriction injury. *Exp. Mol. Med.* **2021**, *53*, 235–249. [CrossRef]
403. Rooney, K.F.; Sewell, R.D. Evaluation of selective actions of dopamine D-1 and D-2 receptor agonists and antagonists on opioid antinociception. *Eur. J. Pharmacol.* **1989**, *168*, 329–336. [CrossRef]
404. Rodgers, H.M.; Yow, J.; Evans, E.; Clemens, S.; Brewer, K.L. Dopamine D1 and D3 receptor modulators restore morphine analgesia and prevent opioid preference in a model of neuropathic pain. *Neuroscience* **2019**, *406*, 376–388. [CrossRef]
405. Khalilzadeh, M.; Hassanzadeh, F.; Aghamiri, H.; Dehpour, A.R.; Shafaroodi, H. Aripiprazole prevents from development of vincristine-induced neuropathic nociception by limiting neural NOS overexpression and NF-kB hyperactivation. *Cancer Chemother. Pharm.* **2020**, *86*, 393–404. [CrossRef]
406. Guertin, P.A.; Ung, R.V.; Rouleau, P.; Steuer, I. Effects on locomotion, muscle, bone, and blood induced by a combination therapy eliciting weight-bearing stepping in nonassisted spinal cord-transected mice. *Neurorehabil. Neural Repair* **2011**, *25*, 234–242. [CrossRef]
407. Wang, Z.; Mei, W.; Wang, Q.; Guo, R.; Liu, P.; Wang, Y.; Zhang, Z.; Wang, L. Role of Dehydrocorybulbine in Neuropathic Pain After Spinal Cord Injury Mediated by P2X4 Receptor. *Mol. Cells* **2019**, *42*, 143–150. [CrossRef]
408. Qu, S.; Le, W.; Zhang, X.; Xie, W.; Zhang, A.; Ondo, W.G. Locomotion is increased in a11-lesioned mice with iron deprivation: A possible animal model for restless legs syndrome. *J. Neuropathol. Exp. Neurol.* **2007**, *66*, 383–388. [CrossRef]
409. Haranishi, Y.; Hara, K.; Terada, T. Antihyperalgesic effects of intrathecal perospirone in a rat model of neuropathic pain. *Pharmacol. Biochem. Behav.* **2020**, *195*, 172964. [CrossRef]
410. Zarrindast, M.R.; Moghaddampour, E. Opposing influences of D-1 and D-2 dopamine receptors activation on morphine-induced antinociception. *Arch. Int. Pharmacodyn. Ther.* **1989**, *300*, 37–50. [PubMed]
411. Verma, A.; Kulkarni, S.K. Modulatory role of D-1 and D-2 dopamine receptor subtypes in nociception in mice. *J. Psychopharmacol.* **1993**, *7*, 270–275. [CrossRef] [PubMed]
412. Ben-Sreti, M.M.; Gonzalez, J.P.; Sewell, R.D. Differential effects of SKF 38393 and LY 141865 on nociception and morphine analgesia. *Life Sci.* **1983**, *33* (Suppl. S1), 665–668. [CrossRef]
413. Zarrindast, M.R.; Nassiri-Rad, S.; Pazouki, M. Effects of dopaminergic agents on antinociception in formalin test. *Gen. Pharm.* **1999**, *32*, 517–522. [CrossRef]
414. Yang, P.; Arnold, S.A.; Habas, A.; Hetman, M.; Hagg, T. Ciliary neurotrophic factor mediates dopamine D2 receptor-induced CNS neurogenesis in adult mice. *J. Neurosci.* **2008**, *28*, 2231–2241. [CrossRef]
415. Naftchi, N.E.; Demeny, M.; Decrescito, V.; Tomasula, J.J.; Flamm, E.S.; Campbell, J.B. Biogenic Amine Concecentrations in Traumatized Spinal Cords of Cats—Effect of Drug Therapy. *J. Neurosurg.* **1974**, *40*, 52–57. [CrossRef]
416. Hedeman, L.S.; Sil, R. Studies in experimental spinal cord trauma. 2. Comparison of treatment with steroids, low molecular weight dextran, and catecholamine blockade. *J. Neurosurg.* **1974**, *40*, 44–51. [CrossRef]
417. Chu, T.H.; Cummins, K.; Stys, P.K. The triple monoamine re-uptake inhibitor DOV 216,303 promotes functional recovery after spinal cord contusion injury in mice. *Neurosci. Lett.* **2018**, *675*, 1–6. [CrossRef]
418. Lahlou, S. Involvement of spinal dopamine receptors in mediation of the hypotensive and bradycardic effects of systemic quinpirole in anaesthetised rats. *Eur. J. Pharmacol.* **1998**, *353*, 227–237. [CrossRef]
419. Pellissier, G.; Demenge, P. Hypotensive and bradycardic effects elicited by spinal dopamine receptor stimulation: Effects of D1 and D2 receptor agonists and antagonists. *J. Cardiovasc. Pharmacol.* **1991**, *18*, 548–555. [CrossRef]
420. Petitjean, P.; Mouchet, P.; Pellissier, G.; Manier, M.; Feuerstein, C.; Demenge, P. Cardiovascular effects in the rat of intrathecal injections of apomorphine at the thoracic spinal cord level. *Eur. J. Pharmacol.* **1984**, *105*, 355–359. [CrossRef]
421. Turtle, J.D.; Henwood, M.K.; Strain, M.M.; Huang, Y.J.; Miranda, R.C.; Grau, J.W. Engaging pain fibers after a spinal cord injury fosters hemorrhage and expands the area of secondary injury. *Exp. Neurol.* **2019**, *311*, 115–124. [CrossRef]
422. Mautes, A.E.; Weinzierl, M.R.; Donovan, F.; Noble, L.J. Vascular events after spinal cord injury: Contribution to secondary pathogenesis. *Phys. Ther.* **2000**, *80*, 673–687. [CrossRef]
423. Davis, J.A.; Bopp, A.C.; Henwood, M.K.; Baine, R.E.; Cox, C.C.; Grau, J.W. Pharmacological transection of brain-spinal cord communication blocks pain-induced hemorrhage and locomotor deficits after spinal cord injury in rats. *J. Neurotrauma* **2020**, *37*, 1729–1739. [CrossRef]
424. Reynolds, J.; Turtle, J.; Leal, G.; Huang, Y.J.; Strain, M.; Grau, J. Inflammatory response to peripheral pain input after SCI is blocked by a spinal transection. *J. Neurotrauma* **2017**, *34*, A6.

425. Fauss, G.N.K.; Strain, M.M.; Huang, Y.-J.; Reynolds, J.A.; Davis, J.A.; Henwood, M.K.; West, C.R.; Grau, J.W. Contribution of Brain Processes to Tissue Loss After Spinal Cord Injury: Does a Pain-Induced Rise in Blood Pressure Fuel Hemorrhage? *Front. Syst. Neurosci.* **2021**, *15*, 733056. [CrossRef] [PubMed]
426. Strain, M.M.; Johnston, D.T.; Baine, R.E.; Reynolds, J.; Huang, Y.J.; Henwood, M.K.; Fauss, G.N.; Davis, J.A.; Miranda, R.C.; West, C.R.; et al. Hemorrhage and locomotor deficits induced by pain input after spinal cord injury are partially mediated by changes in hemodynamics. *J. Neurotrauma* **2021**, *38*, 3406–3430. [CrossRef] [PubMed]
427. Christensen, M.D.; Everhart, A.W.; Pickelman, J.T.; Hulsebosch, C.E. Mechanical and thermal allodynia in chronic central pain following spinal cord injury. *Pain* **1996**, *68*, 97–107. [CrossRef]
428. Hook, M.A.; Liu, G.T.; Washburn, S.N.; Ferguson, A.R.; Bopp, A.C.; Huie, J.R.; Grau, J.W. The impact of morphine after a spinal cord injury. *Behav. Brain Res.* **2007**, *179*, 281–293. [CrossRef]
429. Hook, M.A.; Moreno, G.; Woller, S.; Puga, D.; Hoy, K.; Balden, R.; Grau, J.W. Intrathecal Morphine Attenuates Recovery of Function after a Spinal Cord Injury. *J. Neurotrauma* **2009**, *26*, 741–752. [CrossRef]
430. Dale, E.A.; Ben Mabrouk, F.; Mitchell, G.S. Unexpected benefits of intermittent hypoxia: Enhanced respiratory and nonrespiratory motor function. *Physiology* **2014**, *29*, 39–48. [CrossRef]
431. Allen, L.L.; Seven, Y.B.; Baker, T.L.; Mitchell, G.S. Cervical spinal contusion alters Na^+–K^+–$2Cl^-$ and K^+–Cl^- cation-chloride cotransporter expression in phrenic motor neurons. *Respir. Physiol. Neurobiol.* **2019**, *261*, 15–23. [CrossRef]

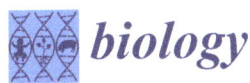

Review

Plasticity in Cervical Motor Circuits following Spinal Cord Injury and Rehabilitation

John R. Walker and Megan Ryan Detloff *

Marion Murray Spinal Cord Research Center, Department of Neurobiology & Anatomy, College of Medicine, Drexel University, Philadelphia, PA 19129, USA; jw3646@drexel.edu
* Correspondence: mrd64@drexel.edu; Tel.: +1-215-991-8986

Simple Summary: Spinal cord injury results in a decreased quality of life and impacts hundreds of thousands of people in the US alone. This review discusses the underlying cellular mechanisms of injury and the concurrent therapeutic hurdles that impede recovery. It then describes the phenomena of neural plasticity—the nervous system's ability to change. The primary focus of the review is on the impact of cervical spinal cord injury on control of the upper limbs. The neural plasticity that occurs without intervention is discussed, which shows new connections growing around the injury site and the involvement of compensatory movements. Rehabilitation-driven neural plasticity is shown to have the ability to guide connections to create more normal functions. Various novel stimulation and recording technologies are outlined for their role in further improving rehabilitative outcomes and gains in independence. Finally, the importance of sensory input, an often-overlooked aspect of motor control, is shown in driving neural plasticity. Overall, this review seeks to delineate the historical and contemporary research into neural plasticity following injury and rehabilitation to guide future studies.

Abstract: Neuroplasticity is a robust mechanism by which the central nervous system attempts to adapt to a structural or chemical disruption of functional connections between neurons. Mechanical damage from spinal cord injury potentiates via neuroinflammation and can cause aberrant changes in neural circuitry known as maladaptive plasticity. Together, these alterations greatly diminish function and quality of life. This review discusses contemporary efforts to harness neuroplasticity through rehabilitation and neuromodulation to restore function with a focus on motor recovery following cervical spinal cord injury. Background information on the general mechanisms of plasticity and long-term potentiation of the nervous system, most well studied in the learning and memory fields, will be reviewed. Spontaneous plasticity of the nervous system, both maladaptive and during natural recovery following spinal cord injury is outlined to provide a baseline from which rehabilitation builds. Previous research has focused on the impact of descending motor commands in driving spinal plasticity. However, this review focuses on the influence of physical therapy and primary afferent input and interneuron modulation in driving plasticity within the spinal cord. Finally, future directions into previously untargeted primary afferent populations are presented.

Keywords: primary afferents; nociceptor; reach-to-grasp; forelimb function; upper extremity function

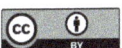

1. Introduction

The negative consequences of spinal cord injury (SCI) arise from far more than the loss of directly damaged grey matter and neural pathways. Unfortunately, these dead and dying neurons release death signals which exacerbate the injury. In response to damaged and dying tissue, the innate and adaptive immune response will become activated as described in detail by Donnelly and Popovich [1]. Monocyte-derived macrophages and activated microglia clear debris from the initial primary insult. However, these immune cells remain long after debris is cleared and provide a continual bombardment of inflammatory cues that initiate secondary injury in areas rostral and caudal to the injury epicenter [2–6]. In an effort to mitigate secondary injury, reactive astrocytes physically limit the spread of inflammation, compensate for a leaky blood brain barrier, and reduce lesion expansion by forming a glial scar [7–9]. However, this physical barrier may also prevent axonal regeneration through the lesion. Reactive astrocytes upregulate signal transducer and activator of transcription 3 (STAT3) and release chondroitin sulfate proteoglycans (CSPGs) and bone morphogenic protein (BMP), inhibiting the growth of neurons and oligodendrocyte maturation and subsequent remyelination efforts [9–16]. Evidence does support astrocytic release of growth promoting factors, such as laminin [7,17]; however, the cumulative effect is detrimental to recovery. Other processes also contribute to the inability of damaged spinal cord axons to regenerate after injury. Wallerian degeneration of the distal axons and myelin results in debris releasing Nogo, OMGp, and MAG, which have all been shown to inhibit regeneration and sprouting [18]. Collectively, these impediments limit the efficacy of spontaneous recovery.

Thus, for the vast majority of individuals, SCI results in permanently lost ascending and descending neuronal connections that are important for normal behavior and function, even with existing treatments and rehabilitation paradigms [19]. Injury-induced damage and failed regeneration necessitates that the remaining central nervous system (CNS) compensates for lost function. Depending on the type and location of injury, damaged and undamaged neurons will show sprouting, new synapse formation, and changes in electrophysiological properties. However, in the case of a complete SCI, in which there are no spared connections, the loss of long descending connections makes volitional control of movement impossible. Therapeutic interventions for individuals with complete SCI are limited to regenerative medicine or the utilization of compensatory devices [20,21]. Some spontaneous plasticity of the spared nervous system provides an avenue for recovery. Evidence for redundant and usually silent interneuron pathways have been shown in injury models, such as in the cross-phrenic phenomenon involved in the recovery of respiratory function [22–24]. Unfortunately, much of the injury-induced plasticity can be maladaptive, taking the form of aberrant sprouting and synaptogenesis as neurons try either to compensate for lost connections or to regenerate through the injury site as they respond to inflammation. Hyperexcitability and inefficiency result from these new connections, making restoration of normal function nearly impossible.

Plasticity is an incredible feature of the CNS, giving it the ability to learn and recover from insult. Without the guidance of rehabilitation, however, it yields limited functional improvements following SCI. Many rehabilitative interventions have been studied for their effects on recovery of function related to alterations in spinal cord anatomy and physiology [25]. Changes in the spinal cord do not just occur with action—i.e., motor output. Instead, rehabilitation- or activity-dependent plasticity of the spinal cord is thought to be afferent driven [26–29]. As the body moves or performs motor tasks, the spinal cord receives input about the quality of the movement from sensory neurons with receptors in the skin, muscles, and joints. Dorsal horn sensory neurons and interneurons receive this afferent input and refine connections, as well as output commands of the motor circuits. Furthermore, projection neurons from spinal cord motor centers provide feedback to supraspinal locations involved in modifying motor behavior (i.e., cerebellum, basal ganglia, motor cortex, etc.) [30–33]. Following an overview of the term "neuroplasticity," this review will focus on the plasticity that occurs naturally following SCI, and how rehabilitative strategies enhance recovery of upper extremity or forelimb function through afferent driven and interneuron-mediated local plasticity in the spinal cord.

2. What Is Neuroplasticity?

Neuroplasticity is defined as the potential for functional and anatomical changes of the nervous system in response to stimuli during learning or in response to injury [34]. Our understanding of neuroplasticity has evolved over decades. Originally, experiments established the importance of circuits in behavior. Subsequent studies revealed how these synapses change with learning and the molecular mechanisms of these changes [35]. Classic experiments from the learning and memory fields described plasticity of the adult nervous system [36]. Receptor changes and the physical addition and/or subtraction of synapses modify synaptic efficiency, thereby driving neuroplasticity. These processes are responsible for learning, memory, and the fine-tuning of motor control. Evidence of neuroplasticity is found in both the spinal cord and the brain. The greatest occurrence of these changes happens during neurodevelopment. Until relatively recently, the dogma prevailed that synaptic connections within the adult nervous system were hardwired and fixed. Now, it is well established that the adult CNS can be modified, especially following injury.

One aspect of neuroplasticity is the strengthening and weakening of synapses in response to input. These synaptic changes are essential for learning, memory, and motor output under normal and pathological conditions. According to Hebbian theory, both pre- and post-synaptic neurons experience changes following repeated and persistent firing [37,38]. Presynaptic release probability, the number and properties of post-synaptic receptors, and the number of active synapses may all be altered [39–41].

In addition to alterations in synaptic strength, researchers have determined that plasticity within learning and memory circuits could occur for varying amounts of time depending upon the composition of pre- and post-synaptic sites. Transient plasticity is known as either short-term facilitation or depression [42,43] (Figure 1).

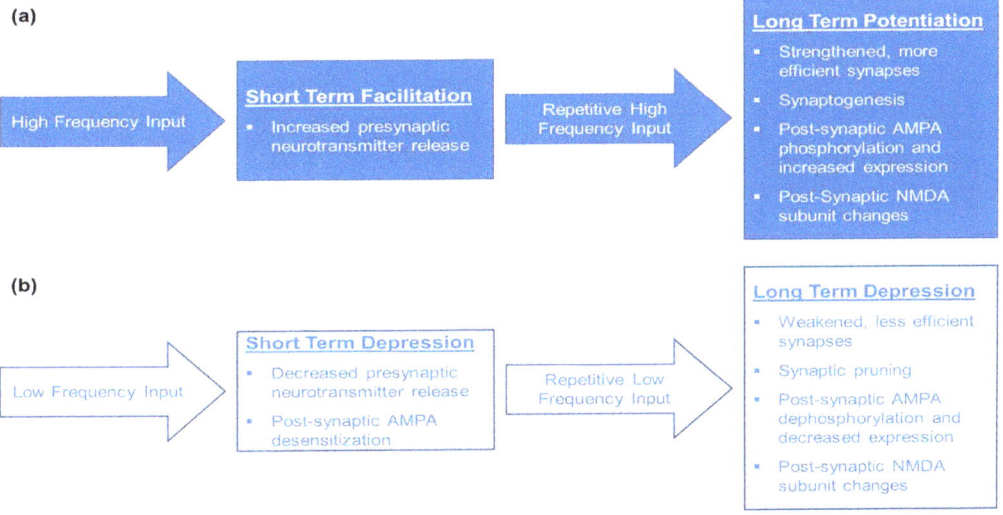

Figure 1. Key Characteristics of Neural Plasticity based on Hebbian learning. (a) Synaptic connections become stronger and more efficient following high frequency and repetitive input. This strengthening is known as either short-term facilitation or long-term potentiation. On a molecular level, single bouts of high frequency input result in increased neurotransmitter release, while repetitive bouts of high frequency input increases synaptogenesis, synaptic efficiency by modulating post-synaptic AMPA and NMDA receptor subunit expression and phosphorylation. These cellular and molecular changes are thought to underlie learning and memory, whether that be for episodic memory or refinement of motor control. (b) Synaptic connections can become weaker and less efficient after low frequency input. An episode of low frequency input results in short-term depression and is associated with decreased presynaptic neurotransmitter release, desensitization of AMPA receptors. Repetitive low frequency input results in long-term depression, which results in weakened, less efficient synapses, pruning of unused synapses, as well as dephosphorylation of AMPA receptors and changes in NMDA receptor subunit composition. Similarly to long-term potentiation, short- and long-term depression are also crucial aspects of learning and memory as unnecessary, redundant, and inefficient connections get pruned away to optimize the function.

Short-term facilitation results from changes in presynaptic neurotransmitter release [42–44] (Figure 2d), while short-term depression occurs when presynaptic neurons lack neurotransmitter vesicles to release into the synaptic cleft (Figure 2b). Postsynaptically, α-Amino-3-hydroxy-5-methyl-4-isoxazolepropionic acid (AMPA) receptors are desensitized [45]. Desensitization occurs when receptors have decreased responsiveness to stimuli. The processes of short-term facilitation and depression are primarily studied in the context of short-term memory and often precede the long-term changes.

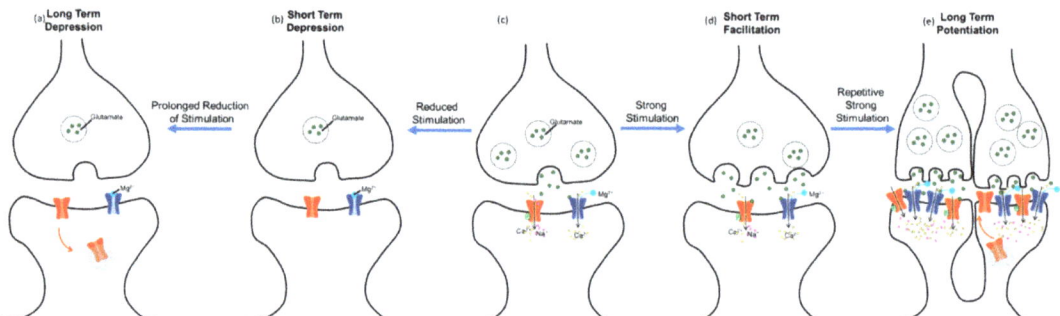

Figure 2. Synaptic Plasticity in Long-Term Potentiation (LTP) and Long-Term Depression (LTD). This figure depicts the cellular mechanisms of LTP and LTD starting from (**c**). During LTP (**c**–**e**), more frequent and greater stimulation releases glutamate form the presynaptic terminal, which binds to and opens AMPARs letting Na^+ and Ca^{2+} enter the post-synaptic dendrite to depolarize the cell. Sufficient depolarization removes the Mg^{2+} from the NMDAR, which is also opened by glutamate, so that the NDMARs can detect the coincidence of activation between the two neurons and allow even greater influx of Ca^{2+} and Na^+. This high concentration of intracellular Ca^{2+} leads to kinase activation, which in turn leads to the phosphorylation of AMPARs. Phosphorylated AMPARs stay open longer when glutamate binds, and more AMPARs are brought to the plasma membrane. Repetition of this process eventually leads to synaptogenesis. During LTD (**a**,**b**), less frequent and smaller release of glutamate binds to fewer receptors leading to a reduced influx of Ca and Na and prevents the removal of the Mg^{2+} plug. Lower Ca levels lead to phosphatase activation and the dephosphorylation of AMPARs, resulting in less time open and the internalization of Inactive AMPARS. LTD often leads to pruning of extraneous synapses.

Longer-lasting plasticity is known as long-term potentiation (LTP) or long-term depression (LTD). LTP occurs when synapses are strengthened and require less stimulation to propagate an action potential [46] (Figure 2e). Conversely, LTD occurs when synaptic strength is decreased, and more stimulation is required to propagate an action potential (Figure 2a). LTP and LTD are the mechanisms of long-term learning and memory. This learning is not limited to episodic memory; these processes also underlie changes in motor control circuitry in the motor cortex, cerebellum, and spinal cord [47–49]. Long-lasting plasticity within the spinal cord will be the focus of this review. The two main mechanisms of LTP in the spinal cord are receptor-mediated plasticity and synaptogenesis of either intact sprouting axons or the regeneration of damaged axons [50–52].

Changes in both AMPA and N-methyl-D-aspartate (NMDA) glutamate receptors on the post-synaptic neuron are a robust method for the nervous system to prioritize different connections.

In AMPA receptor-mediated plasticity, the neurotransmitter glutamate is released from the presynaptic terminal [39,53]. Glutamate then binds to NMDA and AMPA receptors on the post-synaptic neuron. AMPARs open first, allowing an influx of Na^+. A sufficient influx of Na^+ will depolarize the post-synaptic terminal and remove the Mg^{2+} block from NMDARs. This allows an influx of Ca^{2+} to the neuron, and the levels of Ca^{2+} influx are contingent on the degree and frequency of stimulation from presynaptic glutamate release. High stimulation and high Ca^{2+} influx will cause a phosphorylation cascade, resulting in phosphorylated AMPARs and more receptors being expressed on the plasma membrane.

Phosphorylation makes AMPARs reach activation threshold with less stimulation and remain open longer [54]. These changes result in LTP.

Alternatively, lower levels of stimulation and Ca^{2+} influx will result in LTD. Low levels will activate phosphatases which dephosphorylate AMPARs. In this case, dephosphorylated AMPARs are less likely to open and will close sooner. Additionally, fewer receptors will be expressed on the membrane [54]. Although these processes are AMPA receptor-mediated, they are NMDA receptor-dependent because it serves as a coincidence detector for glutamate and depolarization. Alternatively, NMDA receptor-mediated plasticity involves a very similar process [44]. In this case, the NMDARs have subunit changes rather than phosphorylation events that determine their activity levels.

Synaptic sprouting and pruning are two major results of LTP and LTD. Synaptic sprouting, or synaptogenesis, often follows LTP [41,55]. Essentially, synapses experiencing sufficient LTP will split apart, creating two synapses. The post-synaptic density grows until it splits, and the presynaptic density will split to match. The split continues to perforate until the spine separates into multiple spines with multiple synapses. This physical change allows for a greater chance that excitatory post-synaptic potentials will summate into action potentials. Alternatively, LTD will result in pruning of synapses, and inactive synapses will eventually be eliminated [55]. Synaptogenesis and synaptic pruning both play a significant role in plasticity after injury.

3. Neural Plasticity Associated with Reaching and Grasping after SCI

The reach-to-grasp movement is highly synchronous and composed of several observable components, including limb lifting, aiming, and advancing the limb, and followed by opening the digits, pronating the wrist, grasping the object, and supinating to orient the object for release into the mouth [56,57]. In humans, fine motor control of the digits is largely controlled by the descending lateral corticospinal tract (CST), which decussates and crosses midline at the pyramids in the brainstem, and then continues through the dorsolateral white matter of the spinal cord. These lateral CST fibers synapse in cervical motor pools in the spinal cord to control proximal and distal muscles of the limb and digits. The motor pools for the shoulder and arm are located at levels C4-6, and the motor pools of the forearm and digits are located in C7-T1 [58]. In addition to CST control in non-human primates, there is evidence of the involvement of descending rubrospinal and reticulospinal tract (RST) fibers in controlling which upper extremity muscles execute the reach and grasp of a target object [59–62]. Recently, direct excitatory projections from the deep cerebellar nuclei to the ipsilateral cervical spinal cord have been discovered to be involved in the control of the reach-to-grasp movement. Sathymurthy et al. [63] demonstrated direct cerebellospinal connections that were important for reaching and grasping. Mice with silenced ipsilateral cerebellospinal projection neurons took longer to touch the food pellet and failed to successfully grasp it. Rodent models have been extensively studied for reaching and grasping because of the many conserved movements and neuroanatomical substrates across species [64–68]. Forelimb behaviors are reliably measured in the laboratory using a combination of qualitative and quantitative assessments of reach-to-grasp pellet retrieval tasks [56,69], supination tasks [70], digit manipulation [71–73], and grooming behaviors [74]. After SCI, recovery or compensatory reaching and grasping is mediated by several spared systems that respond after injury. Sparing and sprouting of the CST and RST are two of the most well-characterized mechanisms involved in regaining reaching and grasping following SCI that are conserved across species [75–79]. In addition, plasticity of primary afferent fibers is also a key contributor to improved function post-injury. The following sections will focus on discoveries regarding both spontaneous and activity- or rehabilitation-driven plasticity in these pathways that mediate reaching and grasping movements (Figure 3). This review will conclude with our perspective on the specific role of sensory feedback in recovery and rehabilitation.

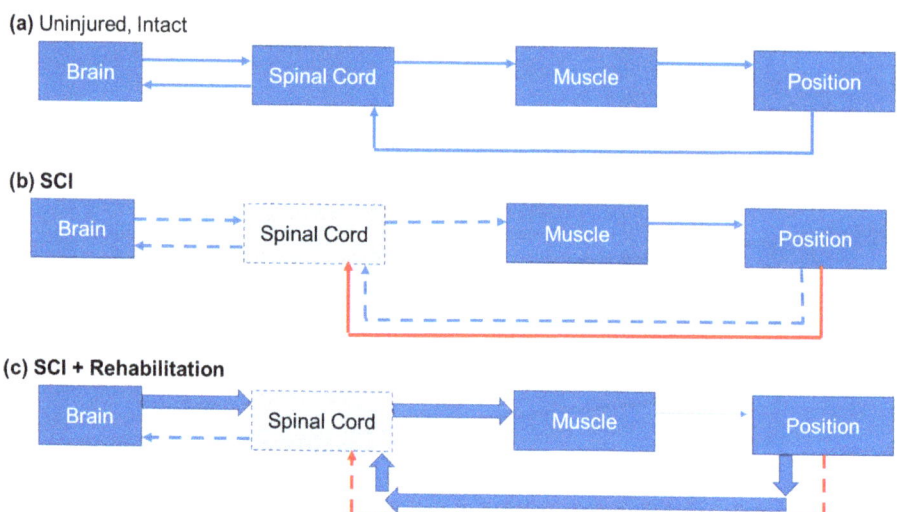

Figure 3. Motor and Sensory Input Through the Spinal Cord. This figure depicts a simplified model of motor output and sensory feedback used to guide movement in the intact CNS (**a**), after SCI (**b**), and during rehabilitation (**c**). (**a**) The final steps of motor planning involve a signal being sent from the motor cortex down to the motoneurons in the spinal cord. These motoneurons send signals to neuromuscular junction causing the appropriate muscle to contract and guide the limb to the final position. Feedback from the periphery regarding the final position gets sent back to the spinal cord. The spinal cord uses this information to refine the local connections and sends that information to brain regions involved in motor refinement, such as the cerebellum. (**b**) After injury, the corticospinal neurons lose some of their connections to the spinal cord (dashed lines), and the cord itself loses motoneurons. This results in a weaker signal to the muscle and mobility problems. Additionally, increased and maladaptive sensory input from primary sensory neurons, like the nociceptor, (red arrows) causes LTP related to central sensitization in chronic pain and noise to enter the system making refinement difficult. The sensory information has weakened connection to the brain. (**c**) Rehabilitation harnesses LTP (Figure 1) by forcing descending input from the brain, and sensory input from the periphery, to strengthen and refine connections withing the cord and motor cortex to regain mobility and decrease nociceptive input.

3.1. Plasticity in Spared Descending Systems

The majority of descending input to upper extremity motoneurons in the cervical spinal cord come from the CST and extensive work has been done to map to its origin in the motor cortex [80,81]. In humans, the CST and the RST are responsible for control of the digits—the CST controls precision gripping, while the RST controls the power grasp [82]. Likewise, CST projections are conserved across species, including rats, non-human primates, and humans [83,84].

There are many examples of CST plasticity after SCI that include sprouting and the indirect control of motoneurons [85]. Weidner, et al. [86] showed that lesions of the corticospinal motor pathway in the high cervical spinal cord of rats led to significant sprouting of the contralateral ventral CST across midline into the ipsilesional medial motor column of Lamina IX and this anatomical plasticity was critical to post-injury gains in function. As in rats, non-human primates with unilateral cervical SCI demonstrated some improvement in reaching and grasping over time that corresponded with changes in the distribution of CST terminals in the spinal cord grey matter compared to intact macaques [87]. These CST axons rostral and caudal to the injury site terminate in Lamina VII, whereas the sprouting fibers synapse near motor pools in Lamina IX. Together, these data suggest that spontaneous plasticity of the spared components of the CST is a compensatory mechanism underlying forelimb motor recovery, as opposed to the restoration and/or regeneration of the damaged motor tract.

Spinal interneurons are key mediators of motor function. They integrate descending motor commands and sensory input from primary afferent fibers to modulate motor neuron activity and motor output [88,89]. There are diverse subpopulations of segmental spinal interneurons, many of which have been discovered in the context of understanding the neural control of locomotion and have been reviewed extensively elsewhere [90–99]. Long projecting propriospinal interneurons that connect cervical and lumbar enlargement are also important for interlimb coordination, especially during locomotion [100]. After SCI, these specialized spinal interneurons are a substrate for spinal plasticity and improved functional recovery. Their long axons allow descending motor commands to bypass lesion sites and reach distal motor pools [101–104].

Interneurons in the cervical cord are involved in many tasks, such as breathing, locomotion, and reach-to-grasp [97,105–108]. An example of propriospinal interneurons involved in the reach are the V2a interneurons, which relay information between motoneurons and the cerebellum to provide an 'internal feedback loop' [109]. The integration of descending and ascending input through these interneurons drives LTP in the spinal cord necessary for recovery. Identification of spinal interneurons that specifically mediate reaching and grasping behaviors will be critical targets for improving therapeutic outcomes.

In humans, anatomical plasticity is often inferred from motor and sensory evoked potential recordings of neural activity, electromyographic (EMG) recordings of motor output, or other neuroimaging techniques. Transmagnetic stimulation (TMS) of different muscle groups has been used to show changes (or the lack thereof) in cortical motor mapping or alterations in root sparing, and to estimate CST innervation of different spinal cord segments following injury [110,111]. Comparisons between stroke and SCI research are useful for understanding the role of upper motor neurons and CNS plasticity. For example, a recent study has shown adaptive strategies of motor unit recruitment from the contralesional RST following stroke that prioritize elbow, wrist, and finger flexion synergy over dextrous digit manipulation, which limits functional recovery [112]. Similarly, muscle groups with spared RST input following SCI have been shown to be stronger than those without [113].

3.2. Neuromodulation to Drive Descending Plasticity after SCI

Because of the importance of dexterity in independence, a major focus of clinical research has been specifically on hand function. Upper extremity function in people with cervical SCI varies greatly. The level and severity of injury determines the loss of function, which dictates the individual's ability to participate in physical rehabilitation. The SCI individual's engagement and the mode of rehabilitation influences the rate and degree of recovery [114,115]. Numerous physical therapy and rehabilitation paradigms exist, such as context-dependent reaching and grasping, object manipulation tasks, strength training and neurostimulation [116–118]. Kinematic analysis of the clinical population has been rigorously performed to categorize several key features of both compensatory and regained upper extremity movement, which shows that existing treatments are not wholly effective at restoring function [119]. Devices are under development to measure improvements in hand motor control remotely [120].

Neuromodulation of spared connections between the CST and RST caudal to an injury has been shown in rodents to precipitate reorganization and functional recovery [121]. A series of studies from the Buford lab [122–124] illustrated the reciprocal control of upper limb flexor and extensor muscles bilaterally. The related firing patterns of the pontomedullary reticular formation may play a role in compensatory neural control of upper extremity function after SCI. Additional connections between RST neurons and propriospinal interneurons within the spinal cord allow for descending input to circumnavigate lesion sites by crossing midline twice [125–127].

Reminiscent of forced-use paradigms popular for post-stroke rehabilitation [128,129], individuals suffering from lost hand dexterity will rely on compensatory movements, which potentially limit complete restoration of hand motor function [130]. In individuals with no remaining motor control of the forearm, brain computer interfaces are a promising alternative strategy for regaining independence. These devices are engineered to either compensate for lost circuitry or to drive anatomical plasticity in efforts to establish new connections or to strengthen existing but weak synaptic circuits. Brain computer interfaces exist that allow for reaching and grasping with robotic arms [131]. Current research is underway to augment these devices to have digit specific movement based on cortical activity [132], as well as to enhance plastic changes through neuromodulation using cortical stimulation, spinal stimulation, and tactile feedback [118,133–136].

3.3. Primary Afferent Plasticity

Primary afferent fibers supply information to spinal cord neurons about proprioception as well as information about object size, shape, and texture that are important for successful grasping of an object [61,137]. Axons from mechanosensitive and proprioceptive neurons ascend supraspinally in the ipsilateral dorsal columns and send collateral axons into motor centers of the spinal cord. Comprehensive reviews of primary afferent input to the spinal cord, as well as its targeting of spinal interneurons, can be found by Gatto et al. [138] as well as Abraira and Ginty [139]. These interneurons in the deep dorsal horn have been shown to regulate sensory input to motor circuits via presynaptic inhibition [138,140,141]. In humans, primary afferent input is integrated with motor commands via presynaptic inhibition in the cord from primary afferents and interneurons [142]. Thus, primary afferent input is one neural substrate that can modulate spinal interneurons involved in the reach-to-grasp movement.

The first example of anatomical plasticity of primary afferent fibers in response to injury was published by Liu and Chambers in 1958 [143]. In this seminal work, the authors demonstrated that dorsal root injury caused collateral sprouting of adjacent dorsal root axons into the dorsal horn of the cat. A series of studies by Murray and Goldberger [144–146] further demonstrated that collateral sprouting of primary afferent fibers resulted in recovery of motor function after either dorsal root or spinal cord injury. Others report sprouting of intact propriospinal interneurons following spinal hemisection as a neural mechanism of locomotor recovery [101–103]. The anatomical changes seen in these experiments were not a regenerative effort of damaged neurons, but rather a growth effort of undamaged and intact neurons that corresponded to improvements in function. Altered primary afferent input may be transmitted to motor neurons through deep dorsal horn interneurons, and membrane properties of these deep dorsal horn interneurons rostral and caudal to SCI demonstrated decreased input resistance and rheobase, indicating a hyperexcitable state [147].

Notably, the primary sensory neurons of the dorsal root ganglia (DRG) do not merely transmit feedback information to motor systems, but certain subclasses, called nociceptors, can transmit pain and temperature information from the peripheral tissues to the superficial or deep dorsal horn of the spinal cord. In addition, these nociceptive neurons extend axon collaterals to grey matter laminae in neighboring spinal cord segments via Lissauer's tract. Detailed descriptions of dorsal horn neuron populations that receive nociceptive afferent input can be found in Peirs et al. [148]. Cutaneous nociceptive primary afferent fibers are analogous to Type III (Aδ) and Type IV (C) primary afferent fibers from the muscle, which innervate slightly deeper into the spinal cord [149]. Importantly, nociceptors can indirectly act on motoneurons at the spinal level. The withdrawal reflex is an example of a nociceptor mediated motor output. This polysynaptic reflex takes afferent input from predominantly Aδ fibers and passes it through a series of interneurons to cause ipsilateral flexion and contralateral extension of the limbs [34]. A recent study showed that C-fibers are responsible for a second, delayed phase of activity in the withdrawal reflex [150]. This suggests that C-fibers are also capable of reaching motoneurons via interneurons. Furthermore, the Type III and IV muscle afferents have been shown to modulate motor unit recruitment when firing during exercise-induced fatigue [151]. This firing has a unique modulatory effect because silent nociceptors become sensitive to stretch in the presence of exercise related metabolites [149]. This evidence shows that nociceptors not only are capable of influencing motor control at the spinal level, but also that different circumstances change how much they are involved.

After experimental SCI, nociceptive primary afferent fibers display a robust and maladaptive increase in their terminal arborizations in the dorsal horn [152,153] and display hyperexcitability and increased spontaneous activity [154]. Analysis of sensation in individuals with cervical SCI suggest that intrinsic changes in primary sensory neurons could, in part, mediate the return of functional sensation, as well as maladaptive allodynia and hyperalgesia, often observed over time following SCI [155]. Of course, these morphological and functional changes in nociceptive primary afferent input are associated with the development of neuropathic pain, but nociceptive information is also supplied for tissue and joint protection via reflex arcs to modulate normal motor circuit function and motor output. Therefore, aberrant plasticity of nociceptive afferents may be detrimental to functional recovery following SCI.

4. Rehabilitation, and Afferent Driven Plasticity for Reaching and Grasping

The current standard of care for tetraplegia after SCI includes a wide range of neuromodulation and physical therapy with varying success [116]. Intraspinal microstimulation and transcutaneous stimulation have been used to augment reaching and grasping after SCI and to have persistent effects, which indicate a promotion in neuroplasticity [117,156]. Other stimulation targets after injury focus on the periphery and exist to aid voluntary movement. These devices provide scaled strength to the hand when volitional movement is detected via tactile pressure sensors to facilitate use of the individual's hand, which promotes both independence and rehabilitation-driven plasticity [157]. Similar devices activate an exoskeleton to aid in arm usage based on EMG recordings of volitional movement [158]. An alternative to task specific training is neurofeedback training using magnetoencephalography. Tetraplegic individuals use this technique to learn to control a virtual hand using the same brain waves they would use to move their own hand. This training led to improvements in grip strength [159]. Efforts to drive LTP and increase synaptic efficiency involve paired associative stimulation in which synchronized stimulation of the cortex with transcranial magnetic stimulation and peripheral nerve electrical stimulation have yielded positive outcomes in forelimb recovery [160,161]. Robotic assistance is also being combined with muscle stimulation to promote recovery and accuracy of the exoskeletal assisted movements [162]. Studies are underway to use multi-modal decoding algorithms to overcome the major hurdle of accurately determining the intended movement based on EMG output [163]. Combinatorial therapies yield the greatest results [164].

Rehabilitative strategies capitalize on the ability of the primary afferent to adapt and change in order to improve function after an injury. These physical therapies can include task specific training, such as repetitively reaching for, grasping, and manipulating objects. Additional therapies include resistance or aerobic training, as well as range-of-motion movements and stretching. Many of these are emulated in the laboratory. It is well established that task specific training improves reaching and grasping behavior after injury [165–168]. Cutaneous afferent input has been shown to significantly improve behavioral restoration and drive CNS plasticity following a lesion of the dorsal column [60]. SCI and subsequent treadmill training alter spinal interneuron excitability [147,169]. In addition, our lab and others have shown that early aerobic exercise can prevent pain development and reduce aberrant changes in nociceptor distribution and density within the superficial dorsal horn [170–172], suggesting a convergence of the nociceptive system and sensorimotor feedback systems within the dorsal horn to influence motor efferent output and behavior.

In 2018, Keller, et al. [173] investigated the EMG patterns in hindlimb muscles of SCI rats that underwent a daily range-of-motion stretching therapy. After several consecutive days of stretching, locomotor ability declined, and EMG recordings revealed increased clonus-like contractions during stretching [173]. This irregular muscle firing due to the stretching may explain the emergence of the irregular stepping patterns. A follow-up study demonstrated that ablation of nociceptors reduced stretching-induced locomotor deficits [174]. Nociceptors are often considered to be isolated in the sensory system, with the only overlap into motor systems occurring in withdrawal reflex circuitry. Even then, the withdrawal reflex is mediated via A fibers (type III fibers), while much of the work here is focused on C-fibers (likely type IV fibers). Collectively, this work shows that nociceptors might play a different and more influential role on motor output after SCI.

Numerous techniques are being used and tested for human rehabilitation after SCI, including a host of task specific and guided movement exercises. At the forefront, is a focus on accessibility and enhancing plasticity. Novel technologies, such as virtual reality (VR), allow individuals with SCI to perform more complex physical therapy independently and from home. VR devices are capable of delivering multiple physical therapy movement routines and accurately tracking associated hand kinematics [175]. Since VR technology only became available a few years ago, there is limited evidence demonstrating that VR therapy may be more beneficial than conventional physical therapy. However, the flexibility and affordability of VR devices and their accuracy in tracking movements will likely drive further research and development of this technology [176].

5. Conclusions

Neuroplasticity is a robust mechanism by which the central nervous system attempts to adapt to a structural or chemical disruption of functional connections between neurons. This adaptation is a prominent feature during neurodevelopment and is found in learning and memory. Following damage to nervous tissue, such as spinal cord injury, spontaneous plasticity may be initiated. Spontaneous plasticity can be maladaptive, as in the case of chronic neuropathic pain, but it can also lead to the recovery of lost function. Sprouting, synaptogenesis, synaptic plasticity, and pruning of connections between afferent fibers, interneurons, and motoneurons of ascending and descending tracts all play a role in mediating meaningful recovery after injury. Minor pathways often compensate for damaged major pathways, but interventions can lead to damaged axons regenerating across the lesion to improve function [14].

One of the major drives of modern neuroscience research is directed towards harnessing the power of neuroplasticity through rehabilitation. The human CNS has limited ability to spontaneously recover, however, many of the underlying mechanisms that allow recovery in other animals are still present. The rehabilitation research field attempts to use physical training to force central drive and primary afferent input into the spinal cord. Significantly, this shows that spontaneous plasticity within segmental spinal cord circuitry can be enhanced by rehabilitation. This gives hope for future research into the field, as rehabilitative techniques are optimized and even combined with pharmacological or neuromodulatory treatments. Not only do future studies need to continue to perfect treatments, but they also need to consider the fundamental changes in the nervous system, especially the spinal cord after injury. Certain cells, such as C-fiber nociceptors, are often neglected when considering movement or modeling motor circuitry. This has changed as alternatives to opioids for chronic pain treatment gain focus. Certainly, further research into the specific role of subclasses of primary afferent feedback after injury, especially nociceptors, is warranted.

Author Contributions: Conceptualization, J.R.W. and M.R.D.; Writing—original draft preparation, J.R.W.; Writing—review and editing, J.R.W. and M.R.D.; Funding acquisition, M.R.D. All authors have read and agreed to the published version of the manuscript.

Funding: This research was funded by the Craig H. Neilsen Foundation, grant number 457508 and by the National Institutes of Health R01 NS097880, both awarded to M.R.D.

Institutional Review Board Statement: Not applicable.

Informed Consent Statement: Not applicable.

Acknowledgments: We gratefully acknowledge Kimberly Dougherty and John Houlé for thoughtful discussions and review of the manuscript.

Conflicts of Interest: The authors declare no conflict of interest.

References

1. Donnelly, D.J.; Popovich, P.G. Inflammation and its role in neuroprotection, axonal regeneration and functional recovery after spinal cord injury. *Exp. Neurol.* **2008**, *209*, 378–388. [CrossRef]
2. Detloff, M.R.; Fisher, L.C.; McGaughy, V.; Longbrake, E.E.; Popovich, P.G.; Basso, D.M. Remote activation of microglia and pro-inflammatory cytokines predict the onset and severity of below-level neuropathic pain after spinal cord injury in rats. *Exp. Neurol.* **2008**, *212*, 337–347. [CrossRef]
3. Gensel, J.C.; Zhang, B. Macrophage activation and its role in repair and pathology after spinal cord injury. *Brain Res.* **2015**, *1619*, 1–11. [CrossRef]
4. Kopper, T.J.; Gensel, J.C. Myelin as an inflammatory mediator: Myelin interactions with complement, macrophages, and microglia in spinal cord injury. *J. Neurosci. Res.* **2018**, *96*, 969–977. [CrossRef]
5. Chhaya, S.J.; Quiros-Molina, D.; Tamashiro-Orrego, A.D.; Houle, J.D.; Detloff, M.R. Exercise-Induced Changes to the Macrophage Response in the Dorsal Root Ganglia Prevent Neuropathic Pain after Spinal Cord Injury. *J. Neurotraum.* **2019**, *36*, 877–890. [CrossRef]
6. Kroner, A.; Almanza, J.R. Role of microglia in spinal cord injury. *Neurosci. Lett.* **2019**, *709*, 134370. [CrossRef] [PubMed]
7. O'Shea, T.M.; Burda, J.E.; Sofroniew, M.V. Cell biology of spinal cord injury and repair. *J. Clin. Investig.* **2017**, *127*, 3259–3270. [CrossRef] [PubMed]
8. Tran, A.P.; Warren, P.M.; Silver, J. New insights into glial scar formation after spinal cord injury. *Cell Tissue Res.* **2021**. [CrossRef]
9. Silver, J.; Miller, J.H. Regeneration beyond the glial scar. *Nat. Rev. Neurosci.* **2004**, *5*, 146–156. [CrossRef] [PubMed]
10. Reier, P.J.; Houle, J.D. The glial scar: Its bearing on axonal elongation and transplantation approaches to CNS repair. *Adv. Neurol.* **1988**, *47*, 87–138. [PubMed]
11. Snow, D.M.; Brown, E.M.; Letourneau, P.C. Growth cone behavior in the presence of soluble chondroitin sulfate proteoglycan (CSPG), compared to behavior on CSPG bound to laminin or fibronectin. *Int. J. Dev. Neurosci.* **1996**, *14*, 331–349. [CrossRef]
12. Fawcett, J.W.; Asher, R.A. The glial scar and central nervous system repair. *Brain Res. Bull.* **1999**, *49*, 377–391. [CrossRef]
13. Herrmann, J.E.; Imura, T.; Song, B.; Qi, J.; Ao, Y.; Nguyen, T.K.; Korsak, R.A.; Takeda, K.; Akira, S.; Sofroniew, M.V. STAT3 is a critical regulator of astrogliosis and scar formation after spinal cord injury. *J. Neurosci.* **2008**, *28*, 7231–7243. [CrossRef]
14. Tom, V.J.; Houle, J.D. Intraspinal microinjection of chondroitinase ABC following injury promotes axonal regeneration out of a peripheral nerve graft bridge. *Exp. Neurol.* **2008**, *211*, 315–319. [CrossRef] [PubMed]
15. Tran, A.P.; Warren, P.M.; Silver, J. The Biology of Regeneration Failure and Success After Spinal Cord Injury. *Physiol. Rev.* **2018**, *98*, 881–917. [CrossRef] [PubMed]
16. O'Reilly, M.L.; Tom, V.J. Neuroimmune System as a Driving Force for Plasticity Following CNS Injury. *Front. Cell Neurosci.* **2020**, *14*, 187. [CrossRef]
17. Anderson, M.A.; Burda, J.E.; Ren, Y.; Ao, Y.; O'Shea, T.M.; Kawaguchi, R.; Coppola, G.; Khakh, B.S.; Deming, T.J.; Sofroniew, M.V. Astrocyte scar formation aids central nervous system axon regeneration. *Nature* **2016**, *532*, 195–200. [CrossRef]
18. Lee, J.K.; Geoffroy, C.G.; Chan, A.F.; Tolentino, K.E.; Crawford, M.J.; Leal, M.A.; Kang, B.; Zheng, B. Assessing spinal axon regeneration and sprouting in Nogo-, MAG-, and OMgp-deficient mice. *Neuron* **2010**, *66*, 663–670. [CrossRef] [PubMed]
19. National Spinal Cord Injury Statistical Center. *Facts and Figures at a Glance*; University of Alabama at Birmingham: Birmingham, AL, USA, 2021.
20. Xiao, Z.; Tang, F.; Zhao, Y.; Han, G.; Yin, N.; Li, X.; Chen, B.; Han, S.; Jiang, X.; Yun, C.; et al. Significant Improvement of Acute Complete Spinal Cord Injury Patients Diagnosed by a Combined Criteria Implanted with NeuroRegen Scaffolds and Mesenchymal Stem Cells. *Cell Transplant.* **2018**, *27*, 907–915. [CrossRef]
21. Flesher, S.N.; Downey, J.E.; Weiss, J.M.; Hughes, C.L.; Herrera, A.J.; Tyler-Kabara, E.C.; Boninger, M.L.; Collinger, J.L.; Gaunt, R.A. A brain-computer interface that evokes tactile sensations improves robotic arm control. *Science* **2021**, *372*, 831–836. [CrossRef]
22. Goshgarian, H.G. Developmental plasticity in the respiratory pathway of the adult rat. *Exp. Neurol.* **1979**, *66*, 547–555. [CrossRef]
23. Zimmer, M.B.; Goshgarian, H.G. GABA, not glycine, mediates inhibition of latent respiratory motor pathways after spinal cord injury. *Exp. Neurol.* **2007**, *203*, 493–501. [CrossRef] [PubMed]
24. Lee, K.Z.; Dougherty, B.J.; Sandhu, M.S.; Lane, M.A.; Reier, P.J.; Fuller, D.D. Phrenic motoneuron discharge patterns following chronic cervical spinal cord injury. *Exp. Neurol.* **2013**, *249*, 20–32. [CrossRef] [PubMed]
25. Hachem, L.D.; Ahuja, C.S.; Fehlings, M.G. Assessment and management of acute spinal cord injury: From point of injury to rehabilitation. *J. Spinal Cord Med.* **2017**, *40*, 665–675. [CrossRef] [PubMed]
26. Wolpaw, J.R.; Lee, C.L.; Carp, J.S. Operantly conditioned plasticity in spinal cord. *Ann. N. Y. Acad. Sci.* **1991**, *627*, 338–348. [CrossRef] [PubMed]
27. Gomes-Osman, J.; Field-Fote, E.C. Cortical vs. afferent stimulation as an adjunct to functional task practice training: A randomized, comparative pilot study in people with cervical spinal cord injury. *Clin. Rehabil.* **2015**, *29*, 771–782. [CrossRef] [PubMed]
28. Field-Fote, E.C. Exciting recovery: Augmenting practice with stimulation to optimize outcomes after spinal cord injury. *Prog. Brain Res.* **2015**, *218*, 103–126. [CrossRef] [PubMed]

29. Schildt, C.J.; Thomas, S.H.; Powell, E.S.; Sawaki, L.; Sunderam, S. Closed-loop afferent electrical stimulation for recovery of hand function in individuals with motor incomplete spinal injury: Early clinical results. In Proceedings of the 2016 38th Annual International Conference of the IEEE Engineering in Medicine and Biology Society (EMBC), Orlando, FL, USA, 16–20 August 2016; pp. 1552–1555. [CrossRef] [PubMed]
30. Fee, M.S. The role of efference copy in striatal learning. *Curr. Opin. Neurobiol.* **2014**, *25*, 194–200. [CrossRef] [PubMed]
31. Alstermark, B.; Ekerot, C.F. The lateral reticular nucleus; integration of descending and ascending systems regulating voluntary forelimb movements. *Front. Comput. Neurosci.* **2015**, *9*, 102. [CrossRef]
32. Person, A.L. Corollary Discharge Signals in the Cerebellum. *Biol. Psychiatry Cogn. Neurosci. Neuroimaging* **2019**, *4*, 813–819. [CrossRef]
33. Van Kemenade, B.M.; Arikan, B.E.; Podranski, K.; Steinstrater, O.; Kircher, T.; Straube, B. Distinct Roles for the Cerebellum, Angular Gyrus, and Middle Temporal Gyrus in Action-Feedback Monitoring. *Cereb. Cortex* **2019**, *29*, 1520–1531. [CrossRef]
34. Kandel, E.; Koster, J.; Mack, S.; Siegelbaum, S. *Principles of Neural Science*, 5th ed.; McGraw-Hill: New York, NY, USA, 2013.
35. Sweatt, J.D. Neural plasticity and behavior—Sixty years of conceptual advances. *J. Neurochem.* **2016**, *139*, 179–199. [CrossRef] [PubMed]
36. Bliss, T.V.; Lomo, T. Long-lasting potentiation of synaptic transmission in the dentate area of the anaesthetized rabbit following stimulation of the perforant path. *J. Physiol.* **1973**, *232*, 331–356. [CrossRef] [PubMed]
37. Hebb, D.O. *The Organization of Behavior: A Neuropsychological Theory*; John Wiley & Sons: New York, NY, USA, 1949.
38. Zenke, F.; Gerstner, W. Hebbian plasticity requires compensatory processes on multiple timescales. *Philos. Trans. R. Soc. Lond. B Biol. Sci.* **2017**, *372*, 20160259. [CrossRef] [PubMed]
39. Diering, G.H.; Huganir, R.L. The AMPA Receptor Code of Synaptic Plasticity. *Neuron* **2018**, *100*, 314–329. [CrossRef]
40. Dittman, J.S.; Ryan, T.A. The control of release probability at nerve terminals. *Nat. Rev. Neurosci.* **2019**, *20*, 177–186. [CrossRef] [PubMed]
41. Harris, K.M. Structural LTP: From synaptogenesis to regulated synapse enlargement and clustering. *Curr. Opin. Neurobiol.* **2020**, *63*, 189–197. [CrossRef] [PubMed]
42. Zucker, R.S.; Regehr, W.G. Short-term synaptic plasticity. *Annu. Rev. Physiol.* **2002**, *64*, 355–405. [CrossRef] [PubMed]
43. Jackman, S.L.; Regehr, W.G. The Mechanisms and Functions of Synaptic Facilitation. *Neuron* **2017**, *94*, 447–464. [CrossRef] [PubMed]
44. Luscher, C.; Malenka, R.C. NMDA receptor-dependent long-term potentiation and long-term depression (LTP/LTD). *Cold Spring Harb. Perspect. Biol.* **2012**, *4*, a005710. [CrossRef]
45. Koike-Tani, M.; Kanda, T.; Saitoh, N.; Yamashita, T.; Takahashi, T. Involvement of AMPA receptor desensitization in short-term synaptic depression at the calyx of Held in developing rats. *J. Physiol.* **2008**, *586*, 2263–2275. [CrossRef] [PubMed]
46. Herring, B.E.; Nicoll, R.A. Long-Term Potentiation: From CaMKII to AMPA Receptor Trafficking. *Annu. Rev. Physiol.* **2016**, *78*, 351–365. [CrossRef] [PubMed]
47. Grasselli, G.; Hansel, C. Cerebellar long-term potentiation: Cellular mechanisms and role in learning. *Int. Rev. Neurobiol.* **2014**, *117*, 39–51. [CrossRef]
48. Wolpaw, J.R. Spinal cord plasticity in acquisition and maintenance of motor skills. *Acta Physiol.* **2007**, *189*, 155–169. [CrossRef]
49. Roth, R.H.; Cudmore, R.H.; Tan, H.L.; Hong, I.; Zhang, Y.; Huganir, R.L. Cortical Synaptic AMPA Receptor Plasticity during Motor Learning. *Neuron* **2020**, *105*, 895–908.e5. [CrossRef]
50. Adkins, D.L.; Boychuk, J.; Remple, M.S.; Kleim, J.A. Motor training induces experience-specific patterns of plasticity across motor cortex and spinal cord. *J. Appl. Physiol.* **2006**, *101*, 1776–1782. [CrossRef]
51. Hoy, K.C.; Huie, J.R.; Grau, J.W. AMPA receptor mediated behavioral plasticity in the isolated rat spinal cord. *Behav. Brain Res.* **2013**, *236*, 319–326. [CrossRef]
52. Ganzer, P.D.; Beringer, C.R.; Shumsky, J.S.; Nwaobasi, C.; Moxon, K.A. Serotonin receptor and dendritic plasticity in the spinal cord mediated by chronic serotonergic pharmacotherapy combined with exercise following complete SCI in the adult rat. *Exp. Neurol.* **2018**, *304*, 132–142. [CrossRef] [PubMed]
53. Lisman, J. Glutamatergic synapses are structurally and biochemically complex because of multiple plasticity processes: Long-term potentiation, long-term depression, short-term potentiation and scaling. *Philos. Trans. R. Soc. Lond. B Biol. Sci* **2017**, *372*, 20160260. [CrossRef]
54. Purkey, A.M.; Dell'Acqua, M.L. Phosphorylation-Dependent Regulation of Ca(2+)-Permeable AMPA Receptors During Hippocampal Synaptic Plasticity. *Front. Synaptic. Neurosci.* **2020**, *12*, 8. [CrossRef] [PubMed]
55. Kulik, Y.D.; Watson, D.J.; Cao, G.; Kuwajima, M.; Harris, K.M. Structural plasticity of dendritic secretory compartments during LTP-induced synaptogenesis. *Elife* **2019**, *8*, e46356. [CrossRef]
56. Whishaw, I.Q.; Pellis, S.M. The structure of skilled forelimb reaching in the rat: A proximally driven movement with a single distal rotatory component. *Behav. Brain Res.* **1990**, *41*, 49–59. [CrossRef]
57. Whishaw, I.Q.; Pellis, S.M.; Gorny, B.; Kolb, B.; Tetzlaff, W. Proximal and distal impairments in rat forelimb use in reaching follow unilateral pyramidal tract lesions. *Behav. Brain Res.* **1993**, *56*, 59–76. [CrossRef]
58. Haines, D.E. *Neuroanatomy: An Atlas of Structures, Sections, and Systems*; Lippincott Williams and Wilkons: Philadelphia, PA, USA, 2000; Volume 5.

59. Pizzimenti, M.A.; Darling, W.G.; Rotella, D.L.; McNeal, D.W.; Herrick, J.L.; Ge, J.; Stilwell-Morecraft, K.S.; Morecraft, R.J. Measurement of reaching kinematics and prehensile dexterity in nonhuman primates. *J. Neurophysiol.* 2007, *98*, 1015–1029. [CrossRef] [PubMed]
60. Qi, H.X.; Gharbawie, O.A.; Wynne, K.W.; Kaas, J.H. Impairment and recovery of hand use after unilateral section of the dorsal columns of the spinal cord in squirrel monkeys. *Behav. Brain Res.* 2013, *252*, 363–376. [CrossRef] [PubMed]
61. Geed, S.; McCurdy, M.L.; van Kan, P.L. Neuronal Correlates of Functional Coupling between Reach- and Grasp-Related Components of Muscle Activity. *Front. Neural. Circuits* 2017, *11*, 7. [CrossRef] [PubMed]
62. Baker, S.N. The primate reticulospinal tract, hand function and functional recovery. *J. Physiol.* 2011, *589*, 5603–5612. [CrossRef] [PubMed]
63. Sathyamurthy, A.; Barik, A.; Dobrott, C.I.; Matson, K.J.E.; Stoica, S.; Pursley, R.; Chesler, A.T.; Levine, A.J. Cerebellospinal Neurons Regulate Motor Performance and Motor Learning. *Cell Rep.* 2020, *31*, 107595. [CrossRef] [PubMed]
64. McKenna, J.E.; Prusky, G.T.; Whishaw, I.Q. Cervical motoneuron topography reflects the proximodistal organization of muscles and movements of the rat forelimb: A retrograde carbocyanine dye analysis. *J. Comp. Neurol.* 2000, *419*, 286–296. [CrossRef]
65. Klein, A.; Sacrey, L.A.; Dunnett, S.B.; Whishaw, I.Q.; Nikkhah, G. Proximal movements compensate for distal forelimb movement impairments in a reach-to-eat task in Huntington's disease: New insights into motor impairments in a real-world skill. *Neurobiol. Dis.* 2011, *41*, 560–569. [CrossRef]
66. Klein, A.; Sacrey, L.A.; Whishaw, I.Q.; Dunnett, S.B. The use of rodent skilled reaching as a translational model for investigating brain damage and disease. *Neurosci. Biobehav. Rev.* 2012, *36*, 1030–1042. [CrossRef]
67. Krisa, L.; Runyen, M.; Detloff, M.R. Translational Challenges of Rat Models of Upper Extremity Dysfunction After Spinal Cord Injury. *Top. Spinal Cord Inj. Rehabil.* 2018, *24*, 195–205. [CrossRef]
68. Gallegos, C.; Carey, M.; Zheng, Y.; He, X.; Cao, Q.L. Reaching and Grasping Training Improves Functional Recovery After Chronic Cervical Spinal Cord Injury. *Front. Cell Neurosci.* 2020, *14*, 110. [CrossRef]
69. Montoya, C.P.; Campbell-Hope, L.J.; Pemberton, K.D.; Dunnett, S.B. The "staircase test": A measure of independent forelimb reaching and grasping abilities in rats. *J. Neurosci. Methods* 1991, *36*, 219–228. [CrossRef]
70. Sindhurakar, A.; Butensky, S.D.; Meyers, E.; Santos, J.; Bethea, T.; Khalili, A.; Sloan, A.P.; Rennaker, R.L., 3rd; Carmel, J.B. An Automated Test of Rat Forelimb Supination Quantifies Motor Function Loss and Recovery After Corticospinal Injury. *Neurorehabil. Neural. Repair.* 2017, *31*, 122–132. [CrossRef] [PubMed]
71. Irvine, K.A.; Ferguson, A.R.; Mitchell, K.D.; Beattie, S.B.; Beattie, M.S.; Bresnahan, J.C. A novel method for assessing proximal and distal forelimb function in the rat: The Irvine, Beatties and Bresnahan (IBB) forelimb scale. *J. Vis. Exp.* 2010, *46*, e2246. [CrossRef] [PubMed]
72. Irvine, K.A.; Ferguson, A.R.; Mitchell, K.D.; Beattie, S.B.; Lin, A.; Stuck, E.D.; Huie, J.R.; Nielson, J.L.; Talbott, J.F.; Inoue, T.; et al. The Irvine, Beatties, and Bresnahan (IBB) Forelimb Recovery Scale: An Assessment of Reliability and Validity. *Front. Neurol.* 2014, *5*, 116. [CrossRef] [PubMed]
73. Ballermann, M.; Metz, G.A.; McKenna, J.E.; Klassen, F.; Whishaw, I.Q. The pasta matrix reaching task: A simple test for measuring skilled reaching distance, direction, and dexterity in rats. *J. Neurosci. Methods* 2001, *106*, 39–45. [CrossRef]
74. Bertelli, J.A.; Mira, J.C. Behavioral evaluating methods in the objective clinical assessment of motor function after experimental brachial plexus reconstruction in the rat. *J. Neurosci. Methods* 1993, *46*, 203–208. [CrossRef]
75. Anderson, K.D.; Gunawan, A.; Steward, O. Quantitative assessment of forelimb motor function after cervical spinal cord injury in rats: Relationship to the corticospinal tract. *Exp. Neurol.* 2005, *194*, 161–174. [CrossRef] [PubMed]
76. Khaing, Z.Z.; Geissler, S.A.; Jiang, S.; Milman, B.D.; Aguilar, S.V.; Schmidt, C.E.; Schallert, T. Assessing forelimb function after unilateral cervical spinal cord injury: Novel forelimb tasks predict lesion severity and recovery. *J. Neurotraum.* 2012, *29*, 488–498. [CrossRef] [PubMed]
77. McCann, M.M.; Fisher, K.M.; Ahloy-Dallaire, J.; Darian-Smith, C. Somatosensory corticospinal tract axons sprout within the cervical cord following a dorsal root/dorsal column spinal injury in the rat. *J. Comp. Neurol.* 2020, *528*, 1293–1306. [CrossRef] [PubMed]
78. Ortiz-Rosario, A.; Berrios-Torres, I.; Adeli, H.; Buford, J.A. Combined corticospinal and reticulospinal effects on upper limb muscles. *Neurosci. Lett.* 2014, *561*, 30–34. [CrossRef]
79. Baker, S.N.; Zaaimi, B.; Fisher, K.M.; Edgley, S.A.; Soteropoulos, D.S. Pathways mediating functional recovery. *Prog. Brain Res.* 2015, *218*, 389–412. [CrossRef]
80. Palmer, E.; Ashby, P. Corticospinal projections to upper limb motoneurones in humans. *J. Physiol.* 1992, *448*, 397–412. [CrossRef]
81. De Noordhout, A.M.; Rapisarda, G.; Bogacz, D.; Gerard, P.; De Pasqua, V.; Pennisi, G.; Delwaide, P.J. Corticomotoneuronal synaptic connections in normal man: An electrophysiological study. *Brain* 1999, *122*, 1327–1340. [CrossRef]
82. Tazoe, T.; Perez, M.A. Cortical and reticular contributions to human precision and power grip. *J. Physiol.* 2017, *595*, 2715–2730. [CrossRef]
83. Schrimsher, G.W.; Reier, P.J. Forelimb motor performance following dorsal column, dorsolateral funiculi, or ventrolateral funiculi lesions of the cervical spinal cord in the rat. *Exp. Neurol.* 1993, *120*, 264–276. [CrossRef]
84. Morecraft, R.J.; Ge, J.; Stilwell-Morecraft, K.S.; McNeal, D.W.; Pizzimenti, M.A.; Darling, W.G. Terminal distribution of the corticospinal projection from the hand/arm region of the primary motor cortex to the cervical enlargement in rhesus monkey. *J. Comp. Neurol.* 2013, *521*, 4205–4235. [CrossRef]

85. Oudega, M.; Perez, M.A. Corticospinal reorganization after spinal cord injury. *J. Physiol.* **2012**, *590*, 3647–3663. [CrossRef] [PubMed]
86. Weidner, N.; Ner, A.; Salimi, N.; Tuszynski, M.H. Spontaneous corticospinal axonal plasticity and functional recovery after adult central nervous system injury. *Proc. Natl. Acad. Sci. USA* **2001**, *98*, 3513–3518. [CrossRef]
87. Nakagawa, H.; Ninomiya, T.; Yamashita, T.; Takada, M. Reorganization of corticospinal tract fibers after spinal cord injury in adult macaques. *Sci. Rep.* **2015**, *5*, 11986. [CrossRef]
88. Armstrong, D.M. Supraspinal contributions to the initiation and control of locomotion in the cat. *Prog. Neurobiol.* **1986**, *26*, 273–361. [CrossRef]
89. Shik, M.L.; Orlovsky, G.N. Neurophysiology of locomotor automatism. *Physiol. Rev.* **1976**, *56*, 465–501. [CrossRef]
90. Dougherty, K.J.; Kiehn, O. Functional organization of V2a-related locomotor circuits in the rodent spinal cord. *Ann. N. Y. Acad. Sci.* **2010**, *1198*, 85–93. [CrossRef] [PubMed]
91. Alaynick, W.A.; Jessell, T.M.; Pfaff, S.L. SnapShot: Spinal cord development. *Cell* **2011**, *146*, 178–178.e1. [CrossRef] [PubMed]
92. Lu, D.C.; Niu, T.; Alaynick, W.A. Molecular and cellular development of spinal cord locomotor circuitry. *Front. Mol. Neurosci.* **2015**, *8*, 25. [CrossRef]
93. Rybak, I.A.; Dougherty, K.J.; Shevtsova, N.A. Organization of the Mammalian Locomotor CPG: Review of Computational Model and Circuit Architectures Based on Genetically Identified Spinal Interneurons(1,2,3). *eNeuro* **2015**, *2*, 1–20. [CrossRef]
94. Flynn, J.R.; Conn, V.L.; Boyle, K.A.; Hughes, D.I.; Watanabe, M.; Velasquez, T.; Goulding, M.D.; Callister, R.J.; Graham, B.A. Anatomical and Molecular Properties of Long Descending Propriospinal Neurons in Mice. *Front. Neuroanat.* **2017**, *11*, 5. [CrossRef] [PubMed]
95. Zholudeva, L.V.; Qiang, L.; Marchenko, V.; Dougherty, K.J.; Sakiyama-Elbert, S.E.; Lane, M.A. The Neuroplastic and Therapeutic Potential of Spinal Interneurons in the Injured Spinal Cord. *Trends Neurosci.* **2018**, *41*, 625–639. [CrossRef] [PubMed]
96. Dobrott, C.I.; Sathyamurthy, A.; Levine, A.J. Decoding Cell Type Diversity Within the Spinal Cord. *Curr. Opin. Physiol.* **2019**, *8*, 1–6. [CrossRef] [PubMed]
97. Zholudeva, L.V.; Abraira, V.E.; Satkunendrarajah, K.; McDevitt, T.C.; Goulding, M.D.; Magnuson, D.S.K.; Lane, M.A. Spinal Interneurons as Gatekeepers to Neuroplasticity after Injury or Disease. *J. Neurosci.* **2021**, *41*, 845–854. [CrossRef]
98. Abraira, V.E.; Kuehn, E.D.; Chirila, A.M.; Springel, M.W.; Toliver, A.A.; Zimmerman, A.L.; Orefice, L.L.; Boyle, K.A.; Bai, L.; Song, B.J.; et al. The Cellular and Synaptic Architecture of the Mechanosensory Dorsal Horn. *Cell* **2017**, *168*, 295–310.e19. [CrossRef] [PubMed]
99. Gatto, G.; Bourane, S.; Ren, X.; Di Costanzo, S.; Fenton, P.K.; Halder, P.; Seal, R.P.; Goulding, M.D. A Functional Topographic Map for Spinal Sensorimotor Reflexes. *Neuron* **2021**, *109*, 91–104.e5. [CrossRef]
100. Pocratsky, A.M.; Shepard, C.T.; Morehouse, J.R.; Burke, D.A.; Riegler, A.S.; Hardin, J.T.; Beare, J.E.; Hainline, C.; States, G.J.; Brown, B.L.; et al. Long ascending propriospinal neurons provide flexible, context-specific control of interlimb coordination. *Elife* **2020**, *9*, e53565. [CrossRef] [PubMed]
101. Bareyre, F.M.; Kerschensteiner, M.; Raineteau, O.; Mettenleiter, T.C.; Weinmann, O.; Schwab, M.E. The injured spinal cord spontaneously forms a new intraspinal circuit in adult rats. *Nat. Neurosci.* **2004**, *7*, 269–277. [CrossRef]
102. Raineteau, O.; Schwab, M.E. Plasticity of motor systems after incomplete spinal cord injury. *Nat. Rev. Neurosci.* **2001**, *2*, 263–273. [CrossRef]
103. Courtine, G.; Song, B.; Roy, R.R.; Zhong, H.; Herrmann, J.E.; Ao, Y.; Qi, J.; Edgerton, V.R.; Sofroniew, M.V. Recovery of supraspinal control of stepping via indirect propriospinal relay connections after spinal cord injury. *Nat. Med.* **2008**, *14*, 69–74. [CrossRef]
104. Benthall, K.N.; Hough, R.A.; McClellan, A.D. Descending propriospinal neurons mediate restoration of locomotor function following spinal cord injury. *J. Neurophysiol.* **2017**, *117*, 215–229. [CrossRef]
105. Morris, R.; Tosolini, A.P.; Goldstein, J.D.; Whishaw, I.Q. Impaired arpeggio movement in skilled reaching by rubrospinal tract lesions in the rat: A behavioral/anatomical fractionation. *J. Neurotraum.* **2011**, *28*, 2439–2451. [CrossRef] [PubMed]
106. Hayashi, M.; Hinckley, C.A.; Driscoll, S.P.; Moore, N.J.; Levine, A.J.; Hilde, K.L.; Sharma, K.; Pfaff, S.L. Graded Arrays of Spinal and Supraspinal V2a Interneuron Subtypes Underlie Forelimb and Hindlimb Motor Control. *Neuron* **2018**, *97*, 869–884.e5. [CrossRef] [PubMed]
107. Whishaw, I.Q.; Gorny, B. Arpeggio and fractionated digit movements used in prehension by rats. *Behav. Brain Res.* **1994**, *60*, 15–24. [CrossRef]
108. Isa, T.; Kinoshita, M.; Nishimura, Y. Role of Direct vs. Indirect Pathways from the Motor Cortex to Spinal Motoneurons in the Control of Hand Dexterity. *Front. Neurol.* **2013**, *4*, 191. [CrossRef]
109. Azim, E.; Jiang, J.; Alstermark, B.; Jessell, T.M. Skilled reaching relies on a V2a propriospinal internal copy circuit. *Nature* **2014**, *508*, 357–363. [CrossRef]
110. Brouwer, B.; Hopkins-Rosseel, D.H. Motor cortical mapping of proximal upper extremity muscles following spinal cord injury. *Spinal Cord* **1997**, *35*, 205–212. [CrossRef]
111. Calancie, B.; Alexeeva, N.; Broton, J.G.; Suys, S.; Hall, A.; Klose, K.J. Distribution and latency of muscle responses to transcranial magnetic stimulation of motor cortex after spinal cord injury in humans. *J. Neurotraum.* **1999**, *16*, 49–67. [CrossRef]
112. McPherson, J.G.; Chen, A.; Ellis, M.D.; Yao, J.; Heckman, C.J.; Dewald, J.P.A. Progressive recruitment of contralesional cortico-reticulospinal pathways drives motor impairment post stroke. *J. Physiol.* **2018**, *596*, 1211–1225. [CrossRef]

113. Sangari, S.; Perez, M.A. Distinct Corticospinal and Reticulospinal Contributions to Voluntary Control of Elbow Flexor and Extensor Muscles in Humans with Tetraplegia. *J. Neurosci.* **2020**, *40*, 8831–8841. [CrossRef]
114. Ditunno, J.F., Jr.; Stover, S.L.; Freed, M.M.; Ahn, J.H. Motor recovery of the upper extremities in traumatic quadriplegia: A multicenter study. *Arch. Phys. Med. Rehabil.* **1992**, *73*, 431–436.
115. Ditunno, J.F., Jr.; Cohen, M.E.; Hauck, W.W.; Jackson, A.B.; Sipski, M.L. Recovery of upper-extremity strength in complete and incomplete tetraplegia: A multicenter study. *Arch. Phys. Med. Rehabil.* **2000**, *81*, 389–393. [CrossRef]
116. Mateo, S.; Di Marco, J.; Cucherat, M.; Gueyffier, F.; Rode, G. Inconclusive efficacy of intervention on upper-limb function after tetraplegia: A systematic review and meta-analysis. *Ann. Phys. Rehabil. Med.* **2020**, *63*, 230–240. [CrossRef] [PubMed]
117. Kasten, M.R.; Sunshine, M.D.; Secrist, E.S.; Horner, P.J.; Moritz, C.T. Therapeutic intraspinal microstimulation improves forelimb function after cervical contusion injury. *J. Neural. Eng.* **2013**, *10*, 044001. [CrossRef] [PubMed]
118. Ajiboye, A.B.; Willett, F.R.; Young, D.R.; Memberg, W.D.; Murphy, B.A.; Miller, J.P.; Walter, B.L.; Sweet, J.A.; Hoyen, H.A.; Keith, M.W.; et al. Restoration of reaching and grasping movements through brain-controlled muscle stimulation in a person with tetraplegia: A proof-of-concept demonstration. *Lancet* **2017**, *389*, 1821–1830. [CrossRef]
119. Mateo, S.; Roby-Brami, A.; Reilly, K.T.; Rossetti, Y.; Collet, C.; Rode, G. Upper limb kinematics after cervical spinal cord injury: A review. *J. Neuroeng. Rehabil.* **2015**, *12*, 9. [CrossRef]
120. Tsai, M.F.; Wang, R.H.; Zariffa, J. Generalizability of Hand-Object Interaction Detection in Egocentric Video across Populations with Hand Impairment. *Annu. Int. Conf. IEEE Eng. Med. Biol. Soc.* **2020**, *2020*, 3228–3231. [CrossRef]
121. Asboth, L.; Friedli, L.; Beauparlant, J.; Martinez-Gonzalez, C.; Anil, S.; Rey, E.; Baud, L.; Pidpruznykova, G.; Anderson, M.A.; Shkorbatova, P.; et al. Cortico-reticulo-spinal circuit reorganization enables functional recovery after severe spinal cord contusion. *Nat. Neurosci.* **2018**, *21*, 576–588. [CrossRef]
122. Davidson, A.G.; Buford, J.A. Bilateral actions of the reticulospinal tract on arm and shoulder muscles in the monkey: Stimulus triggered averaging. *Exp. Brain Res.* **2006**, *173*, 25–39. [CrossRef]
123. Davidson, A.G.; Schieber, M.H.; Buford, J.A. Bilateral spike-triggered average effects in arm and shoulder muscles from the monkey pontomedullary reticular formation. *J. Neurosci.* **2007**, *27*, 8053–8058. [CrossRef]
124. Herbert, W.J.; Davidson, A.G.; Buford, J.A. Measuring the motor output of the pontomedullary reticular formation in the monkey: Do stimulus-triggered averaging and stimulus trains produce comparable results in the upper limbs? *Exp. Brain Res.* **2010**, *203*, 271–283. [CrossRef]
125. Filli, L.; Engmann, A.K.; Zorner, B.; Weinmann, O.; Moraitis, T.; Gullo, M.; Kasper, H.; Schneider, R.; Schwab, M.E. Bridging the gap: A reticulo-propriospinal detour bypassing an incomplete spinal cord injury. *J. Neurosci.* **2014**, *34*, 13399–13410. [CrossRef]
126. Zorner, B.; Bachmann, L.C.; Filli, L.; Kapitza, S.; Gullo, M.; Bolliger, M.; Starkey, M.L.; Rothlisberger, M.; Gonzenbach, R.R.; Schwab, M.E. Chasing central nervous system plasticity: The brainstem's contribution to locomotor recovery in rats with spinal cord injury. *Brain* **2014**, *137*, 1716–1732. [CrossRef]
127. May, Z.; Fenrich, K.K.; Dahlby, J.; Batty, N.J.; Torres-Espin, A.; Fouad, K. Following Spinal Cord Injury Transected Reticulospinal Tract Axons Develop New Collateral Inputs to Spinal Interneurons in Parallel with Locomotor Recovery. *Neural. Plast* **2017**, *2017*, 1932875. [CrossRef] [PubMed]
128. Taub, E.; Wolf, S.L. Constraint Induced Movement Techniques To Facilitate Upper Extremity Use in Stroke Patients. *Top. Stroke Rehabil.* **1997**, *3*, 38–61. [CrossRef] [PubMed]
129. Dos Anjos, S.; Morris, D.; Taub, E. Constraint-Induced Movement Therapy for Lower Extremity Function: Describing the LE-CIMT Protocol. *Phys. Ther.* **2020**, *100*, 698–707. [CrossRef] [PubMed]
130. Schneider, S.; Popp, W.L.; Brogioli, M.; Albisser, U.; Ortmann, S.; Velstra, I.M.; Demko, L.; Gassert, R.; Curt, A. Predicting upper limb compensation during prehension tasks in tetraplegic spinal cord injured patients using a single wearable sensor. *IEEE Int. Conf. Rehabil. Robot.* **2019**, *2019*, 1000–1006. [CrossRef]
131. Bockbrader, M.A.; Francisco, G.; Lee, R.; Olson, J.; Solinsky, R.; Boninger, M.L. Brain Computer Interfaces in Rehabilitation Medicine. *PM R* **2018**, *10*, S233–S243. [CrossRef]
132. Jorge, A.; Royston, D.A.; Tyler-Kabara, E.C.; Boninger, M.L.; Collinger, J.L. Classification of Individual Finger Movements Using Intracortical Recordings in Human Motor Cortex. *Neurosurgery* **2020**, *87*, 630–638. [CrossRef]
133. Zimmermann, J.B.; Jackson, A. Closed-loop control of spinal cord stimulation to restore hand function after paralysis. *Front. Neurosci.* **2014**, *8*, 87. [CrossRef]
134. Benavides, F.D.; Jo, H.J.; Lundell, H.; Edgerton, V.R.; Gerasimenko, Y.; Perez, M.A. Cortical and Subcortical Effects of Transcutaneous Spinal Cord Stimulation in Humans with Tetraplegia. *J. Neurosci.* **2020**, *40*, 2633–2643. [CrossRef]
135. Anderson, K.D.; Bryden, A.M.; Moynahan, M. Risk-benefit value of upper extremity function by an implanted electrical stimulation device targeting chronic cervical spinal cord injury. *Spinal. Cord. Ser. Cases* **2019**, *5*, 68. [CrossRef]
136. Ganzer, P.D.; Colachis, S.C.t.; Schwemmer, M.A.; Friedenberg, D.A.; Dunlap, C.F.; Swiftney, C.E.; Jacobowitz, A.F.; Weber, D.J.; Bockbrader, M.A.; Sharma, G. Restoring the Sense of Touch Using a Sensorimotor Demultiplexing Neural Interface. *Cell* **2020**, *181*, 763–773.e712. [CrossRef] [PubMed]
137. Geed, S.; van Kan, P.L.E. Grasp-Based Functional Coupling Between Reach- and Grasp-Related Components of Forelimb Muscle Activity. *J. Mot. Behav.* **2017**, *49*, 312–328. [CrossRef] [PubMed]
138. Gatto, G.; Smith, K.M.; Ross, S.E.; Goulding, M. Neuronal diversity in the somatosensory system: Bridging the gap between cell type and function. *Curr. Opin. Neurobiol.* **2019**, *56*, 167–174. [CrossRef]

139. Abraira, V.E.; Ginty, D.D. The sensory neurons of touch. *Neuron* **2013**, *79*, 618–639. [CrossRef]
140. Fink, A.J.; Croce, K.R.; Huang, Z.J.; Abbott, L.F.; Jessell, T.M.; Azim, E. Presynaptic inhibition of spinal sensory feedback ensures smooth movement. *Nature* **2014**, *509*, 43–48. [CrossRef]
141. Koch, S.C.; Del Barrio, M.G.; Dalet, A.; Gatto, G.; Gunther, T.; Zhang, J.; Seidler, B.; Saur, D.; Schule, R.; Goulding, M. RORbeta Spinal Interneurons Gate Sensory Transmission during Locomotion to Secure a Fluid Walking Gait. *Neuron* **2017**, *96*, 1419–1431.e5. [CrossRef]
142. Knikou, M.; Chaudhuri, D.; Kay, E.; Schmit, B.D. Pre- and post-alpha motoneuronal control of the soleus H-reflex during sinusoidal hip movements in human spinal cord injury. *Brain Res.* **2006**, *1103*, 123–139. [CrossRef]
143. Liu, C.N.; Chambers, W.W. Intraspinal sprouting of dorsal root axons; development of new collaterals and preterminals following partial denervation of the spinal cord in the cat. *AMA Arch. Neurol. Psychiatry* **1958**, *79*, 46–61. [CrossRef]
144. Goldberger, M.E.; Murray, M. Restitution of function and collateral sprouting in the cat spinal cord: The deafferented animal. *J. Comp. Neurol.* **1974**, *158*, 37–53. [CrossRef] [PubMed]
145. Murray, M.; Goldberger, M.E. Restitution of function and collateral sprouting in the cat spinal cord: The partially hemisected animal. *J. Comp. Neurol.* **1974**, *158*, 19–36. [CrossRef]
146. Polistina, D.C.; Murray, M.; Goldberger, M.E. Plasticity of dorsal root and descending serotoninergic projections after partial deafferentation of the adult rat spinal cord. *J. Comp. Neurol.* **1990**, *299*, 349–363. [CrossRef]
147. Rank, M.M.; Galea, M.P.; Callister, R.; Callister, R.J. Is more always better? How different 'doses' of exercise after incomplete spinal cord injury affects the membrane properties of deep dorsal horn interneurons. *Exp. Neurol.* **2018**, *300*, 201–211. [CrossRef]
148. Peirs, C.; Dallel, R.; Todd, A.J. Recent advances in our understanding of the organization of dorsal horn neuron populations and their contribution to cutaneous mechanical allodynia. *J. Neural. Transm.* **2020**, *127*, 505–525. [CrossRef] [PubMed]
149. Laurin, J.; Pertici, V.; Dousset, E.; Marqueste, T.; Decherchi, P. Group III and IV muscle afferents: Role on central motor drive and clinical implications. *Neuroscience* **2015**, *290*, 543–551. [CrossRef] [PubMed]
150. Kimura, S.; Honda, M.; Tanabe, M.; Ono, H. Noxious stimuli evoke a biphasic flexor reflex composed of A delta-fiber-mediated short-latency and C-fiber-mediated long-latency withdrawal movements in mice. *J. Pharmacol. Sci.* **2004**, *95*, 94–100. [CrossRef] [PubMed]
151. Zajac, A.; Chalimoniuk, M.; Maszczyk, A.; Golas, A.; Lngfort, J. Central and Peripheral Fatigue During Resistance Exercise—A Critical Review. *J. Hum. Kinet* **2015**, *49*, 159–169. [CrossRef]
152. Ondarza, A.B.; Ye, Z.; Hulsebosch, C.E. Direct evidence of primary afferent sprouting in distant segments following spinal cord injury in the rat: Colocalization of GAP-43 and CGRP. *Exp. Neurol.* **2003**, *184*, 373–380. [CrossRef]
153. Detloff, M.R.; Quiros-Molina, D.; Javia, A.S.; Daggubati, L.; Nehlsen, A.D.; Naqvi, A.; Ninan, V.; Vannix, K.N.; McMullen, M.K.; Amin, S.; et al. Delayed Exercise Is Ineffective at Reversing Aberrant Nociceptive Afferent Plasticity or Neuropathic Pain After Spinal Cord Injury in Rats. *Neurorehabil. Neural. Repair.* **2016**, *30*, 685–700. [CrossRef] [PubMed]
154. Bedi, S.S.; Yang, Q.; Crook, R.J.; Du, J.; Wu, Z.; Fishman, H.M.; Grill, R.J.; Carlton, S.M.; Walters, E.T. Chronic spontaneous activity generated in the somata of primary nociceptors is associated with pain-related behavior after spinal cord injury. *J. Neurosci.* **2010**, *30*, 14870–14882. [CrossRef]
155. Kramer, J.K.; Taylor, P.; Steeves, J.D.; Curt, A. Dermatomal somatosensory evoked potentials and electrical perception thresholds during recovery from cervical spinal cord injury. *Neurorehabil. Neural. Repair* **2010**, *24*, 309–317. [CrossRef]
156. Inanici, F.; Samejima, S.; Gad, P.; Edgerton, V.R.; Hofstetter, C.P.; Moritz, C.T. Transcutaneous Electrical Spinal Stimulation Promotes Long-Term Recovery of Upper Extremity Function in Chronic Tetraplegia. *IEEE Trans. Neural. Syst. Rehabil. Eng.* **2018**, *26*, 1272–1278. [CrossRef]
157. Osuagwu, B.A.C.; Timms, S.; Peachment, R.; Dowie, S.; Thrussell, H.; Cross, S.; Shirley, R.; Segura-Fragoso, A.; Taylor, J. Home-based rehabilitation using a soft robotic hand glove device leads to improvement in hand function in people with chronic spinal cord injury:a pilot study. *J. Neuroeng. Rehabil.* **2020**, *17*, 40. [CrossRef]
158. McDonald, C.G.; Sullivan, J.L.; Dennis, T.A.; O'Malley, M.K. A Myoelectric Control Interface for Upper-Limb Robotic Rehabilitation Following Spinal Cord Injury. *IEEE Trans. Neural. Syst. Rehabil. Eng.* **2020**, *28*, 978–987. [CrossRef]
159. Foldes, S.T.; Boninger, M.L.; Weber, D.J.; Collinger, J.L. Effects of MEG-based neurofeedback for hand rehabilitation after tetraplegia: Preliminary findings in cortical modulations and grip strength. *J. Neural. Eng.* **2020**, *17*, 026019. [CrossRef] [PubMed]
160. Roy, F.D.; Yang, J.F.; Gorassini, M.A. Afferent regulation of leg motor cortex excitability after incomplete spinal cord injury. *J. Neurophysiol.* **2010**, *103*, 2222–2233. [CrossRef] [PubMed]
161. Rodionov, A.; Savolainen, S.; Kirveskari, E.; Makela, J.P.; Shulga, A. Restoration of hand function with long-term paired associative stimulation after chronic incomplete tetraplegia: A case study. *Spinal. Cord Ser. Cases* **2019**, *5*, 81. [CrossRef]
162. Dunkelberger, N.; Schearer, E.M.; O'Malley, M.K. A review of methods for achieving upper limb movement following spinal cord injury through hybrid muscle stimulation and robotic assistance. *Exp. Neurol.* **2020**, *328*, 113274. [CrossRef] [PubMed]
163. Corbett, E.A.; Sachs, N.A.; Kording, K.P.; Perreault, E.J. Multimodal decoding and congruent sensory information enhance reaching performance in subjects with cervical spinal cord injury. *Front. Neurosci.* **2014**, *8*, 123. [CrossRef] [PubMed]
164. Lu, X.; Battistuzzo, C.R.; Zoghi, M.; Galea, M.P. Effects of training on upper limb function after cervical spinal cord injury: A systematic review. *Clin. Rehabil.* **2015**, *29*, 3–13. [CrossRef]
165. Hurd, C.; Weishaupt, N.; Fouad, K. Anatomical correlates of recovery in single pellet reaching in spinal cord injured rats. *Exp. Neurol.* **2013**, *247*, 605–614. [CrossRef]

166. Garcia-Alias, G.; Truong, K.; Shah, P.K.; Roy, R.R.; Edgerton, V.R. Plasticity of subcortical pathways promote recovery of skilled hand function in rats after corticospinal and rubrospinal tract injuries. *Exp. Neurol.* **2015**, *266*, 112–119. [CrossRef] [PubMed]
167. Fenrich, K.K.; May, Z.; Torres-Espin, A.; Forero, J.; Bennett, D.J.; Fouad, K. Single pellet grasping following cervical spinal cord injury in adult rat using an automated full-time training robot. *Behav. Brain Res.* **2016**, *299*, 59–71. [CrossRef]
168. Fenrich, K.K.; Hallworth, B.W.; Vavrek, R.; Raposo, P.J.F.; Misiaszek, J.E.; Bennett, D.J.; Fouad, K.; Torres-Espin, A. Self-directed rehabilitation training intensity thresholds for efficient recovery of skilled forelimb function in rats with cervical spinal cord injury. *Exp. Neurol.* **2021**, *339*, 113543. [CrossRef]
169. Garcia-Ramirez, D.L.; Ha, N.T.B.; Bibu, S.; Stachowski, N.J.; Dougherty, K.J. Spinal cord injury alters spinal Shox2 interneurons by enhancing excitatory synaptic input and serotonergic modulation while maintaining intrinsic properties in mouse. *J. Neurosci.* **2021**, *41*, 5833–5848. [CrossRef]
170. Detloff, M.R.; Smith, E.J.; Quiros Molina, D.; Ganzer, P.D.; Houle, J.D. Acute exercise prevents the development of neuropathic pain and the sprouting of non-peptidergic (GDNF- and artemin-responsive) c-fibers after spinal cord injury. *Exp. Neurol.* **2014**, *255*, 38–48. [CrossRef]
171. Nees, T.A.; Tappe-Theodor, A.; Sliwinski, C.; Motsch, M.; Rupp, R.; Kuner, R.; Weidner, N.; Blesch, A. Early-onset treadmill training reduces mechanical allodynia and modulates calcitonin gene-related peptide fiber density in lamina III/IV in a mouse model of spinal cord contusion injury. *Pain* **2016**, *157*, 687–697. [CrossRef] [PubMed]
172. Sliwinski, C.; Nees, T.A.; Puttagunta, R.; Weidner, N.; Blesch, A. Sensorimotor Activity Partially Ameliorates Pain and Reduces Nociceptive Fiber Density in the Chronically Injured Spinal Cord. *J. Neurotraum.* **2018**, *35*, 2222–2238. [CrossRef] [PubMed]
173. Keller, A.V.; Rees, K.M.; Seibt, E.J.; Wood, B.D.; Wade, A.D.; Morehouse, J.; Shum-Siu, A.; Magnuson, D.S.K. Electromyographic patterns of the rat hindlimb in response to muscle stretch after spinal cord injury. *Spinal. Cord* **2018**, *56*, 560–568. [CrossRef]
174. Keller, A.V.; Hainline, C.; Rees, K.; Krupp, S.; Prince, D.; Wood, B.D.; Shum-Siu, A.; Burke, D.A.; Petruska, J.C.; Magnuson, D.S.K. Nociceptor-dependent locomotor dysfunction after clinically-modeled hindlimb muscle stretching in adult rats with spinal cord injury. *Exp. Neurol.* **2019**, *318*, 267–276. [CrossRef]
175. De Los Reyes-Guzman, A.; Lozano-Berrio, V.; Alvarez-Rodriguez, M.; Lopez-Dolado, E.; Ceruelo-Abajo, S.; Talavera-Diaz, F.; Gil-Agudo, A. RehabHand: Oriented-tasks serious games for upper limb rehabilitation by using Leap Motion Controller and target population in spinal cord injury. *NeuroRehabilitation* **2021**, *48*, 365–373. [CrossRef] [PubMed]
176. De Miguel-Rubio, A.; Rubio, M.D.; Alba-Rueda, A.; Salazar, A.; Moral-Munoz, J.A.; Lucena-Anton, D. Virtual Reality Systems for Upper Limb Motor Function Recovery in Patients With Spinal Cord Injury: Systematic Review and Meta-Analysis. *JMIR Mhealth Uhealth* **2020**, *8*, e22537. [CrossRef] [PubMed]

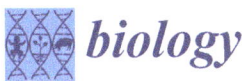

Article

Delivery of the 5-HT$_{2A}$ Receptor Agonist, DOI, Enhances Activity of the Sphincter Muscle during the Micturition Reflex in Rats after Spinal Cord Injury

Jaclyn H. DeFinis, Jeremy Weinberger and Shaoping Hou *

Marion Murray Spinal Cord Research Center, Department of Neurobiology & Anatomy, Drexel University College of Medicine, Philadelphia, PA 19129, USA; jhd43@drexel.edu (J.H.D.); jw3396@drexel.edu (J.W.)
* Correspondence: sh698@drexel.edu; Tel.: +1-215-991-8411; Fax: +1-215-843-9082

Simple Summary: Spinal cord injury often disrupts connections between the brain and spinal cord leading to a plethora of health complications, including bladder dysfunction. Spinal cord injured patients are left with symptoms such as a leaky bladder (the inability to hold their urine), frequent urinary tract infections, and potential kidney failure. However, previous studies have shown that manipulation of serotoninergic receptors can improve urinary performance following spinal cord injury. In the current study, we sought to explore how stimulation of a specific serotonergic receptor subtype can significantly enhance bladder function in spinal cord injured rats. To do so, we utilized spinal cord injured female rats that underwent various bladder performance evaluations combined with pharmacological intervention of a specific serotonergic subtype. Additionally, the primary site of action was investigated to determine effects elicited during various administration routes (e.g., directly into the cord, into the femoral vein, or into the skin). Stimulation of this receptor subtype, regardless of delivery route, improved activity of the external urethral sphincter and detrusor-sphincter coordination in spinal cord injured rats. Collectively, the results of these experiments have the potential to provide vital guidance for the development of therapeutic strategies to alleviate urinary dysfunction following spinal cord injury.

Abstract: Traumatic spinal cord injury (SCI) interrupts spinobulbospinal micturition reflex pathways and results in urinary dysfunction. Over time, an involuntary bladder reflex is established due to the reorganization of spinal circuitry. Previous studies show that manipulation of serotonin 2A (5-HT$_{2A}$) receptors affects recovered bladder function, but it remains unclear if this receptor regulates the activity of the external urethral sphincter (EUS) following SCI. To elucidate how central and peripheral serotonergic machinery acts on the lower urinary tract (LUT) system, we employed bladder cystometry and EUS electromyography recordings combined with intravenous or intrathecal pharmacological interventions of 5-HT$_{2A}$ receptors in female SCI rats. Three to four weeks after a T10 spinal transection, systemic and central blockage of 5-HT$_{2A}$ receptors with MDL only slightly influenced the micturition reflex. However, delivery of the 5-HT$_{2A}$ receptor agonist, DOI, increased EUS tonic activity and elicited bursting during voiding. Additionally, subcutaneous administration of DOI verified the enhancement of continence and voiding capability during spontaneous micturition in metabolic cage assays. Although spinal 5HT$_{2A}$ receptors may not be actively involved in the recovered micturition reflex, stimulating this receptor subtype enhances EUS function and the synergistic activity between the detrusor and sphincter to improve the micturition reflex in rats with SCI.

Keywords: micturition; external urethral sphincter; spinal cord injury; serotonin; electromyogram

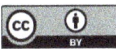

1. Introduction

The lower urinary tract (LUT) has two main functions, the storage and periodic elimination of urine. These two processes are dependent upon coordinated activity between the smooth muscle of the bladder detrusor and the striated external urethral sphincter (EUS). In normal conditions, this synergy is accomplished through a complex neural control system involving multiple neurotransmitters and neuropeptides at the brain, spinal cord, and peripheral levels. Among the many neuromodulators of micturition, serotonin (5-hydroxytrpytamine, 5-HT) has gained significant attention over the years as numerous anatomical [1–3] and pharmacological investigations [4,5] provide important evidence of 5-HT in the central pathways controlling bladder function [6]. Supraspinal serotonergic pathways mainly originate from the caudal raphe nuclei within the brainstem [7] and distribute terminals to sensory, motor, and autonomic regions of the spinal cord [8]. Additionally, previous studies have demonstrated that 5-HT$_{2A}$ receptors are expressed in the lower spinal cord [9], suggesting that these receptors have a modulatory role in pelvic visceral function.

Traumatic spinal cord injury (SCI) often interrupts spinobulbospinal micturition reflex pathways and results in LUT dysfunction. Following SCI, the bladder is initially areflexic but then partially recovers over time due to the reestablishment of an involuntary spinal micturition reflex pathway [10]. However, this partial recovery entails the emergence of detrusor-sphincter dyssynergia (DSD) and bladder hyperreflexia (or overactivity) which causes inefficient voiding and incontinence. Additionally, a large volume of residual urine remains in the bladder which increases the risk of infection and even life-threatening renal failure [11]. The most common treatments used to empty the bladder or treat overactivity are intermittent catheterization [12], antimuscarinic medications [13], and the neuromuscular blocker onabotulinumtoxin A (BTX-A) [14,15]. However, some treatment strategies have been met with serious health complications. Intermittent catheterization often leads to recurrent urinary tract infections and re-hospitalization, and antimuscarinic medications can have varying effects, such as tachycardia and impairment in cognition depending on what muscarinic receptor they are acting upon [11,16]. Additionally, patients who have undergone BTX-A injections have reported minor side effects, including urinary retention, urinary tract infection, and hematuria [17]. Therefore, limited effective treatment options are available to SCI individuals who suffer from lower urinary tract dysfunction.

The mechanisms that underlie and regulate micturition function after SCI are not well understood. Thus, there is an urgent need to elucidate such mechanisms of the recovered bladder reflex following SCI. Although disrupted supraspinal 5-HT projections no longer transport serotonin to the spinal cord, a small amount of serotonin remains detectable below the lesion [18]. This residual neurotransmitter was believed to be produced solely by sparse intraspinal 5-HT neurons [19]. That is, until recent investigations demonstrated that SCI enables spinal aromatic L-amino acid decarboxylase (AADC) cells distal to the lesion to acquire an enhanced ability to produce 5-HT from its immediate precursor, 5-hydroxytryptophan [20]. This change in spinal AADC cells is thought to be initiated by the loss of inhibition from descending 5-HT projections, which together with an upregulation of 5-HT$_{2A}$ receptors, increases the excitability of spinal motoneurons. In fact, expression of a variety of 5-HT receptors persists in the injured spinal cord [21].

Though previous studies reported that activation of 5-HT$_{2A}$ receptors affects bladder contractions to reduce residual urine and increase voiding efficiency in urethane-anesthetized SCI rats [22], it remains unclear if 5-HT$_{2A}$ receptors regulate activity of the EUS and coordination of detrusor and sphincter activity following SCI. Further, various 5-HT receptor subtypes were recently found to be expressed within the peripheral organs of the LUT [23,24]. It has been suggested that 5-HT$_{2A}$ subtypes can function as postjunctional receptors to peripherally induce detrusor contractions, whereas 5-HT$_7$ causes relaxation of the bladder neck [25]. This implies that these receptors may have contrasting roles in micturition function depending on where they are localized. It is thus necessary to differentiate the central vs. peripheral role of the 5-HT system with respect to micturition function. In the present study, we utilized pharmacological interventions of spinal 5-HT$_{2A}$ receptors combined with bladder and EUS reflex assessments as well as metabolic cage assays in conscious SCI rats to answer these questions. The results of these experiments have the potential to provide vital guidance for the development of therapeutic strategies to alleviate urinary dysfunction following SCI.

2. Materials and Methods

2.1. Animals

A total of 23 female adult Wistar rats (weigh 200–250 g, Charles River, Wilmington, MA, USA) were used. Animals were housed in sets of three per cage to provide social enrichment. Rats with a spinal cord transection (n = 7) were employed for metabolic cages. Some of these rats (n = 6, one suffered a leg injury after testing so it was excluded from subsequent experiments) were later used, together with other SCI rats (n = 6), for micturition reflex assays. Naïve rats (n = 10) were used to collect spinal cord tissue for molecular analyses. Institutional Animal Care and Use Committee and National Institute of Health guidelines on animal care were strictly followed to minimize the number of animals used and any potential suffering. Humane consideration for the well-being of animals was incorporated into the experimental design and conduct. All experimental procedures were reviewed by a local animal care committee to ensure compliance (Project identification code: 1045137).

2.2. Spinal Cord Surgery

Rats underwent a complete spinal cord transection at the 10th thoracic level (T10) to remove supraspinal control of micturition. Animals were anesthetized with 2% isoflurane and a partial laminectomy was performed at the T8 vertebrae to expose the dorsal spinal cord. The spinal cord was completely transected at T10 using a No. 11 blade. Lesion completeness was verified visually at the time of surgery. Overlying musculature and skin were then closed. Animals were administered Lactated Ringer's solution (Baxter Healthcare, Deerfield, IL, USA), cefazolin (10 mg/kg), and buprenex (0.1 mg/kg; Reckitt Benckiser, Slough, United Kingdom) post-operatively. Bladders were manually expressed at least three times per day until sacrifice.

2.3. Metabolic Cages

Three weeks after SCI, rats (n = 7) were placed in a metabolic cage apparatus (Braintree Scientific, Chicago, IL, USA) to record spontaneous voiding patterns. It is important to note that prior to being placed in cages, bladders were manually expressed to ensure that they were empty at the beginning of the recording. After being placed into cages, animals were allowed 3 h for acclimation before the administration of drugs or vehicle. Then, animals were subcutaneously (s.c) injected with 300 µL of either saline or the 5-HT$_{2A}$ agonist 2,5-dimethoxy-4-iodoamphetamine (DOI, 60 µg/kg). Urine output was measured on a pressure sensor connected to a computer for the recording of micturition frequency, expelled volume per void of urine, and voiding interval. Data was collected and stored using Windaq-148 software (Dataq Instruments, Akron, OH, USA). This procedure was repeated three times with either saline or DOI injections. The following micturition variables were assessed: (i) total urine expelled, (ii) volume of urine expelled per void, (iii) voiding frequency, and (iv) total water consumed. These variables were evaluated at both a 3 and 6 h time point following drug or vehicle administration. In each rat, parameter values from three different experiments were averaged together to determine the mean value, which was further used to statistically analyze the data using a paired t-test.

2.4. Bladder Cystometry and EUS Electromyography (EMG) Recordings

Three to four weeks after SCI, rats were anesthetized with 2% isoflurane and an incision was made in the lower abdomen to expose the bladder. The apex of the bladder dome was punctured using a 20-gauge needle. One end of a catheter (PE-60; Clay Adams, New York, NY, USA) was inserted into the bladder [26]. The abdominal wall was then sutured closed with the other end of the catheter protruding from the sutured area to allow for infusion of saline into the bladder. To obtain EUS electromyography (EMG) recordings, the pubic symphysis was removed to expose the urethra and EUS. Two fine-wire electrodes (AstroNova, West Warwick, RI, USA) with exposed tips were percutaneously inserted on both sides of the EUS. Alternatively, two internal electrodes were placed on both sides of the EUS via the opening of the pubic symphysis. In rats receiving intravenous (i.v.) delivery of pharmacological agents (n = 6), a separate cannula (PE-10) filled with saline was implanted in the right femoral vein. In rats receiving intrathecal (i.t.) delivery of drugs or vehicle (n = 6), an ITC 32G catheter (ReCathCo, Allison Park, PA, USA) was placed underneath the dura at the 1st/2nd lumbar spinal cord level (L1/2) and the tip of the catheter was further advanced to the L6/S1 level [27]. In both i.v. and i.t. delivery, rats received injections of gradually increased doses of MDL and then increasing doses of DOI followed by blockage with MDL.

After disconnecting with isoflurane, rats were placed into a restraining cage (KN-326, Natsume, Tokyo, Japan and given time to regain consciousness before recordings. The bladder catheter was connected to a pressure transducer (Transbridge, WPI, Sarasota, FL, USA) and a microinjection pump (SP2001, WPI). Electrodes were connected to an alternating amplifier (P511, AstroNova, West Warwick, RI, USA) and a recording system (Windaq, DATAQ Instruments, Akron, OH, USA) at a sample frequency of 10 kHz. Room temperature saline was slowly infused into the bladder (0.1 mL/min) and at least 1 h adaptation time was ensured before starting the recording. Adaptation was confirmed visually by the appearance of consistent voids as evident in bladder pressure and stabilization of EUS EMG activity. During the recordings, at least 4 continuous stable micturition cycles pre- and post- drug delivery were collected per rat. Experiments lasted no longer than 4 h. Afterwards, the recorded cystometry and EMG traces were opened in Dataq Browser software for analysis. Urodynamic parameters including the voiding amplitude of intravesical pressure (VA), the voiding interval between two sequential voiding events (VI), the voiding volume (VV), bladder contraction duration (CD), and non-voiding contractions (NVCs) were measured. NVCs were defined as rhythmic intravesical pressure increases that were at least 5 mmHg from baseline without a release of fluid from the urethra [28]. Additionally, various EUS EMG parameters were also evaluated including, EUS tonic and bursting activity which occur before and during voiding, respectively. To measure the tonic activity, the root mean square (RMS) and maximum amplitude (MA) of EMG activity were evaluated during 5 s of the filling phase right before a void occurred. The duration of EUS bursting activity during voiding was measured. In these SCI rats, EUS bursting activity occurred ~40–50% of the time while others displayed high-amplitude tonic activity during voiding. In each rat, the parameter values in 4 voiding cycles were averaged to determine the mean value for statistical analysis. The post-drug/saline parameters for each rat were normalized by basal values as a percentage and then a Friedman's test followed by Dunn's multiple comparisons was used. Immediately after the recordings, some rats were overdosed with euthasol to harvest fresh tissues for molecular analysis.

2.5. Drugs

The 5-HT$_{2A}$ agonist DOI or antagonist (R-(+)-α-(2,3-dimethoxyphenyl)-1-[2-(4-fluorophenylethyl)]-4-piperidinemethanol (MDL) were dissolved in saline. The doses of drugs (Tables 1 and 2) were chosen on the basis of previously described data [22] as well as our own pilot experiments. In metabolic cage assays, DOI (60 μg/kg; 300 μL) was s.c. administered whereas injections of saline (vehicle) served as a control. For cystometry and EUS EMG recordings, saline was delivered i.v. (100 μL) first and increased doses of drugs with equivalent volumes subsequently followed. In rats with i.t. drug administration, a volume of 10 μL was injected for saline or each drug dose. Urodynamic data were collected after each dose of a drug was delivered. The interval was at least 30 min between adjacent doses. For administration of the 2nd drug (DOI), we waited at least 1 h after the last dose of the 1st drug (MDL) was delivered to allow sufficient time for washout. Data were then collected again during basal and saline conditions followed by drug delivery.

Table 1. Normalized parameters of bladder cystometry and EUS EMG activity in SCI rats (*i.v.* administration).

Drugs	Doses (/kg)	Bladder CMG				EUS EMG		VV
		VA	CD	VI	# NVCs	RMS	MA	
MDL (n = 6) (5HT$_{2A}$ receptor antagonist)	Saline	1.11 ± 0.10	0.96 ± 0.05	1.00 ± 0.05	1.31 ± 0.31	0.95 ± 0.06	0.82 ± 0.12	0.95 ± 0.09
	20 µg	1.01 ± 0.19	0.93 ± 0.05	1.07 ± 0.14	1.25 ± 0.70	0.87 ± 0.02	0.71 ± 0.09	1.00 ± 0.15
	0.1 mg	0.97 ± 0.06	0.98 ± 0.06	1.22 ± 0.11 *	1.56 ± 0.86	0.96 ± 0.09	0.81 ± 0.10	1.15 ± 0.10
	0.5 mg	1.04 ± 0.04	0.95 ± 0.06	1.10 ± 0.07	0.88 ± 0.79	1.11 ± 0.16	1.00 ± 0.37	1.09 ± 0.14
DOI (n = 6) (5HT$_{2A}$ receptor agonist)	Saline	1.11 ± 0.10	0.96 ± 0.05	1.00 ± 0.05	1.31 ± 0.31	0.95 ± 0.06	0.82 ± 0.12	0.95 ± 0.09
	5.0 µg	1.08 ± 0.04	0.98 ± 0.04	1.34 ± 0.11	1.00 ± 0.84	1.03 ± 0.14	0.69 ± 0.97	1.23 ± 0.15
	20 µg	1.06 ± 0.08	1.12 ± 0.04	1.73 ± 0.17 *	2.19 ± 1.59	1.13 ± 0.13	0.84 ± 0.21	1.32 ± 0.12 *
	0.1 mg	1.00 ± 0.08	1.01 ± 0.04	1.51 ± 0.30	1.31 ± 0.80	1.53 ± 0.24 *	1.64 ± 0.55	1.24 ± 0.17

* $p < 0.05$; VA, voiding amplitude of intravesical pressure, CD, contraction duration, VI, voiding interval, VV, voiding volume, NVCs, non-voiding contractions, RMS, root mean square, MA, maximum amplitude of tonic activity; # non-normalized data.

Table 2. Normalized parameters of bladder cystometry and EUS EMG activity in SCI rats (*i.t.* administration).

Drugs	Doses (/kg)	Bladder CMG				EUS EMG		VV
		VA	CD	VI	# NVCs	RMS	MA	
MDL (n = 6) (5HT$_{2A}$ receptor antagonist)	Saline	1.23 ± 0.11	1.01 ± 0.01	1.12 ± 0.11	0.29 ± 0.15	0.97 ± 0.19	0.92 ± 0.07	0.81 ± 0.03
	2 µg	1.13 ± 0.10	0.97 ± 0.01	1.12 ± 0.11	0.20 ± 0.13	1.09 ± 0.06	0.95 ± 0.08	0.78 ± 0.03
	10 µg	1.22 ± 0.18	1.08 ± 0.09	1.34 ± 0.20	0.29 ± 0.15	0.98 ± 0.05	0.74 ± 0.11	1.07 ± 0.09
	50 µg	0.81 ± 0.08	0.83 ± 0.05	1.19 ± 0.15	0.58 ± 0.26	1.11 ± 0.05	1.46 ± 0.30	0.95 ± 0.09
DOI (n = 6) (5HT$_{2A}$ receptor agonist)	Saline	0.94 ± 0.03	1.09 ± 0.04	1.24 ± 0.14	1.08 ± 0.60	1.01 ± 0.03	1.17 ± 0.20	0.95 ± 0.10
	0.5 µg	1.03 ± 0.09	1.14 ± 0.05	1.42 ± 0.46	0.79 ± 0.64	1.01 ± 0.03	1.05 ± 0.09	0.88 ± 0.12
	2 µg	1.21 ± 0.13	1.13 ± 0.08	3.27 ± 1.04 *	2.70 ± 1.77	1.14 ± 0.17	1.12 ± 0.28	1.14 ± 0.18
	10 µg	1.12 ± 0.11	1.09 ± 0.05	3.98 ± 1.58 *	3.33 ± 2.41	1.46 ± 0.21	1.96 ± 0.31	1.33 ± 0.18 *

* $p < 0.05$; VA, voiding amplitude of intravesical pressure, CD, contraction duration, VI, voiding interval, VV, voiding volume, NVCs, non-voiding contractions, RMS, root mean square, MA, maximum amplitude of tonic activity; # non-normalized data.

2.6. Fresh Tissue Harvesting and Protein Isolation

Anesthetized rats were perfused with HEPES buffer and approximately 0.5 cm spinal cord segments at T4/5 above the injury as well as L1/2 and L6/S1 below the injury, where neurons control the LUT, were extracted from naïve (n = 4) and SCI rats (n = 8). Sections were immediately frozen in dry ice and stored in −80 °C. Spinal cords were homogenized in 1 ml of RIPA buffer with Pierce™ protease and phosphatase inhibitors (1 tablet/10 mL RIPA buffer, Thermo Scientific, Waltham, MA, USA). The homogenized spinal cords were centrifuged at 4700 rpm for 90 s, and supernatants were obtained and stored at −80 °C. Following homogenization, standard protein concentrations were established with a Bradford protein assay, and plates were read on an Infinite® 200 Pro microplate reader (Tecan, Männerdorf, Switzerland) at 595 nm using the i-control software package.

2.7. Western Blot

A total of 30 µg of each spinal cord sample was denatured using 2× Laemmli buffer containing 5% β-mercaptoethanol at 95 °C for 5 min and loaded onto a Mini-PROTEAN® TGX Stain-Free™ Protein Gel (Bio-Rad, Hercules, CA, USA). All gels ran for 15 min at 80 V, followed by an additional 30 min at 200 V. Following separation, the samples were transferred onto a polyvinylidene difluoride membrane (Bio-Rad) using the Trans-Blot® Turbo™ machine (Bio-Rad). After transfer, membranes were incubated with primary antibody against the 5-HT$_{2A}$ receptor (rabbit, 1:500, Immunostar, Hudson, WI, USA) and glyceraldehye-3-phosphate dehydrogenase (GAPDH, mouse, 1:2000, Cell Signaling Technology, Danvers, MA, USA) overnight at 4 °C. Membranes were then probed with an anti-rabbit or mouse HRP-linked secondary antibody (1:10,000, Cell Signaling). Membranes were then developed with the Clarity™ Western ECL substrate kit (Bio-Rad) and imaged using HyBlot CL™ autoradiography film (Denville, Metuchen, NJ, USA). Receptor expression was normalized to the corresponding protein density of GAPDH. Following normalization, data was averaged and further compared between naïve and SCI groups with a student's t-test ($p < 0.05$).

2.8. RNA Extraction/Quantitative Real-Time PCR

Anesthetized rats (n = 6 naïve and 9 SCI) were decapitated and immediately fresh spinal cord tissue at T4/5, L1/2, and L6/S1 segments (approximately 0.5 cm) was dissected. Total RNA was extracted with an E.Z.N.A. Kit II (Omega Bio-Tek, Norcross, GA, USA) according to the manufacturer's instructions. RNA concentration and the 260/280 nm absorbance ratio were assessed using a Nanodrop spectrophotometer (Thermo Fisher). RNA was reverse transcribed into cDNA using the iScript reverse transcription supermix (Bio-Rad). Quantitative real-time PCR was performed with SYBR Green PCR Master Mix on a CFX Connect Real-Time PCR detection system (Bio-Rad). Primer sequences used were 5-HT$_{2A}$ forward: 5′-AGAAGCCACCTTGTGTGTGA-3′, reverse: 5′-TTGCTCATTGCTGATGGACT-3′; GAPDH forward: 5′-CCATCCCAGACCC CATAAC-3′, reverse: 5′-GCAGCGAACTTTATTGATGG-3′. Expression levels for each amplified gene were calculated using the comparative ΔCt method, where ΔCt = Ct (experimental gene) − Ct (reference gene) for each biological replicate. GAPDH was chosen as a reference gene. For each mRNA measured in qPCR, gene expression values were averaged across biological replicates. The data was further statistically analyzed using a student's t-test to compare gene expression between naïve and SCI rats ($p < 0.05$).

2.9. Statistical Analyses

Statistical analyses were performed in GraphPad Prism 8 (GraphPad Software, San Deigo, CA, USA). Significance throughout all experiments was set at $p < 0.05$. Data are represented as mean ± SEM. All groups (intact vs. SCI) and drugs (saline, MDL, DOI) were kept blind to the observer as to avoid biases during molecular and urodynamic analyses. Detailed analyses are listed separately under each experiment described above.

3. Results

3.1. 5-HT$_{2A}$ Protein and Gene Expression Is Sustained in the Spinal Cord Following SCI

Protein expression of 5-HT$_{2A}$ receptors was measured with western blot. No difference was observed between naïve and SCI rats in terms of protein expression levels of this receptor above and below the level of injury (Naïve T4/5, 0.24 ± 0.05; SCI T4/5, 0.18 ± 0.03; Naïve L1/2, 0.33 ± 0.08; SCI L1/2, 0.19 ± 0.05; Naïve L6/S1, 0.33 ± 0.09; SCI L6/S1, 0.21 ± 0.04; all $p > 0.05$, Unpaired t-test). This included two important segments, L1/2 and L6/S1, which are related to micturition control (Figure 1A, B). In line with the aforementioned results, mRNA levels of 5-HT$_{2A}$ receptors measured with qPCR were not altered (Naïve T4/5, 7.08 ± 0.62; SCI T4/5, 6.41 ± 0.68; Naïve L1/2, 7.28 ± 0.85; SCI L1/2, 6.13 ± 0.65; Naïve L6/S1, 7.30 ± 0.79; SCI L6/S1, 5.89 ± 0.59; all $p > 0.05$) in SCI rats (Figure 1C). Therefore, the results suggest that expression of 5-HT$_{2A}$ receptors is sustained in the spinal cord after SCI.

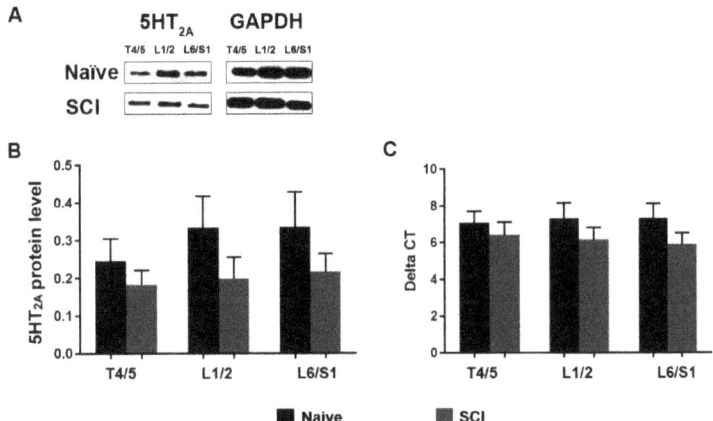

Figure 1. Spinal 5-HT$_{2A}$ receptor expression remains unchanged after SCI. (**A**), Western blots show that there is no difference between naïve and SCI rats in terms of protein expression levels of the 5-HT$_{2A}$ receptor above (T4/5) and below the level of injury (L1/2, L6/S1) (Student's t-test, all $p > 0.05$). (**B,C**), Quantitative PCR analysis reveals that mRNA levels of this receptor were not altered at any of the aforementioned segments in SCI rats (all $p > 0.05$). GAPDH served as a control.

3.2. I.v. Drug Delivery and its Effects on Bladder and EUS Reflexes

Three to four weeks after T10 spinal cord transection, animals were utilized for bladder cystometry and EUS EMG assays. Firstly, a serial dose of the 5-HT$_{2A}$ receptor antagonist MDL was administered i.v. to determine the function of these receptors in the recovered micturition reflex (Table 1). Following administration of the antagonist, there were no dramatic changes in cystometry and EMG parameters except a significantly prolonged VI ($p < 0.05$, Friedman's test followed by Dunn's) following injection of the middle dose of the drug. However, some obvious responses were detected after the 5-HT$_{2A}$ receptor agonist DOI was administered. The mid (20 µg/kg) dose of the drug was able to increase the VI ($p < 0.05$) and induce a larger VV ($p < 0.01$). The occurrence of NVCs had no significant changes after administration of any of the drugs (all $p > 0.05$). Notably, the high dose of DOI (0.1 mg/kg) produced a significant increase in tonic EUS activity (RMS $p < 0.01$) and there was also a trend for an increase in the MA value. It also induced non-specific activity of the EUS along with high amplitude contraction during continuous infusion of saline into the bladder (Figure 2A). More importantly, DOI was able to trigger a bursting pattern in the EUS in 4 rats that did not have any such events during baseline or saline delivery. It is important to note that corresponding bladder high frequency oscillations (HFO) did not often accompany bursting in these animals (Figure 2B). Ensuing administration with the mid dose of MDL (0.1 mg/kg) abolished the effects of DOI on the EUS, including decreased EUS tonic activity in the filling phase and masked bursting during voiding. Specifically, the results illustrate that systemic blockage of 5-HT$_{2A}$ receptors with MDL has subtle effects while activation of this receptor subtype with DOI increases EUS tonic activity and elicits bursting to facilitate voiding in SCI rats.

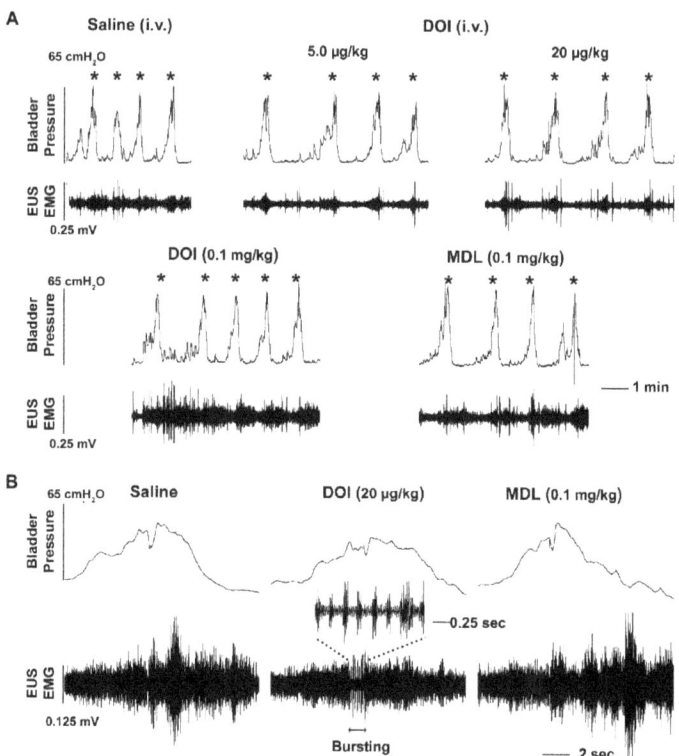

Figure 2. Intravenous (i.v.) administration of DOI to stimulate 5-HT$_{2A}$ receptors improves the micturition reflex during bladder cystometry and sphincter EMG in SCI rats. (**A**), Stimulating 5-HT$_{2A}$ receptors with the middle dose of DOI (20 µg/kg) prolongs the VI ($p < 0.05$, Friedman's test followed by Dunn's) between voiding contractions (asterisks). The high dose of DOI (0.1 mg/kg) increases EUS tonic activity in the filling phase ($p < 0.01$). Ensuing injection of MDL (0.1 mg/kg) eliminates the provoked effects. (**B**), Representative traces show no EUS bursting activity during voiding when saline is delivered. However, the middle dose of DOI triggers EUS bursting activity during voiding. Injection of MDL following the high dose of DOI masks the triggered bursting EUS activity during voiding.

3.3. I.t. Drug Delivery and Its Effects on Bladder and EUS Reflexes

To clarify whether the effects produced from 5-HT$_{2A}$ receptor manipulation on the urinary system were working through central mechanisms, we administered drugs i.t. during bladder cystometry and EUS EMG assays in SCI rats (Table 2). As a result, central delivery of the 5-HT$_{2A}$ antagonist MDL did not trigger significant responses in bladder and EUS reflexes. When DOI was administered, both the middle and high doses significantly prolonged the VI (both $p < 0.05$, Friedman's test followed by Dunn's). The high dose increased the VV ($p < 0.05$). Particularly, there was a trend for the high dose of DOI to induce an increase in EUS tonic activity in both the RMS (1.4 fold) and MA (1.6 fold) values, although not statistically significant. During voiding, EUS bursting activity accompanied by bladder detrusor HFO were elicited in 4 animals that did not have such events originally. The middle dose of DOI increased the duration of EUS bursting (saline 1.6 ± 0.9, DOI 3.8 ± 1.5 s) in 2 rats that had such activity during baseline recordings. This suggests that DOI can improve the synergistic activity of the sphincter and detrusor (Figure 3). In addition, there was a trend that suggests the number of NVCs increases after the middle and high doses of DOI injections, which could be related to the dramatically prolonged VI seen with these two doses. After administration with the middle dose of MDL, the effects of DOI on the EUS were completely abolished. This was apparent by the presence of reduced EUS tonic activity and the disappearance of bursting (Figure 4). MDL also shortened the VI of bladder voiding contractions. This suggests that activation of 5-HT$_{2A}$ receptors, by central administration of DOI, largely affects activity of the EUS, leading to improved micturition function in SCI rats.

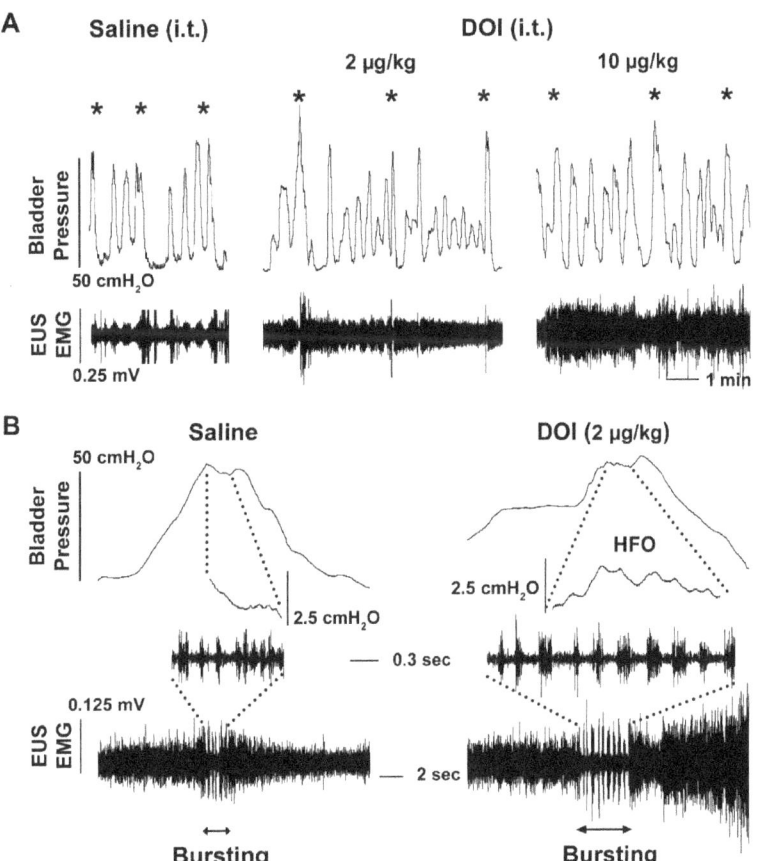

Figure 3. Intrathecal (i.t.) administration of DOI to stimulate 5-HT$_{2A}$ receptors affects the micturition reflex during bladder cystometry and sphincter EMG in SCI rats. (**A**), Representative tracers show that stimulating 5-HT$_{2A}$ receptors with the middle (2 µg/kg) and high (10 µg/kg) doses of DOI prolongs the VI (both $p < 0.05$, Friedman's test followed by Dunn's) between voiding contractions (asterisks) and induces an increase in EUS tonic activity. (**B**), Importantly, the middle dose of DOI increases the duration of EUS bursting that consists of more regularly occurring active and silent periods along with bladder HFO, indicating an enhancement of detrusor-sphincter coordination during voiding.

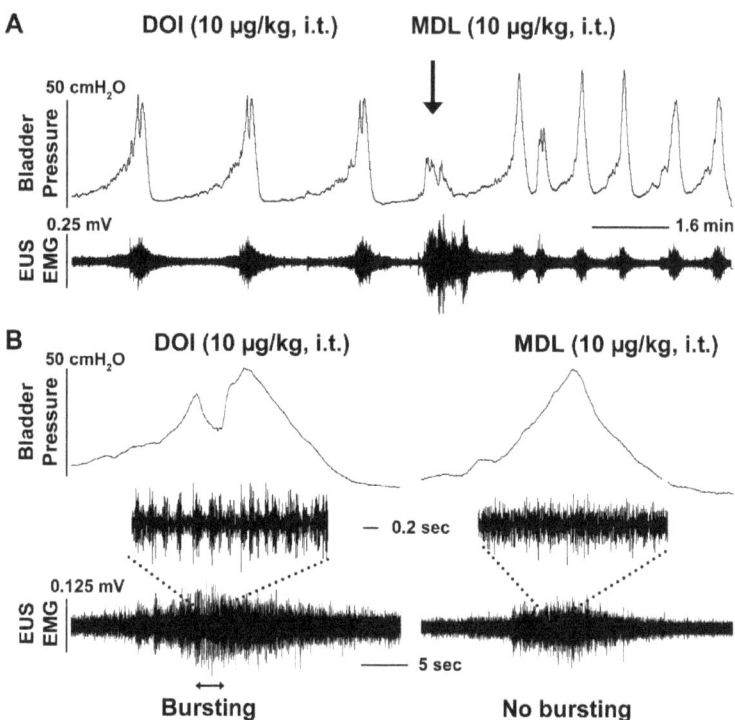

Figure 4. Intrathecal (i.t.) administration of MDL abolishes DOI induced excitatory effects on the EUS reflex in SCI rats. A representative cystometry and EMG trace demonstrates that MDL, a 5-HT$_{2A}$ receptor antagonist (10 µg/kg), shortens the VI ($p < 0.05$, Friedman's test followed by Dunn's) (**A**) and masks bursting EUS activity (**B**), leading to the occurrence of detrusor-sphincter dyssynergia.

3.4. S.c. Delivery of DOI Improves Spontaneous Micturition Performance Following SCI

SCI rats were s.c. administered DOI in metabolic cage assays. During the 6 h time period following drug delivery, DOI significantly increased the VI (saline 52.19 ± 7.36, DOI 82.60 ± 8.93; Paired *t*-test, $p < 0.05$) and VV per void (saline 0.8 ± 0.13, DOI 1.04 ± 0.17, $p < 0.05$) but decreased the voiding frequency (saline 7.63 ± 1.33, DOI 5.11 ± 0.95, $p < 0.05$) (Figure 5). It is important to note that urodynamic parameters were examined out to 12 hr post-drug delivery. However, it was found that only significant changes in urinary performance could be detected at a maximum of 6 h post-drug administration. There was no significant change in the total VV. Total water intake was not significantly different between drug and saline controls (both $p > 0.05$). This implies that DOI can improve spontaneous micturition function by increasing continence and voiding capability.

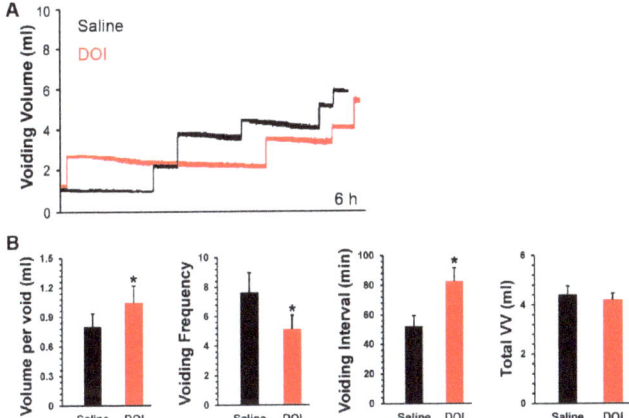

Figure 5. Stimulating 5-HT$_{2A}$ receptors with DOI delivery improves spontaneous micturition function in SCI rats. Representative traces show volume-frequency patterns of urination in metabolic cage assays after 5-HT$_{2A}$ receptor stimulation with DOI within a 6-h time period. Saline injections served as a control. In each "step-like" curve of these traces (**A**), the vertical lines represent the VV per void and the horizontal lines illustrate the VI. After s.c. injection of the 5-HT$_{2A}$ receptor agonist DOI (60 μg/kg, 300 μL), (**B**) there was a significant increase in the VV per void and VI in comparison to saline controls (Paired *t*-test, all * $p < 0.05$).

4. Discussion

The present study examined the contribution of 5-HT$_{2A}$ receptors in the micturition reflex after SCI, with a particular focus on the function of these receptors in the EUS. Blocking spinal 5-HT$_{2A}$ receptors with central delivery of MDL did not have a meaningful impact on bladder and sphincter activity. This denotes that endogenous spinal 5-HT, which has been shown to be present at low levels in the cord after injury, [18] may not modulate recovered micturition function via spinal receptors following SCI. However, systemic or central stimulation of 5-HT$_{2A}$ receptors with DOI induced similar effects that increased EUS tonic activity in the filling phase and triggered bursting during voiding. This indicates that DOI enhances synergistic activity between the detrusor and sphincter to improve voiding capability. Thus, DOI elicits its effects mainly through spinal receptors regardless of delivery route. Though spinal 5-HT$_{2A}$ receptors may not play a role in the established involuntary spinal micturition reflex after SCI, our results suggest that stimulation of these receptors mainly acts on motoneurons controlling the EUS to improve coordination of bladder and sphincter activity while also mitigating DSD to enhance micturition function.

Serotonergic regulation of LUT function has been explored since the 1960s when dense supraspinal 5-HT innervation to autonomic nuclei was observed in the lower spinal cord [29,30], including the dorsal horn and Onuf's nucleus which contains the motoneurons that control EUS function [7,31]. Although SCI interrupts descending neuronal pathways, previous studies have demonstrated the ability of the injured spinal cord to produce monoamines, such as serotonin, caudal to the level of injury [20]. Further, the expression of various serotonergic receptors within the lumbosacral cord has been examined [32,33] as well as an indication for their role in micturition function [34–38]. Accordingly, it is possible that these spinally located 5-HT receptors also serve to modulate pelvic visceral function after SCI. In line with this, our results have confirmed that neither the protein nor mRNA levels of 5-HT$_{2A}$ receptors significantly decreased above or below the level of injury. However, previous studies reported that their expression is upregulated in motoneurons following SCI [39]. This contradiction could be due to the fact that our tissue samples were collected from spinal segments as opposed to specific populations of individual neurons. Nevertheless, spinal 5-HT$_{2A}$ receptor expression is sustained in the cord of SCI rats.

Serotonergic receptors lie within both the central and peripheral nervous systems. Despite the fact that 5-HT$_{2A}$ receptors are widely distributed throughout the brain and spinal cord [9,31,40], this subtype is also present in the smooth muscle and urothelium of the bladder [24]. This implies that systemic drug administration may have both peripheral and central-mediated effects. The middle dose of MDL increased the VI when it was i.v. injected but did not do so in i.t. delivery, suggesting this minor effect may be mediated peripherally. In opposition to this, delivery of DOI both i.v. or i.t. elicited similar effects on the micturition reflex. The role of DOI in bladder function following SCI has previously been studied and dramatic effects on the facilitation of voiding were reported. Yet, it is unknown if this drug acts on motoneurons controlling the EUS muscle with regards to the coordination of the detrusor and sphincter for micturition function.

In the present study, DOI was able to elicit EUS bursting and bladder HFO. This indicates that stimulating spinal 5-HT$_{2A}$ receptors, irrespective of delivery route, largely triggers its effects through central mechanisms that control the sphincter muscle. The EUS is continuously relaxed during voiding in humans whereas it is phasically relaxed in rats. Bursting EUS activity and bladder HFO occur during the expulsion phase in rats. SCI rats mainly show increased EUS tonic activity with little or no bursting and virtually no bladder HFO during voiding [41]. EUS bursting consists of both high frequency spikes that are deemed active periods (AP) and quiescent periods known as silent periods (SP), which alternate in such a way to allow for relaxation and contraction of the EUS, respectively, and are essential for efficient voiding [42]. HFO are thought to be generated by EUS bursting activity since these two patterns often occur synergistically [43]. Here we reported that stimulation of spinal 5-HT$_{2A}$ receptors with DOI provoked EUS bursting. Subsequently, delivery of MDL to block these receptors eliminated the aforementioned effects, confirming mediation by spinal 5-HT$_{2A}$ receptors. Similar to results from previous studies in which 5-HT$_{2A}$ receptors exert excitatory control of the EUS in spinal cord intact rats [44], our results verified that activation of spinal 5-HT$_{2A}$ receptors in SCI rats triggers EUS bursting which originates from simultaneous firing of Onuf's motoneurons. Nevertheless, it has been assumed that propriospinal neurons in the L3/4 spinal cord contribute to the emergence of EUS bursting and bladder-EUS coordination [45]. If this is the case, DOI may indirectly affect Onuf's motoneurons or does so via propriospinal neurons that express 5-HT$_{2A}$ receptors.

Stimulation of spinal 5-HT$_{2A}$ receptors with DOI increased EUS tonic activity in the filling phase during reflex assessments. Since EUS tonic activity reflects the capability of continence and DOI prolonged this activity between bladder contractions (e.g., prolonged VI), our data implies that DOI augments the ability to prevent leakage. This was also confirmed in spontaneous micturition assays by metabolic cages and s.c. administration of DOI in SCI rats. Because DOI did not affect the amplitude of bladder contractions, it is reasonable to conclude that the general impact of DOI on the micturition reflex is primarily caused by the agonist's effects on motoneurons controlling the EUS rather than on parasympathetic preganglionic neurons regulating the bladder. In addition to its effects on the EUS, stimulation of 5-HT$_{2A}$ receptors with DOI was able to significantly increase the voiding volume with both i.v. and i.t. delivery. This implies that the drug improved voiding efficiency by either (1) reducing the residual volume of urine that remains in the bladder following a contraction, (2) increasing bladder capacity, or (3) both. Based on previous reports, delivery of DOI peripherally or centrally increases the voiding volume while reducing the residual volume of urine [22,39]. Therefore, it seems likely that the increase in the voiding volume illustrated in the current experiments is due to improved voiding efficiency. It appears that DOI can produce similar effects in LUT performance when administered intravenously, intrathecally, and even subcutaneously. Thus, administration of DOI mainly stimulates centrally located 5-HT$_{2A}$ receptors and contributes to detrusor-sphincter synergy to enhance voiding capability in SCI rats. Additionally, it is known that DOI also has an affinity for 5-HT$_{2C}$ receptors [46,47]. Previous studies have shown that central 5-HT$_{2C}$ receptors mainly inhibit the micturition reflex [4]. With this in mind, we administered MDL, which is a selective antagonist for 5-HT$_{2A}$ receptors [48], directly following the high dose of DOI. This ultimately blocked changes that DOI induced on urinary function (e.g., EUS bursting and bladder HFO), and therefore, further supports the notion that DOI improves micturition performance via 5-HT$_{2A}$ and not $_{2C}$ receptors.

Urethane is currently the most widely used anesthetic to study micturition physiology. In fact, the majority of studies that examine the role of 5-HT receptors have been completed with the use of urethane or some other anesthetic [22,37,49]. The widespread use of this anesthetic is largely due to the fact that it spares the micturition reflex and is long-lasting [50]. Although urethane preserves vital parameters, such as bladder HFO and EUS bursting, it can interfere with the actions of glutamate and its analogs in the micturition pathway [51]. In addition, urethane was found to suppress sympathetic outflow to the bladder, and thus alter bladder capacity [52]. Notably, things become more complicated when applying anesthetics to SCI animals that already display several urinary complications (e.g., no bursting periods and emergence of non-voiding contractions) [53]. Therefore, the present study sought to avoid analgesic-related confounds by using awake rats for bladder cystometry and EUS EMG recordings.

Although most SCI patients have incomplete injuries as opposed to complete [54,55], a complete spinal cord transection model was deemed the most appropriate for the purposes of this study. The overall goal of this research was to determine the role of 5-HT$_{2A}$ receptors in the recovered involuntary micturition reflex following SCI, specifically as it pertains to EUS activity since this has not been thoroughly examined. If an incomplete injury was to be used in the current experiments, it would be almost impossible to differentiate whether the agonist or antagonist were acting at both supraspinal and spinal levels that control bladder and EUS reflexes due to sparing. Accordingly, to focus on spinal serotonergic mechanisms, it was necessary to disrupt all supraspinal control. However, future experiments may be conducted in a contusion model to determine the efficacy of the effects seen within the current experiments with DOI. Additionally, we used female rats instead of males due to the ease of bladder care. Since male rats have a long and narrow urethra [56], bladder care is very difficult in these animals directly following injury. Importantly, our previous work has shown that both males and females manifest similar urinary complications, such as DSD and bladder hyperreflexia, following SCI. However, future experiments should be conducted in male SCI rats to confirm that there are no apparent sex differences in terms of the role that 5-HT$_{2A}$ receptors play in the recovered bladder reflex.

In clinical studies, it was established that duloxetine, a 5-HT and norepinephrine reuptake inhibitor, was able to significantly reduce stress-related urinary incontinence episodes in women [57]. Duloxetine is proposed to improve continence by increasing the bioavailability of 5-HT and norepinephrine at presynaptic neurons in Onuf's nucleus of the sacral cord, which in turn, is thought to increase EUS activity. This suggests that serotonergic mechanisms also exist in the human spinal cord, and stimulating these pathways enhances LUT performance not only following SCI but across a broad range of conditions that elicit urinary complications. Nevertheless, it is important to note that the effects of each drug used within our study do not discern what population of cells these receptors are acting upon. Thus, sites of action should be further explored by whole cell patch clamp recordings in future studies.

5. Conclusions

Endogenous spinal 5-HT may not modulate recovered micturition function via 5-HT$_{2A}$ receptors following SCI. Nonetheless, both systemic and central stimulation of these receptors with DOI can induce similar effects to increase EUS tonic activity in the filling phase and trigger bursting during voiding. It indicates that DOI enhances coordination of detrusor and sphincter activity to improve micturition function in SCI rats.

Author Contributions: S.H. and J.H.D. designed the experiments. J.H.D. and J.W. carried out the experiments and analyzed the data. J.H.D. and S.H. prepared the figures. J.H.D. and S.H. wrote the paper. All authors have read and agreed to the published version of the manuscript.

Funding: The support for this project was provided by NIH NINDS R01NS099076 to S. Hou and NIDDK F31DK123840-01 to J.H.D.

Institutional Review Board Statement: The study was conducted according to the guidelines of the National Institute of Health (NIH), and approved by the Institutional Animal Care and Use Committee (IACUC) of Drexel University College of Medicine (protocol code: 20550, date of approval: 09/07/2016).

Informed Consent Statement: Not applicable.

Data Availability Statement: The data that support the findings of this study are available from the corresponding author, (Shaoping Hou, PhD), upon reasonable request.

Acknowledgments: The authors are grateful for Dong Wang and Yuan Qiao's technical assistance. The support for this project was provided by NIH NINDS R01NS099076 to S. Hou and NIDDK F31DK123840-01 to J.H.D.

Conflicts of Interest: The authors declare no competing interests.

References

1. Nadelhaft, I.; Vera, P.L. Central nervous system neurons infected by pseudorabies virus injected into the rat urinary bladder following unilateral transection of the pelvic nerve. *J. Comp. Neurol.* **1995**, *359*, 443–456. [CrossRef] [PubMed]
2. Sugaya, K.; Roppolo, J.R.; Yoshimura, N.; Card, J.P.; de Groat, W.C. The central neural pathways involved in micturition in the neonatal rat as revealed by the injection of pseudorabies virus into the urinary bladder. *Neurosci. Lett.* **1997**, *223*, 197–200. [CrossRef]
3. Vizzard, M.A.; Erickson, V.L.; Card, J.P.; Roppolo, J.R.; de Groat, W.C. Transneuronal labeling of neurons in the adult rat brainstem and spinal cord after injection of pseudorabies virus into the urethra. *J. Comp. Neurol.* **1995**, *355*, 629–640. [CrossRef] [PubMed]
4. Mbaki, Y.; Ramage, A.G. Investigation of the role of 5-HT2 receptor subtypes in the control of the bladder and the urethra in the anaesthetized female rat. *Br. J. Pharmacol.* **2008**, *155*, 343–356. [CrossRef] [PubMed]
5. Norouzi-Javidan, A.; Javanbakht, J.; Barati, F.; Fakhraei, N.; Mohammadi, F.; Dehpour, A.R. Effect of 5-HT7 receptor agonist, LP-211, on micturition following spinal cord injury in male rats. *Am. J. Transl. Res.* **2016**, *8*, 2525–2533. [PubMed]
6. De Groat, W.C. Influence of central serotonergic mechanisms on lower urinary tract function. *Urology* **2002**, *59*, 30–36. [CrossRef]
7. Bowker, R.M.; Westlund, K.N.; Coulter, J.D. Origins of serotonergic projections to the spinal cord in rat: An immunocytochemical-retrograde transport study. *Brain Res.* **1981**, *226*, 187–199. [CrossRef]
8. Ahn, J.; Saltos, T.M.; Tom, V.J.; Hou, S. Transsynaptic tracing to dissect supraspinal serotonergic input regulating the bladder reflex in rats. *Neurourol. Urodyn.* **2018**, *37*, 2487–2494. [CrossRef]
9. Thor, K.B.; Nickolaus, S.; Helke, C.J. Autoradiographic localization of 5-hydroxytryptamine1A, 5-hydroxytryptamine1B and 5-hydroxytryptamine1C/2 binding sites in the rat spinal cord. *Neuroscience* **1993**, *55*, 235–252. [CrossRef]
10. de Groat, W.C.; Yoshimura, N. Plasticity in reflex pathways to the lower urinary tract following spinal cord injury. *Exp. Neurol.* **2012**, *235*, 123–132. [CrossRef] [PubMed]
11. Taweel, W.A.; Seyam, R. Neurogenic bladder in spinal cord injury patients. *Res. Rep. Urol.* **2015**, *7*, 85–99. [CrossRef]
12. Romo, P.G.B.; Smith, C.P.; Cox, A.; Averbeck, M.A.; Dowling, M.; Beckford, C.; Manohar, P.; Duran, S.; Cameron, A.P. Non-surgical urologic management of neurogenic bladder after spinal cord injury. *World J. Urol.* **2018**, *36*, 1555–1568. [CrossRef] [PubMed]
13. Madersbacher, H.; Murtz, G.; Stohrer, M. Neurogenic detrusor overactivity in adults: A review on efficacy, tolerability and safety of oral antimuscarinics. *Spinal Cord* **2013**, *51*, 432–441. [CrossRef]
14. Al Taweel, W.; Alzyoud, K.M. The effect of spinal cord-injury level on the outcome of neurogenic bladder treatment using OnabotulinumtoxinA. *Urol. Ann.* **2015**, *7*, 320–324. [CrossRef] [PubMed]
15. Schurch, B.; Schmid, D.M.; Stohrer, M. Treatment of neurogenic incontinence with botulinum toxin A. *N. Engl. J. Med.* **2000**, *342*, 665. [CrossRef]
16. Jamil, F. Towards a catheter free status in neurogenic bladder dysfunction: A review of bladder management options in spinal cord injury (SCI). *Spinal Cord* **2001**, *39*, 355–361. [CrossRef] [PubMed]
17. Leu, R.; Stearns, G.L. Complications of Botox and their Management. *Curr. Urol. Rep.* **2018**, *19*, 90. [CrossRef] [PubMed]
18. Magnusson, T. Effect of chronic transection on dopamine, noradrenaline and 5-hydroxytryptamine in the rat spinal cord. *Naunyn Schmiedebergs Arch. Pharmacol.* **1973**, *278*, 13–22. [CrossRef]
19. Newton, B.W.; Hamill, R.W. The morphology and distribution of rat serotoninergic intraspinal neurons: An immunohistochemical study. *Brain Res. Bull.* **1988**, *20*, 349–360. [CrossRef]
20. Wienecke, J.; Ren, L.Q.; Hultborn, H.; Chen, M.; Møller, M.; Zhang, Y.; Zhang, M. Spinal cord injury enables aromatic L-amino acid decarboxylase cells to synthesize monoamines. *J. Neurosci.* **2014**, *34*, 11984–12000. [CrossRef]

21. Sawynok, J.; Reid, A. Spinal supersensitivity to 5-HT1, 5-HT2 and 5-HT3 receptor agonists following 5,7-dihydroxytryptamine. *Eur. J. Pharmacol.* **1994**, *264*, 249–257. [CrossRef]
22. Chen, J.; Gu, B.; Wu, G.; Tu, H.; Si, J.; Xu, Y.; Andersson, K.E. The effect of the 5-HT2A/2C receptor agonist DOI on micturition in rats with chronic spinal cord injury. *J. Uro.* **2013**, *189*, 1982–1988. [CrossRef] [PubMed]
23. D'Agostino, G.; Condino, A.M.; Franceschetti, G.P.; Tonini, M. Characterization of prejunctional serotonin receptors modulating [3H]acetylcholine release in the human detrusor. *J. Pharmacol. Exp. Ther.* **2006**, *316*, 129–135. [CrossRef]
24. Ochodnicky, P.; Humphreys, S.; Eccles, R.; Poljakovic, M.; Wiklund, P.; Michel, M.C. Expression profiling of G-protein-coupled receptors in human urothelium and related cell lines. *BJU Int.* **2012**, *110*, 293–300. [CrossRef] [PubMed]
25. Matsumoto-Miyai, K.; Yoshizumi, M.; Kawatani, M. Regulatory Effects of 5-Hydroxytryptamine Receptors on Voiding Function. *Adv. Ther.* **2015**, *32*, 3–15. [CrossRef] [PubMed]
26. Yoshiyama, M.; Nezu, F.M.; Yokoyama, O.; de Groat, W.C.; Chancellor, M.B. Changes in micturition after spinal cord injury in conscious rats. *Urology* **1999**, *54*, 929–933. [CrossRef]
27. Kadekawa, K.; Nishijima, S.; Sugaya, K.; Miyazato, M.; Saito, S. Mechanisms by which the serotonergic system inhibits micturition in rats. *Life Sci.* **2009**, *85*, 592–596. [CrossRef] [PubMed]
28. Mitsui, T.; Shumsky, J.S.; Lepore, A.C.; Murray, M.; Fischer, I. Transplantation of neuronal and glial restricted precursors into contused spinal cord improves bladder and motor functions, decreases thermal hypersensitivity, and modifies intraspinal circuitry. *J. Neurosci.* **2005**, *25*, 9624–9636. [CrossRef] [PubMed]
29. Dahlstroem, A.; Fuxe, K. Evidence for the Existence of Monoamine-Containing Neurons in the Central Nervous System. I. Demonstration of Monoamines in the Cell Bodies of Brain Stem Neurons. *Acta Physiol. Scand. Suppl.* **1964**, *232*, 1–55.
30. Dahlstroem, A.; Fuxe, K. Evidence for the Existence of Monoamine Neurons in the Central Nervous System. Ii. Experimentally Induced Changes in the Intraneuronal Amine Levels of Bulbospinal Neuron Systems. *Acta Physiol. Scand. Suppl.* **1965**, *247*, 1–36.
31. Xu, C.; Giuliano, F.; Sun, X.Q.; Brisorgueil, M.-J.; Leclerc, P.; Vergé, D.; Conrath, M. Serotonin 5-HT2A and 5-HT5A receptors are expressed by different motoneuron populations in rat Onuf's nucleus. *J. Comp. Neurol.* **2007**, *502*, 620–634. [CrossRef]
32. Helton, L.; Thor, K.B.; Baez, M. 5-Hydroxytryptamine$_{2a}$, 5-Hydroxytryptamine$_{2B}$, 5-Hydroxytryptamine$_{2C}$ receptor mRNA expression in the spinal cord of rat, cat, monkey, and human. *Neuroreport* **1994**, *5*, 2617–2620. [CrossRef]
33. Kong, X.Y.; Wienecke, J.; Hultborn, H.; Zhang, M. Robust upregulation of serotonin 2A receptors after chronic spinal transection of rats: An immunohistochemical study. *Brain Res.* **2010**, *1320*, 60–68. [CrossRef]
34. Chang, H.Y.; Cheng, C.L.; Chen, J.-J.J.; de Groat, W.C. Roles of glutamatergic and serotonergic mechanisms in reflex control of the external urethral sphincter in urethane-anesthetized female rats. *Am. J. Physiol. Regul. Integr. Comp. Physiol.* **2006**, *291*, R224–R234. [CrossRef]
35. Chang, H.Y.; Cheng, C.L.; Chen, J.-J.J.; de Groat, W.C. Serotonergic drugs and spinal cord transections indicate that different spinal circuits are involved in external urethral sphincter activity in rats. *Am. J. Physiol Renal Physiol* **2007**, *292*, F1044–F1053. [CrossRef]
36. Cheng, C.L.; de Groat, W.C. Role of 5-HT1A receptors in control of lower urinary tract function in anesthetized rats. *Am. J. Physiol. Renal. Physiol.* **2010**, *298*, F771–F778. [CrossRef]
37. Dolber, P.C.; Gu, B.; Zhang, X.; Fraser, M.O.; Thor, K.B.; Reiter, J.P. Activation of the external urethral sphincter central pattern generator by a 5-HT(1A) receptor agonist in rats with chronic spinal cord injury. *Am. J. Physiol. Regul. Integr. Comp. Physiol.* **2007**, *292*, R1699–R1706. [CrossRef]
38. Ramage, A.G. The role of central 5-hydroxytryptamine (5-HT, serotonin) receptors in the control of micturition. *Br. J. Pharmacol.* **2006**, *147*, S120–S131. [CrossRef]
39. Cao, N.; Ni, J.; Wang, X.; Tu, H.; Gu, B.; Si, J.; Wu, G.; Andersson, K.E. Chronic spinal cord injury causes upregulation of serotonin (5-HT)2A and 5-HT2C receptors in lumbosacral cord motoneurons. *BJU Int.* **2018**, *121*, 145–154. [CrossRef]
40. Doly, S.; Madeira, A.; Fischer, J.; Brisorgueil, M.J.; Daval, G.; Bernard, R.; Vergé, D.; Conrath, M. The 5-HT2A receptor is widely distributed in the rat spinal cord and mainly localized at the plasma membrane of postsynaptic neurons. *J. Comp. Neurol.* **2004**, *472*, 496–511. [CrossRef]
41. Kruse, M.N.; Belton, A.L.; de Groat, W.C. Changes in bladder and external urethral sphincter function after spinal cord injury in the rat. *Am. J. Physiol.* **1993**, *264*, R1157–R1163. [CrossRef] [PubMed]
42. Kakizaki, H.; Fraser, M.O.; De Groat, W.C. Reflex pathways controlling urethral striated and smooth muscle function in the male rat. *Am. J. Physiol.* **1997**, *272*, R1647–R1656. [CrossRef] [PubMed]
43. Maggi, C.A.; Giuliani, S.; Santicioli, P.; Meli, A. Analysis of factors involved in determining urinary bladder voiding cycle in urethan-anesthetized rats. *Am. J. Physiol.* **1986**, *251*, R250–R257. [CrossRef]
44. Danuser, H.; Thor, K.B. Spinal 5-HT2 receptor-mediated facilitation of pudendal nerve reflexes in the anaesthetized cat. *Br. J. Pharmacol.* **1996**, *118*, 150–154. [CrossRef]
45. Karnup, S.V.; de Groat, W.C. Propriospinal Neurons of L3-L4 Segments Involved in Control of the Rat External Urethral Sphincter. *Neuroscience* **2020**, *425*, 12–28. [CrossRef]
46. Hoyer, D. Molecular pharmacology and biology of 5-HT1C receptors. *Trends Pharmacol. Sci.* **1988**, *9*, 89–94. [CrossRef]
47. Lopez-Gimenez, J.F.; Vilaró, M.T.; Palacios, J.M.; Mengod, G. Multiple conformations of 5-HT2A and 5-HT 2C receptors in rat brain: An autoradiographic study with [125I](+/-)DOI. *Exp. Brain Res.* **2013**, *230*, 395–406. [CrossRef] [PubMed]

48. Lopez-Gimenez, J.F.; Mengod, G.; Palacios, J.M.; Vilaró, M.T. Selective visualization of rat brain 5-HT2A receptors by autoradiography with [3H]MDL 100,907. *Naunyn Schmiedebergs Arch. Pharmacol.* **1997**, *356*, 446–454. [CrossRef]
49. Wang, X.; Cao, N.; Ni, J.; Si, J.; Gu, B.; Karl-Erik, A. Effect of 5-HT2A receptor antagonist ketanserin on micturition in male rats. *Neurosci. Lett.* **2018**, *687*, 196–201. [CrossRef]
50. Brouillard, C.B.J.; Crook, J.J.; Lovick, T.A. Suppression of Urinary Voiding "on Demand" by High-Frequency Stimulation of the S1 Sacral Nerve Root in Anesthetized Rats. *Neuromodulation* **2019**, *22*, 703–708. [CrossRef]
51. Yoshiyama, M.; Roppolo, J.R.; De Groat, W.C. Alteration by urethane of glutamatergic control of micturition. *Eur. J. Pharmacol.* **1994**, *264*, 417–425. [CrossRef]
52. Morikawa, K.; Ichihashi, M.; Kakiuchi, M.; Yamauchi, T.; Kato, H.; Ito, Y.; Gomi, Y. Effects of various drugs on bladder function in conscious rats. *Jpn. J. Pharmacol.* **1989**, *50*, 369–376. [CrossRef]
53. Hou, S.; Rabchevsky, A.G. Autonomic consequences of spinal cord injury. *Compr. Physiol.* **2014**, *4*, 1419–1453. [PubMed]
54. Van Middendorp, J.J.; Goss, B.; Urquhart, S.; Atresh, S.; Williams, R.P.; Schuetz, M. Diagnosis and prognosis of traumatic spinal cord injury. *Global. Spine J.* **2011**, *1*, 1–8. [CrossRef]
55. Wyndaele, M.; Wyndaele, J.J. Incidence, prevalence and epidemiology of spinal cord injury: What learns a worldwide literature survey? *Spinal Cord* **2006**, *44*, 523–529. [CrossRef] [PubMed]
56. Abelson, B.; Sun, D.; Que, L.; Nebel, R.A.; Baker, D.; Popiel, P.; Amundsen, C.L.; Chai, T.; Close, C.; DiSanto, M.; et al. Sex differences in lower urinary tract biology and physiology. *Biol. Sex. Differ.* **2018**, *9*, 45. [CrossRef] [PubMed]
57. Li, J.; Yang, L.; Pu, C.; Tang, Y.; Yun, H.; Han, P. The role of duloxetine in stress urinary incontinence: A systematic review and meta-analysis. *Int. Urol. Nephrol.* **2013**, *45*, 679–686. [CrossRef]

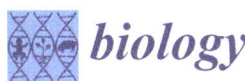

Article

What Makes a Successful Donor? Fecal Transplant from Anxious-Like Rats Does Not Prevent Spinal Cord Injury-Induced Dysbiosis

Emma K. A. Schmidt [1], Pamela J. F. Raposo [2,3], Karen L. Madsen [4], Keith K. Fenrich [1,2], Gillian Kabarchuk [1] and Karim Fouad [1,2,3,*]

1. Neuroscience and Mental Health Institute, University of Alberta, Edmonton, AB T6G 2R3, Canada; ekschmid@ualberta.ca (E.K.A.S.); fenrich@ualberta.ca (K.K.F.); kabarchu@ualberta.ca (G.K.)
2. Faculty of Rehabilitation Medicine, University of Alberta, Edmonton, AB T6G 2R3, Canada; praposo@ualberta.ca
3. Department of Physical Therapy, University of Alberta, Edmonton, AB T6G 2R3, Canada
4. Division of Gastroenterology, Faculty of Medicine and Dentistry, University of Alberta, Edmonton, AB T6G 2R3, Canada; karen.madsen@ualberta.ca
* Correspondence: karim.fouad@ualberta.ca; Tel.: +1-(780)-492-5971

Simple Summary: Spinal cord injury disrupts the composition of gut bacteria and increases the prevalence of anxiety-like and depressive-like behaviours. We have previously shown that a fecal transplant from uninjured donor rats prevents both injury-induced microbiota changes and the development of anxiety-like behaviour. In the present study, we aimed to determine whether donor selection would influence the efficacy of a fecal transplant after spinal cord injury. We found that a fecal transplant from uninjured donor rats with increased anxiety-like behaviour was not only ineffective in preventing injury-induced microbiota changes, but it also increased intestinal permeability and anxiety-like behaviour of the recipient rats. The results of this study emphasize the importance of optimal donor selection for successful fecal transplant treatment following spinal cord injury.

Abstract: Spinal cord injury (SCI) causes gut dysbiosis and an increased prevalence of depression and anxiety. Previous research showed a link between these two consequences of SCI by using a fecal transplant from healthy rats which prevented both SCI-induced microbiota changes and the subsequent development of anxiety-like behaviour. However, whether the physical and mental state of the donor are important factors in the efficacy of FMT therapy after SCI remains unknown. In the present study, rats received a fecal transplant following SCI from uninjured donors with increased baseline levels of anxiety-like behaviour and reduced proportion of *Lactobacillus* in their stool. This fecal transplant increased intestinal permeability, induced anxiety-like behaviour, and resulted in minor but long-term alterations in the inflammatory state of the recipients compared to vehicle controls. There was no significant effect of the fecal transplant on motor recovery in rehabilitative training, suggesting that anxiety-like behaviour did not affect the motivation to participate in rehabilitative therapy. The results of this study emphasize the importance of considering both the microbiota composition and the mental state of the donor for fecal transplants following spinal cord injury.

Keywords: spinal cord injury; fecal microbiota transplant; inflammation; anxiety; rehabilitation

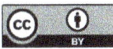

1. Introduction

Spinal cord injury (SCI) causes damage to the spinal cord and disrupts the physical and mental well-being of individuals with SCI [1]. In addition to motor and sensory deficits, SCI can cause impairments in autonomic, immune and bowels functions as well as disturb the composition of the gut microbiota (termed dysbiosis) [2–5]. In a rat model of SCI, we have previously prevented SCI-induced dysbiosis by transferring fecal matter from uninjured donor rats into recipient rats immediately after SCI. This fecal microbiota transplant (FMT) from uninjured, non-anxious-like rats not only successfully re-established a healthy microbiota composition after injury, but also improved symptoms of anxiety-like behaviour [2].

Clinically, FMT is defined as the administration of fecal matter solution from a healthy donor into the intestinal tract of a recipient [6,7]. The use of FMT in clinical trials has most commonly been to treat *Clostridium difficile* infections and irritable bowel disease, however case reports have demonstrated beneficial results of an FMT for individuals with Parkinson's disease, multiple sclerosis, Tourette syndrome, autism and epilepsy [8–14]. Unfortunately, the definition of a healthy donor is less straightforward. Currently, donors are selected primarily to exclude known pathogens and mitigate the risk of transferring infectious diseases [15–18]. While ensuring recipient safety is a priority above all, research on optimal donor selection beyond the exclusion of transmissible pathogens is still at an early stage [15,19]. Although the choice of donor does not influence the efficacy of FMT to treat *Clostridium difficile* infections (currently the only FDA approved use of FMT [20]), it is unknown how critical donor selection is to treat diseases and disorders with more complex host-microbiota interaction, such as SCI [9,21].

In the present study, we aimed to determine whether the mental state of FMT donor rats would influence the therapeutic benefits of FMT after SCI. Rats who displayed naturally reduced baseline activity levels and increased anxiety-like behaviour (referred to as *anxious* donors) were selected as FMT donors. Notably these rats were uninjured and had similar alpha diversity to uninjured, non-anxious-like rats, which is important since a diverse microbial diversity has been shown to be an indicator of FMT success for treatment of ulcerative colitis and *Clostridium difficile* infections [19,22]. We therefore hypothesized that FMT from *anxious* rats would yield similar therapeutic benefits as FMT from non-*anxious* rats as in our previous research [2]. Here, rats in the experimental groups received either vehicle or FMT treatment for 3 days following a cervical contusion SCI and underwent 7 weeks of rehabilitative training in a reaching task targeting their impaired forearm. Fecal matter and plasma were collected throughout the experiment, and anxiety- and depressive-like behaviours were assessed at the end of the rehabilitation period. The inherently increased anxiety-like behaviour of the FMT donors was associated with a decreased abundance of *Lactobacillus* in their stool and thus in the FMT solution. Contrary to our hypothesis, FMT from *anxious* donors did not prevent SCI-induced gut dysbiosis and even resulted in some negative side effects. Rats which received the FMT displayed chronically increased anxiety-like behaviour, long-term alterations in local and systemic inflammation, and increased intestinal permeability. These results indicate that donor selection is critical for successful FMT following SCI and possibly other CNS injuries and diseases as well.

2. Materials and Methods

2.1. Animals

40 female adult Lewis rats (Charles River) were group housed (n = 5 per cage, experimental groups housed separately to avoid coprophagy) on a 12 h light-dark cycle and received ad libitum access to standard rat chow and water. During training periods, rats were food restricted to 10 g per rat per day (to encourage reaching for training pellets). Behavioural testing and all analyses were performed by an experimenter blinded to the experimental groups. Three groups of rats were used: SCI + vehicle (n = 15), SCI + FMT (n = 15), and FMT donors (n = 10). The two cages which displayed the highest baseline anxiety-like behaviour in the open field were chosen as uninjured age and sex matched fecal donors and were not trained in the single pellet grasping (SPG) training. SCI + vehicle and SCI + FMT groups were chosen to average each group's pre-injury success rate in the SPG task. Data from previous experiments that were used to compare elevated plus maze

behaviour and *Lactobacillus* levels were taken from genetically comparable rats from the same supplier with the same weight, handled the same amount, and received the same diet.

This study was approved by a local animal care and use committee (Health Sciences) at the University of Alberta and in accordance with the guidelines of the Canadian Council for Animal Care.

2.2. Experimental Timeline

Prior to SCI, rats in the two experimental groups were pre-trained on the SPG task and underwent baseline testing on the open field, von frey and gap tests. The von frey test was also performed 7 days post SCI. Final behavioural testing was performed at the end of the rehabilitative training period between 63 and 77 days post injury. The FMT donors were handled daily to control for the potential effect of handling during rehabilitative training. Immediately following SCI and for two consecutive days thereafter, rats were gavaged with FMT or vehicle solution. Following 7 weeks of rehabilitative training on the SPG task, rats underwent behavioural testing. Fecal matter was collected for 16S rRNA analysis at baseline, on the day of injury (6–12 h after), 3, 7, 14 and 56 days post-SCI. Blood was collected to measure inflammatory plasma analytes at baseline, 3, 21 and 77 days post-SCI (Figure 1).

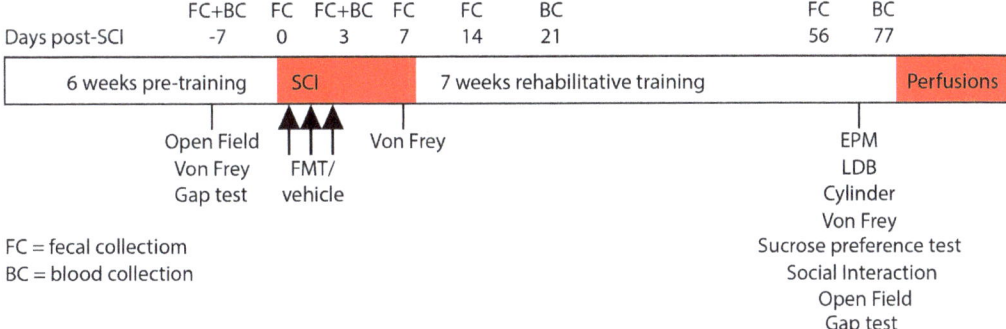

Figure 1. Experimental Timeline.

2.3. Single Pellet Grasping Training

The SPG protocols and equipment were used as previously described [23]. Rats were first acclimatized to the SPG double-window enclosure and each rat's preferred paw was established by manually counting the number of left and right reaching attempts for a sucrose pellet. Once the preferred paw was established, the pellet dispenser was positioned so the rat could only reach the pellet with its preferred paw. Rats were trained to reach for a pellet on one side of the enclosure and then travel to the opposite end where another pellet was dispensed, etc. Training consisted of 10 min per rat per day, 5 days a week for 6 weeks prior to SCI. Rehabilitative training began 10 days following SCI and continued for 7 weeks. Training sessions were video recorded and analyzed offline. The total number of attempts made (rat reached towards the pellet) and number of successes (rat successfully reached, grasped and consumed the pellet) were quantified. Success rate was defined as the total number of successful attempts divided by the total number of attempts multiplied by 100. Once before SCI and again at the end of the rehabilitative period, rats were tested on a modified single pellet grasping gap test that prevents compensatory scooping strategies.

2.4. Spinal Cord Injury

SCI cervical contusions were performed as previously described [2]. Rats were anesthetized with isoflurane (5% induction; 2.5% maintenance; 50:50 air/oxygen mixture) and the dorsal neck was shaved and disinfected with 10% chlorhexidine digluconate

(Sigma-Aldrich, St. Louis, MO, USA). The Infinite Horizons impactor (Precision Systems & Instrumentation) was used to deliver a 125 kdyn unilateral contusion 1.25 mm lateral to the midline (on the side of the preferred paw) at an angle of 15 degrees (towards midline) at cervical level 5. Synthetic braided sutures were used to suture the muscles and the skin was closed using 9 mm stainless steel clips. Buprenorphine was injected immediately after SCI and again 8 h after (0.03 mg/kg; subcutaneous; WDDC). Saline was injected (4 mL, subcutaneous) post operatively and bladders were manually expressed until voiding was re-established (within 2 days post SCI).

2.5. Behavioural Testing

2.5.1. Light Dark Box

Rats were placed in the light component of a customized light-dark box apparatus (dark compartment 0 lux; light compartment 100 lux; each chamber 30 cm long × 30 cm wide × 30 cm high) and allowed to freely explore for 10 min while video recorded from above. The time spent in the light component was analyzed as measures of anxiety-like behaviour.

2.5.2. Elevated Plus Maze

Rats were placed in the center of the elevated plus maze apparatus (2 closed arms: each 50 cm long × 10 cm wide × 50 cm high, and 2 open arms: each 50 cm long × 10 cm wide × 1 cm high) and video recorded from above for 10 min. Customized tracking software (https://github.com/cdoolin/rat-apps, accessed on 1 September 2020) was used to quantify the percent time spent in the open arms and the total distance travelled. This test was used only once to avoid one-trial tolerance [24].

2.5.3. Sucrose Preference Test

Rats were exposed to two water bottles in their home cage: one with a 2% sucrose solution and one with regular drinking water. The percentage of sucrose water consumed over 48 h was calculated as a measure of anhedonia. The location of the bottles was switched at 24 h to avoid side preference.

2.5.4. Open Field

Rats were placed in the center of an open field arena (100 cm long × 80 cm wide × 30 cm high) and video recorded from above for 5 min. Offline video analysis was performed using customized tracking software (https://github.com/cdoolin/rat-apps, accessed on 1 September 2020) to quantify the total distance travelled.

2.5.5. Cylinder

Rats were placed in an acrylic cylinder (21 cm diameter × 23 cm high) with mirrors located behind so that the rat could be observed from all sides using one camera. Each rat was video recorded for 3 min and offline analysis was used to quantify the number of left and right paw placements made on the side of the cylinder. Forepaw asymmetry was expressed as the percentage of ipsilesional paw placements.

2.5.6. Von Frey Test

Rats were acclimatized to the testing chamber 5 min per rat the day before testing (IITC Life Science, Woodland Hills, CA, USA). Tactile sensitivity was assessed on both forepaws (when the animal was weight-bearing on its forepaws). A rigid probe connected to the automated Von Frey apparatus was applied in increasing pressure until the rat displayed a defined nociceptive response (paw retraction, licking) and the maximum pressure that elicited a withdrawal was recorded. This was repeated 3 times per paw, with a minimum of 3 min between measures. The average of the 3 measures per paw was used for analysis.

2.5.7. Social Interaction

The test rat was placed in the open field apparatus with an unfamiliar, uninjured rat for 10 min while video recorded from above. The time spent in active interaction (sniffing, nipping, grooming, following, mounting, kicking, boxing, wrestling, jumping on, and crawling) was recorded as a measure of anxiety-like behaviour [25].

2.6. Fecal Collection and Transplantation

Fecal samples were collected as previously described [2]. During the dark cycle, rats were placed into individual sterile cages. Fecal pellets were immediately collected, placed into sterile eppendorf tubes and stored in a $-80\ °C$ freezer until further processing. For the fecal transplant solution, pellets were collected from uninjured FMT donors (pooled from all 10 rats as pooling samples from multiple donors has been shown to be more effective [26]) and immediately processed to make the transplant solution. The fresh fecal matter was diluted 1:10 in sterile PBS (10%), L-cysteine HCL (0.05%), glycerol (20%) and sterile water (60%) and passed through a 100 µm filter. The solution was frozen at $-20\ °C$ and thawed at room temperature for 12 h prior to use (the use of frozen fecal matter for oral FMT has proven to be effective [27]). The SCI + vehicle group received the filtered solution that did not contain fecal matter. Then, 2 h after SCI and for 2 consecutive days after, rats were gavaged with 500 µL of either FMT or vehicle solution.

2.7. 16S rRNA Sequencing

DNA was extracted as previously described [28]. Fecal microbial DNA was extracted with AquaStool solution (Multitarget Pharmaceuticals LLC, Colorado Springs, CO, USA) as per the manufacturer instructions. Briefly, 100 mg of rat fecal pellet was homogenized in the AquaStool solution with 0.1 mm beads at 0.6 m/s for 40 s. AquaRemove was added to remove potential PCR inhibitors per manufacturer's instruction followed by ethanol/NaCl precipitation for further purification. DNA Samples were sent to Genome Quebec (McGill University, Montreal, QC, Canada) for Illumina Miseq sequencing. V3-V4 region of universal 16S rRNA primers with 341 forward primer: 5′-TCG TCG GCA GCG TCA GAT GTG TAT AAG AGA CAG CCT ACG GGN GGC WGC AG-3′ and 805 reverse primer: 5′-GTC TCG TGG GCT CGG AGA TGT GTA TAA GAG ACA GGA CTA CHV GGG TAT CTA ATC C-3′ were used.

Demultiplexed paired-end sequences were merged and performed quality control implementation (mean sequence quality score ≥ 30) and features table construction (amplicon sequences variants, ASVs) via DADA2 [29] plugin in QIIME2 (version 2019.10) [30]. An even sequence depth of 9452 reads per sample was used to conduct microbiome diversity and composition analyses. Taxonomy assignments from the phylum to genus levels were conducted by a pre-trained Naive Bayes classifier [30] (Silva 132 99% OTUs database) and the q2-feature-classifier function in QIIME2. Alpha-diversity of Shannon index and community balance of Pielou's evenness index, and beta-diversity analysis (unweighted unifrac emperor distance) were conducted using the QIIME2.

2.8. Blood Collection

The area over the tarsal joint was shaved and the saphenous vein was punctured using a sterile needle. Blood was collected into a microvette CB300 capillary tube (Sarstedt Inc., Nümbrecht, Germany) and immediately centrifuged for 5 min at 3000 rpm. Plasma was then pipetted into sterile microcentrifuge tubes and stored at $-80\ °C$ freezer until further processing.

2.9. Cytokine Analysis

Frozen plasma samples were sent to Eve Technologies (Calgary, AB, Canada) and diluted 2-fold for the Rat Cytokine 27-Plex discovery assay. Cytokines and chemokines measured were: Eotaxin, EGF, Fractalkine, IFN-gamma, IL-1a, IL-1b, IL-2, IL-4, IL-5, IL-6, IL-10, IL-12(p70), IL-13, IL-17A, IL-18, IP-10, GRO/KC, TNF-alpha, G-CSF, GM-CSF, MCP-

1, Leptin, LIX, MIP-1alpha, MIP-2, RANTES, and VEGF. GRO/KC values are not reported as they were out of range in our samples. For heatmap visualization, plasma analytes were expressed as a change from baseline $(x_2 - x_1/x_1)$.

2.10. Intestinal Permeability Assay

Once the uninjured FMT donor rats had completed all of their baseline testing and fecal collections, they were used to assess intestinal permeability. These rats were randomly divided into an SCI + vehicle group (n = 5) and an SCI + FMT group (n = 5) and received identical treatment as the original treatment groups (2 h after SCI and for 2 consecutive days after, rats were gavaged with 500 µL of either FMT or vehicle solution). The day before injury and again 7 days following SCI, rats were fasted for 4 h and then gavaged with 0.6 g/kg FITC dextran (4 kD, Sigma-Aldrich) diluted in sterile PBS. Blood was collected 4 h later via the saphenous vein and plasma was collected as described above. Plasma samples were diluted 1:10 with sterile PBS and transferred to an opaque-bottom 96-well plate. Samples were run in duplicates and a PBS blank and standard curve measurements were measured on the same plate. Fluorescence was determined at 530 nm with an excitation at 485 nm on a plate reader (SpectraMax, Molecular Devices, San Jose, CA, USA). Intestinal permeability was quantified as a fold change from baseline levels.

2.11. Perfusion and Tissue Cutting

At the end of rehabilitative training and all final behavioural assessments (78 days after SCI), rats were euthanized with sodium pentobarbital (240 mg/kg). Rats were transcardially perfused with saline containing 0.02 g heparin/L followed by 4% paraformaldehyde in 0.1 M phosphate-buffered saline (PBS) and 5% sucrose. Spinal cords were extracted and post-fixed in 4% paraformaldehyde 4 °C for 4 h and transferred to a 30% sucrose solution for 5 days. A 1 cm block around the lesion site was embedded in O.C.T. (Sakura Finetek, Torrance, CA, USA), mounted onto filter paper and frozen at -40 °C in 2-methylbutane. A NX70 cryostat (Fisher Scientific, Waltham, MA, USA) was used to section the cord at a thickness of 25 µm. Every second section was kept and staggered across eight slides and stored at -20 °C.

2.12. Lesion Analysis

Frozen slides were thawed for 1 h at 37 °C and washed in TBS (2 × 10 min). Slides were placed into 0.5% cresyl violet for 3 min, rinsed with filtered water and serially dehydrated in EtOH (2 min in 50%, 75%, and 99%). Slides were then placed in xylene (2 × 2 min) and coverslipped with Permount™. Images of the entire lesion extension were taken with an epifluorescence microscope (Leica DM6000B, camera Leica DFC350 FX, Wetzlar, Germany) at 5× magnification and analyzed using ImageJ (National Institute of Health, Bethesda, MD, USA). Lesion size was calculated as the percent of damaged tissue divided by the total area of the spinal cord cross section.

2.13. Analysis of IBA1 Staining

Sections were thawed at 37 °C for 1 h and rehydrated in PBS (2 × 10) minutes followed by PBS with 0.3% Triton™ X-100 (PBS-T) (1 × 10 min). Blocking buffer consisting of 5% normal donkey serum in PBS-T was applied 1 h at room temperature. Sections were incubated overnight at room temperature in rabbit-anti-IBA1 (1:500, Wako, Cape Charles, VA, USA) antibody (to visualize microglia/macrophages) with blocking buffer. The next day, sections were washed with PBS (3 × 10 min) and incubated with donkey-anti-rabbit AF488-conjugated (1:500, Life Technologies, Carlsbad, CA, USA) antibody in the blocking buffer solution for 2 h. Sections were then rinsed in PBS (2 × 10 min) and cover slipped with Fluoromount™. Images were captured with an epifluorescence microscope (Leica DM6000B, camera Leica DFC350 FX, Wetzlar, Germany) and analyzed using ImageJ (National Institute of Health, Bethesda, MD, USA). Then, 5× magnification images were taken to visualize the entire spinal cord cross section 0.25 cm rostral to the lesion, at the lesion epicenter, and 0.25 cm caudal to the lesion. The area of IBA+ immunoreactivity was divided by the total area of each individual spinal cord cross section and expressed as a percentage of IBA1+ area using thresholding.

2.14. Statistical Analysis

Statistical analyses were performed using GraphPad Prism 8 (San Diego, CA, USA) and an alpha value of 5% or less was considered significant. Normality was analyzed using the D'Agostino-Pearson omnibus test. Data at a single time point were analyzed using an unpaired parametric *t*-test for two groups and an ordinary one-way ANOVA for three groups (non-parametric tests were used for data that did not pass normality). Data with multiple time points were analyzed using an ordinary repeated measures two-way ANOVA followed by Sidak's multiple comparison test.

3. Results

3.1. Fecal Microbiota Transplant from Anxious Donors

Although the rats used in the present experiment are genetically identical siblings, there is a natural variability in their baseline levels of anxiety-like behaviour, which can be further influenced by environmental stressors. To determine how important optimal donor selection is, the two cages of rats who naturally displayed decreased baseline activity in the open field (as an indicator of anxiety-like behaviour [31,32]) were chosen as the FMT donors. Compared to SCI + vehicle and SCI + FMT groups at baseline (prior to SCI), FMT donors travelled significantly less distance in the open field ($p = 0.0052$) (Figure 2A). This altered behavioural phenotype was associated with significantly reduced levels of *Lactobacillus* in the FMT donor's stool compared to the experimental groups (SCI + Vehicle and SCI + FMT) at baseline ($p = 0.0006$) (Figure 2B). Reflecting the lack of *Lactobacillus* in the donor stool, the FMT solution also contained a lack of *Lactobacillus* (Figure 2B). FMT donors displayed a similar alpha diversity (the bacterial variance within the samples) as the experimental groups, which was also reflected in the FMT solution (Figure 2C). Compared to previously successful FMT donors (which, when transferred to rats after SCI, prevented both SCI-induced dysbiosis and anxiety-like behaviour [2]), *anxious* FMT donors spent significantly less time in the open arms of the elevated plus maze, confirming their increased anxiety-like phenotype ($p = 0.0002$) (Figure 2D). The robustness of behaviour in the elevated plus maze of non-*anxious* uninjured rats throughout different cohorts of animals is shown in Supplementary Figure S1. Not only did *anxious* FMT donors spend significantly less time in the open arms compared to previous non-*anxious* donors, they also displayed significant increased anxiety-like behaviour compared to two separate groups (from different experiments) of uninjured animals run in the elevated plus maze ($p = 0.0006$). Anxious FMT donors also displayed significantly lower proportions of *Lactobacillus* compared to the non-*anxious* FMT donors described in our previous study ($p < 0.0001$; [2]) (Figure 2E). These data suggest that, although the FMT donors were uninjured and had a diverse microbiota composition, they had an increased anxiety-like phenotype and reduced proportion of the genus *Lactobacillus*, a commonly prescribed probiotic [33–35].

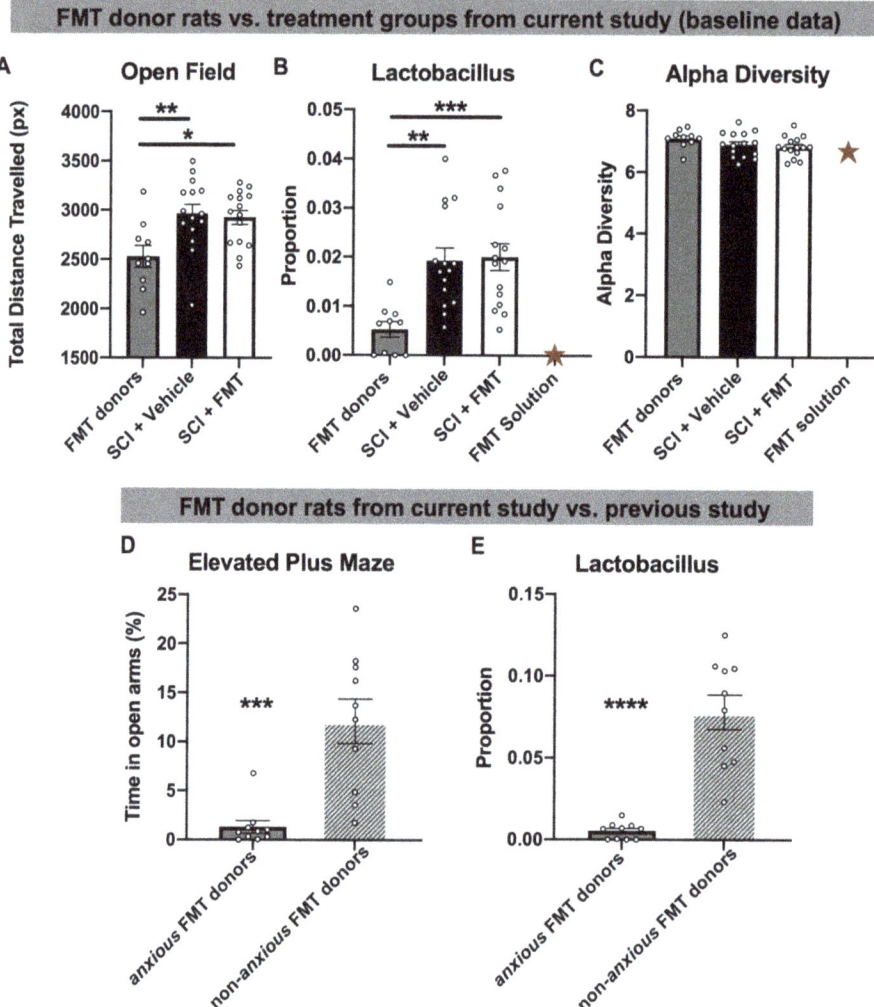

Figure 2. Uninjured FMT donor rats displayed altered baseline levels of anxiety-like behaviour and proportions of fecal *Lactobacillus*. (**A**) Fecal microbiota transplant (FMT) donors travelled significantly less distance in the open field compared to the SCI + vehicle and SCI + FMT treatment groups in the present experiment (measured at baseline prior to SCI). (**B**) Fecal matter from FMT donors had significantly decreased baseline proportions of *Lactobacillus*, which is also reflected in the decreased amount of *Lactobacillus* found in the FMT solution. (**C**) All groups had similar baseline levels of alpha diversity, including the FMT solution. (**D**) FMT donors in the current study displayed significantly increased anxiety-like behaviour in the elevated plus maze (indicated by the percent of time spent in the open arms) and (**E**) had significantly less fecal proportion of *Lactobacillus* relative to successful FMT donor rats from previous experiments. * $p < 0.05$, ** $p < 0.01$, *** $p < 0.001$, **** $p < 0.0001$. Gold star represents the FMT solution (A single value and therefore not included in statistical analysis). Error bars represent standard error mean.

3.2. FMT from Anxious Rats Did Not Prevent Dysbiosis after SCI

Fecal samples were collected prior to injury, on the day of injury, then 3, 7, 14 and 56 days after SCI for 16S rRNA sequencing. The differences in microbial abundance between the fecal samples was visualized using beta diversity plots. On the day of injury, 3- and 14-days post-SCI there was a deviation in the samples away from baseline values, confirming our previous results that a cervical SCI induces acute dysbiosis. At 7- and 56-days post-SCI, the samples clustered closely with baseline values (Figure 3A). When looking at the beta diversity of the two treatment groups across all time points, there was no difference between FMT or vehicle treated groups (Figure 3B). Although SCI resulted in acute dysbiosis visualized in the beta diversity plots, there was no significant effect of injury or FMT on the alpha diversity (which does not necessarily correlate with changes of individual bacteria; Figure 3C). Next, we looked at the four most abundant bacteria at the Phylum level: Bacteroidetes, Firmicutes, Cyanobacteria and Proteobacteria. There was no effect of SCI or FMT in the proportion of Bacteroidetes or Firmicutes (Figure 3D,E). The proportion of Proteobacteria was increased on the day of injury and 3 days post injury (Figure 3F) and the proportion of Cyanobacteria was increased 3 days post-SCI ($p < 0.0001$ for both) (Figure 3G), however there were no significant effects of FMT treatment. The proportion of the genus *Lactobacillus*, a common bacteria present in probiotics [34], was reduced chronically after SCI in both FMT treated and untreated groups ($p < 0.0001$) (Figure 3H). There was no significant difference between groups in any bacteria at the genus level (Supplementary Figures S2 and S3). These results indicate that the FMT from *anxious* donor rats was not successful in preventing SCI-induced dysbiosis.

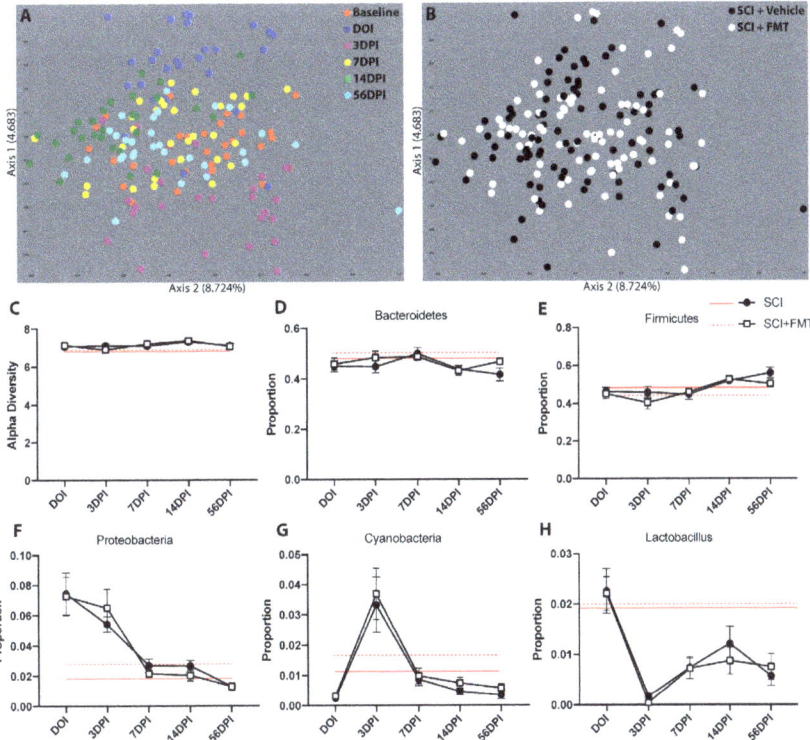

Figure 3. FMT from *anxious* donors did not prevent gut dysbiosis following SCI. (**A**) PCoA plot of beta diversity shows the diversity between fecal samples over time on the day of injury (DOI), 3-, 7-, 14- and 56-days post-injury (DPI). (**B**) The same PCoA plot is shown with the colors representing the groups instead of timepoints. Axis 1 and 2 explain 4.683% and 8.724% of the variance between samples, respectively. (**C**) There was no effect of injury or treatment on the alpha diversity. The four most abundant operational taxonomic units at the phylum level also show no differences between experimental groups in the proportion of (**D**) Bacteroidetes, (**E**) Firmicutes, (**F**) Proteobacteria and (**G**) Cyanobacteria. (**H**) The proportion of the genus *Lactobacillus* was reduced after SCI but not affected by FMT. Red lines represent baseline values. Error bars represent standard error mean.

3.3. FMT from Anxious Rats Did Not Affect Functional Recovery from SCI

10 days following SCI, rats began 7 weeks of rehabilitative therapy in the SPG task which targeted their impaired forepaw (Figure 4A). There was no difference between FMT or vehicle treated rats in the number of attempts made to reach for the pellet, indicating that the FMT did not influence participation in rehabilitation (Figure 4C). There was a significant decrease in success rate following SCI, which gradually improved for both vehicle and FMT groups throughout the rehabilitation period (Figure 4D). To prevent compensatory pellet-scooping strategies, rats were tested in a modified task where a gap was introduced between the pellet and the training chamber (Figure 4B). There was a trend for FMT rats to perform better in the gap test at the end of the rehabilitation period, however this did not reach statistical significance ($p = 0.089$) (Figure 4E). FMT treatment did not alter mechanical sensitivity, however both groups experienced reduced sensitivity of the ipsilesional forepaw at 7 and 63 days post injury (Figure 4F). At the end of the rehabilitative training period, rats were tested in the cylinder task to measure forepaw asymmetry and in the open field to assess locomotor activity; there were no differences between groups in either of these tests (Figure 4G,H). Although there was no significant treatment effect in the efficacy of rehabilitative training or motor recovery following SCI, treatment with FMT from *anxious* donors resulted in a chronic (77 days post injury) decrease in the percentage area of IBA+ immunoreactivity caudal to ($p = 0.046$), but not rostral to or at, the lesion site compared to vehicle controls (Figure 5A–F). This decreased area of IBA+ cells was not due to differences in injury size, as the lesion extension and area were similar between groups (Figure 5G–I).

3.4. FMT from Anxious Donors Increased Anxiety-Like Behaviour

At the end of rehabilitative training, rats were tested for depressive- and anxiety-like behaviours. Rats that received an FMT from *anxious* donors spent significantly less time in the open arms of the elevated plus maze ($p = 0.0341$), although both groups travelled a similar total distance (Figure 6A–C). The magnitude of differences between groups in the open arms is less than that observed between *anxious* and non-*anxious* FMT donors (Figure 2D). Furthermore, SCI + vehicle rats displayed less anxiety-like behaviour than untreated SCI control rats in our previous study [2], which may be due to the daily rehabilitative training received in the present study. There was also a trend for the SCI + FMT group to spend less time in the light component of the light-dark box (Figure 6D) and they drank significantly less sucrose solution ($p < 0.0001$) (Figure 6E) compared to vehicle controls. Both FMT and vehicle groups spent a similar amount of time interacting in the social interaction test (Figure 6F).

3.5. Temporal Profile of Plasma Analytes Following Spinal Cord Injury

To determine the effect of both SCI and the FMT on acute and chronic systemic inflammation, plasma analytes were measured before SCI, then 3, 21 and 77 days after injury. There was an overall trend of increased levels of all plasma analytes at 3- and 21-days post SCI, and a drastic downregulation by 77 days in both experimental groups (Figure 7). Looking at the concentrations of each plasma analyte over time, rats which received the FMT displayed significantly increased concentration of LIX at 77 days ($p = 0.009$), reduced levels of RANTES at 21 days ($p = 0.012$) and higher levels of RANTES by 77 days post injury ($p = 0.023$) (Figure 8B). There was no significant treatment effect in any of the other chemokines, cytokines or other analytes measured (growth factors, glycoproteins and the hormone leptin) (Figure 8A,C).

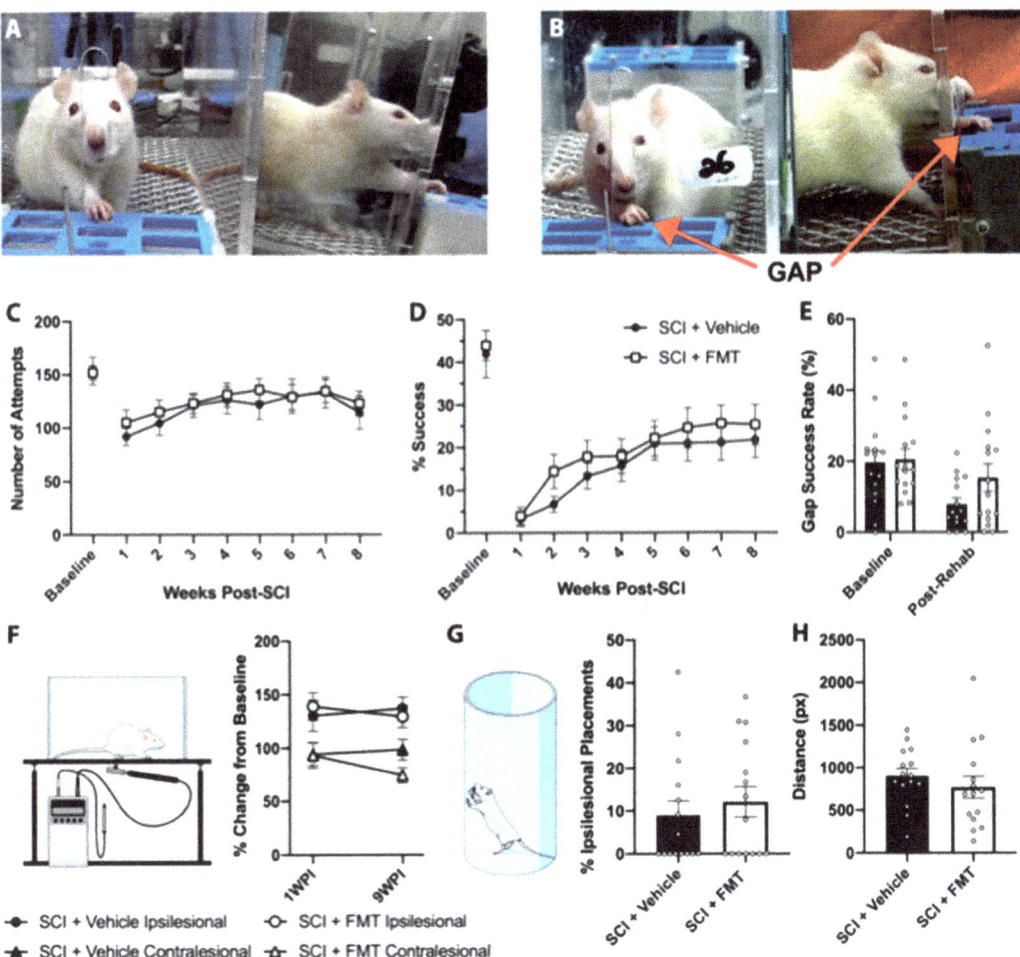

Figure 4. FMT from *anxious* rats did not significantly affect motor recovery following spinal cord injury. (**A**) Image of a rat in the regular single pellet grasping apparatus, reaching through a narrow opening for a food pellet. (**B**) Image of a rat reaching in the single pellet grasping apparatus that has been modified to include a gap between the pellet and the opening of the chamber (to eliminate compensatory pellet scooping behaviour). (**C**) There was no difference between FMT and vehicle groups in the number of attempts or (**D**) the success rate in rehabilitative training. (**E**) The success rate in the modified gap task was measured once at baseline and again at the end of the rehabilitation period. There were no significant differences between FMT and vehicle treated groups in the von frey test (quantified as the force required to elicit a withdrawal response, expressed as a percentage of baseline values) (**F**) the cylinder test (**G**) or the distance travelled in the open field (**H**). Error bars represent standard error mean.

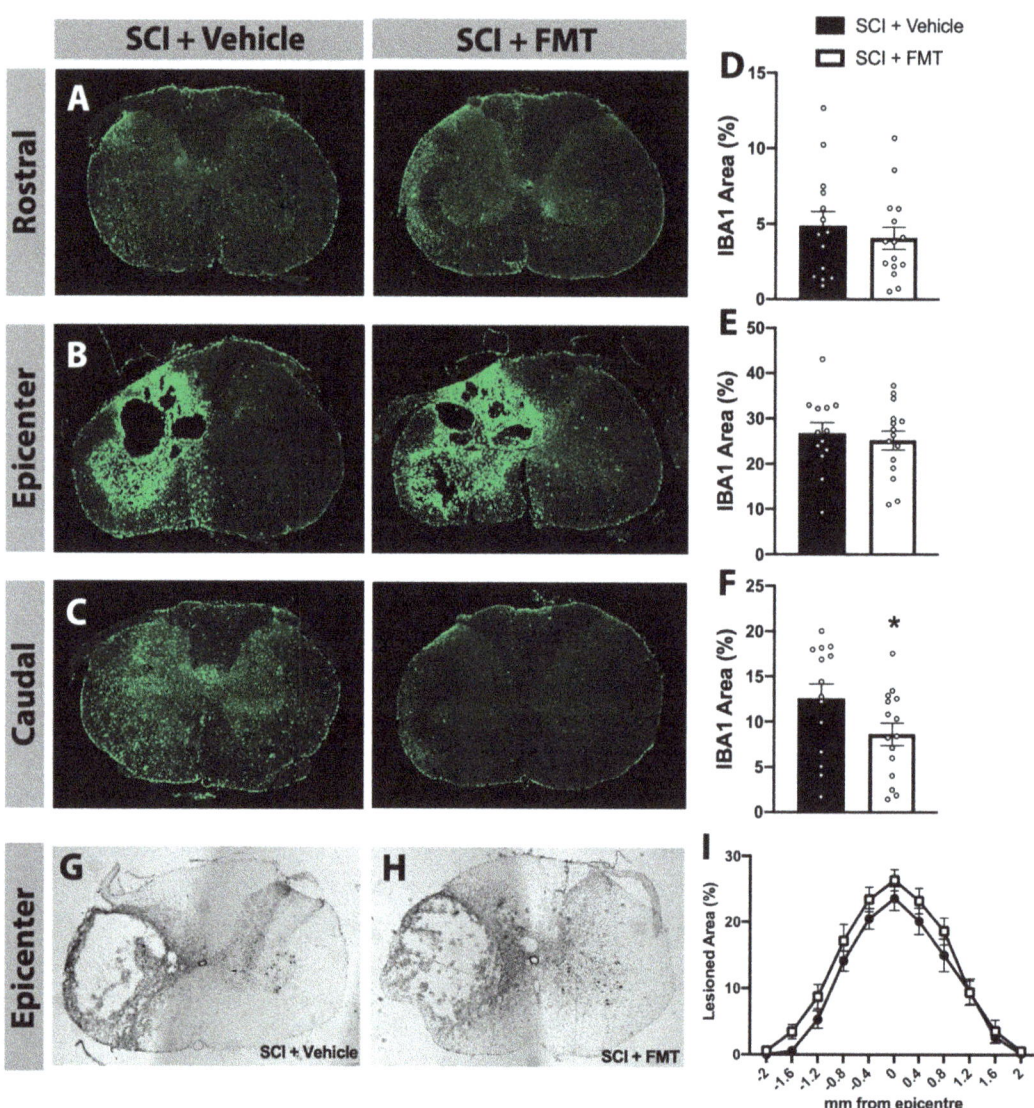

Figure 5. FMT from *anxious* donors reduced the area of IBA1+ cells caudal to the injury. Representative images of IBA1+ positive cells in the cervical spinal cord immediately rostral to the injury (**A**), at the injury epicenter (**B**) and immediately caudal to the injury (**C**). The percentage of IBA1+ area per spinal cord cross section rostral to, at and caudal to the lesion is quantified in (**D**–**F**), respectively. Immediately caudal to the injury, SCI + FMT rats displayed significantly reduced IBA1+ area compared to vehicle controls. Representative cross sections of the maximum injury site for SCI + Vehicle and SCI + FMT groups are shown in (**G**,**H**), respectively. (**I**) Quantification of the rostral (negative measurements) to caudal (positive measurements) extension of the lesion area was expressed as a percentage of lesioned tissue. * $p < 0.05$. Error bars represent standard error mean.

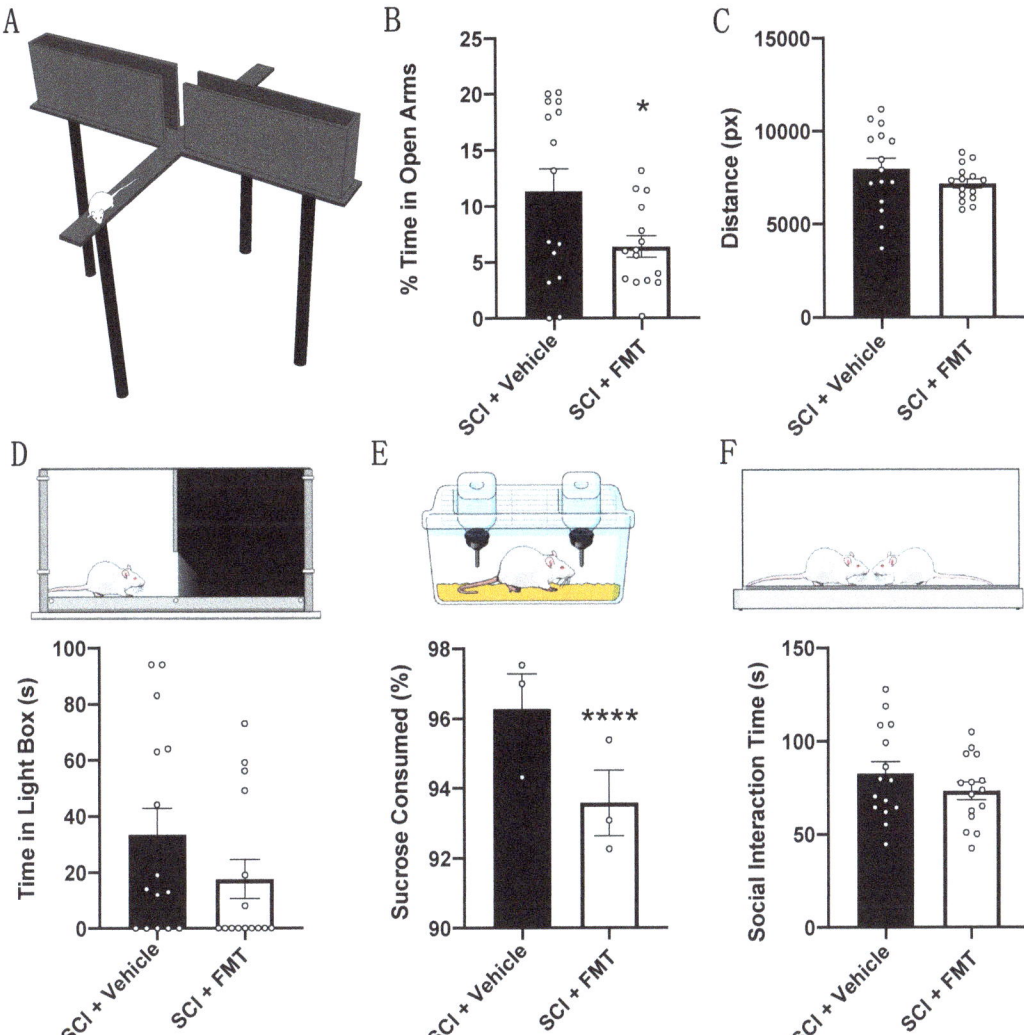

Figure 6. FMT from *anxious* donors resulted in a chronic increase in anxiety-like behaviour after SCI. At the end of rehabilitative training, rats were tested for anxiety-like and depressive-like behaviours. (**A**) Schematic of a rat in the open arm of the elevated plus maze. (**B**) SCI + FMT rats spent significantly less time in the open arms compared to untreated rats. (**C**) Both groups of rats travelled a similar amount of distance in the elevated plus maze. (**D**) SCI + FMT rats spent less time in the light-component of the light-dark box and (**E**) drank less sucrose water than untreated rats (each data point represents a cage containing 5 rats, each of which were considered for statistical analyses). (**F**) Both fecal transplant treated and untreated rats spent a similar amount of time interacting in the social interaction test. * $p < 0.05$, **** $p < 0.0001$. Error bars represent standard error mean.

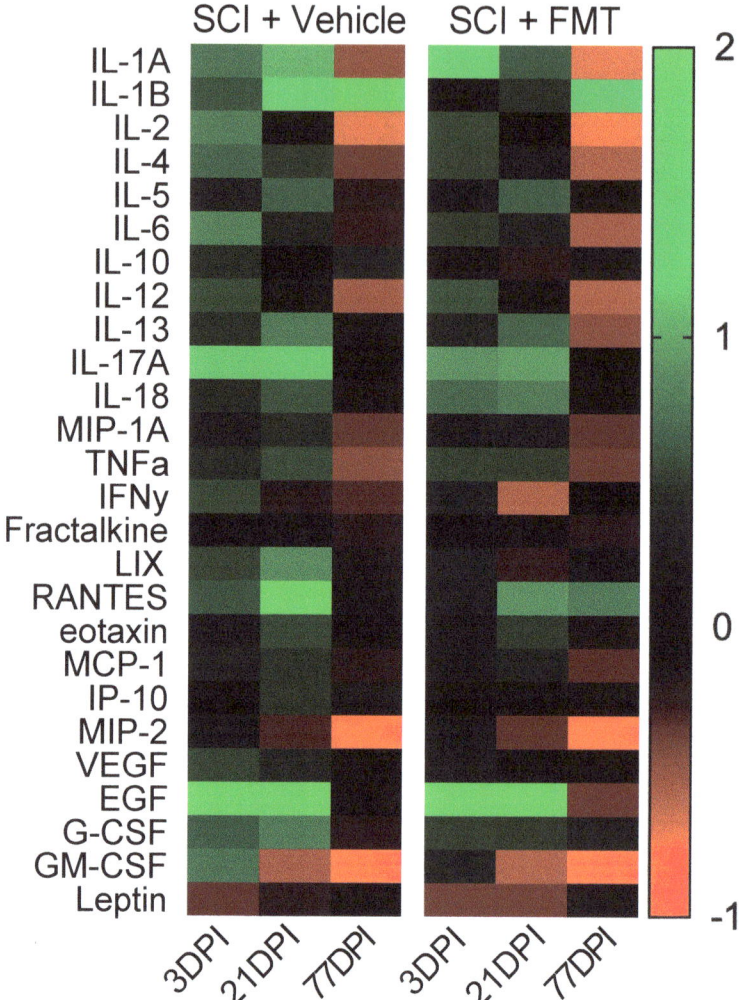

Figure 7. Heatmap of plasma markers over time following SCI. Plasma markers (cytokines, chemokines, growth factors, glycoproteins and hormones) were expressed as a change from baseline values and plotted over time (positive numbers represent an increase from baseline values and negative numbers represent a decrease from baseline values). Values above 2 were set at 2 for visualization purposes (RANTES and EGF were affected).

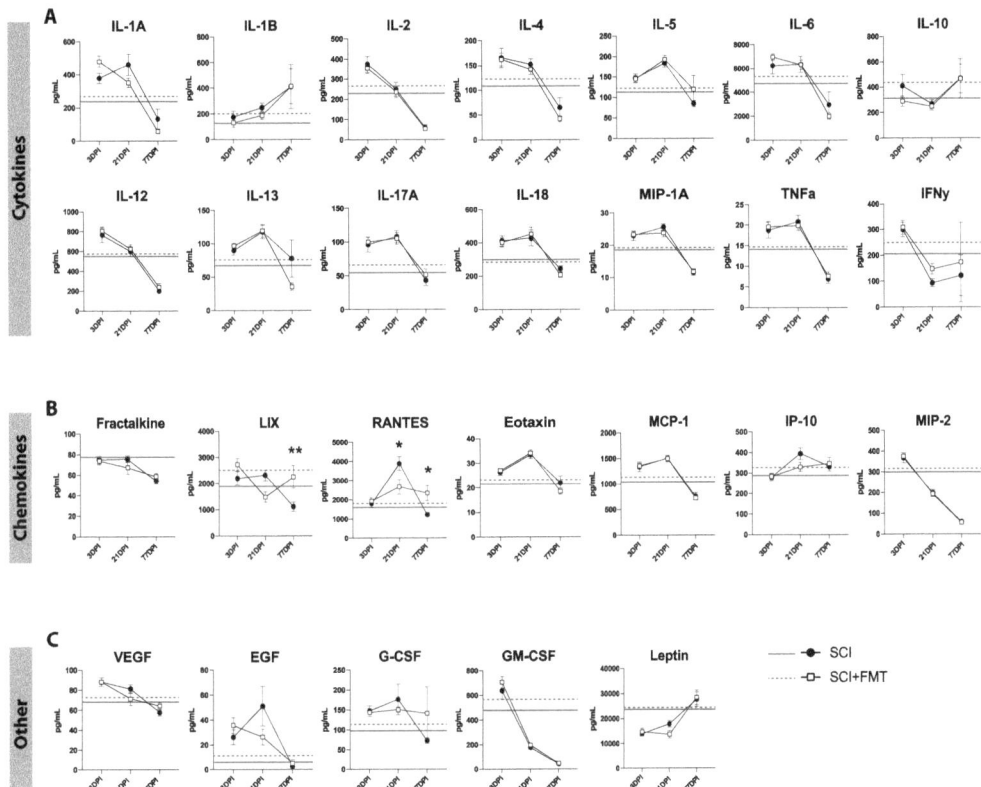

Figure 8. SCI induced time-dependent changes in plasma cytokines and chemokines. (**A**) Temporal profile of plasma cytokines 3 days post injury (3DPI), 21 days post injury (21DPI) and days post injury (77DPI) for SCI + Vehicle and SCI + FMT groups. (**B**) Temporal profile of plasma chemokines show that SCI + FMT rats have significantly increased levels of LIX and RANTES at 77 days compared to vehicle controls. (**C**) Profile of other plasma markers (growth factors, glycoproteins and hormones) over time after injury. Red lines represent baseline values. * $p < 0.05$. ** $p < 0.01$. Error bars represent standard error mean.

3.6. FMT from Anxious Donors Increased Intestinal Permeability

Increased intestinal barrier permeability has previously been shown in mice 7 days following a thoracic SCI, which can allow bacterial and other matter to translocate across the impaired epithelial tight junctions [4,36]. To test whether a cervical contusion SCI in rats also triggers an increase in intestinal permeability, rats were gavaged with FITC-dextran and the concentration of FITC was measured in blood 4 h later (Figure 9A). This test was performed before SCI and again 7 days later and expressed as a fold change from baseline to account for individual differences. SCI alone did not alter intestinal permeability, however FMT from *anxious* donors increased intestinal permeability by nearly 20% compared to baseline (SCI + Vehicle vs. SCI + FMT $p = 0.043$) (Figure 9B). This increased intestinal permeability was not due to differences in lesion size (Figure 9C). To determine whether differences in intestinal permeability between groups was associated with changes in systemic inflammation at the same time, plasma cytokines/chemokines were analyzed in these rats 7 days post injury. There was no difference between FMT or vehicle controls in plasma concentrations of cytokines, chemokines, or other growth factors, glycoproteins and hormones (Figure 9D–F).

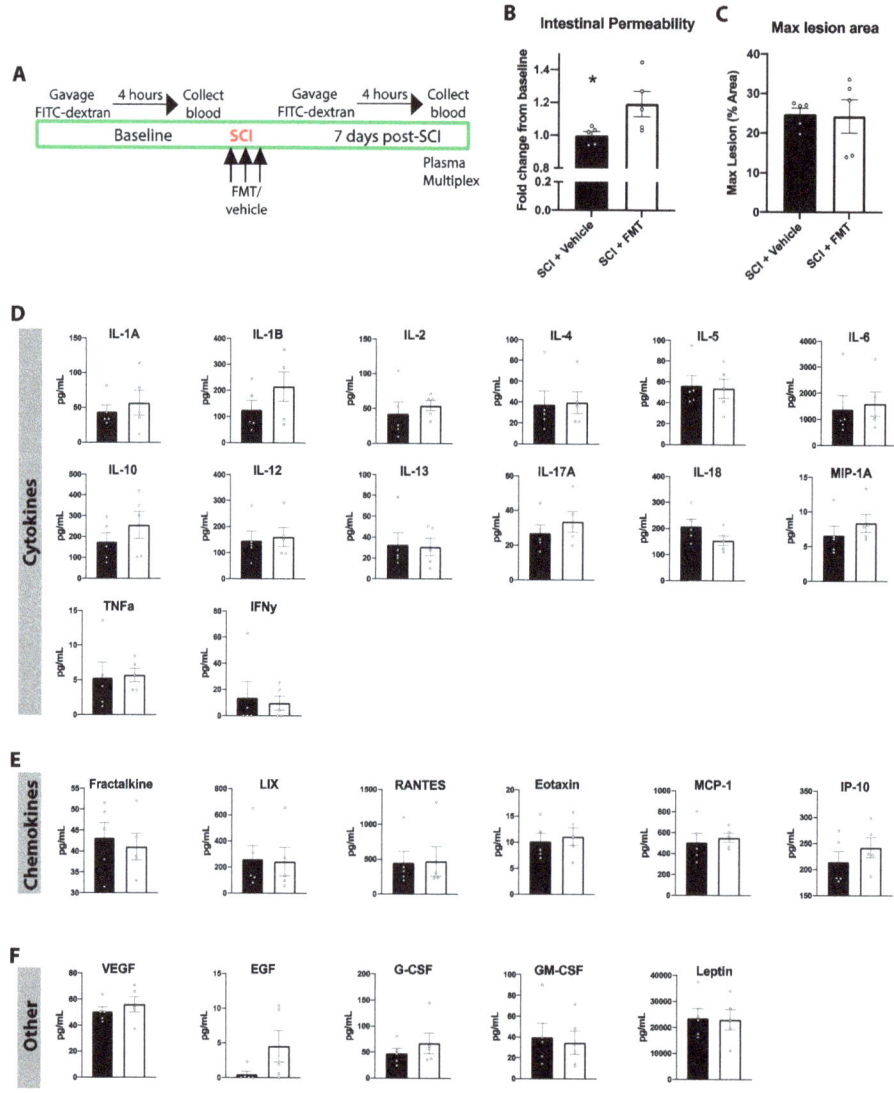

Figure 9. FMT from *anxious* donors increased intestinal permeability. (**A**) The FITC-dextran test for intestinal permeability was performed at baseline prior to spinal cord injury and again 7 days after injury. (**B**) SCI + FMT rats displayed significantly increased intestinal permeability relative to vehicle controls. (**C**) There were no differences between groups in the maximum lesion size. 7 days following injury, plasma was extracted and analyzed for levels of various cytokines (**D**), chemokines (**E**) and other growth factors, glycoproteins and hormones (**F**). * $p < 0.05$. Error bars represent standard error mean.

4. Discussion

The use of healthy human stool to treat diseases has been documented in Chinese medicine for over 1700 years [37]. However, the first report of FMT treatment in modern Western medicine was not until 1958 [38], and it was not until 2013 that FMT was included in the treatment guidelines for recurrent *Clostridium difficile* infections [39]. The popularity of FMT as a treatment is increasing rapidly for various other diseases, such as: irritable bowel disease, irritable bowel syndrome, obesity, autism, Parkinson's disease, multiple sclerosis, metabolic syndrome, stroke and SCI [2,8,14,40–48]. Aside from excluding donors with known fecal matter pathogens, the selection of FMT donor does not appear to influence the success of treatment for *Clostridium difficile* infection [9,21]. However, the same is not necessarily true for other disorders, especially those with more complicated microbiota-disease interactions such as SCI. Donor selection criteria beyond the exclusion of known pathogens is therefore a crucial area of research that is still in its infancy [15,19].

Previously we have shown that FMT from uninjured, non-*anxious* rats prevented both acute dysbiosis and the development of anxiety-like behaviour following SCI [2]. Contrary to our hypothesis, here we show that optimal donor selection is essential for successful (i.e., prevents SCI-induced dysbiosis) FMT treatment following SCI. Critically, the FMT donor rats in the present study were uninjured, free of pathogens and are genetically compatible to the recipients and would likely have passed screening criteria used clinically for FMT donors. In FMT trials, potential donors undergo a preliminary interview to rule out potential risk factors such as drug use and medical history [15,19,49–51]. Individuals who pass the preliminary interview then undergo blood and stool testing to exclude the risk for transferring infectious diseases [15,19,50,51]. Although a history of psychiatric conditions is a risk factor for potential FMT donors [52], it is often not considered for donor screening [15,19,49–51]. This is particularly relevant for studies on the efficacy of FMT for depression and anxiety. While there are relatively few human studies on FMT for treating psychiatric disorders, the existing results show short-term success but inconsistent long-term improvement [53–57]. The results of the present study in rats suggest that even minor behavioural abnormalities can impact the success of FMT and may help explain the inconsistent long-term results of FMT treatment for psychiatric disorders. Indeed, multiple animal studies show that the behaviour of the FMT donor can be transferred to the recipient [58–62].

In the present study, the FMT donors had increased baseline levels of anxiety-like behaviour which was associated with a significant reduction in the proportion of *Lactobacillus* in their stool. Although a causal relationship between gut bacteria and the development of mental health disorders has not been shown, many studies have found a strong association between the two. For example, humans diagnosed with major depressive disorder have reduced levels of *Lactobacillus* compared to controls [63]. Furthermore, *Lactobacillus* is one of the most frequently used probiotic bacteria and has been shown to improve anxiety and depression in multiple preclinical studies [64–66] and clinical trials [67–69]. In a recent double-blind, randomized, placebo controlled study, treatment with the probiotic *Lactobacillus* was shown to significantly reduce kynurenine concentrations in patients with major depressive disorder [70]. The kynurenine pathway can be activated by inflammation and is thought to play a significant role in the pathogenesis of depression [71,72]. Reducing kynurenine concentrations by blocking indoleamine 2,3-dioxygenase (the rate-limiting enzyme in the kynurenine pathway of tryptophan metabolism [73]) has also been shown to block lipopolysaccharide (LPS) induced depressive-like behaviour in rodents [74]. The kynurenine pathway may therefore be an important player in the microbiota-immune-brain axis involved in the pathogenesis of depression and anxiety following SCI. The lack of *Lactobacillus* present in the FMT donor stool may indicate alterations in the kynurenine pathway and be, at least, partly responsible for the unsuccessful FMT. However, there were no significant differences between FMT and vehicle groups in the proportion of *Lactobacillus* following SCI at the time points measured. More detailed sequencing may be required to detect differences at the species level, as there are over 260 metabolically unique *Lactobacillus* strains and only some species are used in probiotics [34,75]. Nonetheless, sequencing at the Phylum level indicated a global acute shift in the microbiota composition on the day of injury and 3 days post-SCI which returned to baseline by 35 days, similar to previously reported [2]. However, in the present study, using FMT from *anxious* donors with low levels of *Lactobacillus* was unsuccessful in preventing SCI-induced dysbiosis.

Although the FMT from *anxious* donors used in the present study did not improve SCI-induced dysbiosis, there were some long-term effects on inflammation and anxiety-like behaviour. There is a strong link between increased inflammation and the development of mental health disorders [76,77]. In rodent models of SCI, increased local (brain and spinal cord tissue) and systemic inflammation have been associated with the development of anxiety and depressive-like behaviours [78,79]. Here, rats that received the FMT from *anxious* donors displayed increased anxiety-like behaviour, which may suggest an increased inflammatory phenotype. In support of this, FMT from *anxious* donors resulted in increased intestinal permeability measured 7 days after SCI. As a potential confound to this test, the intestinal permeability assay was run in rats with increased baseline levels of anxiety-like behaviour. Since stress itself can alter intestinal permeability, this may explain why we did not observe a change in intestinal permeability following SCI in control rats. Nonetheless, FMT from *anxious* donors increased the gut permeability of FMT recipient rats, which can allowed bacterial matter such as LPS to translocate across the impaired epithelial tight junctions [4,80]. Once in circulation, LPS triggers a strong immune response that can reach the central nervous system and last for months after exposure [81,82]. Recently, we showed that systemic injection of LPS following cervical SCI in rats induced a chronic increase in anxiety-like behaviour in the elevated plus maze [83]. Furthermore, rats that received LPS displayed enhanced recovery in rehabilitative training and a paradoxical reduction in microglial and astrocyte density around the lesion site [83]. Similar findings were observed in the present study; although not statistically significant, FMT treated rats displayed improved motor recovery in the modified gap test. Additionally, in line with our previous research, we found that the increased anxiety-like behaviour did not interfere with willingness of the rats to participate in rehabilitative training (as evidenced by their similar attempt rates across groups) [83]. Furthermore, rats that received the FMT also displayed significantly reduced area of IBA1+ cells caudal to the lesion site. These parallels between LPS and treatment with FMT from *anxious* donors provide credence to the hypothesis that the long-term side effects of FMT from *anxious* donors are a result of endotoxin translocation from a permeable intestinal barrier [36]. Although we did not measure systemic LPS, the chemokines LIX and RANTES (both of which are upregulated by LPS) were significantly increased in FMT treated rats 77 days after injury. RANTES mediates the trafficking of immune cells such as T cells, monocytes, natural killer cells and mast cells, whereas LIX is best known for recruiting neutrophils [84,85]; both chemokines are associated with a variety of inflammatory disorders. Therefore, increased concentrations of LIX and RANTES may suggest a chronic systemic inflammatory state compared to vehicle controls, however, further evidence would be required to substantiate this claim. In both groups, we observed a significant increase in both pro-inflammatory and anti-inflammatory cytokines and chemokines at 3 and 21 days after SCI. This is likely due to the acute systemic inflammatory response initiated following trauma to the spinal cord [86,87]. By 77 days, both FMT and vehicle groups displayed a drastic downregulation in the majority of inflammatory cytokines, which may reflect a symptom of SCI-induced immune depression [88]. This immune depression is hypothesized to be triggered by sympathetic dysregulation associated with upper thoracic and cervical SCIs and generally takes time to develop following injury [89,90].

5. Conclusions

In conclusion, these results highlight the importance of optimal donor selection for successful FMT treatment following SCI. Although the FMT donors were otherwise healthy and pathogen free, they displayed naturally increased anxiety-like behaviour and reduced proportions of *Lactobacillus*. FMT from these *anxious* donors did not prevent SCI-induced dysbiosis and had some negative side effects including increased intestinal permeability, increased anxiety-like behaviour, and minor yet chronic alterations in both local and systemic inflammation. Future work should investigate whether specific bacteria (such as *Lactobacillus*) are required for successful FMT as well as the optimal timing and dosage of treatment. While recipient safety must prevail above all, vigilant donor selection beyond the exclusion of known pathogens is essential to improve the success of FMT as shown here in the context of SCI.

Supplementary Materials: The following are available online at https://www.mdpi.com/2079-7737/10/4/254/s1, Figure S1: Percent time in the open arms of the elevated plus maze compared between anxious FMT donors, non-anxious FMT donors, and two other cohorts of rats from previous experiments. Figures S2 and S3: Microbiota changes at the genus level.

Author Contributions: Conceptualization, K.F. and E.K.A.S.; methodology, E.K.A.S., P.J.F.R., K.L.M., K.K.F. and K.F.; formal analysis, E.K.A.S., G.K., and K.L.M.; resources, K.F. and K.L.M.; data curation, E.K.A.S.; writing—original draft preparation, E.K.A.S.; writing—review and editing, E.K.A.S., P.J.F.R., K.K.F. and K.F.; visualization, E.K.A.S.; supervision, K.F.; project administration, E.K.A.S. and P.J.F.R.; funding acquisition, K.F. All authors have read and agreed to the published version of the manuscript.

Funding: This research was funded by the Craig Neilsen Foundation, grant number NPRG 542589.

Institutional Review Board Statement: This study received research ethics approval from the University of Alberta Research Ethics Board, Project Name: "Repairing the injured spinal cord", AUP00000254, 22 December 2020.

Informed Consent Statement: Not applicable.

Data Availability Statement: The data presented in this study are openly available from at https://scicrunch.org/odc-sci, accessed on 1 September 2020 (DOI: 10.34945/F5XW2P).

Conflicts of Interest: The authors declare no conflict of interest.

References

1. Simpson, L.A.; Eng, J.J.; Hsieh, J.T.; Dalton, L. Wolfe And The Spinal Cord Injury Spinal Cord Injury Rehabilitation Evidence Scire Research Team The Health and Life Priorities of Individuals with Spinal Cord Injury: A Systematic Review. *J. Neurotrauma* **2012**, *29*, 1548–1555. [CrossRef] [PubMed]
2. Schmidt, E.K.A.; Torres-Espin, A.; Raposo, P.J.F.; Madsen, K.L.; Kigerl, K.A.; Popovich, P.G.; Fenrich, K.K.; Fouad, K. Fecal transplant prevents gut dysbiosis and anxiety-like behaviour after spinal cord injury in rats. *PLoS ONE* **2020**, *15*, e0226128. [CrossRef] [PubMed]
3. Sun, X.; Jones, Z.B.; Chen, X.-M.; Zhou, L.; So, K.-F.; Ren, Y. Multiple organ dysfunction and systemic inflammation after spinal cord injury: A complex relationship. *J. Neuroinflamm.* **2016**, *13*, 260. [CrossRef] [PubMed]
4. Kigerl, K.A.; Hall, J.C.; Wang, L.; Mo, X.; Yu, Z.; Popovich, P.G. Gut dysbiosis impairs recovery after spinal cord injury. *J. Exp. Med.* **2016**, *213*, 2603–2620. [CrossRef]
5. Jogia, T.; Ruitenberg, M.J. Traumatic Spinal Cord Injury and the Gut Microbiota: Current Insights and Future Challenges. *Front. Immunol.* **2020**, *11*, 704. [CrossRef] [PubMed]
6. Bakken, J.S.; Borody, T.; Brandt, L.J.; Brill, J.V.; Demarco, D.C.; Franzos, M.A.; Kelly, C.; Khoruts, A.; Louie, T.; Martinelli, L.P.; et al. Treating *Clostridium difficile* Infection With Fecal Microbiota Transplantation. *Clin. Gastroenterol. Hepatol.* **2011**, *9*, 1044–1049. [CrossRef]
7. Smits, L.P.; Bouter, K.E.; de Vos, W.M.; Borody, T.J.; Nieuwdorp, M. Therapeutic Potential of Fecal Microbiota Transplantation. *Gastroenterology* **2013**, *145*, 946–953. [CrossRef]
8. Xu, D.; Chen, V.L.; Steiner, C.A.; Berinstein, J.A.; Eswaran, S.; Waljee, A.K.; Higgins, P.D.; Owyang, C. Efficacy of Fecal Microbiota Transplantation in Irritable Bowel Syndrome: A Systematic Review and Meta-Analysis. *Am. J. Gastroenterol.* **2019**, *114*, 1043–1050. [CrossRef]
9. Kassam, Z.; Lee, C.H.; Yuan, Y.; Hunt, R.H. Fecal Microbiota Transplantation for *Clostridium difficile* Infection: Systematic Review and Meta-Analysis. *Am. J. Gastroenterol.* **2013**, *108*, 500–508. [CrossRef]
10. Kang, D.-W.; Park, J.G.; Ilhan, Z.E.; Wallstrom, G.; LaBaer, J.; Adams, J.B.; Krajmalnik-Brown, R. Reduced Incidence of Prevotella and Other Fermenters in Intestinal Microflora of Autistic Children. *PLoS ONE* **2013**, *8*, e68322. [CrossRef]
11. He, Z.; Cui, B.-T.; Zhang, T.; Li, P.; Long, C.-Y.; Ji, G.-Z.; Zhang, F.-M. Fecal microbiota transplantation cured epilepsy in a case with Crohn's disease: The first report. *World J. Gastroenterol.* **2017**, *23*, 3565–3568. [CrossRef]
12. Zhao, H.; Shi, Y.; Luo, X.; Peng, L.; Yang, Y.; Zou, L. The Effect of Fecal Microbiota Transplantation on a Child with Tourette Syndrome. *Case Rep. Med.* **2017**, *2017*, 6165239. [CrossRef] [PubMed]
13. Borody, T.; Leis, S.; Campbell, J.; Torres, M.; Nowak, A. Fecal Microbiota Transplantation (FMT) in Multiple Sclerosis (MS). *Am. J. Gastroenterol.* **2011**, *106*, S352. [CrossRef]
14. Huang, H.; Xu, H.; Luo, Q.; He, J.; Li, M.; Chen, H.; Tang, W.; Nie, Y.; Zhou, Y. Fecal microbiota transplantation to treat Parkinson's disease with constipation: A Case Report. *Medicine* **2019**, *98*, e16605. [CrossRef]
15. Duvallet, C.; Zellmer, C.; Panchal, P.; Budree, S.; Osman, M.; Alm, E.J. Framework for rational donor selection in fecal microbiota transplant clinical trials. *PLoS ONE* **2019**, *14*, e0222881. [CrossRef] [PubMed]
16. Paramsothy, S.; Kamm, M.A.; Kaakoush, N.O.; Walsh, A.J.; Van Den Bogaerde, J.; Samuel, D.; Leong, R.W.L.; Connor, S.; Ng, W.; Paramsothy, R.; et al. Multidonor intensive faecal microbiota transplantation for active ulcerative colitis: A randomised placebo-controlled trial. *Lancet* **2017**, *389*, 1218–1228. [CrossRef]

17. Bafeta, A.; Yavchitz, A.; Riveros, C.; Batista, R.; Ravaud, P. Methods and Reporting Studies Assessing Fecal Microbiota Transplantation: A Systematic Review. *Ann. Intern. Med.* **2017**, *167*, 34–39. [CrossRef] [PubMed]
18. Van Nood, E.; Vrieze, A.; Nieuwdorp, M.; Fuentes, S.; Zoetendal, E.G.; De Vos, W.M.; Visser, C.E.; Kuijper, E.J.; Bartelsman, J.F.W.M.; Tijssen, J.G.P.; et al. Duodenal Infusion of Donor Feces for Recurrent *Clostridium difficile*. *N. Engl. J. Med.* **2013**, *368*, 407–415. [CrossRef]
19. Barnes, D.; Park, K.T. Donor Considerations in Fecal Microbiota Transplantation. *Curr. Gastroenterol. Rep.* **2017**, *19*, 10. [CrossRef] [PubMed]
20. Food and Drug Administration Enforcement Policy Regarding Investigational New Drug Requirements for Use of Fecal Microbiota for Transplantation to Treat *Clostridium difficile* Infection Not Responsive to Standard Therapies. Available online: https://www.fda.gov/regulatory-information/search-fda-guidance-documents/enforcement-policy-regarding-investigational-new-drug-requirements-use-fecal-microbiota (accessed on 1 September 2020).
21. Osman, M.; Stoltzner, Z.; O'Brien, K.; Ling, K.; Koelsch, E.; Dubois, N.; Amaratunga, K.; Smith, M.; Kassam, Z. Donor Efficacy in Fecal Microbiota Transplantation for Recurrent *Clostridium difficile*: Evidence From a 1,999-Patient Cohort. *Open Forum Infect. Dis.* **2016**, *3*, 841. [CrossRef]
22. Kump, P.; Wurm, P.; Gröchenig, H.P.; Wenzl, H.; Petritsch, W.; Halwachs, B.; Wagner, M.; Stadlbauer, V.; Eherer, A.; Hoffmann, K.M.; et al. The taxonomic composition of the donor intestinal microbiota is a major factor influencing the efficacy of faecal microbiota transplantation in therapy refractory ulcerative colitis. *Aliment. Pharmacol. Ther.* **2018**, *47*, 67–77. [CrossRef]
23. Torres-Espín, A.; Forero, J.; Schmidt, E.K.; Fouad, K.; Fenrich, K.K. A motorized pellet dispenser to deliver high intensity training of the single pellet reaching and grasping task in rats. *Behav. Brain Res.* **2018**, *336*, 67–76. [CrossRef]
24. File, S.E. One-trial tolerance to the anxiolytic effects of chlordiazepoxide in the plus-maze. *Psychopharmacology* **1990**, *100*, 281–282. [CrossRef] [PubMed]
25. File, S.E.; Hyde, J. Can social interaction be used to measure anxiety? *Br. J. Pharmacol.* **1978**, *62*, 19–24. [CrossRef]
26. Kazerouni, A.; Wein, L.M. Exploring the Efficacy of Pooled Stools in Fecal Microbiota Transplantation for Microbiota-Associated Chronic Diseases. *PLoS ONE* **2017**, *12*, e0163956. [CrossRef] [PubMed]
27. Youngster, I.; Mahabamunuge, J.; Systrom, H.K.; Sauk, J.; Khalili, H.; Levin, J.; Kaplan, J.L.; Hohmann, E.L. Oral, frozen fecal microbiota transplant (FMT) capsules for recurrent *Clostridium difficile* infection. *BMC Med.* **2016**, *14*, 134. [CrossRef]
28. Laffin, M.; Fedorak, R.; Zalasky, A.; Park, H.; Gill, A.; Agrawal, A.; Keshteli, A.; Hotte, N.; Madsen, K.L. A high-sugar diet rapidly enhances susceptibility to colitis via depletion of luminal short-chain fatty acids in mice. *Sci. Rep.* **2019**, *9*, 12294. [CrossRef]
29. Callahan, B.J.; Mcmurdie, P.J.; Rosen, M.J.; Han, A.W.; Johnson, A.J.A.; Holmes, S.P. DADA2: High-resolution sample inference from Illumina amplicon data. *Nat. Methods* **2016**, *13*, 581–583. [CrossRef]
30. Bolyen, E.; Rideout, J.R.; Dillon, M.R.; Bokulich, N.A.; Abnet, C.C.; Al-Ghalith, G.A.; Alexander, H.; Alm, E.J.; Arumugam, M.; Asnicar, F.; et al. Reproducible, interactive, scalable and extensible microbiome data science using QIIME 2. *Nat. Biotechnol.* **2019**, *37*, 852–857. [CrossRef] [PubMed]
31. Russell, P.A. Relationships Between Exploratory Behaviour And Fear: A Review. *Br. J. Psychol.* **1973**, *64*, 417–433. [CrossRef]
32. Gould, T.D.; Dao, D.T.; Kovacsics, C.E. The Open Field Test. In *Mood and Anxiety Related Phenotypes in Mice*; Humana Press: Totowa, NJ, USA, 2009; Volume 42, pp. 1–20.
33. Sanders, M.E.; Klaenhammer, T.R. Invited Review: The Scientific Basis of Lactobacillus acidophilus NCFM Functionality as a Probiotic. *J. Dairy Sci.* **2001**, *84*, 319–331. [CrossRef]
34. Maragkoudakis, P.A.; Zoumpopoulou, G.; Miaris, C.; Kalantzopoulos, G.; Pot, B.; Tsakalidou, E. Probiotic potential of Lactobacillus strains isolated from dairy products. *Int. Dairy J.* **2006**, *16*, 189–199. [CrossRef]
35. Lebeer, S.; Vanderleyden, J.; De Keersmaecker, S.C.J. Genes and Molecules of Lactobacilli Supporting Probiotic Action. *Microbiol. Mol. Biol. Rev.* **2008**, *72*, 728–764. [CrossRef] [PubMed]
36. Ghosh, S.S.; Wang, J.; Yannie, P.J.; Ghosh, S. Intestinal Barrier Dysfunction, LPS Translocation, and Disease Development. *J. Endocr. Soc.* **2020**, *4*, bvz039. [CrossRef]
37. Zhang, F.; Luo, W.; Shi, Y.; Fan, Z.; Ji, G. Should We Standardize the 1,700-Year-Old Fecal Microbiota Transplantation? *Am. J. Gastroenterol.* **2012**, *107*, 1755. [CrossRef] [PubMed]
38. Eiseman, B.; Silen, W.; Bascom, G.S.; Kauvar, A.J. Fecal enema as an adjunct in the treatment of pseudomembranous enterocolitis. *Surgery* **1958**, *44*, 854–859. [PubMed]
39. Surawicz, C.M.; Brandt, L.J.; Binion, D.G.; Ananthakrishnan, A.N.; Curry, S.R.; Gilligan, P.H.; McFarland, L.V.; Mellow, M.; Zuckerbraun, B.S. Guidelines for Diagnosis, Treatment, and Prevention of *Clostridium difficile* Infections. *Am. J. Gastroenterol.* **2013**, *108*, 478–498. [CrossRef] [PubMed]
40. Sun, M.-F.; Zhu, Y.-L.; Zhou, Z.-L.; Jia, X.-B.; Xu, Y.-D.; Yang, Q.; Cui, C.; Shen, Y.-Q. Neuroprotective effects of fecal microbiota transplantation on MPTP-induced Parkinson's disease mice: Gut microbiota, glial reaction and TLR4/TNF-α signaling pathway. *Brain Behav. Immun.* **2018**, *70*, 48–60. [CrossRef] [PubMed]
41. Xue, L.-J.; Yang, X.-Z.; Tong, Q.; Shen, P.; Ma, S.-J.; Wu, S.-N.; Zheng, J.-L.; Wang, H.-G. Fecal microbiota transplantation therapy for Parkinson's disease: A Preliminary Study. *Medicine* **2020**, *99*, e22035. [CrossRef]
42. Imdad, A.; Nicholson, M.R.; Tanner-Smith, E.E.; Zackular, J.P.; Gomez-Duarte, O.G.; Beaulieu, D.B.; Acra, S. Fecal transplantation for treatment of inflammatory bowel disease. *Cochrane Database Syst. Rev.* **2018**, *11*, CD012774. [CrossRef]

43. Borody, T.J.; Eslick, G.D.; Clancy, R.L. Fecal microbiota transplantation as a new therapy: From Clostridioides difficile infection to inflammatory bowel disease, irritable bowel syndrome, and colon cancer. *Curr. Opin. Pharmacol.* **2019**, *49*, 43–51. [CrossRef] [PubMed]
44. Chen, R.; Xu, Y.; Wu, P.; Zhou, H.; Lasanajak, Y.; Fang, Y.; Tang, L.; Ye, L.; Li, X.; Cai, Z.; et al. Transplantation of fecal microbiota rich in short chain fatty acids and butyric acid treat cerebral ischemic stroke by regulating gut microbiota. *Pharmacol. Res.* **2019**, *148*, 104403. [CrossRef] [PubMed]
45. Marotz, C.A.; Zarrinpar, A. Treating Obesity and Metabolic Syndrome with Fecal Microbiota Transplantation. *Yale J. Biol. Med.* **2016**, *89*, 383–388. [PubMed]
46. De Groot, P.F.; Frissen, M.N.; De Clercq, N.C.; Nieuwdorp, M. Fecal microbiota transplantation in metabolic syndrome: History, present and future. *Gut Microbes* **2017**, *8*, 253–267. [CrossRef] [PubMed]
47. Kang, D.-W.; Adams, J.B.; Gregory, A.C.; Borody, T.; Chittick, L.; Fasano, A.; Khoruts, A.; Geis, E.; Maldonado, J.; McDonough-Means, S.; et al. Microbiota Transfer Therapy alters gut ecosystem and improves gastrointestinal and autism symptoms: An open-label study. *Microbiome* **2017**, *5*, 10. [CrossRef]
48. Makkawi, S.; Camara-Lemarroy, C.; Metz, L. Fecal microbiota transplantation associated with 10 years of stability in a patient with SPMS. *Neurol. Neuroimmunol. Neuroinflamm.* **2018**, *5*, e459. [CrossRef] [PubMed]
49. Bibbò, S.; Settanni, C.R.; Porcari, S.; Bocchino, E.; Ianiro, G.; Cammarota, G.; Gasbarrini, A. Fecal Microbiota Transplantation: Screening and Selection to Choose the Optimal Donor. *J. Clin. Med.* **2020**, *9*, 1757. [CrossRef]
50. Woodworth, M.H.; Carpentieri, C.; Sitchenko, K.L.; Kraft, C.S. Challenges in fecal donor selection and screening for fecal microbiota transplantation: A review. *Gut Microbes* **2017**, *8*, 225–237. [CrossRef] [PubMed]
51. Wilson, B.C.; Vatanen, T.; Cutfield, W.S.; O'Sullivan, J.M. The Super-Donor Phenomenon in Fecal Microbiota Transplantation. *Front. Cell. Infect. Microbiol.* **2019**, *9*, 2. [CrossRef]
52. Cammarota, G.; Ianiro, G.; Tilg, H.; Rajilić-Stojanović, M.; Kump, P.; Satokari, R.; Sokol, H.; Arkkila, P.; Pintus, C.; Hart, A.; et al. European consensus conference on faecal microbiota transplantation in clinical practice. *Gut* **2017**, *66*, 569–580. [CrossRef]
53. Mizuno, S.; Masaoka, T.; Naganuma, M.; Kishimoto, T.; Kitazawa, M.; Kurokawa, S.; Nakashima, M.; Takeshita, K.; Suda, W.; Mimura, M.; et al. Bifidobacterium-Rich Fecal Donor May Be a Positive Predictor for Successful Fecal Microbiota Transplantation in Patients with Irritable Bowel Syndrome. *Digestion* **2017**, *96*, 29–38. [CrossRef]
54. Kurokawa, S.; Kishimoto, T.; Mizuno, S.; Masaoka, T.; Naganuma, M.; Liang, K.-C.; Kitazawa, M.; Nakashima, M.; Shindo, C.; Suda, W.; et al. The effect of fecal microbiota transplantation on psychiatric symptoms among patients with irritable bowel syndrome, functional diarrhea and functional constipation: An open-label observational study. *J. Affect. Disord.* **2018**, *235*, 506–512. [CrossRef]
55. Mazzawi, T.; Lied, G.A.; Sangnes, D.A.; El-Salhy, M.; Hov, J.R.; Gilja, O.H.; Hatlebakk, J.G.; Hausken, T. The kinetics of gut microbial community composition in patients with irritable bowel syndrome following fecal microbiota transplantation. *PLoS ONE* **2018**, *13*, e0194904. [CrossRef]
56. Paramsothy, S.; Borody, T.J.; Lin, E.; Finlayson, S.; Walsh, A.J.; Samuel, D.; Van Den Bogaerde, J.; Leong, R.W.L.; Connor, S.; Ng, W.; et al. Donor Recruitment for Fecal Microbiota Transplantation. *Inflamm. Bowel Dis.* **2015**, *21*, 1600–1606. [CrossRef] [PubMed]
57. Huang, H.L.; Chen, H.T.; Luo, Q.L.; Xu, H.M.; He, J.; Li, Y.Q.; Zhou, Y.L.; Yao, F.; Nie, Y.Q.; Zhou, Y.J. Relief of irritable bowel syndrome by fecal microbiota transplantation is associated with changes in diversity and composition of the gut microbiota. *J. Dig. Dis.* **2019**, *20*, 401–408. [CrossRef]
58. Li, N.; Wang, Q.; Wang, Y.; Sun, A.; Lin, Y.; Jin, Y.; Li, X. Fecal microbiota transplantation from chronic unpredictable mild stress mice donors affects anxiety-like and depression-like behavior in recipient mice via the gut microbiota-inflammation-brain axis. *Stress* **2019**, *22*, 592–602. [CrossRef] [PubMed]
59. Lv, W.-J.; Wu, X.-L.; Chen, W.-Q.; Li, Y.-F.; Zhang, G.-F.; Chao, L.-M.; Zhou, J.-H.; Guo, A.; Liu, C.; Guo, S.-N. The Gut Microbiome Modulates the Changes in Liver Metabolism and in Inflammatory Processes in the Brain of Chronic Unpredictable Mild Stress Rats. *Oxidative Med. Cell. Longev.* **2019**, *2019*, 7902874. [CrossRef]
60. Siopi, E.; Chevalier, G.; Katsimpardi, L.; Saha, S.; Bigot, M.; Moigneu, C.; Eberl, G.; Lledo, P.-M. Changes in Gut Microbiota by Chronic Stress Impair the Efficacy of Fluoxetine. *Cell Rep.* **2020**, *30*, 3682–3690.e6. [CrossRef] [PubMed]
61. Kelly, J.R.; Borre, Y.; Brien, C.O.; Patterson, E.; El Aidy, S.; Deane, J.; Kennedy, P.J.; Beers, S.; Scott, K.; Moloney, G.; et al. Transferring the blues: Depression-associated gut microbiota induces neurobehavioural changes in the rat. *J. Psychiatr. Res.* **2016**, *82*, 109–118. [CrossRef] [PubMed]
62. Zhao, W.; Hu, Y.; Li, C.; Li, N.; Zhu, S.; Tan, X.; Li, M.; Zhang, Y.; Xu, Z.; Ding, Z.; et al. Transplantation of fecal microbiota from patients with alcoholism induces anxiety/depression behaviors and decreases brain mGluR1/PKC ε levels in mouse. *BioFactors* **2020**, *46*, 38–54. [CrossRef]
63. Aizawa, E.; Tsuji, H.; Asahara, T.; Takahashi, T.; Teraishi, T.; Yoshida, S.; Ota, M.; Koga, N.; Hattori, K.; Kunugi, H. Possible association of Bifidobacterium and Lactobacillus in the gut microbiota of patients with major depressive disorder. *J. Affect. Disord.* **2016**, *202*, 254–257. [CrossRef]
64. Liu, W.-H.; Chuang, H.-L.; Huang, Y.-T.; Wu, C.-C.; Chou, G.-T.; Wang, S.; Tsai, Y.-C. Alteration of behavior and monoamine levels attributable to Lactobacillus plantarum PS128 in germ-free mice. *Behav. Brain Res.* **2016**, *298*, 202–209. [CrossRef] [PubMed]
65. Liang, S.; Wang, T.; Hu, X.; Luo, J.; Li, W.; Wu, X.; Duan, Y.; Jin, F. Administration of Lactobacillus helveticus NS8 improves behavioral, cognitive, and biochemical aberrations caused by chronic restraint stress. *Neuroscience* **2015**, *310*, 561–577. [CrossRef] [PubMed]

66. Bravo, J.A.; Forsythe, P.; Chew, M.V.; Escaravage, E.; Savignac, H.M.; Dinan, T.G.; Bienenstock, J.; Cryan, J.F. Ingestion of Lactobacillus strain regulates emotional behavior and central GABA receptor expression in a mouse via the vagus nerve. *Proc. Natl. Acad. Sci. USA* **2011**, *108*, 16050–16055. [CrossRef] [PubMed]
67. Slykerman, R.F.; Hood, F.; Wickens, K.; Thompson, J.M.D.; Barthow, C.; Murphy, R.; Kang, J.; Rowden, J.; Stone, P.; Crane, J.; et al. Effect of Lactobacillus rhamnosus HN001 in Pregnancy on Postpartum Symptoms of Depression and Anxiety: A Randomised Double-blind Placebo-controlled Trial. *EBioMedicine* **2017**, *24*, 159–165. [CrossRef] [PubMed]
68. Lew, L.-C.; Hor, Y.-Y.; Yusoff, N.A.A.; Choi, S.-B.; Yusoff, M.S.; Roslan, N.S.; Ahmad, A.; Mohammad, J.A.; Abdullah, M.F.I.; Zakaria, N.; et al. Probiotic Lactobacillus plantarum P8 alleviated stress and anxiety while enhancing memory and cognition in stressed adults: A randomised, double-blind, placebo-controlled study. *Clin. Nutr.* **2019**, *38*, 2053–2064. [CrossRef] [PubMed]
69. Wallace, C.J.K.; Milev, R. Erratum to: The effects of probiotics on depressive symptoms in humans: A systematic review. *Ann. Gen. Psychiatry* **2017**, *16*, 18. [CrossRef] [PubMed]
70. Rudzki, L.; Ostrowska, L.; Pawlak, D.; Małus, A.; Pawlak, K.; Waszkiewicz, N.; Szulc, A. Probiotic Lactobacillus Plantarum 299v decreases kynurenine concentration and improves cognitive functions in patients with major depression: A double-blind, randomized, placebo controlled study. *Psychoneuroendocrinology* **2019**, *100*, 213–222. [CrossRef]
71. Ogyu, K.; Kubo, K.; Noda, Y.; Iwata, Y.; Tsugawa, S.; Omura, Y.; Wada, M.; Tarumi, R.; Plitman, E.; Moriguchi, S.; et al. Kynurenine pathway in depression: A systematic review and meta-analysis. *Neurosci. Biobehav. Rev.* **2018**, *90*, 16–25. [CrossRef]
72. Savitz, J. Role of Kynurenine Metabolism Pathway Activation in Major Depressive Disorders. In *Inflammation-Associated Depression: Evidence, Mechanisms and Implications*; Dantzer, R., Capuron, L., Eds.; Springer International Publishing: Cham, Switzerland, 2016; Volume 31, pp. 249–267. ISBN 978-3-319-51151-1.
73. Savitz, J. The kynurenine pathway: A finger in every pie. *Mol. Psychiatry* **2020**, *25*, 131–147. [CrossRef]
74. O'Connor, J.; Lawson, M.; André, C.; Moreau, M.; Lestage, J.; Castanon, N.; Kelley, K.; Dantzer, R. Lipopolysaccharide-induced depressive-like behavior is mediated by indoleamine 2,3-dioxygenase activation in mice. *Mol. Psychiatry* **2008**, *14*, 511–522. [CrossRef]
75. Zheng, J.; Wittouck, S.; Salvetti, E.; Franz, C.M.A.P.; Harris, H.M.B.; Mattarelli, P.; O'Toole, P.W.; Pot, B.; Vandamme, P.; Walter, J.; et al. A taxonomic note on the genus Lactobacillus: Description of 23 novel genera, emended description of the genus Lactobacillus Beijerinck 1901, and union of Lactobacillaceae and Leuconostocaceae. *Int. J. Syst. Evol. Microbiol.* **2020**, *70*, 2782–2858. [CrossRef]
76. Raison, C.L.; Capuron, L.; Miller, A.H. Cytokines sing the blues: Inflammation and the pathogenesis of depression. *Trends Immunol.* **2006**, *27*, 24–31. [CrossRef]
77. Miller, A.H.; Raison, C.L. The role of inflammation in depression: From evolutionary imperative to modern treatment target. *Nat. Rev. Immunol.* **2016**, *16*, 22–34. [CrossRef]
78. Do Espírito Santo, C.C.; da Silva Fiorin, F.; Ilha, J.; Duarte, M.M.M.F.; Duarte, T.; Santos, A.R.S. Spinal cord injury by clip-compression induces anxiety and depression-like behaviours in female rats: The role of the inflammatory response. *Brain Behav. Immun.* **2019**, *78*, 91–104. [CrossRef] [PubMed]
79. Maldonado-Bouchard, S.; Peters, K.; Woller, S.A.; Madahian, B.; Faghihi, U.; Patel, S.; Bake, S.; Hook, M.A. Inflammation is increased with anxiety- and depression-like signs in a rat model of spinal cord injury. *Brain Behav. Immun.* **2016**, *51*, 176–195. [CrossRef]
80. Drewe, J.; Beglinger, C.; Fricker, G. Effect of ischemia on intestinal permeability of lipopolysaccharides: Lipopolysaccharide Absorption. *Eur. J. Clin. Investig.* **2001**, *31*, 138–144. [CrossRef]
81. Lu, Y.-C.; Yeh, W.-C.; Ohashi, P.S. LPS/TLR4 signal transduction pathway. *Cytokine* **2008**, *42*, 145–151. [CrossRef]
82. Qin, L.; Wu, X.; Block, M.L.; Liu, Y.; Breese, G.R.; Hong, J.-S.; Knapp, D.J.; Crews, F.T. Systemic LPS causes chronic neuroinflammation and progressive neurodegeneration. *Glia* **2007**, *55*, 453–462. [CrossRef] [PubMed]
83. Schmidt, E.; Raposo, P.; Vavrek, R.; Fouad, K. Inducing inflammation following subacute spinal cord injury in female rats: A double-edged sword to promote motor recovery. *Brain Behav. Immun.* **2021**, *93*, 55–65. [CrossRef] [PubMed]
84. Appay, V.; Rowland-Jones, S.L. RANTES: A versatile and controversial chemokine. *Trends Immunol.* **2001**, *22*, 83–87. [CrossRef]
85. Mei, J.; Liu, Y.; Dai, N.; Favara, M.; Greene, T.; Jeyaseelan, S.; Poncz, M.; Lee, J.S.; Worthen, G.S. CXCL5 Regulates Chemokine Scavenging and Pulmonary Host Defense to Bacterial Infection. *Immunity* **2010**, *33*, 106–117. [CrossRef]
86. Bloom, O.; Herman, P.E.; Spungen, A.M. Systemic inflammation in traumatic spinal cord injury. *Exp. Neurol.* **2020**, *325*, 113143. [CrossRef] [PubMed]
87. Gris, D.; Hamilton, E.F.; Weaver, L.C. The systemic inflammatory response after spinal cord injury damages lungs and kidneys. *Exp. Neurol.* **2008**, *211*, 259–270. [CrossRef]
88. Allison, D.J.; Ditor, D.S. Immune dysfunction and chronic inflammation following spinal cord injury. *Spinal Cord* **2014**, *53*, 14–18. [CrossRef] [PubMed]
89. Riegger, T.; Conrad, S.; Liu, K.; Schluesener, H.J.; Adibzahdeh, M.; Schwab, J.M. Spinal cord injury-induced immune depression syndrome (SCI-IDS): SCI-IDS. *Eur. J. Neurosci.* **2007**, *25*, 1743–1747. [CrossRef] [PubMed]
90. Zhang, Y.; Guan, Z.; Reader, B.; Shawler, T.; Mandrekar-Colucci, S.; Huang, K.; Weil, Z.; Bratasz, A.; Wells, J.; Powell, N.D.; et al. Autonomic Dysreflexia Causes Chronic Immune Suppression after Spinal Cord Injury. *J. Neurosci.* **2013**, *33*, 12970–12981. [CrossRef]

MDPI
St. Alban-Anlage 66
4052 Basel
Switzerland
Tel. +41 61 683 77 34
Fax +41 61 302 89 18
www.mdpi.com

Biology Editorial Office
E-mail: biology@mdpi.com
www.mdpi.com/journal/biology

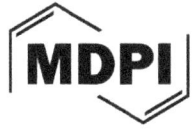

www.ingramcontent.com/pod-product-compliance
Lightning Source LLC
LaVergne TN
LVHW070453100526
838202LV00014B/1717